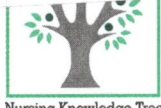

Nursing Knowledge Tree
An Initiative by CBS Nursing Division

NATIONAL HEALTH PROGRAMMES AND POLICIES 2020-21

Second Edition

Compiled by

Samta Soni

Lecturer
Government College of Nursing
Jaipur, Rajasthan

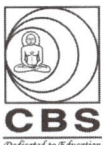

CBS
Dedicated to Education

CBS Publishers & Distributors Pvt Ltd

• New Delhi • Bengaluru • Chennai • Kochi • Kolkata • Lucknow
• Mumbai • Hyderabad • Nagpur • Patna • Pune • Vijayawada

NATIONAL HEALTH PROGRAMMES AND POLICIES 2020–21

ISBN: 978-93-90619-13-9

Second Edition: 2022

First Edition: 2018

Published by **Satish Kumar Jain** and produced by **Varun Jain** for

CBS Publishers & Distributors Pvt Ltd

4819/XI Prahlad Street, 24 Ansari Road, Daryaganj, New Delhi 110 002, India.
Ph: +91-11-23289259, 23266861, 23266867   Website: www.cbspd.com
Fax: 011-23243014
e-mail: delhi@cbspd.com; cbspubs@airtelmail.in.

Corporate Office: 204 FIE, Industrial Area, Patparganj, Delhi 110 092
 Ph: +91-11-4934 4934   Fax: 4934 4935
e-mail: feedback@cbspd.com; bhupesharora@cbspd.com

Branches

- **Bengaluru:** Seema House 2975, 17th Cross, K.R. Road, Banasankari 2nd Stage, Bengaluru 560 070, Karnataka
  Ph: +91-80-26771678/79   Fax: +91-80-26771680   e-mail: bangalore@cbspd.com
- **Chennai:** 7, Subbaraya Street, Shenoy Nagar, Chennai 600 030, Tamil Nadu
  Ph: +91-44-26680620, 26681266   Fax: +91-44-42032115   e-mail: chennai@cbspd.com
- **Kochi:** 68/1534, 35, 36-Power House Road, Opp. KSEB, Cochin-682018, Kochi, Kerala
  Ph: +91-484-4059061-65   Fax: +91-484-4059065   e-mail: kochi@cbspd.com
- **Kolkata:** 6/B, Ground Floor, Rameswar Shaw Road, Kolkata-700 014, West Bengal
  Ph: +91-33-22891126, 22891127, 22891128   e-mail: kolkata@cbspd.com
- **Lucknow:** Basement, Khushnuma Complex, 7-Meerabai Ma Rg, (Behind Jawahar Bhawan), Lucknow-226001, Uttar Pradesh
  Ph: +0522-4000032   e-mail: tiwari.lucknow@cbspd.com
- **Mumbai:** PWD Shed, Gala No. 25/26, Ramchandra Bhatt Marg, Next to J.J. Hospital Gate No. 2, Opp. Union Bank of India, Noor Baug, Mumbai-400009
  Ph: +91-22-66661880/89   Fax: +91-22-24902342   e-mail: mumbai@cbspd.com

Representatives

- **Hyderabad**   +91-9885175004   • **Patna**   +91-9334159340
- **Pune**   +91-9623451994   • **Vijayawada**   +91-9000660880

Printed at: SDR Printers, Trans Delhi Signature City, Ghaziabad, UP, India

Preface to the Second Edition

I am happy to present the Second Edition of the book, *National Health Programmes and Policies* before the readers. This edition has been thoroughly revised and updated, and the uniqueness of the content lies in the fact that it has maintained its pace with the changing scenario. It is precisely and timely updated, with new editions incorporating the latest changes in magnitude of the problems and strategies or programs implemented to control them. All data and recent references have been updated and upgraded as per the present changes accordingly.

Changes in the programmes have been included, findings of various review committees are incorporated, and some chapters have been extensively revised. The main focus of this edition is to describe the various National Health Programmes of India, and policies related to health, like—nutrition policy, children policy, etc. This has been a continuous process from the inception of this title. I have tried my level best to present this title with all the recent changes and revisions. It will serve as best source for the nursing and healthcare fraternities to make out policy formulation and its implementation.

Hope, this compendium will be your best companion. All the very best for your future endeavours.

Samta Soni

Preface to the First Edition

I am happy to hand over this book to learners. This book is intended to have a wider look on programmes and policies. It will also assist the readers in gaining perfection in all manners.

The idea behind writing this book culminated as a result of my teaching 'Health Policy and Programmes' to the BSc and MSc nursing students. However, I started compiling some parts of this book more than 5 years ago as class-notes for my students, and the actual writing of the book began in 2014 and was completed in 2017.

The primary focus of this book is to describe the various National Health Programmes of India, and the policies related to health, like—nutrition policy, children policy, etc.

The purpose of this book is to compile all information useful for nurses, nursing students and health professionals regarding policy formulation and implementation. The content of the book is an interactive outcome of student-teacher and student-student collaborations. I wish to thank my students whom I taught and also many times learned. Their questions in class and their answers revealed in assessment papers, and oral presentations, helped me to shape the book. Most of the candidates were from Master of Nursing, especially community health degree.

This book is designed as a reference source regarding National Health Planning, Health Institutes, Health Acts and Health Days.

All the best!

Samta Soni

Acknowledgments

I would like to express my gratitude to many people who observe me through this book; to all those who provided support, talked things over, read, wrote, offered comments, and assisted in the editing, proofreading and design.

Above all I want to thank my Mother, without her, none of this would be possible, my family, friends and students, who supported and encouraged me in spite of all the time it took me away from them. It was a long and difficult journey for them.

Last but not the least, my special thanks are due to Mr Satish Kumar Jain (Chairman) and Mr Varun Jain (Managing Director), M/s CBS Publishers and Distributors Pvt Ltd for their wholehearted support in publication of this book. I have no words to describe the role, efforts, inputs and initiatives undertaken by Mr Bhupesh Aarora [Sr. Vice President – Health Science Division (Publishing and Marketing)] for helping and motivating me.

I sincerely thank the entire CBS team for bringing out the book with utmost care and attractive presentation. I would like to thank Ms Nitasha Arora (Publishing Head & Content Strategist – PGMEE & Nursing), andDr Anju Dhir (Product Manager cum Commissioning Editor – Medical) for their editorial support. I would also extend my thanks to Mr Shivendu Bhushan Pandey (Sr. Manager & Team Lead), Mr Manoj K Yadav (Production Manager), Mr Ashutosh Pathak (Sr. Proofreader cum Team Coordinator) and all the production team members for devoting laborious hours in designing and typesetting the book.

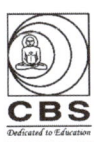
CBS
Dedicated to Education

CBS Nursing Knowledge Tree

Extends its Tribute to

Florence Nightingale

"

For glorifying the role of women as nurses,
For holding the title of " The Lady with the Lamp,"
For working tirelessly for humanity—
Florence Nightingale will always be
remembered for her
selfless and memorable services to the
human race.

Florence Nightingale
(May 1820 – August 1910)

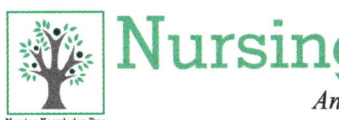

Nursing Knowledge Tree

An Initiative by CBS Nursing Division

"Coming together is a beginning. Keeping together is progress. Working together is success."

It gives us immense pleasure to share with you that the Nursing Knowledge Tree—An Initiative by CBS Nursing Division, has successfully established itself in the field of nursing as we have been able to stand as a strong contender by sharing approximately 50% of the market share. This growth could not have been possible without your invaluable contribution as our reader, author, reviewer, contributor and recommender, and your outstanding support for the growth of our titles as a whole. You people are the pillars of our series and we are so glad that you all have strengthened our basic foundation.

Nursing Knowledge Tree has been a pioneer and specialist in publishing best quality books for nursing education. Keeping in mind the changing trends in nursing education, we, at Nursing Knowledge Tree, have taken up a mission to bring student-friendly and syllabus-based books written by Subject Experts PAN India.

Our Noteworthy Achievements:

- Our nationally-acclaimed titles
  - *PGIMER NINE Clinical Nursing Procedures*—**Sandhya Ghai**
  - *Target High Staff Nurse Entrance Examination*—**Muthuvenkatachalam S, Ambili M Venugopal**
  - *CBS Nursing Drug Guide*—**Yogesh Gulati/Rakesh Sharma**
  - *Textbook of Nursing Foundations*—**Harindarjeet Goyal**
  - *Essentials of Biochemistry*—**Harbans Lal**
  - *Textbook of Nursing Education*—**Ratna Prakash**
  - *Nursing Research in 21st Century*—**Sukhpal Kaur and Amarjeet Singh**
  - *Essentials of Applied Microbiology*—**D R Arora and Brij Bala Arora**
  - *Textbook of Pediatric Nursing*—**Meharban Singh and Raman Kalia**
- Liaised with the topmost institutes of the country, like **AIIMS, NIMHANS, PGIMER NINE, CMC-Vellore, Manipal University, JIPMER, RAK-Delhi**, etc.
- Published **100+ Quality Nursing Books** and more than **50 New Books** on various subjects for Nursing Undergraduates, Postgraduates and Nursing superspecialty are under process and will be releasing in 2021.
- Increased our social presence by participating in more than **200+ National Conferences, CME's, College Exhibitions & Webinars** in previous years.
- We have come out with **Nursing Next Live**, an EdTech platform, the Next Level of Nursing Education, where we bring learning to people, instead of people going for learning. Through NNL App we are providing various study modules/plans covering All Subjects/All Topics, Video Lectures, Question Banks, E-notes and a Variety of Tests. Students can choose the plan according to their needs and requirements.
- We are excited to announce that we are coming out with our new initiative—**Nursing Next Live Social**, where nursing faculties can share as well as gain knowledge, with the aim to revolutionize the way the nursing segment connects. It's going to be India's first networking platform for Nursing Segment.

Our Journey towards providing Quality Nursing Education is Incomplete without YOU ! Join Us Now !

We specialize in publishing nursing books of superior quality, going ahead we see us publishing more and more quality content and it will only be possible when intellectuals from across the nation come together. Keeping pace with the advancements, we want to strengthen the nursing sector, which was long neglected, and establish a strong foundation when it comes to quality content for the segment.

We are determined to bring about changes in the Nursing Education system and with your support and contributions, we will do it for sure. We will be delighted if you join hands with us in the form of Author, Contributor or Reviewer and take the vision of quality education for nursing students ahead.

Let's join hands together and share our ideas and knowledge. Be the part of this Revolution. We are looking forward to your cooperation in future as well. Share your CVs at **bhupesharora@nursingnextlive.in** or scan the given QR code and fill the form or you can talk to me directly at +9555353330.

With Best Wishes
Mr Bhupesh Aarora
Sr. Vice President – Health Science Division
(Publishing and Marketing)

References

Books

1. Park K. Preventive and Social Medicine, 24th edition
2. A framework for Community Health Nursing Education, WHO, SEARO
3. Public Health Nursing, 9th Edition, Stanhope and Lancaster
4. McKenzie JF, Pinger, RR Kotecki JE, et al. An Introduction to Community Health
5. Eldredge LK, Markham, CM, Robert AC. Planning Health Promotion Programs: An Intervention Mapping Approach, 4th Edition
6. Karen (Kay) M. Perrin. Essential of Planning and Evaluation for Public Health

Websites

1. www.mygov.in
2. www.nhm.gov.in
3. www.vikaspedia.in
4. www.ddnews.gov.in
5. www.icds.wcd.gov.in
6. www.tbcindia.gov.in
7. www.thenortheast today.com
8. www.semanticscholar.org
9. www.iapb.org
10. www.idsp.nic.in
11. www.researchgate.net
12. www.mohfw.gov.in
13. www.nihfw.nic.in
14. www.indiacelebrating.com
15. www.planningcommission.gov.in
16. www.cbhidghs.nic.in
17. www.india.gov.in
18. www.cehat.org
19. www.nhp.gov.in
20. www.pitt.edu
21. www.who.int > Countries > India
22. www.archive.india.gov.in > Citizens > Health
23. www.medindia.net/indian_health_act/acts.asp
24. www.icmr.nic.in
25. www.ninindia.org
26. www.india.com/topic/national-health-institute
27. www.nioh.org
28. www.aiihph.gov.in
29. www.nie.gov.in

Contents

SECTION I: NATIONAL HEALTH PROGRAMMES

SECTION II: HEALTH RELATED POLICIES IN INDIA

SECTION III: NATIONAL HEALTH DAYS

SECTION IV: HEALTH-RELATED ACTS

SECTION V: NATIONAL HEALTH INSTITUTES

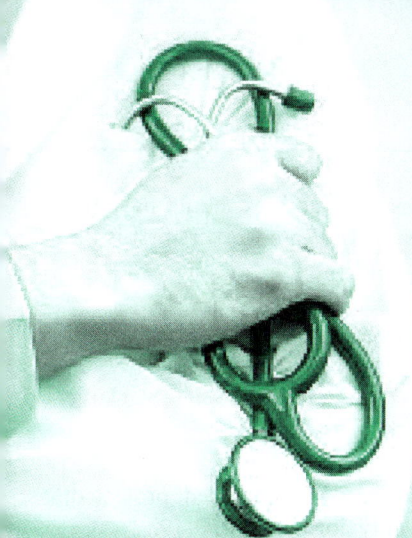

Appendices

1

YEAR OF THE HEALTH AND CARE WORKERS

INTRODUCTION

2021 has been designated as the International Year of Health and Care Workers (YHCW) in appreciation and gratitude for their unwavering dedication in the fight against the COVID-19 pandemic. WHO is launching a year-long campaign, under the theme—**Protect. Invest. Together.** It highlights the urgent need to invest in health workers for shared dividends in health, jobs, economic opportunity and equity.

AIMS

- Ensure the world's health and care workers are prioritized for the COVID-19 vaccine in the first 100 days of 2021.
- Recognize and commemorate all health and care workers who have lost their lives during the pandemic.
- Mobilize commitments from Member States, International Financing Institutions, bilateral and philanthropic partners to protect and invest in health and care workers to accelerate the attainment of the SDGs and COVID-19 recovery.
- Engage Member States and all relevant stakeholders in dialogue on a care compact to protect health and care workers' rights, decent work and practice environments.
- Bring together communities, influencers, political and social support in solidarity, advocacy and care for health and care workers.

OBJECTIVES

- PROTECT our health and care workers
  - Health and care workers have protected the world during COVID-19: We have a moral obligation to protect them.

- Health workers delivering new COVID-19 health care innovations and vaccines should have the requisite support and enabling work environment. Vaccinating health and care workers first is the right thing to do and the smart thing to do.
- INVEST in the people who invest in us
  - The world is facing a global shortage of health workers. We must invest in education, jobs and decent work to protect the world from disease and achieve universal health coverage.
  - Globally, 70% of the health and social workforce are women. Nurses and midwives represent a large portion of this. We need to invest in gender equity.
- TOGETHER, we can make it happen
  - We all have a role to play to ensure that our health and care workforces are supported, protected, motivated and equipped to deliver safe health care at all times, not only during COVID-19.

INTERNATIONAL LEAD POISONING PREVENTION WEEK

INTRODUCTION

25 to 31 October is International Lead Poisoning Prevention Week.

The aim of International Lead Poisoning Prevention Week is to draw attention to the health impacts of lead exposure, highlight efforts by countries and partners to prevent childhood lead exposure, and accelerate efforts to phase out the use of lead in paint.

Even though there is wide recognition of the harmful effects of lead and many countries have taken action, exposure to lead, particularly in childhood, remains the key concern to health care providers and public health officials worldwide.

WHO, the UN Environment Programme (UNEP), governments, civil society organizations, health partners, industry and others will organize activities and events during the Eighth International Lead Poisoning Prevention Week.

This week of action is an initiative of the Global Alliance to Eliminate Lead Paint (the Lead Paint Alliance), which is jointly led by UNEP and WHO.

OBJECTIVES OF INTERNATIONAL LEAD POISONING PREVENTION WEEK

- Raise awareness about health effects of lead exposure.
- Highlight the efforts of countries and partners to prevent lead exposure, particularly in children.
- Urge further action to eliminate lead paint through regulatory action at country level.

CALL FOR ACTION

Lead exposure from paint is entirely preventable. Paints for a range of uses can be manufactured without the addition of lead compounds. WHO calls on all countries that have not yet done so to establish the necessary legally binding measures to stop the use of lead in paint.

3

WORLD FOOD SAFETY DAY

INTRODUCTION

7th June is World Food Safety Day. The second World Food Safety Day (WFSD) was celebrated on 7th June 2020 to draw attention and inspire action to help prevent, detect and manage foodborne risks, contributing to food security, human health, economic prosperity, agriculture, market access, tourism and sustainable development.

Food safety is a shared responsibility between governments, producers and consumers. Everybody has a role to play from farm to table to ensure the food we consume is safe and will not cause damages to our health. Through the World Food Safety Day, WHO pursues its efforts to mainstream food safety in the public agenda and reduce the burden of foodborne diseases globally.

Under the theme "Food safety, everyone's business", the action-oriented campaign will promote global food safety awareness and call upon countries and decision makers, the private sector, civil society, UN organizations and the general public to take action.

Food safety is a shared responsibility between governments, producers and consumers. Everybody has a role to play from farm to table to ensure the food we consume is safe and will not cause damages to our health. Through the World Food Safety Day, WHO pursues its efforts to mainstream food safety in the public agenda and reduce the burden of foodborne diseases globally.

CALLS TO ACTION

- Ensure it's safe—Government must ensure safe and nutritious food for all.
- Grow it safe—Agriculture and food producers need to adopt good practices.
- Keep it safe—Business operators must make sure food is safe.
- Eat it safe: All consumers have a right to safe, healthy and nutritious food.
- Team up for safety—Food Safety is a shared responsibility.

WORLD HEARING DAY

INTRODUCTION

World Hearing Day is held on 3rd March each year to raise awareness on how to prevent deafness and hearing loss, and promote ear and hearing care across the world.

Each year, WHO decides the theme and develops evidence-based advocacy materials such as brochures, flyers, posters, banners, infographics and presentations, among others. These materials are shared with partners in government and civil society around the world as well as WHO regional and country offices.

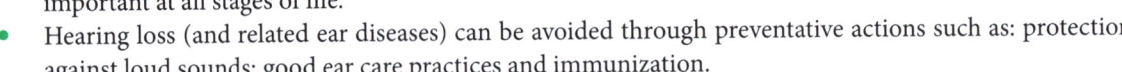

World Hearing Day
3 March 2021

At its headquarters in Geneva, WHO organizes an annual World Hearing Day event. In recent years, an increasing number of Member States and other partner agencies have joined World Hearing Day by hosting a range of activities and events in their countries. WHO invites all stakeholders to join this global initiative.

- Good hearing and communication are important at all stages of life.
- Hearing loss (and related ear diseases) can be avoided through preventative actions such as: protection against loud sounds; good ear care practices and immunization.
- Hearing loss (and related ear diseases) can be addressed when it is identified in a timely manner and appropriate care sought.
- People at risk of hearing loss should check their hearing regularly.
- People having hearing loss (or related ear diseases) should seek care from a health care provider.

POLICY REQUIRED

- The number of people living with unaddressed hearing loss and ear diseases is unacceptable.
- Timely action is needed to prevent and address hearing loss across the life course.
- Investing in cost effective interventions will benefit people with hearing loss and bring financial gains to the society.
- Governments must act to integrate person-centered ear and hearing care within national health plans for universal health coverage.

5

PRADHAN MANTRI BHARTIYA JANAUSHADHI PARIYOJANA

INTRODUCTION

Pradhan Mantri Bhartiya Janaushadhi Pariyojana (PMBJP) is a campaign launched by the Department of Pharmaceuticals to provide quality medicines at affordable prices to the masses. PMBJP stores have been set up to provide generic drugs, which are available at lesser prices but are equivalent in quality and efficacy as expensive branded drugs. It was launched by the Department of Pharmaceuticals in November 2008 under the name Janaushadhi Campaign. Bureau of Pharma PSUs of India (BPPI) is the implementation agency for PMBJP.

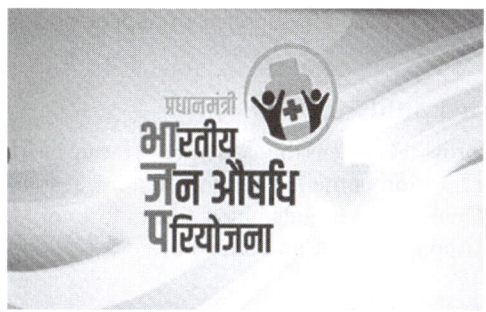

VISION

To bring down the healthcare budget of every citizen of India through providing Quality Generic Medicines at Affordable Prices.

MISSION

- Create awareness among the public regarding generic medicines.
- Create demand for generic medicines through medical practitioners.
- Create awareness through education and awareness program that high price need not be synonymous with high quality.
- Provide all the commonly used generic medicines covering all the therapeutic groups.
- Provide all the related health care products too under the scheme.

OBJECTIVE

Making quality medicines available at affordable prices for all, particularly the poor and disadvantaged, through exclusive outlets "Janaushadhi Medical Store" so as to reduce out of pocket expenses in healthcare.

ABOUT JANAUSHADHI STORE (JAS)

- Janaushadhi stores have been opened across the country.
- The normal working hours of JAS are 8 am to 8 pm.
- All therapeutic medicines are made available from Janaushadhi Stores.
- In addition to medicines and surgical items supplied by BPPI, Janaushadhi stores also sell allied medical products commonly sold in chemist shops so as to improve the viability of the Janaushadhi store.
- OTC (Over-the-counter) products can be purchased by any individual without a prescription. A prescription from a registered medical practitioner is necessary for the purchase of scheduled drugs.
- Bureau of Pharma Public Sector Undertakings of India (BPPI) has been established under the Department of Pharmaceuticals, Govt. of India, with the support of all the CPSUs for co-coordinating procurement, supply and marketing of generic drugs through the Janaushadhi Stores.
- The quality, safety and efficacy of medicines are ensured by getting each batch of medicines procured from CPSUs as well as private suppliers tested from NABL approved laboratories and conforming to

the required standards before the same are supplied to Supers stockists/Janaushadhi Stores from the Warehouse of BPPI.

Locate your Nearest Janaushadhi Store

Janaushadhi Sugam Mobile App provides citizens the assistance to locate nearby Janaushadhi kendra, direction guided through Google Map for location of the Janaushadhi kendra, search Janaushadhi generic medicines, analyze product comparison of Generic and Branded medicine in form of MRP and overall Savings, etc.

Janaushadhi Sugam Mobile App is available on both Android & I-phone platforms.

Who can Open a Janaushadhi Store

State Governments or any organization/reputed NGOs/Trusts/Private hospitals/Charitable institutions/ Doctors/Unemployed pharmacist/ individual entrepreneurs are eligible to apply for new Janaushadhi stores. The applicants shall have to employ one B Pharma/D Pharma degree holder as Pharmacist in their proposed stores.

Requirements for Opening a Janaushadhi Stores by Organizations/Individuals other than Government Nominated

- Applications shall be submitted to BPPI either online or offline.
- Own space or hired space duly supported by proper lease agreement.
- Minimum required space conforming to standards as approved by the BPPI i.e. 120 sq. ft.
- Drug license in the name of "Pradhan Mantri Bhartiya Janaushadhi Kendra" and other permissions to run a drug store. Compliance with all statutory requirements for storage of drugs shall be ensured by the applicant.
- For individuals, Aadhaar and PAN Card are mandatory.
- For Institutions/NGO/Charitable Institute/Hospital, etc. documents include Aadhaar Card, PAN card, Certificate of Incorporation and Registration certificate.
- For Government/Govt Nominated Agency documents include Details of Department who has allocated the space, along with supporting documents/sanction order, PAN card and Aadhaar Card.
- Proof of securing a pharmacist with computer knowledge (name of the pharmacist, Registration with the State Council, etc. needs to be furnished).
- Financial capacity to run the Store supported by audited accounts for the last three years (Bank Statements for the last 03 years or sanction letter from Bank for extending loan in case of individuals).

Procedure for Opening a Janaushadhi Store

Bureau of Pharma Public Sector Undertakings of India (BPPI) writes to all the State Governments with a request to open Janaushadhi Stores in their states. The State Government, Department of Health would make recommendations in favor of the operating agency who would run the Stores and also instruct the District Hospital Authority to provide the minimum space conforming to standards as approved by BPPI in the Hospital premises. The location of the store should be at such a place which is easily accessible to the OPD patients, preferably at the entry of the hospital and given to the agency free of cost. The State Government needs to issue suitable instructions to the Hospitals/Doctors for prescribing generic medicines.

Other entities may approach BPPI either on the basis of the advertisement issued by BPPI or suo moto with a complete application along with the supporting documents mentioned in fulfilling requirements specified above. An agreement is to be entered into between BPPI and the operating agency before the JAS starts functioning and BPPI makes arrangements for the dispatch of medicine.

6

PRADHAN MANTRI MATRU VANDANA YOJANA (PMMVY)

INTRODUCTION

Pradhan Mantri Matru Vandana Yojana (PMMVY) is a Maternity Benefit Programme that is implemented in all the districts of the country in accordance with the provision of the National Food Security Act, 2013.

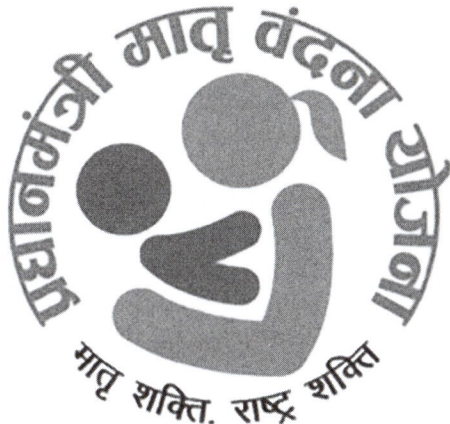

OBJECTIVES

- Providing partial compensation for the wage loss in terms of cash incentives so that the woman can take adequate rest before and after delivery of the first living child.
- The cash incentive provided would lead to improved health seeking behavior amongst the Pregnant Women and Lactating Mothers (PW and LM).

TARGET BENEFICIARIES

- All Pregnant Women and Lactating Mothers, excluding PW&LM who are in regular employment with the Central Government or the State Governments or PSUs or those who are in receipt of similar benefits under any law for the time being in force.
- All eligible Pregnant Women and Lactating Mothers who have their pregnancy on or after 01.01.2017 for first child in family.
- The date and stage of pregnancy for a beneficiary would be counted with respect to her LMP date as mentioned in the MCP card.
- Case of Miscarriage/Still Birth:
    - A beneficiary is eligible to receive benefits under the scheme only once.
    - In case of miscarriage/still birth, the beneficiary would be eligible to claim the remaining installment(s) in the event of any future pregnancy.

- Thus, after receiving the 1st installment, if the beneficiary has a miscarriage, she would only be eligible for receiving 2nd and 3rd installment in the event of future pregnancy subject to fulfillment of eligibility criterion and conditionalities of the scheme. Similarly, if the beneficiary has a miscarriage or stillbirth after receiving 1st and 2nd installments, she would only be eligible for receiving 3rd installment in the event of future pregnancy subject to fulfillment of eligibility criterion and conditionalities of the scheme.
- Case of Infant Mortality: A beneficiary is eligible to receive benefits under the scheme only once. That is, in case of infant mortality, she will not be eligible for claiming benefits under the scheme, if she has already received all the installments of the maternity benefit under PMMVY earlier.
- Pregnant and Lactating AWWs/AWHs/ASHA may also avail the benefits under the PMMVY subject to fulfillment of scheme conditionalities.

BENEFITS UNDER PMMVY

- Cash incentives in three installments, i.e. first installment of ₹1000/- on early registration of pregnancy at the Anganwadi Center (AWC)/approved Health facility as may be identified by the respective administering State/UT, second installment of ₹2000/- after six months of pregnancy on receiving at least one ante-natal check-up (ANC) and third installment of ₹2000/- after childbirth is registered and the child has received the first cycle of BCG, OPV, DPT and Hepatitis-B, or its equivalent/substitute.
- The eligible beneficiaries would receive the incentive given under the Janani Suraksha Yojana (JSY) for Institutional delivery and the incentive received under JSY would be accounted towards maternity benefits so that on an average a woman gets ₹6000/-.

REGISTRATION UNDER THE SCHEME

- The eligible women desirous of availing maternity benefits are required to register under the scheme at the Anganwadi Center (AWC)/approved Health facility depending upon the implementing department for that particular State/UT.
- For registration, the beneficiary shall submit the prescribed application Form 1 - A , complete in all respects, along with the relevant documents and undertaking/consent duly signed by her and her husband, at the AWC/approved Health facility. While submitting the form, the beneficiary will be required to submit her and her husband's Aadhaar details with their written consents, her/husband/family member's Mobile Number and her Bank/Post Office account details.
- The prescribed form (s) can be obtained from the AWC/ approved Health facility free of cost. The form(s) can also be downloaded from the website of Ministry of Women and Child Development.
- The beneficiary would be required to fill up the prescribed scheme forms for registration and claim of the installment and submit the same at the Anganwadi Center/approved Health facility. The beneficiary should obtain acknowledgment from Anganwadi Worker/ASHA/ANM for record and future reference.
- For registration and claim of first installment, duly filled Form 1 - A along with copy of MCP Card (Mother and Child Protection Card), Proof of Identity of Beneficiary and her Husband (Aadhaar Card or permitted Alternate ID Proof of both and Bank/Post Office Account details of the beneficiary is required to be submitted.
- For claiming second installment, beneficiary is required to submit duly filled up Form 1 - B after six months of pregnancy, along with the copy of MCP Card showing at least one ANC.

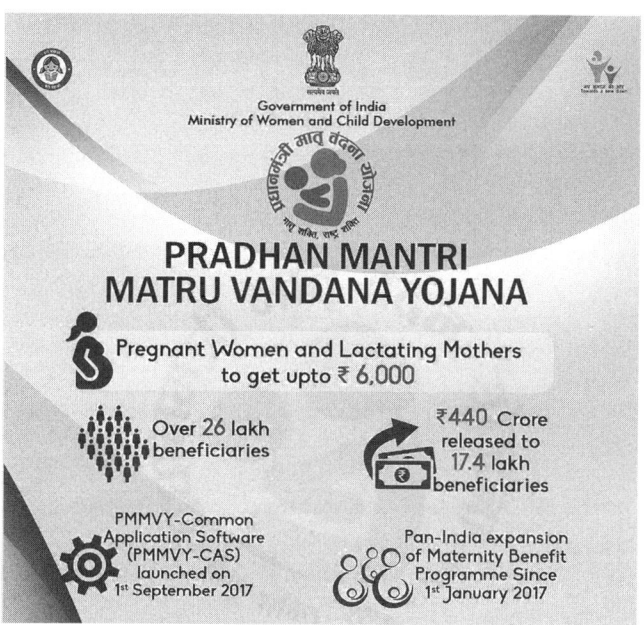

- For claiming third installment, beneficiary is required to submit duly filled up Form 1 - C along with copy of childbirth registration and copy of MCP card showing that the child has received first cycle of immunization or its equivalent/substitute.

- In case a beneficiary has complied the conditionalities stipulated under the scheme but could not register/ submit claims within the stipulated time, can submit claim(s) - A beneficiary can apply, at any point of time but not later than 730 days of pregnancy, even if she had not claimed any of the installments earlier but fulfills eligibility criterion and conditionalities for receiving benefits. In cases where LMP date is not recorded in MCP card, viz. a beneficiary is coming for claim of third installment under the scheme, the claim in such cases must be submitted within 460 days from the date of birth of the child beyond which period no claim shall be entertained.

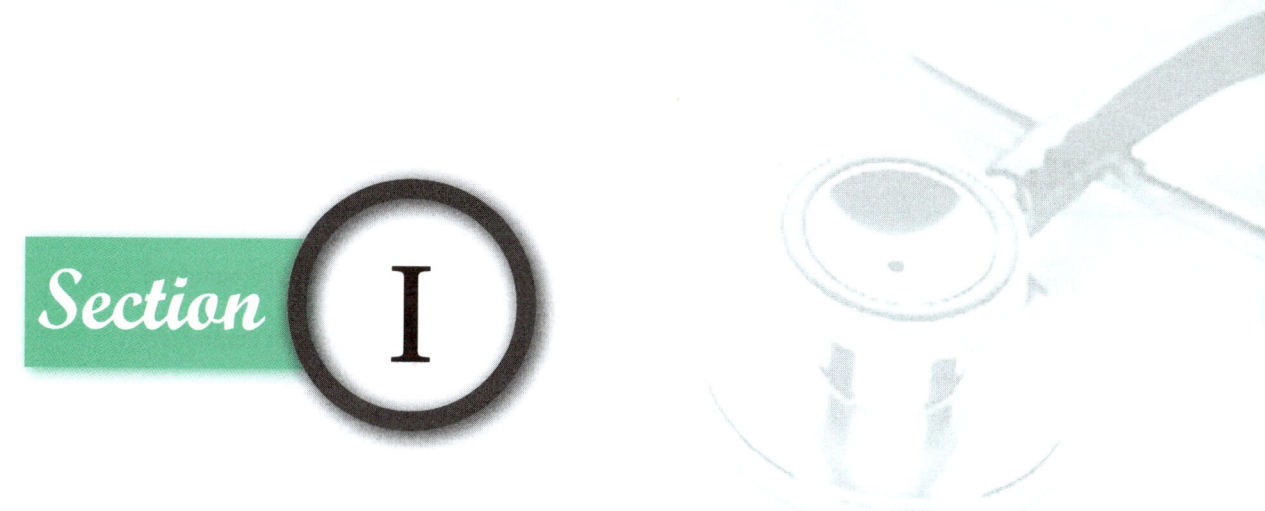

Section I

NATIONAL HEALTH PROGRAMMES

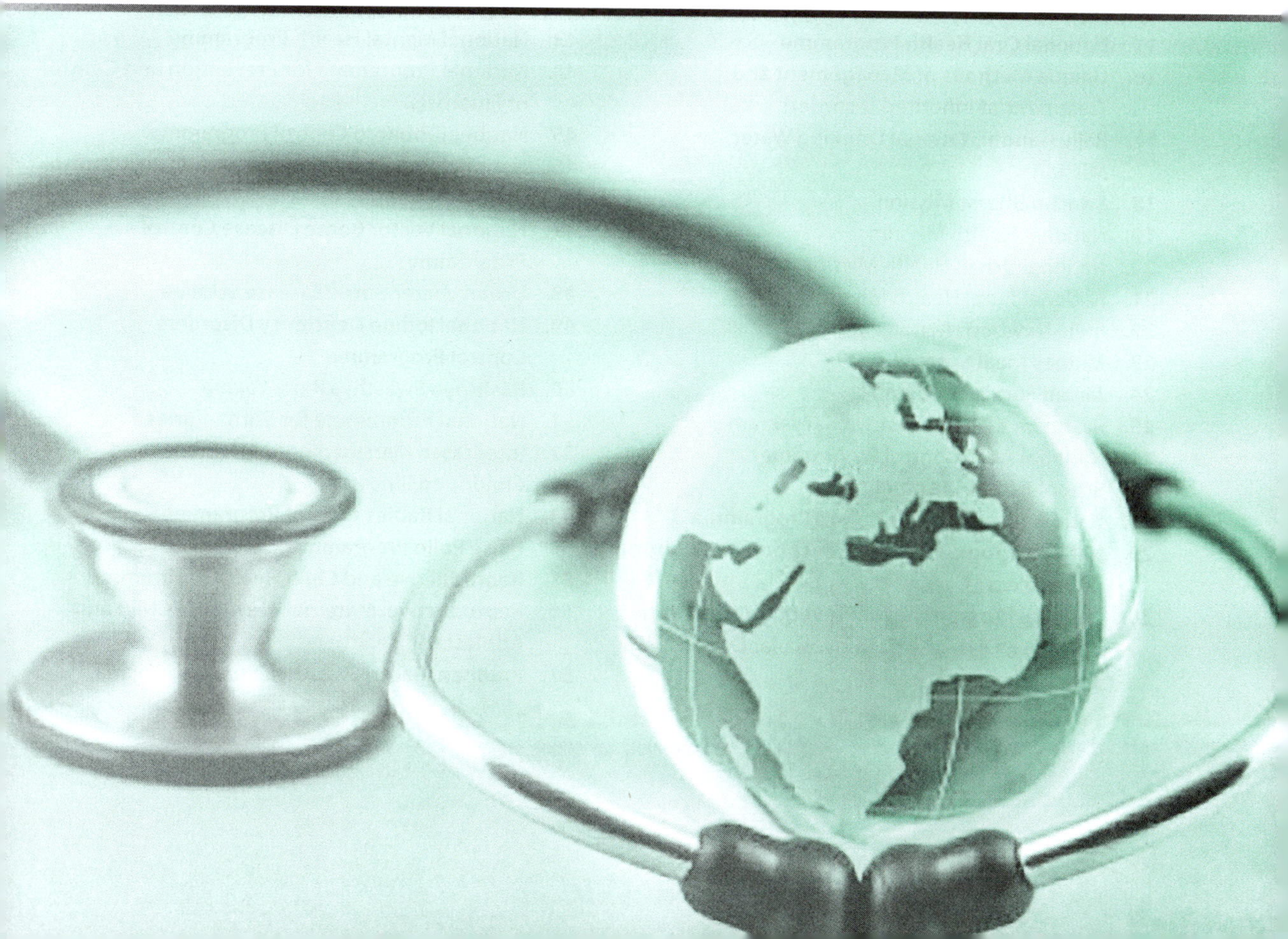

Contents

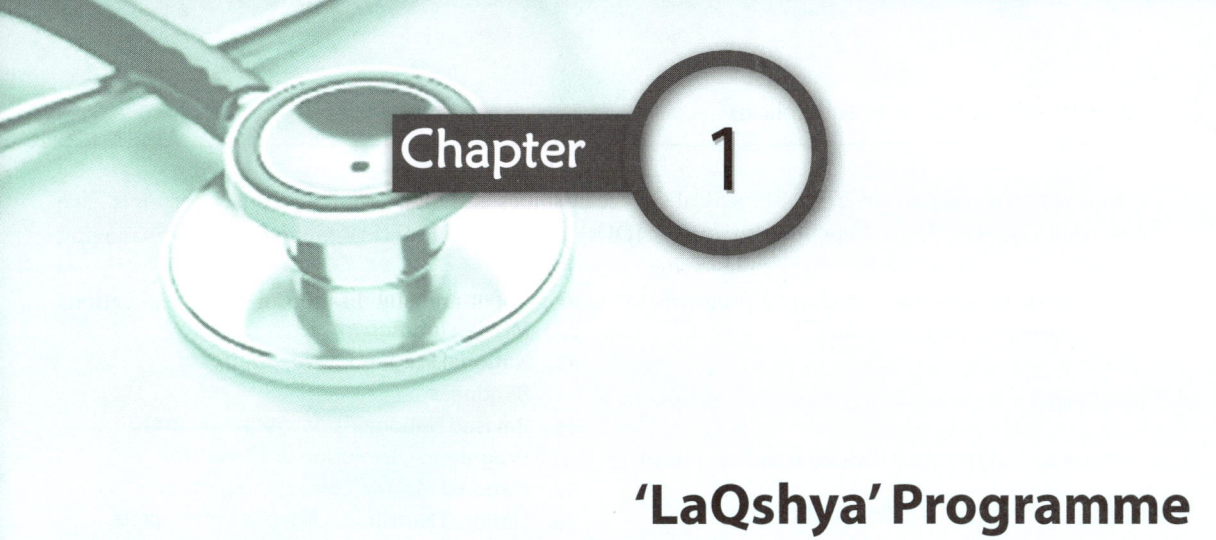

Chapter 1

'LaQshya' Programme

INTRODUCTION

After launch of the National Health Mission (NHM), there has been a substantial increase in the number of institutional deliveries. However, this increase in the numbers has not resulted into commensurate improvements in the key maternal and newborn health indicators. A transformational change in the processes related to the care during the delivery, which essentially relates to intrapartum and immediate postpartum care is required to achieve tangible results within short period of time. Prerequisite of such approach would also hinge upon the health system's preparedness for prompt identification and management of maternal and newborn complications.

'LaQshya' Programme (Labor Room and Quality Improvement Initiative) of the Ministry of Health and Family Welfare (MoHFW) aims at improving quality of care in labor room and maternity operation theater (OT).

GOAL

To reduce preventable maternal and newborn mortality, morbidity and stillbirths associated with the care around delivery in labor room and maternity OT and ensure respectful maternity care.

OBJECTIVES

- To reduce maternal and newborn mortality and morbidity due to antepartum hemorrhage (APH), postpartum hemorrhage (PPH), retained placenta, preterm, preeclampsia and eclampsia, obstructed labor, puerperal sepsis, newborn asphyxia, and sepsis, etc.
- To improve quality of care during the delivery and immediate postpartum care, stabilization of complications and ensure timely referrals, and enable an effective two-way follow-up system.
- To enhance satisfaction of beneficiaries visiting the health facilities and provide Respectful Maternity Care (RMC) to all pregnant women attending the public health facility.

STRATEGIES

- Reorganizing/aligning labor room and maternity OT layout and workflow as per 'Labor Room Standardization Guidelines' and 'Maternal and Newborn Health Toolkit' issued by the MoHFW, Government of India (GoI).

- Ensuring that at least all government medical college hospitals and high case-load district hospitals have dedicated obstetric High Dependency Units (HDUs) as per GoI MoHFW Guidelines, for managing complicated pregnancies that require life-saving critical care.
- Ensuring strict adherence to clinical protocols for management and stabilization of the complications before referral to higher centers.

ACTIVITIES

Activities under LaQshya are divided into four phases (Fig. 1).

Preparatory Phase—2 Months

- Launch and dissemination of the scheme.
- Identification of members for national mentoring group and operationalization of the group.
- National level orientation workshop of national resource team and state nodal officers.
- Issue of the instructions to the state and district stakeholders.
- Formation of state mentoring group.
- Identification and listing of facilities to be included in the initiative.
- State level training of trainers (ToT) of the quality coaches.
- Formation of quality circles at the labor rooms and operation theaters.
- Assigning states to development partners.

Assessment Phase—2 Months

- Orientation of quality circles on Quality Improvement and Clinical Protocols.
- Assessment of the Labor Rooms and Maternity OT against National Quality Standards.
- Planning for expansion of Labor rooms as per 'Guidelines for Standardization of Labor Rooms at Delivery Points' and upgradation of the maternity OT.
- Preparation of time bound action plan, based on the identified gaps.
- Planning for creation of obstetrics HDU as per recommendations of 'Guidelines for Obstetrics HDU and ICU'.
- Collation of requirements and resource allocation through the PIP process under the NHM.
- Mapping of referral facilities (type of facility, distance and travel time, contact details, availability of services including facility for the blood transfusion, availability of other specialties such as physician, surgeon, pathology and biochemistry lab and ultrasound facility, nearest tertiary care institution).

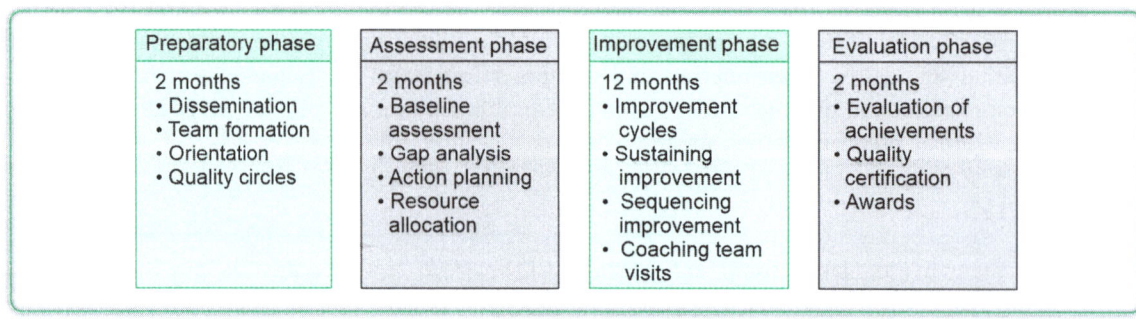

Figure 1: Activities under LaQshya

- Ensuring availability of updated version of clinical protocols for end users and training of labor room and OT staff.
- Training of the staff in recording of data elements for monitoring of the indicators and implementation of Quality Management System.
- Ensuring availability of drugs and supplies.
- Development of resource package for monthly campaigns.
- Initiation of Patients' Satisfaction Survey among all patients reporting in the labor room and operation theater.
- Development of IT platform for the initiative or integration with existing IT platform.

Improvement Phase—12 Months

- Launch of rapid improvement cycles. Each cycle includes one month of improvement and subsequent month of consolidation and sustenance.
- Ensuring adherence to clinical protocols and peer-mentoring.
- Establish standard operating procedures for labor rooms and maternity OT.
- Quality circle understands the issues regarding selected theme of alternate month and tries to improve the processes using quality improvement methodology (Plan – Do – Check –Act [PDCA]) cycle, and sustain them.
- Preparatory visit, followed by monthly visits—Visits in the second month of each improvement cycle would be in last week for performance review through objective indicators. Support for the forthcoming campaign would also be extended during this visit.
- Documentation and photography of the improvement.
- Observation and assessment of processes, refresher and hands-on training, demonstrations and hand-holding.
- Information, Education and Communication (IEC) campaign for each improvement cycle—This includes reading material/brochure on the theme, short videos, presentations, etc. disseminated through social media/dedicated IT platform.
- Collection and reporting of indicators linked with quality objectives of each cycle from quality circle to State Mentoring Group and SQAC.
- Structural augmentation include rearranging the layout and human resource deployment and skill upgradation in the labor room and OT will go parallel.
- Concurrent evaluation of quality indicators by SQAC and MH Division/National Health Systems Resource Center (NHSRC) and feedback to quality circles.
- Analysis of patients' feedback and taking actions for addressing the beneficiaries' concerns.

Evaluation Phase—2 Months

- Evaluation of the quality objectives and indicators.
- External assessment and quality certification of labor rooms and maternity OT.
- Awards to best performing quality circles and coaching teams.
- National level dissemination of achievements.
- Development of strategy for sustenance and scaling-up.

IMPLEMENTATION

- The 'LaQshya' Programme will be implemented by all Medical College Hospitals, District Hospitals and First Referral Unit (FRU), and Community Health Centers (CHCs) and will benefit every pregnant woman and newborn getting delivered in public health institutions.

- Under the initiative, a multipronged strategy has been adopted such as improving infrastructure up-gradation, ensuring the availability of essential equipment, providing adequate human resources, capacity building of health care workers and improving quality processes in the labor room.
- The quality improvement in the labor room and maternity OT will be assessed through National Quality Assurance Standards (NQAS).

TARGETS

Immediate (0–4 Months)

- 80% of the selected labor rooms and maternity OTs assess their quality and staff competence using defined NQAS checklists and Objective Structured Clinical Examination (OSCE).
- 80% of labor rooms and maternity OTs have setup functional quality circles and facility level quality teams.

Short Term (Up to 8 Months)

- 80% of labor room and OT quality circles are oriented to latest labor room protocols, quality improvement processes and Respectful Maternity Care (RMC).
- 50% of deliveries take place in presence of the birth companions.
- 60% of deliveries are conducted using safe birth checklist and safe surgery checklist in labor room and maternity OT respectively.
- 60% of the deliveries are conducted using real-time partograph.
- 30% increase in breastfeeding within one hour of delivery.
- 80% labor rooms and Maternity OTs take microbiological samples from defined areas every month.
- 30% reduction in surgical site infection rate in planned surgery in the Maternity OT.

Intermediate Term (Up to 12 Months)

- 30% increase in antenatal corticosteroid administration in case of preterm labor.
- 30% reduction in preeclampsia, eclampsia and Pregnancy induced hypertension (PIH) related mortality.
- 30% reduction in Antepartum hemorrhage/Postpartum hemorrhage (APH/PPH) related mortality.
- 20% reduction in newborn asphyxia related admissions in Special Newborn Care Units (SNCUs) for inborn deliveries.
- 20% reduction in newborn sepsis rate in SNCUs for inborn deliveries.
- 20% reduction in stillbirth rate.
- 80% of all beneficiaries are either satisfied or highly satisfied.
- 60% of the labor rooms are reorganized as per 'Guidelines for Standardization of Labor Rooms at Delivery Points'.
- 80% of labor rooms have staffing as per defined norms.
- 100% compliance to administration of oxytocin, immediately after birth.
- 30% improvement in OSCEs score of labor room staff.
- 100% maternal death, neonatal death audit and clinical discussion on maternal near miss and neonatal complications.
- 80% labor room and OTs are reporting zero stock-outs of drugs and consumables.

Long Term (Up to 18 Months)

- 60% of labor rooms achieve quality certification against the NQAS.
- 50% of labor rooms are linked to obstetrics high dependency units/intensive care units (HDU/ICU).

- 15% improvement in short term and intermediate targets.
  After 18 months, this initiative would be continued through sustained mentoring.

INTERVENTIONS

- Ensuring availability of optimal and skilled human resources as per case-load and prevalent norms through rational deployment and skill upgradation.
- Ensuring skill assessment of all staff of labor room (LR) and maternal OT through OSCE testing as per Dakshata guidelines for delivery of 'zero-defect' quality obstetric and newborn care. Enhance proficiency of labor room and operation theater staff for management of the complications through skill-lab training, simulations and drills. Ensuring that staff working in the labor room and maternity OT are not shifted from maternity duty to other departments/wards frequently.
- Sensitizing care-providers for delivery of respectful maternity care and close monitoring of language, behavior and conduct of the labor room, OT and HDU Staff.
- Creating an enabling environment for natural birthing process.
- Implementation of Clinical Guidelines, Labor Room Clinical Pathways, Referral Protocols, safe birth checklist (in labor room and obstetric OT) and surgical safety check-list.
- Ensuring round the clock availability of blood transfusion services, diagnostic services, drugs and consumables.
- Ensuring availability of triage area and functional newborn care area.
- Ensuring systematic facility-level audit of all cases of maternal/neonatal deaths, stillbirth, and maternal near miss, etc. including with their mentor teams through clinical discussions, peer reviews in teaching institutes, video conference, or other distance mode mechanisms for continuous improvement and learning.
- Operationalization of 'C' Section audit and corrective and preventive actions for ensuring that 'C' Sections are undertaken judiciously in those cases having robust clinical indications.
- Instituting an ongoing system of capturing of beneficiaries' independent feedback through mechanism 'Mera–Aspataal' or manual recording, or Grievance Redressal Help Desk and take action to address concerns, for continual enhancement in their satisfaction.
- Ensuring availability of essential support services such as 24 × 7 running water, electricity, housekeeping, linen and laundry, security, equipment maintenance, laboratory services, dietary services, biomedical waste (BMW) management, etc.
- Use of digital technology for record keeping and monitoring for maternity wing management information system (MIS), including use of electronic partograph. Piloting of technology for managing care, such as computer on wheel, Computerized Physician Order Entry.
- Use aggressive information, education and communication (IEC), user friendly training material and IT-enabled tools. Facilitating branding of all high case load facilities meeting quality standards to improve visibility and awareness.
- Using quality tools for prioritization, and gap closure such as PDCA, Root Cause Analysis, Run Charts, Pareto Chart and Mistake Proofing for achieving desired targets.
- **Rapid improvement events:** Six cycles of two months each as defined below will need to be rigorously supervised and ensured. This will enable competency in all critical skills needed. For each area, a targeted campaign would be launched for a two-month duration, with the first month for the roll-out, followed by sustaining such efforts during the subsequent month (Period for one event – 2 months). Suggested list of the themes for campaigns is given as follows:
  - **Cycle 1:** Real-time partograph generation including shift to electronic partograph and usage of safe birth check-list and surgical safety check-list and strengthening documentation practices for generating robust data for driving improvement.

- **Cycle 2:** Presence of birth companion during delivery, respectful maternity care and enhancement of patients' satisfaction.
- **Cycle 3:** Assessment, triage and timely management of complications including strengthening of referral protocols.
- **Cycle 4:** Management of labor as per protocols including AMTSL and rational use of oxytocin.
- **Cycle 5:** Essential and emergency care of newborn and pre-term babies including management of birth asphyxia and timely initiation of breastfeeding as well as KMC for preterm newborn.
- **Cycle 6:** Infection prevention including biomedical waste management.

INCENTIVES

The quality improvement in labor room and maternity OT will be assessed through NQAS. Every facility achieving 70% score on NQAS will be certified as LaQshya certified facility. Furthermore, branding of LaQshya certified facilities will be done as per the NQAS score. Facilities scoring more than 90%, 80% and 70% will be given Platinum, Gold and Silver badge accordingly. Facilities achieving NQAS certification, defined quality indicators and 80% satisfied beneficiaries will be provided incentive of ₹6 lakh, ₹3 lakh and ₹2 lakh for Medical College Hospital, District Hospital and FRUs, respectively.

Digital Innovation

- LaQshya Web portal—All LaQshya related data will be uploaded on the portal for prompt report generation as well as visualization of dashboard to monitor progress in key maternal newborn indicators at various levels (Facility, District, State and National).
- Safe Delivery App—Job aid as well as training tool for health workers.

Certification, Incentives and Branding

- Quality improvement in labor room and maternity OT will be assessed through NQAS. Every facility achieving 70% score on NQAS will be certified as **LaQshya Certified Facility**.
- Furthermore, branding of LaQshya certified facilities will be done as per the NQAS score. Facilities scoring more than 90%, 80% and 70% will be given Platinum, Gold and Silver badge accordingly.
- Facilities achieving NQAS certification, defined quality indicators and 80% satisfied beneficiaries will be provided incentive of ₹6 lakhs, ₹3 lakhs and ₹2 lakhs for Medical College Hospital, District Hospital and FRUs respectively.

Way Forward

- New innovations for escalating quality of health care services for mothers and newborn.
- Increased satisfaction of beneficiaries and positive birthing experience.
- Increased demand of services from beneficiaries of public health facilities.
- LaQshya certification of all health facilities.
- Sustained efforts to achieve sustainable development goal (SDG) targets and goals related to maternal newborn health.
- Maintain and accelerate unprecedented progress—end all preventable maternal, newborn and child deaths.

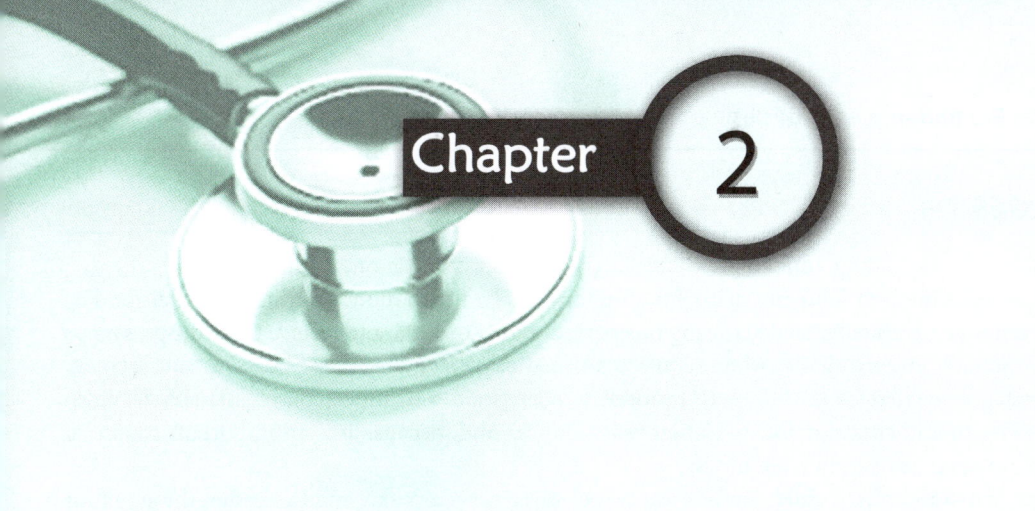

Chapter 2

MAA

INTRODUCTION

MAA—"Mother's Absolute Affection" is a nationwide programme of the Ministry of Health and Family Welfare in an attempt to bring undiluted focus on promotion of breastfeding and provision of counselling services for supporting breastfeeding through health systems. The programme has been named 'MAA' to signify the support a lactating mother requires from family members and at health facilities to breastfed successfully (Fig. 1).

GOAL

The 'MAA' Programme is to revitalize efforts toward promotion, protection and support of breastfeding practices through health systems to achieve higher breastfeding rates.

OBJECTIVES

- Building and enabling environment for breastfeeding through awareness generation activities, targeting pregnant and lactating mothers, family members and society in order to promote optimal breastfeding practices.

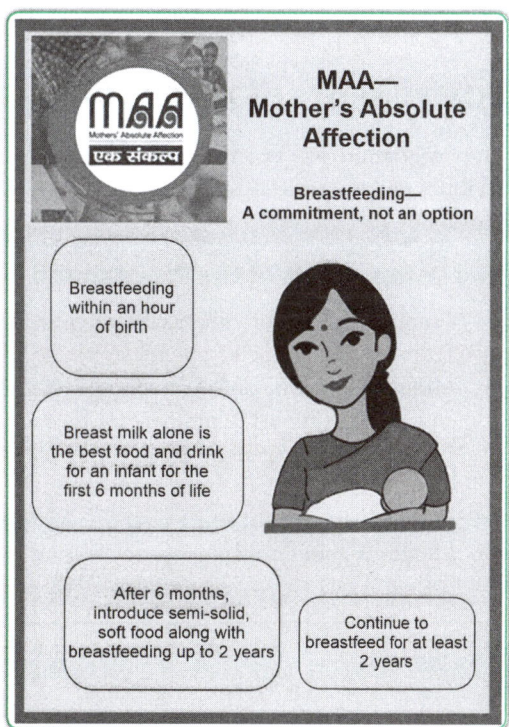

Figure 1: Mother's Absolute Affection

- Breastfeding to be positioned as an important intervention for child survival and development.
- Reinforcing lactation support services at public health facilities through trained healthcare providers and through skilled community health workers.
- To incentivize and recognize those health facilities that show high rates of breastfeding along with processes in place of lactation management.

KEY MESSAGES

- Early initiation of breastfeding; immediately after birth, preferably within one hour.
- Breast-milk alone is the best food and drink for an infant for the first 6 months of life. No other food or drink, not even water, is usually needed during this period. But allow infant to receive ORS, drops, syrups of vitamins, minerals and medicines when required for medical reasons.
- After 6 months of age, babies should be introduced to semi-solid, soft food (complementary feeding) but breastfeding should continue for up to two years and beyond, because it is an important source of nutrition, energy and protection from illness.
- From the age of 6–8 months, a child needs to eat two to three times per day and thereafter, three to four times per day starting at 9 months—in addition to breastfeding. Depending on the child's appetite, one or two nutritious snacks, such as fruit, home-made energy dense food, may be needed between meals. The baby should be fed small amounts of food that steadily increase in variety and quantity as he/she grows.
- During an illness, children need additional fluids and encouragement to eat regular meals, and breastfeding infants need to be breastfed more often. After an illness, children need to be offered more food than usual, to replenish the energy and nourishment lost due to the illness.

COMPONENTS OF MAA PROGRAMME

The Programme will be implemented at three levels: Macro-level through mass media; meso-level in health facilities and micro-level at communities. An overview (Figs 2 and 3) of the components of the programme is as follows:

Key Components of the Programme

- Communication for enhanced awareness and demand generation through mass media and mid media.
- Training and capacity enhancement of nurses at government institutions, and all Auxiliary Nurse Midwives (ANMs) and Accredited Social Health Activists (ASHAs). They will provide information and counselling support to mothers for breastfeding.
- Community engagement by ASHAs for breastfeding promotion, who will conduct mothers' meetings. Breastfeding mothers requiring more support will be referred to a health facility or the ANM sub-center or the Village Health and Nutrition Day (VHND)—organized every month at the village level.
- Monitoring and impact assessment is an integral part of MAA Programme. Progress will be measured

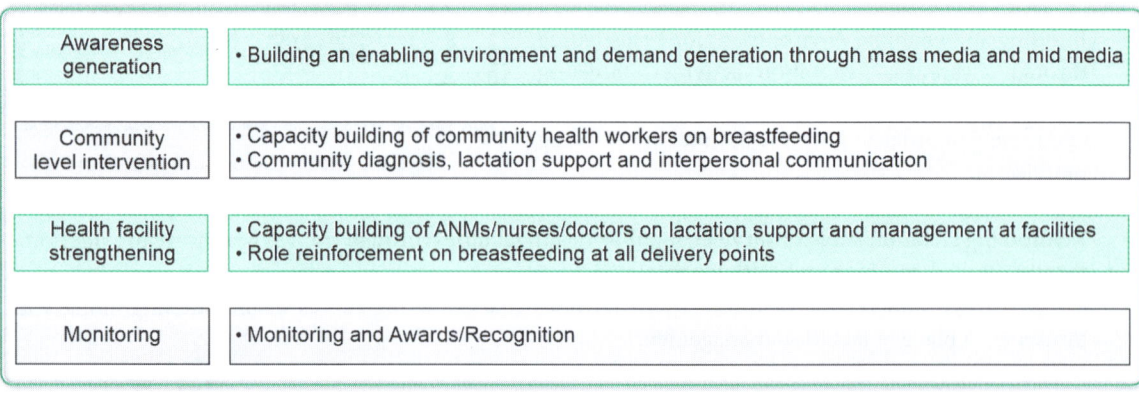

Figure 2: Overview of MAA programme

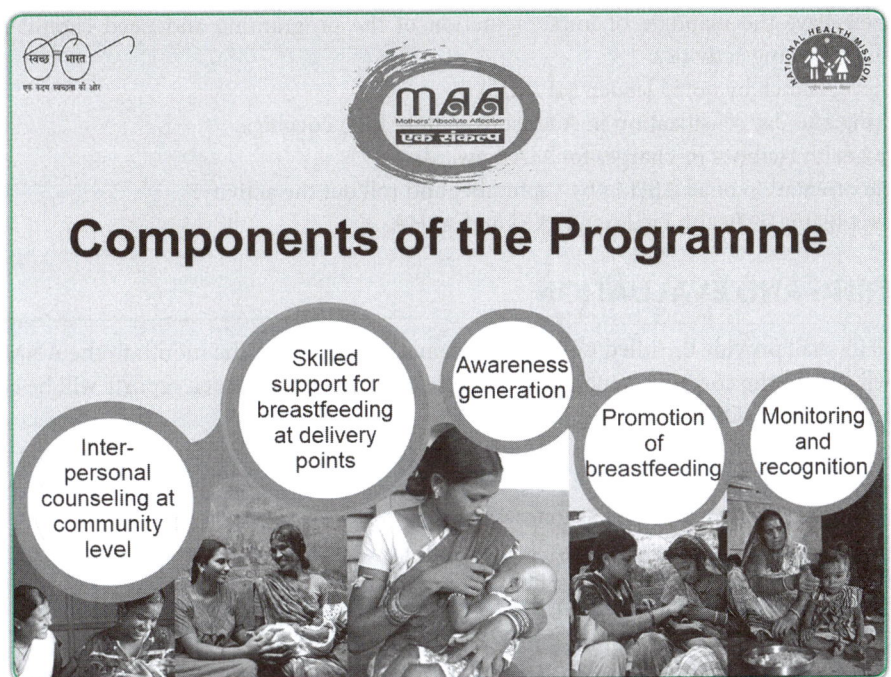

Figure 3: Components of MAA programme

against key indicators, such as availability of skilled persons at delivery points for counselling, improvement in breastfeding practices and number of accredited health facilities.

- Recognition and team awards will be given to facilities showing good performance, based on evaluation against predecided criteria.

PROGRAMME IMPLEMENTATION

The following implementation mechanism is suggested for successful roll out of the MAA Programme:

A, MAA coordination committee formed at state level, may oversee the implementation of suggestive activities as follows:

- Disbursal of guidelines (translated if needed) and funds to districts.
- Adaptation of Information, Education and Communication (IEC) material as per local needs.
- Preparing state and district plans for trainings.
- Identifying Infant and Young Child Feeding (IYCF) master trainers and chalking out training strategy.
- Conducting intersectoral meeting with Women and Child Development (WCD) department and lead development partners for implementation.
- Preparing monitoring plan for monthly reporting.
- Identifying monitors for conducting monitoring to provide awards, in consultation with National Resource Center.
- Printing of IEC material at state/district level.
- Conducting meeting to orient district and block-level health officials on roll out of MAA programme.

Districts largely have the mandate of implementation of the programme and need careful planning for conducting the following activities:

- District level launch by noted leader/MP/MLA.
- Conducting one-day sensitization in August to achieve high coverage.
- Sensitize health facilities in-charges for MAA awards.
- Complete orientation of all ASHAs by September and roll out the activity.
- Plan for reporting by health facilities, ANM and ASHA.

MONITORING AND EVALUATION

- Each ASHA shall provide the filled monitoring formats at the end of the month to the ANM.
- ANM will submit the compiled report to the Block Medical Officer. Block reports will be compiled and submitted to District Official.
- District and States would submit monthly reports on progress of trainings, monitoring and visits at monthly basis.
- The key monitorable indicators are as follows:
  - Number and % of ASHAs for whom sensitization on IYCF was conducted in block meetings.
  - Number of districts that conducted launch of MAA programme.
  - Number of mothers' meetings held.
  - Number and % of pregnant and lactating mothers who attended mother's meetings.
  - Number and % of ASHAs having IYCF info kit.
  - Number and % of ASHAs provided incentive for mothers' meetings.
  - Number and % of ANMs for whom one-day sensitization was undertaken.
  - Number and % of ANMs and nurses trained on 4-day trainings.
  - Number and % of delivery points, where healthcare providers have been oriented using one-day sensitization module.
  - Number of facilities received MAA awards (at state level).
  - A state wide evaluation survey would be undertaken after one year of implementation of MAA programme.

Chapter 3

National AYUSH Mission

INTRODUCTION

Department of AYUSH, Ministry of Health and Family Welfare, Government of India has launched National AYUSH Mission (NAM) during 12th Plan for implementing through States/UTs. The basic objective of NAM is to promote AYUSH medical systems through cost effective AYUSH services, strengthen educational systems, and facilitate the enforcement of quality control of Ayurveda, Siddha and Unani and Homeopathy (ASU and H) drugs and sustainable availability of ASU and H raw-materials. It envisages flexibility of implementation of the programmes which will lead to substantial participation of the State Governments/UT. The NAM contemplates establishment of a National Mission as well as corresponding Missions at the State level. NAM is likely to improve significantly the Department's outreach in terms of planning, supervision and monitoring of the schemes.

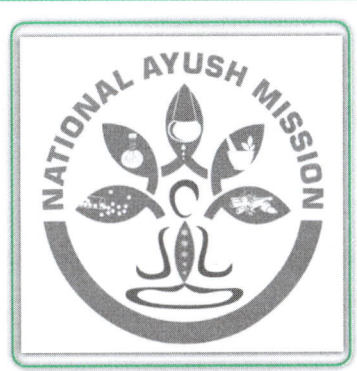

VISION

- To provide cost effective and equitable AYUSH health care throughout the country by improving access to the services.
- To revitalize and strengthen the AYUSH systems making them prominent medical streams in addressing the health care of the society.
- To improve educational institutions capable of imparting quality AYUSH education.
- To promote the adoption of quality standards of AYUSH drugs and making available the sustained supply of AYUSH raw-materials.

OBJECTIVES

- To provide cost effective AYUSH services, with a universal access through upgrading AYUSH Hospitals and Dispensaries, co-location of AYUSH facilities at Primary Health Centers (PHCs), Community Health Centers (CHCs) and District Hospitals (DHs).

- To strengthen institutional capacity at the state level by upgrading AYUSH educational institutions, State Govt. ASU and H Pharmacies, Drug Testing Laboratories and ASU and H enforcement mechanism.
- Support cultivation of medicinal plants by adopting Good Agricultural Practices (GAPs) so as to provide sustained supply of quality raw-materials and support certification mechanism for quality standards, Good Agricultural/Collection/Storage Practices.
- Support setting up of clusters through convergence of cultivation, warehousing, value addition and marketing and development of infrastructure for entrepreneurs.

COMPONENTS OF THE MISSION

Mandatory Components

- AYUSH Services
- AYUSH Educational Institutions
- Quality Control of ASU and H Drugs
- Medicinal Plants

Flexible Components

- Out of the total state envelop available, 20% funds will be earmarked for flexible funds which can be spent on any of the items given below with the stipulation that not more than 5% of the envelope is spent on any of the components:
  - AYUSH Wellness Centers including Yoga and Naturopathy.
  - Tele-medicine.
  - Sports medicine through AYUSH.
  - Innovations in AYUSH including Public Private Partnership.
  - Interest subsidy component for Private AYUSH Educational Institutions.
  - Reimbursement of testing charges.
  - IEC activities.
  - Research and Development in areas related to medicinal plants.
  - Voluntary certification scheme: Project-based.
  - Market promotion, market intelligence and buy back interventions.
  - Crop insurance for medicinal plants.
- The financial assistance from Government of India shall be supplementary in the form of contractual engagements, infrastructure development, capacity building and supply of medicines to be provided from Department of AYUSH. This will ensure better implementation of the programme through effective coordination and monitoring. States shall ensure to make available all the regular manpower posts filled in the existing facilities. The procurement of medicines will be made by the States/UTs as per the existing guidelines of the scheme.

SUPPORTING FACILITIES UNDER MISSION

- In order to strengthen the AYUSH infrastructure both attached Central and State levels, financial assistance for setting up of the Programme Management Units (PMUs) will be provided. The PMU will consist of management and technical professionals both at Central and State level and will be essentially on contract or through service providers.

- The PMU staff will be engaged from the open market on contractual basis or outsourcing and the expenditure on their salary will be met out of admissible administrative and managerial cost for the mission period. This PMU will provide the technical support for the implementation of National AYUSH Mission in the state through its pool of skilled professionals like MBA, CA, accounts and technical specialist, etc. All appointments would be contractual and Central Government's liability will be limited only to the extent of Central share admissible for administrative and management costs on salary head for the mission period.

- In addition to the manpower cost for PMU, the States/UTs can avail the financial assistance for such administrative costs like office expenditure, traveling expenditure, contingency, Annual Maintenance Cost (AMC) of infrastructure including equipment', computer, software for health management information system (HMIS), Training and Capacity Building for concerned personnel under each component, audit, monitoring and evaluation, project preparation consultancy and additional manpower for AYUSH Hospitals and Dispensaries. A total 4% of the net funds available for the state is earmarked for State/UTs administrative costs under the mission.

RESOURCE ALLOCATION FRAMEWORK

- **For AYUSH Services, Educational Institutions and Quality Control of ASU and H Drugs:** For special Category states (NE States and three hilly States of Himachal Pradesh, Uttarakhand, Jammu and Kashmir), Grant-in-aid component will be 90% from Govt. of India and remaining 10% is proposed to be the State contribution toward all components under the scheme. For other States/UTs, the sharing pattern will be 75%:25%.

- For medicinal plants: This component will be financed 100% by Central Government in North Eastern State and hilly States of Himachal Pradesh, Uttarakhand and Jammu and Kashmir whereas in other states it will be shared in the ratio of 90:10 between Center and States.

- The resource pool to the States from the Government of India under the mission shall be determined on the basis of following:
  - Population with 70% weightage and 2 as multiplying factor for Empowered Action Group (EAG) States, Island UTs and Hilly States.
  - Backwardness determined on the basis of proxy indicator of per capita income will have 15% weightage.
  - Performance to be determined on inverse proportion of percentage of UCs due and pending as on 31st March of previous financial year will have 15% weightage.

- Components of National AYUSH Mission will have certain core activities that are essential and other activities that are optional. For core/essential items 80% of the resource pool allocated to the States can be used. For optional items, the remaining 20% of resource pool allocated to the States can be used in a flexible manner, with the restriction that this 20% of resource pool can be spent on any of the items allowed with constraints that not more than 5% of the envelope is spent on any of the components:

- The amount of release against the central share will be: Entitled Central Share – (Unspent balance of the Grant-in Aid released in previous years + interest accrued).

ACTION PLAN

- Indication of tentative State allocation by Department of AYUSH, Government of India - 31st, December.
- Budget Provision by the State Government along with matching State Share - 31st March.

- Preparation of State Annual Action Plan by Executive Committee of the State AYUSH Society – 30th April.
- The receipt of State Annual Action Plan in the Department of AYUSH, Government of India – 1st week of May.

Monitoring and Evaluation

- Dedicated MIS monitoring and evaluation cell would be established at Center/State level. It is, therefore, proposed to have a HMIS Cell at National level with three HMIS Managers and one HMIS Manager at State level.
- The concurrent evaluation of the AYUSH Mission shall be carried out to know the implementation progress and bottlenecks and scope for improvement. Third party evaluation will also be carried out after two years of Mission implementation.

Expected Outcomes

- Improvement in AYUSH education through enhanced number of AYUSH Educational Institutions upgraded.
- Better access to AYUSH services through increased number of AYUSH Hospital and Dispensaries coverage, availability of drugs and manpower.
- Sustained availability of quality raw-materials for AYUSH Systems of Medicine.
- Improved availability of quality ASU and H drugs through increase in the number of quality Pharmacies and Drug Laboratories and enforcement mechanism of ASU and H drugs.

AYUSH HEALTH AND WELLNESS CENTER

Recently, the Union Cabinet has approved the inclusion of AYUSH Health and Wellness Centers (AYUSH HWCs) in the National AYUSH Mission (NAM).

- AYUSH HWC is a component of the Ayushman Bharat.

Background

- The National Health Policy 2017 advocated for mainstreaming the potential of AYUSH systems (Ayurveda, Yoga and Naturopathy, Unani, Siddha, Sowa-rigpa and Homeopathy) within a pluralistic system of integrative healthcare.
- In 2018, the Government of India decided that 1.5 lakh health and wellness centers would be created by transforming existing sub-health centers and primary health centers to deliver comprehensive primary health care. So, it was decided that the Ministry of AYUSH would operationalize 10% of the total sub-health centers as HWCs under Ayushman Bharat.

Key Points

- **Cost and time:**
  - **Expenditure:** ₹3399.35 Crore (with a ratio of almost 2:1 between the center and the states respectively).
  - **Times:** Within a period of five-years from 2019–20 to 2023–24.
- AYUSH HWCs operating under NAM will have the following objectives:
  - To establish a holistic wellness model based on AYUSH principles and practices focusing on preventive, promotive, curative, rehabilitative and palliative healthcare by integration with the existing public health care system.

- To provide informed choice to the public in need, by making the AYUSH services available.
- To spread community awareness about lifestyle, yoga, medicinal plants and provision of medicines for selected conditions as per strength of AYUSH systems.
- After consulting with the States/UTs, Ministry of Health and Family Welfare and other ministries involved, the Ministry of AYUSH has proposed two models for operationalization of AYUSH HWCs:
  - Upgradation of existing AYUSH dispensaries.
  - Upgradation of existing Sub Health Centers (SHCs).
- **Benefits:**
  - Enhanced accessibility to achieve universal health coverage for affordable treatment.
  - Reduced burden on secondary and tertiary health care facilities.
  - Reduced out of pocket expenditure due to self-care model.
  - Integration of AYUSH in implementation of Sustainable Development Goal (SDG) 3 (Good Health and Well-being), as mandated by the NITI Aayog.
  - Validated holistic wellness model in target areas.

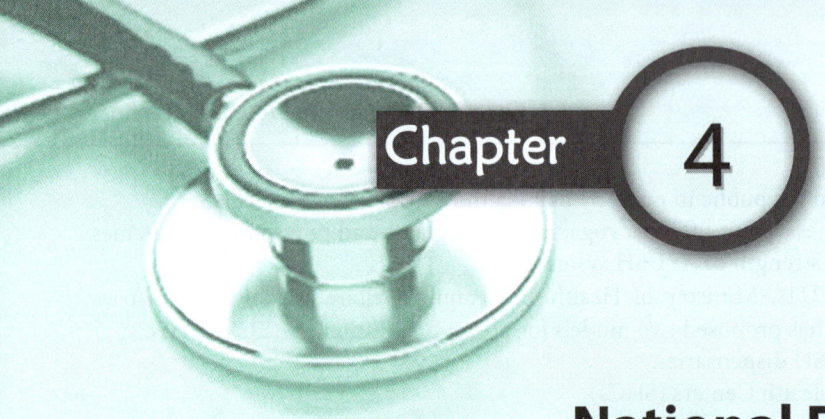

Chapter 4

National Framework for a Gender-responsive Approach to TB in India

INTRODUCTION

Tuberculosis (TB) affects an estimated 10 million people globally every year, of which around 3.2 million are women. India has the world's highest annual incidence of TB as well as the highest TB-related mortality. Although more men are affected by TB, women and transgender persons experience the disease differently.

Gender differences and inequalities play a significant role in how people of all genders access and receive healthcare in the public and private sectors. There is adequate evidence to indicate that gender is a significant influencer of the epidemiology, risk factors, probability of diagnosis, access to healthcare, treatment adherence and overall impact of TB on communities.

A gendered approach to TB care and prevention is a felt need in the Revised National Tuberculosis Control Programme (RNTCP) for which a framework has been developed.

GOAL

To adopt and implement a gender-responsive approach to TB in India.

OBJECTIVES

- To aim for equitable, rights-based TB services for women, men and transgender persons by adopting a gender-specific programmatic approach at all levels.
- To mobilize, empower and engage women, men and transgender persons in the TB response at the health system and community levels.

OVERALL GUIDING PRINCIPLES

- **Nondiscrimination:** Treat all people with TB fairly, regardless of age, sex, sexual orientation, gender identity, ethnicity, religion, class, occupation, disability and mode of transmission.
- **Informed choice:** Enable people with TB to make well-considered, voluntary decisions by providing a full range of information and options related to their healthcare.
- **Informed consent:** Provide sufficient information about medical procedures and tests to ensure that these are understood, and respect the individual's autonomy in making fully informed decisions.

- **Confidentiality:** Ensure that all medical records and information are kept confidential. Only healthcare professionals with a direct role in the management of care seekers or people with TB should have access to such records, on a need-to-know basis.
- **Respect for all:** Each programme stakeholder and beneficiary must be treated with respect and dignity.
- **Access for all:** Make services accessible to as many people as possible with regard to availability, affordability and acceptability.
- **Working in partnership:** Build partnerships between government and civil society (including community- based organizations, women's groups, TB Champion and survivor led networks), and among all social sectors, both public and private.
- **Linking prevention, treatment and care:** Build comprehensive programmes by linking TB prevention, treatment and care services, as well as other related health services needed by people with TB or TB symptoms.
- **Promoting the rights of individuals and groups:** Promote, respect and enforce the human rights of people with TB, including the right to adequate health information.
- **Fostering accountability:** Foster the accountability of all staff, including programme managers and decision makers, for the achievement of gender-related goals and objectives.
- **Empowering communities:** Contribute to the creation of an enabling environment for people with TB by empowering individuals and communities through outreach and community education about TB and related gender inequalities.

BASIC STEPS FOR GENDER RESPONSIVE PROGRAMMING

- Assess provider knowledge on gender responsive programming and existing gender-sensitive practices.
- Build capacity of providers on the gender perspective and providing comprehensive person-centric care.
- Conduct baseline assessment of facilities, infrastructure and linkages in the context of gender-responsive programming.
- Promote active involvement of people affected by TB of all genders in all aspects of the design, planning and delivery of programmes. The participation of people affected by TB and survivors must be supported through capacity building and mentoring. Accordingly, all the activities outlined under the National Strategic Plan (NSP) heads— Detect, Treat, Prevent and Build—incorporate components of community engagement.

ABOUT THE FRAMEWORK

The framework reflects the interactions between TB and gender at various levels, and aims to:
- Outline the influences and impact of gender on the TB burden and response, based on available literature and data.
- Define actions which would help move towards a gender-responsive approach.
- Provide guidance to implement these actions.

The framework is in keeping with the NSP for TB for 2017–2025 and is intended to spark dialogue at all levels within the TB programme and among key stakeholders, thereby strengthening the collective understanding of TB and gender.

GENDER AS A DETERMINANT FOR TB

- **Gender Differences in Incidence of TB:** A higher proportion of the 27.4 lakh diagnosed with TB in India are men and the ratio is approximately 2:1 (Global TB Report 2018) between men and women.

Multiple studies on the incidence of TB across the country indicate that more men report microbiologically confirmed pulmonary TB and women are more likely to have clinically diagnosed pulmonary TB and extrapulmonary forms of TB. Research shows that the prevalence of HIV-TB co-infection is higher among women and among transgender persons who live in overcrowded houses and consume alcohol. Pregnant women and women in the postpartum period face a higher risk of TB and TB is one of the leading non-obstetric causes of maternal mortality in low-income countries like India.

- **Gender differences in exposure, risks and vulnerability:** Women are especially constrained by social norms which prevent prioritizing of their nutrition, health and wellbeing. Undernutrition, their role as caretakers and the use of solid fuel for cooking puts women at risk for TB. While alcoholism and smoking among women is poorly accepted, these behaviors may be condoned or even encouraged as a result of the prevailing gender norms for men. Smoking and alcohol consumption are therefore specific gender-linked barriers to TB diagnosis and treatment for men. Men are at greater risk of developing TB due to their employment in mining, quarrying, metals and construction industries. Transgender persons often have low literacy, low education levels and are poor. A high proportion of transgender persons are known to smoke, consume alcohol and use drugs. All these factors make them vulnerable to TB.

- **Gender differences in health seeking and health system factors:** While the fear of loss of income and the consequences of absence from work hinder care seeking in men, women face difficulties due to perceived stigma, prioritization of household chores, lack of money or financial dependence. Poor health literacy and fear of criminalization hinders transgender persons from seeking care. Besides gender differences, influencing care-seeking, health system factors such as limited access, lower index of suspicion of TB for women and provision of inadequate information to care-seekers also significantly affect the access to services across all genders.

- **Gender differences in treatment outcomes:** Traditionally, women tend to have better adherence and treatment outcomes as compared to men. The pressure to get back to work and lifestyle habits such as smoking or consumption of alcohol influence discontinuation of treatment in men. Migrant workers, mostly men, often face difficulties in adherence to treatment in the face of extreme poverty and issues of daily survival. Stigma and discrimination are major impediments to treatment adherence, mainly among unmarried women, newly married women and the elderly.

INTERVENTIONS

The framework deals with interventions under the heads of Detect, Treat, Prevent and Build. It also outlines potential gender-responsive interventions under public and private sectors as well as by and with communities.

- **Detect:** Actions proposed will include training of RNTCP staff in the public sector and private providers on gender differences along the diagnostic pathway between women, men and transgender persons. The programme will ensure that Active Case Finding (ACF) teams are trained on gender-responsive questioning and that the fundamental principle of 'do no harm' is conveyed during training. The programme will also strengthen the involvement of TB Champions and survivor led networks to improve care-seeking behavior among all groups, especially women and transgender persons.

- **Treat:** Key actions will include orienting health workers on adopting a respectful attitude, respecting the need for confidentiality, improving treatment literacy and providing gender-responsive counseling. Private sector providers will be trained on the need for gendered adherence support and TB Champions and survivor-led networks will be involved for the provision of gendered psychosocial support.

- **Prevent:** Women and caregivers will be involved to strengthen contact screening and chemoprophylaxis; periodic screening of health workers for TB will be undertaken; involvement of communities in prevention drives will be strengthened.
- **Build:** The emphasis will be on building the capacity of the programme and the private sector to provide gendered, comprehensive, and patient-centric care. Promoting gender representativeness among survivor-led networks will be a priority.

  The framework will guide the programme to mobilize, empower and engage women, men and transgender persons in the TB response at the health system and community levels. Once implemented, the framework envisages a gender-responsive programme which will catalyze and accelerate efforts to end TB in India.

HOW TO USE THIS FRAMEWORK?

This framework is intended for programme managers, healthcare providers at the district, state and national levels in the RNTCP as well as for civil society and community representatives, programme managers and healthcare providers involved in provision and evaluation of TB care services in the not-for-profit and private sectors. This framework can be used to:

- Understand the elements of a gender responsive approach to TB.
- Give training to health providers and staff on how to provide gender-responsive care and support along the care cascade.
- Assess and improve the gender sensitivity of services and service providers.

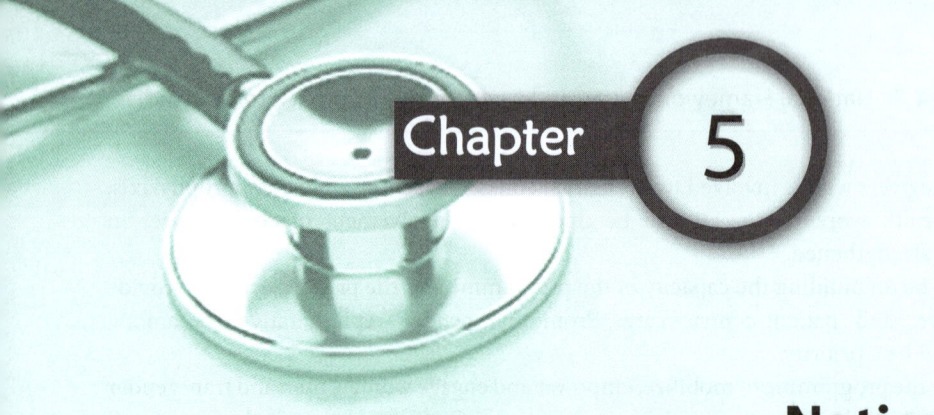

Chapter 5

National Iron Plus Initiative for Anemia Control

INTRODUCTION

A nemia is a serious public health challenge in India with more than 50% prevalence among the vulnerable groups such as pregnant women, infants, young children and adolescents. Iron deficiency is the most common form of nutritional anemia. National Iron Plus Initiative was launched by the Adolescent Division of the Ministry of Health and Family Welfare (MoHFW), Government of India (Fig. 1).

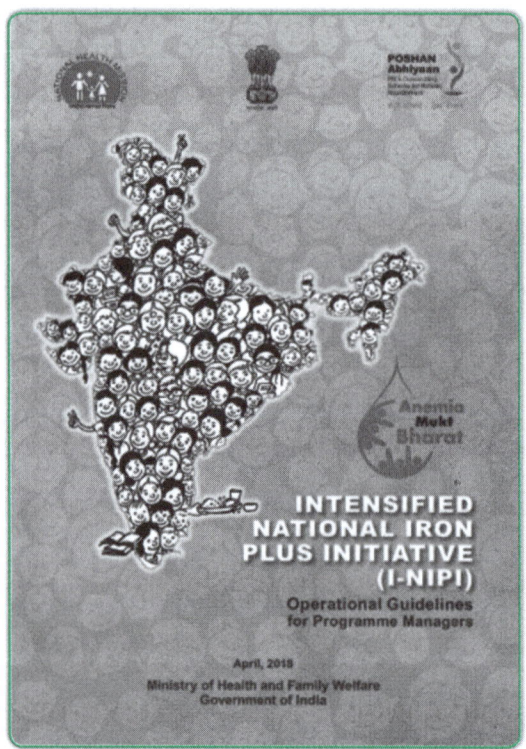

Figure 1: National Iron Plus Initiative

OBJECTIVE

The reduction of anemia is one of the important objectives of the POSHAN Abhiyaan launched in March 2018. Complying with the targets of POSHAN Abhiyaan and National Nutrition Strategy set by NITI Aayog, the Anemia Mukt Bharat strategy has been designed to reduce prevalence of anemia by 3 percentage points per year among children, adolescents and women in the reproductive age group (15–49 years), between the year 2018 and 2022.

AIMS

- To reach the following age groups for supplementation of iron and folic acid.
- Taking cognizance of ground realities discussed above, the Ministry of Health and Family Welfare took a policy decision to develop the National Iron+ Initiative.
- This initiative will bring together existing programmes (IFA supplementation for: pregnant and lactating women and; children in the age group of 6–60 months) and introduce new age groups.
- Thus National Iron+ Initiative will reach the following age groups for supplementation or preventive programming:
  - Bi-weekly iron supplementation for preschool children 6 months to 5 years.
  - Weekly supplementation for children from 1st to 5th grade in Govt. and Govt. aided schools.
  - Weekly supplementation for out of school children (5–10 years) at Anganwadi Centers.
  - Weekly supplementation for adolescents (10–19 years).
  - Pregnant and lactating women.
  - Weekly supplementation for women in reproductive age.

  Establishing a continuum of care, the National Iron Plus Initiative also defines a minimum service of packages for treatment and management of anemia across levels of care. Platforms and services at each level have also been mapped out and service providers' roles and responsibilities detailed.

BENEFICIARIES AND TARGETS

The strategy is estimated to reach out to 450 million beneficiaries with specific anemia prevalence targets for year 2022 (Table 1) to be achieved among various population groups.

Table 1: Anemia Mukt Bharat beneficiaries and anemia reduction targets for different age groups for 2022

Age group	Estimated beneficiaries (in millions)
Children (6–59 months)	124
Children (5–9 years)	134
Adolescent boys (10–19 years)	47
Adolescent girls (10–19 years)	68
Women of reproductive age (20–24 years)	17
Pregnant women	30
Lactating women	27
Total beneficiaries	~450 million

Beneficiary estimations are as per Census 2011 estimations for 2017.

Estimated number of beneficiaries will be annually revised and updated. While all women of reproductive age should ideally be covered, the estimated number of beneficiaries are the women aged 20–24 years from Mission Parivar Vikas Yojana who will be initially covered in Anemia Mukt Bharat (Table 2).

The Anemia Mukt Bharat strategy will be implemented in all villages, blocks, and districts of all the States/UTs of India through existing delivery platforms as envisaged in the National Iron Plus Initiative (NIPI) and Weekly Iron Folic Acid Supplementation (WIFS) programme.

Table 2: Anemia Mukt Bharat anemia reduction targets for 2022

Age group	Anemia prevalence (%)	
	Baseline (NFHS 4)	National target 2022 (at 3 percentage points per annum from baseline)
Children (6–59 months)	58	40
Adolescent girls (15–19 years)	54	36
Adolescent boys (15–19 years)	29	11
Women of reproductive age	53	35
Pregnant women	50	32
Lactating women	58	40

STRATEGY FOR IMPLEMENTATION

A snapshot of the Anemia Mukt Bharat 6 × 6 × 6 strategy is depicted in Figures 2A and B as follows:

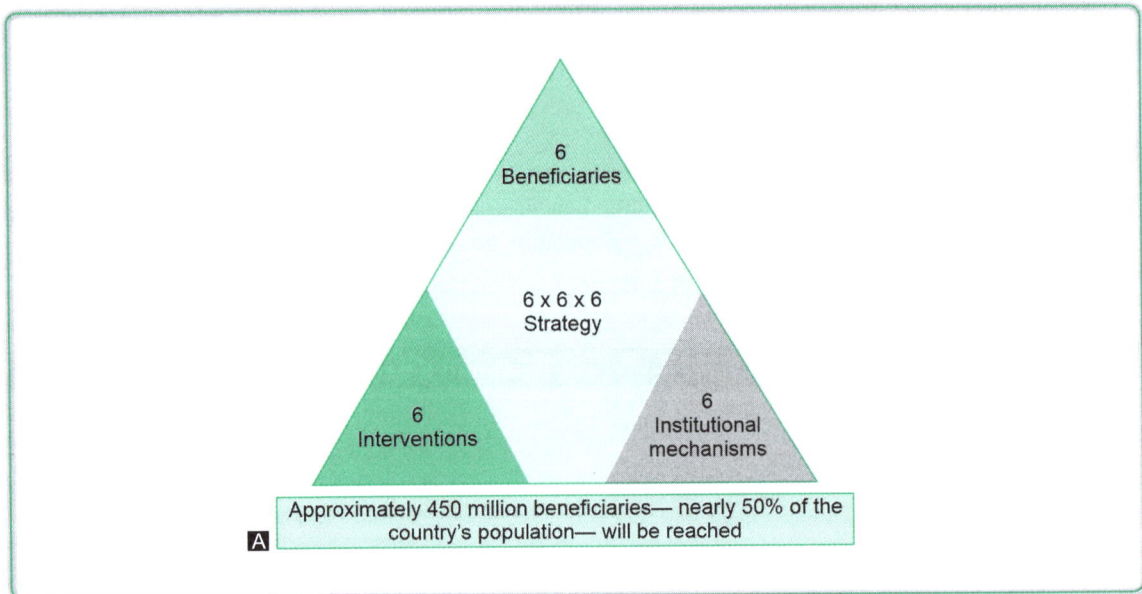

Figure 2A:

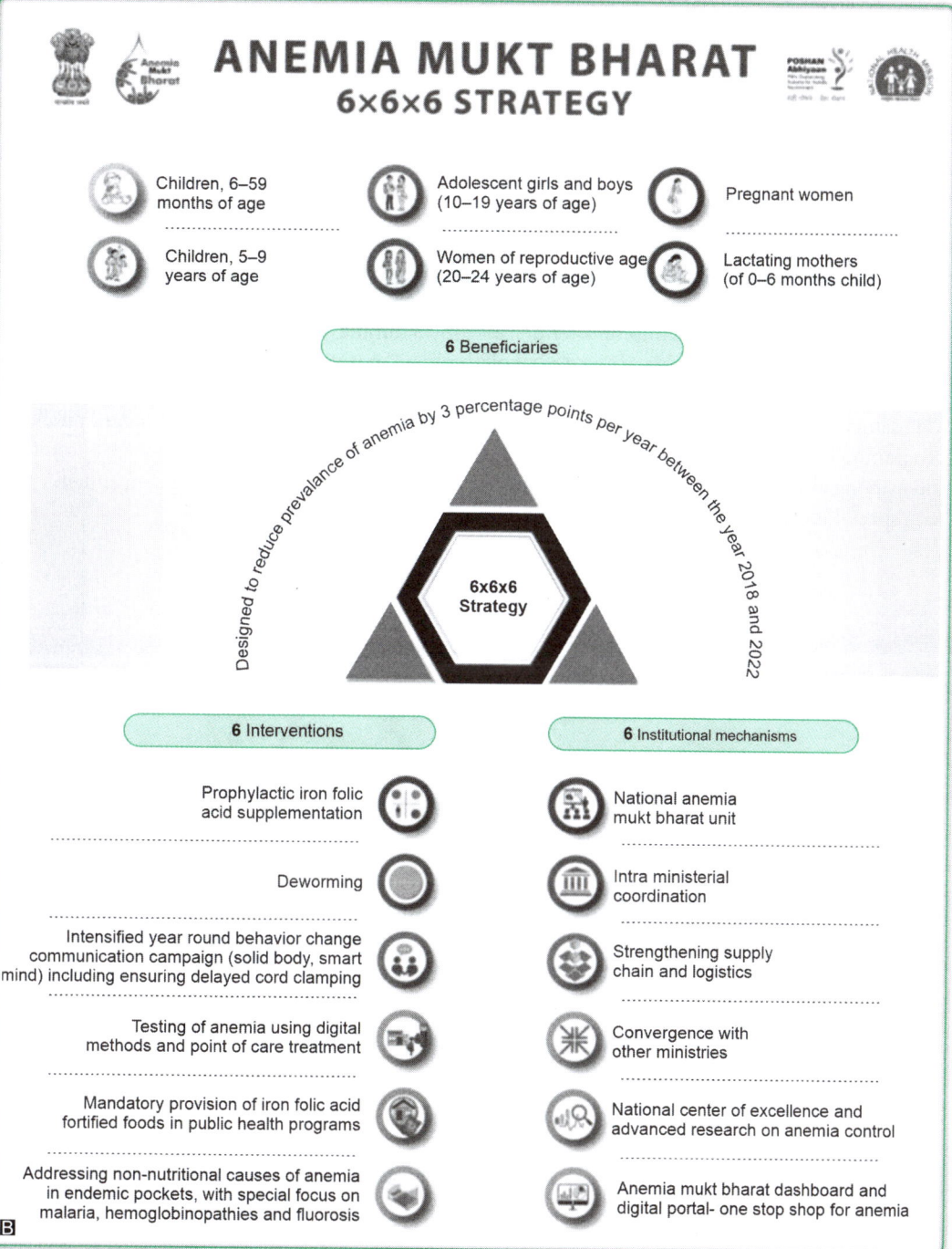

Figures 2A and B: Anemia Mukt Bharat

INTERVENTIONS

The Anemia Mukt Bharat strategy (Fig. 3) is a universal strategy and will focus on the following interventions:
- Prophylactic Iron and Folic Acid supplementation.
- Deworming.
- Intensified year-round Behavior Change Communication Campaign (Solid Body, Smart Mind) focusing on four key behaviors.
  - Improving compliance to Iron Folic Acid supplementation and deworming.
  - Appropriate infant and young child feeding practices.
  - Increase in intake of iron-rich food through diet diversity/quantity/frequency and/or fortified foods with focus on harnessing locally available resources.
  - Ensuring delayed cord clamping after delivery (by 3 minutes) in health facilities.
- Testing and treatment of anemia, using digital methods and point of care treatment, with special focus on pregnant women and school-going adolescents.
- Mandatory provision of Iron and Folic Acid fortified foods in government-funded public health programmes.
- Intensifying awareness, screening and treatment of non-nutritional causes of anemia in endemic pockets, with special focus on malaria, and hemoglobinopathies.

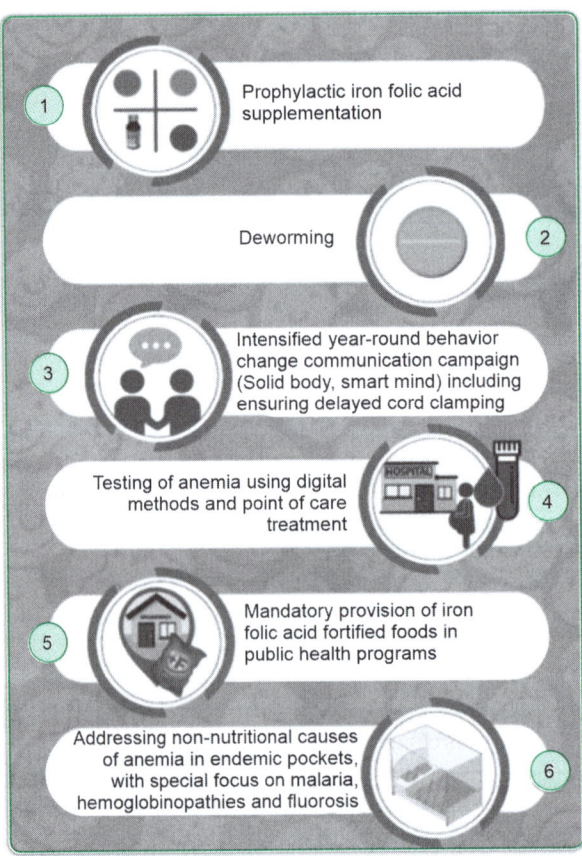

Figure 3: Anemia Mukt Bharat strategy

Prophylactic Iron Folic Acid Supplementation

Prophylactic Iron Folic Acid supplementation is given to children, adolescents, women of reproductive age and pregnant women, irrespective of anemia. It is a key continued intervention under Anemia Mukt Bharat (Table 3).

Table 3: Prophylactic dose and regime for iron folic acid supplementation

Age group	Dose and regime
Children 6–59 months of age	Biweekly, 1 mL Iron and Folic Acid syrup, each mL of Iron and Folic Acid syrup containing 20 mg elemental Iron + 100 mcg of Folic Acid Bottle (50 mL) to have an 'auto-dispenser' and information leaflet as per MoHFW guidelines in the mono-carton
Children 5–9 years of age	Weekly, 1 Iron and Folic Acid tablet, each tablet containing 45 mg elemental Iron + 400 mcg Folic Acid, sugar-coated, pink color
School-going adolescent girls and boys, 10–19 years of age Out-of-school adolescent girls, 10–19 years of age	Weekly, 1 Iron and Folic Acid tablet, each tablet containing 60 mg elemental iron + 500 mcg Folic Acid, sugar-coated, blue color
Women of reproductive age (non-pregnant, non-lactating) 20–24 years	Weekly, 1 Iron and Folic Acid tablet, each tablet containing 60 mg elemental Iron + 500 mcg Folic Acid, sugar-coated, red color
Pregnant women and lactating mothers (of 0–6 months child)	Daily, 1 Iron and Folic Acid tablet starting from the fourth month of pregnancy (that is from the second trimester), continued throughout pregnancy (minimum 180 days during pregnancy) and to be continued for 180 days, post-partum. Each tablet containing 60 mg elemental Iron + 500 mcg Folic Acid, sugar-coated, red color

Note 1: *Prophylaxis with iron should be withheld in case of acute illness (fever, diarrhea, pneumonia, etc.), and in a known case of thalassemia major/history of repeated blood transfusion. In case of SAM children, IFA supplementation should be continued as per SAM management protocol.*
Note 2: *All women in the reproductive age group in the pre-conception period and up to the first trimester of the pregnancy are advised to have 400 mcg of Folic Acid tablets, daily to reduce the incidence of neural tube defects in the fetus.*

Deworming

Dose and regime of deworming for different age groups are given in Table 4.

Table 4: Dose and regime for deworming

Age group	Dose and regime
Children 12–59 months of age	Biannual dose of 400 mg albendazole (½ tablet to children 12–24 months and 1 tablet to children 24–59 months)
Children 5–9 years of age	Biannual dose of 400 mg albendazole (1 tablet)
School-going adolescent girls and boys 10–19 years of age Out-of-school adolescent girls 10–19 years of age	Biannual dose of 400 mg albendazole (1 tablet)
Women of reproductive age (non-pregnant, non-lactating) 20–49 years	Biannual dose of 400 mg albendazole (1 tablet)
Pregnant women	One dose of 400 mg albendazole (1 tablet), after the first trimester, preferably during the second trimester

Promotion and monitoring of delayed clamping of the umbilical cord for at least 3 minutes (or until cord pulsations ceases) for newborns across all health facilities will be carried out for improving the infant's iron reserves up to 6 months after birth. Simultaneously, all birth attendants should make an effort to ensure early initiation of breastfeeding within 1 hour of birth.

THERAPEUTIC MANAGEMENT OF ANEMIA

Therapeutic management of anemia for children, adolescents and pregnant women are given in Tables 5 to 7 respectively.

Table 5: Anemia management protocol for children

Target group A	Children 6–59 months
Who will screen and place of screening	ANM: VHND/sub-center/session site RSBK team: AWC/school Medical Officer: health facility
Periodicity	RBSK/ANM: as per scheduled microplan MO: opportunistic
If hemoglobin is 7–10.9 g/dL (mild and moderate anemia)	
First level of treatment (at all levels of care)	mg of iron/kg/day for 2 months • For children 6–12 months (6–10.9 kg): 1 mL IFA syrup, once a day • For children 1–3 years (11–14.9 kg): 1.5 mL IFA syrup, once a day • For children 3–5 years (15–19.9 kg): 2 mL IFA syrup, once a day Line listing for all anemic children to be maintained by the ANM/ASHA/AWW
Follow-up	• Every month by ANM at VHND • Hb estimation after 2 months for completing 2 months of treatment to document Hb $\geq$ = 11 g/dL • Monitoring by ASHA for compliance of IFA syrup every 14 days for a period of 2 months If hemoglobin levels have improved to normal level, discontinue the treatment, but continue with the prophylactic IFA dose
If no improvement after first level of treatment	In case the child has not responded to the treatment of anemia with daily dose of iron for 2 months, refer the child to the FRU/DH medical officer/pediatrician/physician for further investigation
If hemoglobin is <7 g/dL (severe anemia)	
Treatment	• Refer urgently to District Hospital/First Referral Unit • Management of severe anemia in children of 6–59 months is to be done by the medical officer at the First Referral Unit/District Hospital based on investigation
Target group B	Children 5–9 years
Who will screen and place of screening	RSBK teams will screen in-school and out-of-school children for anemia. All children with clinical signs and symptoms of anemia will be referred to SC/PHC for Hb estimation and further management
Periodicity	• Once a year • Opportunistic screening, e.g., routine Hb assessment of sick children presented to health facility
If hemoglobin is 8–11.4 g/dL (mild and moderate anemia)	

Contd...

Target group B	Children 5–9 years
First level of treatment (at all levels of care)	3 mg of iron/kg/day for 2 months Line listing of all anemic cases to be maintained in the school register for Iron Folic Acid supplementation and given to the ANM/LHV/Multipurpose Health Worker for designated area
Follow-up	• Class teacher/Nodal teacher at school to orient parents during Parent Teacher Meeting (PTM) for compliance of treatment • Parents to ensure follow-up of child after 30 days and 60 days at nearest SC/health facility • Follow-up by ANM/LHV/MPW of designated area, as feasible. • Hb estimation after completing 2 months of treatment to document Hb $\geq$ = 11.5 g/dL • If hemoglobin levels have improved to normal level, discontinue the treatment, but continue with the prophylactic IFA dose
If no improvement after first level of treatment	In case the child has not responded to the treatment of anemia with daily dose of iron for 2 months, refer the child to the FRU/DH medical officer/pediatrician/physician for further investigation
If hemoglobin is <8 g/dL (severe anemia)	
Treatment	• Refer urgently to District Hospital/First Referral Unit • Management of severe anemia in children of 5–9 years is to be done by the medical officer at the First Referral Unit/District Hospital based on investigation

Table 6: Anemia management protocol for adolescents

Target group	All school-going adolescents 10–19 years in government/government-aided schools
Who will screen and place of screening	In school premises by RSBK team
Periodicity	Annually
Mild and moderate anemia (Hb cut-off as per Table 1)	
First level of treatment (at all levels of care)	Two IFA tablets (each with 60 mg elemental iron and 500 mcg folic acid), once daily, for 3 months, orally after meals
Follow-up	• Line listing of all anemic cases to be maintained in the school register for Iron Folic Acid supplementation and given to the ANM/LHV/MPHW of designated area • Follow-up by ANM/LHV/MPHW of designated area, as feasible for the state • Parents to ensure follow-up of adolescent after 45 days to 90 days at the nearest sub-center/health facility> • If hemoglobin levels have improved to normal level, discontinue the treatment, but continue with the prophylactic IFA dose
If no improvement after first level of treatment	If no improvement after three months of treatment (i.e., still in mild/moderate category), ANM/MO of nearest facility to refer adolescent to First Referral Unit (FRU)/District Hospital (DH)
If hemoglobin is <8 g/dL (severe anemia)	
First dose of treatment	Management of severe anemia in adolescents 10–19 years is to be done by the medical officer at FRU/DH based on investigation and subsequent diagnosis

Table 7: Anemia management protocol for pregnant women

Target group	Pregnant women registered for antenatal care
Who will screen and place of screening	Health service provider at any ANC contact, including Pradhan Mantri Surakshit Matritva Abhiyan (PMSMA)
Periodicity	At every ANC contact
If hemoglobin is 10–10.9 g/dL (mild anemia)	
First level of treatment (at all levels of care)	• Two tablets of Iron and Folic Acid tablet (60 mg elemental Iron and 500 mcg Folic Acid) daily, orally given by the health provider during the ANC contact • Parental iron (IV Iron Sucrose or Ferric Carboxymaltose (FCM) may be considered as the first line of management in pregnant women who are detected to be anemic late in pregnancy or in whom compliance is likely to be low (high chance of lost to follow-up)
Follow-up	• Every 2 months for compliance of treatment by health provider during the contact • If hemoglobin levels have come up to normal level, discontinue the treatment and continue with the prophylactic IFA dose
If no improvement after first level of treatment	If no improvement in hemoglobin (<1 g/dL increase) after one month of treatment, refer to First Referral Unit (FRU)/District Hospital (DH) by health provider The case to be referred to FRU/DH for further investigations for cause of anemia and may be managed with IV Iron Sucrose/FCM
If hemoglobin is 7–9.9 g/dL (moderate anemia)	
First level of treatment (at all levels of care)	Two tablets of Iron and Folic Acid tablet (60 mg elemental Iron and 500 mcg Folic Acid) daily, orally given by the health provider during the ANC contact • Parental iron (IV Iron Sucrose or FCM) may be considered as the first line of management in pregnant women who are detected to be anemic late in pregnancy or in whom compliance is likely to be low (high chance of lost to follow-up)
Follow-up	• Every 2 months for compliance of treatment by health provider at regular ANC clinics/PMSMA/VHND platform. • The contact is to be utilized by the health provider to also conduct hemoglobin estimation of the anemic cases every month. If hemoglobin levels have come up to normal level, discontinue the treatment and continue with the prophylactic IFA dose.
If no improvement after first level of treatment	If no improvement in hemoglobin (<1 g/dL increase) after two months of treatment, refer to First Referral Unit (FRU)/District Hospital (DH) by health provider The case to be referred to FRU/DH for further investigations for cause of anemia and may be managed with IV Iron Sucrose/FCM
If hemoglobin is 5.0–6.9 g/dL (severe anemia)	
First level of treatment	Management of severe anemia in pregnant women will be done by the medical officer at PHC/CHC/FRU/DH The treatment will be done using IV Iron Sucrose/Ferric Carboxymaltose (FCM) by the medical officer *Immediate hospitalization recommended in the third trimester of pregnancy at a health facility where round-the-clock specialist care is available*

Contd...

Target group	Pregnant women registered for antenatal care
Follow-up after first level of treatment	After the first level of treatment, monthly or as prescribed by the medical officer
Treatment protocol if no improvement	As prescribed by the medical officer
Note	For severely anemic pregnant women with hemoglobin less than 5 g/dL, immediate hospitalization irrespective of period of gestation where round-the-clock specialist care is available. This is to be done till normal level of hemoglobin is achieved.

Management protocol for severe anemia mentioned is contraindicated for patients with thalassemia major and sickle cell disease. Treatment of anemia through folic acid is recommended in thalassemia major cases.

Chapter 6

National Nutrition Mission

INTRODUCTION

Rashtriya Poshan Abhiyaan (National Nutrition Mission) is a flagship programme of the Ministry of Women and Child Development (MWCD), Government of India, which ensures convergence with various programmes i.e., Anganwadi Services, Pradhan Mantri Matru Vandana Yojana (PMMVY), Scheme for Adolescent Girls (SAG) of MWCD, Janani Suraksha Yojana (JSY), National Health Mission (NHM), Swachh-Bharat Mission, Public Distribution System (PDS), Department of Food and Public Distribution, Mahatma Gandhi National Rural Employment Guarantee Scheme (MGNREGS) and Ministry of Drinking Water and Sanitation.

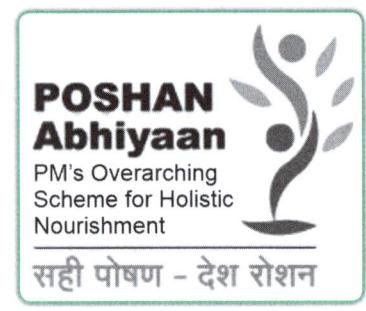

GOAL

To achieve improvement in nutritional status of children from 0 to 6 years, adolescent girls, pregnant women and lactating mothers in a time bound manner during the next three years beginning 2017–18.

TARGETS

- Poshan Abhiyaan, the world's largest nutrition programme expected to benefit 10 crore people, was launched in 2018 by government.
- Aims to reduce stunting, underweight, and low birth weight, each by 2% per year; and anemia among young children, adolescents and women each by 3% per year until 2022. A special target for stunting is set at 25% by 2022.
- The National Nutrition Mission (NNM) (Fig. 1) has been set up with a three-year budget of ₹9046.17 crore commencing from 2017–18.
- The NNM is a comprehensive approach towards raising nutrition level in the country on a war footing.
- It will comprise mapping of various schemes contributing towards addressing malnutrition, including a very robust convergence mechanism, ICT based Real Time Monitoring system, incentivizing States/UTs for meeting the targets, incentivizing Anganwadi Workers (AWWs) for using IT based tools, eliminating registers used by AWWs, introducing measurement of height of children at the Anganwadi Centers (AWCs), Social Audits, setting-up Nutrition Resource Centers, involving masses through Jan Andolan for their participation on nutrition through various activities among others.

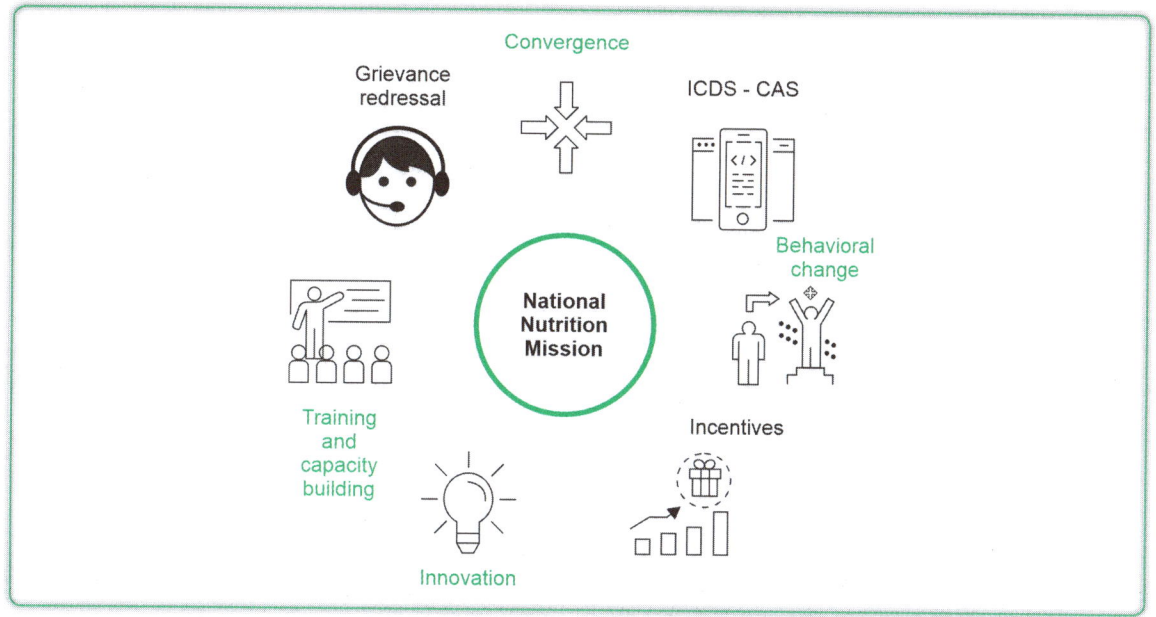

Figure 1: National Nutrition Mission

MONITORING

As a part of its mandate, NITI Aayog is required to submit implementation status reports of POSHAN Abhiyaan every six months to the PMO.

NATIONAL NUTRITION MISSION AND NITI AAYOG

NITI Aayog has played a critical role in shaping the Poshan Abhiyaan. The National Nutrition Strategy, released by NITI Aayog in September 2017, presented a microanalysis of the problems persisting within this area and chalked out an in-depth strategy for course correction. Most of the recommendations presented in the strategy document have been subsumed within the design of the Poshan Abhiyaan and now that the Abhiyaan is launched, NITI Aayog has been entrusted with the task of closely monitoring the Poshan Abhiyaan and undertaking periodic evaluations.

With the overarching aim to build a people's movement (Jan Andolan) around malnutrition, Poshan Abhiyaan intends to significantly reduce malnutrition in the next three years.

For implementation of Poshan Abhiyaan, the four-point strategy/pillars of the mission are:

- Intersectoral convergence for better service delivery.
- Use of technology information and communication technology (ICT) for real time growth monitoring and tracking of women and children.
- Intensified health and nutrition services for the first 1000 days.
- Jan Andolan.

As a part of its mandate, NITI Aayog is required to submit implementation status reports of Poshan Abhiyaan every six months to the PMO. The first bi-annual report was prepared and presented at third National Nutrition Council on India's Nutrition Challenges (which is housed within NITI) in November 2018.

The task of implementation of Poshan Abhiyaan is to be carried out through the Technical Support Unit (TSU) established at NITI Aayog which, in addition to the M and E, will also provide research, policy and technical support to the Abhiyaan.

Integrated child development services (ICDS) system strengthening is depicted below in Figure 2:

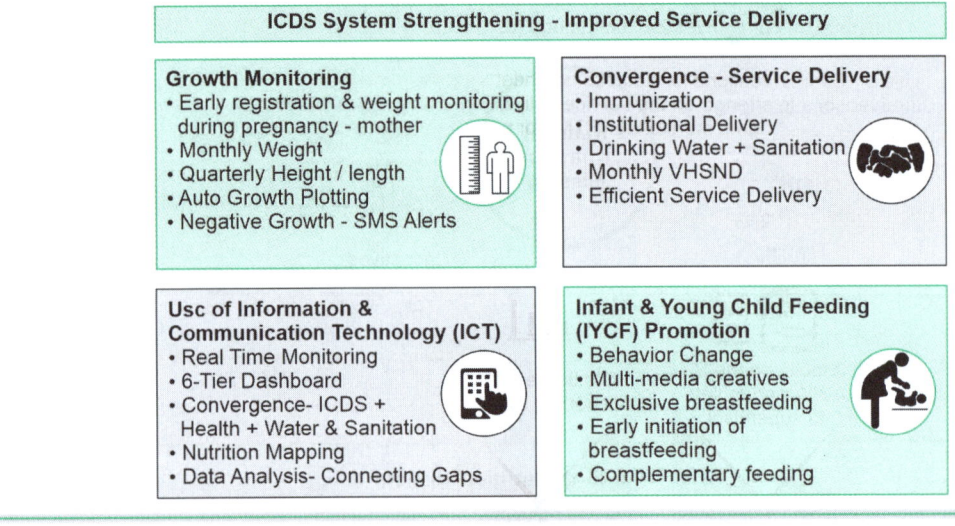

Figure 2: ICDS system strengthening

KEY PROPOSALS

The NNM, as an apex body, monitors, supervises, fixes targets and guides the nutrition-related interventions across the Ministries. The key proposals of NNM are given as follows:

- Mapping of various schemes contributing towards addressing malnutrition.
- Introducing a very robust convergence mechanism.
- ICT based Real-Time Monitoring system.
- Incentivizing states/UTs for meeting the targets.
- Incentivizing Anganwadi Workers (AWWs) for using IT-based tools.
- Eliminating registers used by AWWs.
- Introducing measurement of the height of children at the Anganwadi Centers (AWCs).
- Social audits.
- Setting-up Nutrition Resource Centers, involving masses through Jan Andolan for their participation in nutrition through various activities, among others.

Key Facts

- Poshan Abhiyaan addresses three aspects—the food that should be given to rein in stunting, undernourishment, low birth weight and anemia; the delivery system required for it; and monitoring of the entire process.
- Under the mission, the government is targeting a reduction of 2% a year in stunting, undernutrition and low birth weight among 100 million people. Also, it aims to reduce anemia among young children, women and adolescent girls by 3% a year.

- The mission includes several components like an information and communications technology (ICT)-based real-time monitoring (RTM) (Fig. 3) system, incentivizing of states and Union territories to meet their targets, social audits, and setting up of nutrition resource centers.

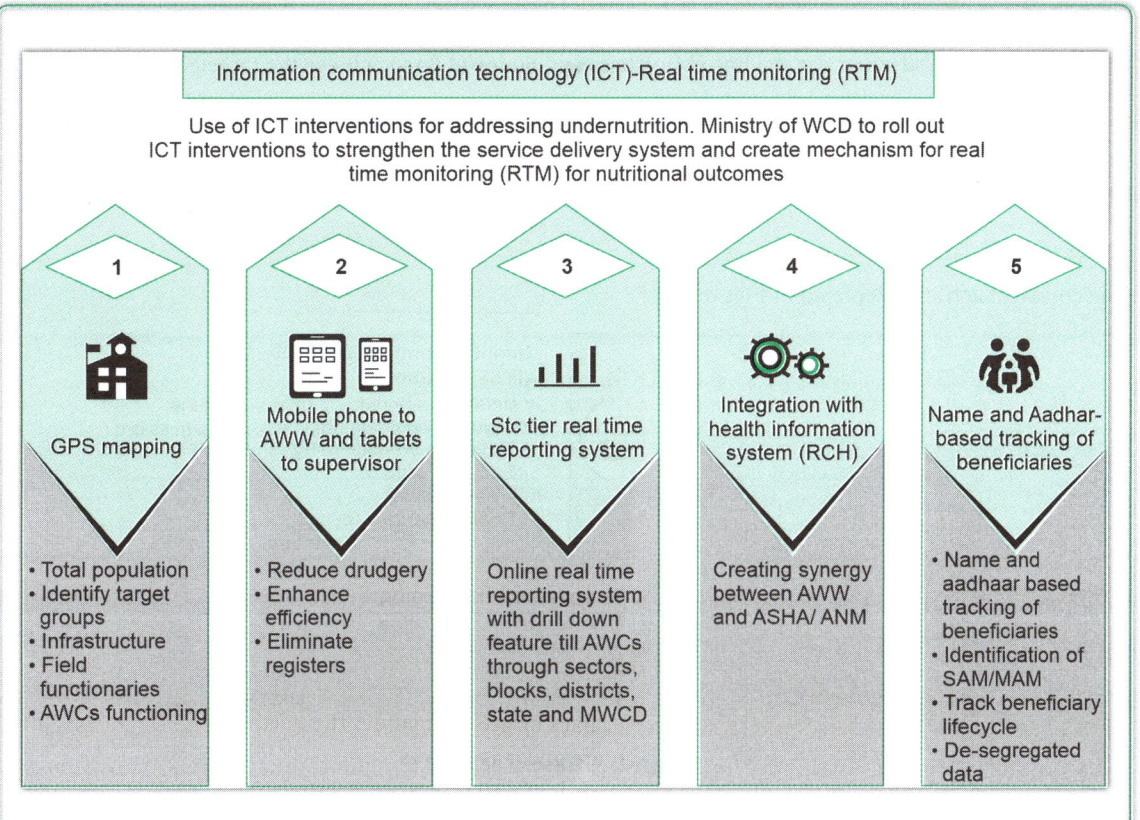

Figure 3: ICT- RTM

POSHAN MAAH

Month of September 2018 was celebrated as Rashtriya Poshan Maah. The activities in Poshan Maah focused on Social Behavioral Change and Communication (SBCC). The broad themes were: antenatal care, optimal breastfeeding (early and exclusive), complementary feeding, anemia, growth monitoring, girl-education, diet, right age of marriage, hygiene and sanitation, eating healthy-food fortification.

More than 12.2 Crore women, 6.2 Crore men and over 13 Crore children (male and female) were reached through the various activities undertaken during Poshan Maah. It is worth mentioning that 30.6 Crore people were reached in 30 days. Poshan Maah has given a major impetus to the Abhiyaan.

MAJOR IMPACT

The programme through the targets strives to reduce the level of stunting, under-nutrition, anemia and low birth weight babies.

NNM targets to reduce stunting, under- nutrition, anemia (among young children, women and adolescent girls) and reduce low birth weight by 2%, 2%, 3% and 2% per annum respectively. Although the target to reduce stunting is at least 2% p.a., mission strives to achieve reduction in stunting from 38.4% (NFHS-4) to 25% by 2022 (Mission 25 by 2022).

It will create synergy, ensure better monitoring, issue alerts for timely action, and encourage States/UTs to perform, guide and supervise the line (Ministries and States/UTs) to achieve the targeted goals.

Benefits and Coverage

More than 10 crore people were benefitted by this programme. All the states and districts were covered in a phased manner, i.e., 315 districts in 2017–18, 235 districts in 2018–19 and remaining districts in 2019–20.

Course of Action

The course of action is depicted in Figure 4.

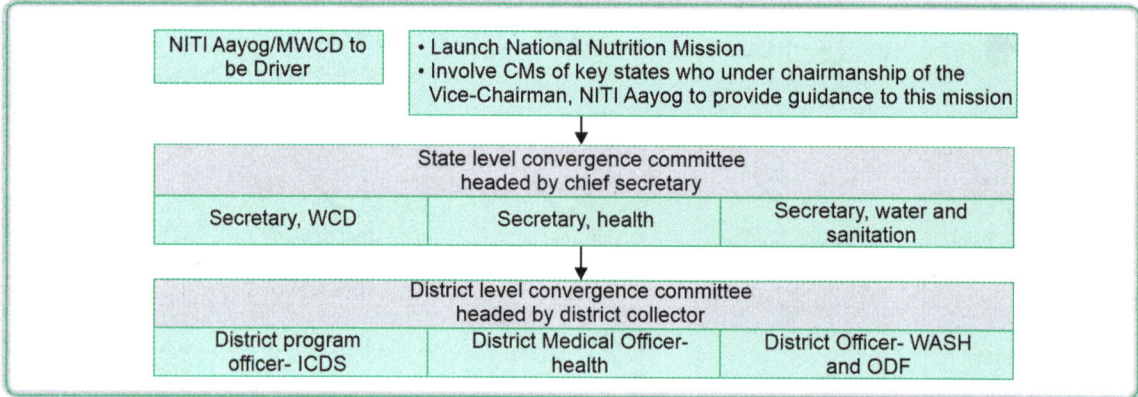

Figure 4: Course of action

Abbreviations: WASH, water, sanitation and hygiene; ODF, open defecation free; WCD, women and child development

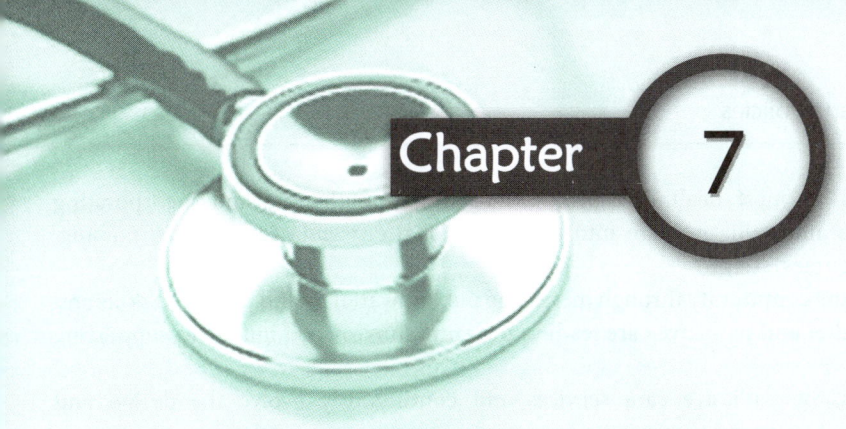

Chapter 7

National Programme for Palliative Care

INTRODUCTION

The Ministry of Health and Family Welfare, Government of India constituted an expert group on Palliative care which submitted its report 'Proposal of Strategies for Palliative Care in India' in November, 2012. On the basis of the Report, an EPC note for 12th Five-Year Plan was formulated. No separate budget is allocated for the implementation of National Palliative Care Programme. However, the Palliative Care is part of the 'Mission Flexipool' under National Health Mission (NHM).

A Performance Improvement Planning (PIP) model, a framework of operational and financial guidelines for the states, has been designed. On the basis of a model PIP, the states/UTs may prepare their proposals related to palliative care and incorporate them in their respective PIPs to seek financial support under NHM.

BENEFICIARIES

The terminal cases of Cancer, AIDS, etc.

How to Avail

On the basis of a model PIP (Guidelines), the states/UTs may prepare their proposals related to Palliative Care and incorporate them in their respective PIPs to seek financial support under NHM.

DETAILS OF SCHEME

Goal: Availability and accessibility of rational, quality pain relief and palliative care to the needy, as an integral part of Health Care at all levels, in alignment with the community requirements.

Objectives

- Improve the capacity to provide palliative care service delivery within government health programmes such as the National Programme for Prevention and Control of Cancer, Cardiovascular Disease, Diabetes, and Stroke; National Programme for Health Care of the Elderly; the National AIDS Control Programme; and the National Rural Health Mission.
- Refine the legal and regulatory systems and support implementation to ensure access and availability of Opioids for medical and scientific use while maintaining measure for preventing diversion and misuse.

- Encourage attitudinal shifts amongst healthcare professionals by strengthening and incorporating principles of long term care and palliative care into the educational curricula (of medical, nursing, pharmacy and social work courses).
- Promote behavior change in the community through increasing public awareness and improved skills and knowledge regarding pain relief and palliative care leading to community owned initiatives supporting health care system.
- Develop national standards for palliative care services and continuously evolve the design and implementation of the national programme to ensure progress toward the vision of the programme.

(**Note:** NHM flexi-pool has mandate for the activities for district level and below and hence the PIPs should be for seeking financial assistance for district palliative care unit and activities as well as state palliative care cell for implementing the programme).

IMPLEMENTATION MECHANISM

It is envisaged that activities would be initiated through National Programme for Prevention and Control of Cancer, cardiovascular diseases, Diabetes and Stroke. The integration of national programmes is attempted under the common umbrella for synergistic activities. Thus, strategies proposed will provide essential funding to build capacity within the key health programmes for non-communicable diseases, including cancer, HIV/AIDS, and efforts targeting elderly populations. Working across ministries of health and finance, the programme will also ensure that the national law and regulations allow for access to medical and scientific use of opioids.

The regulatory aspects, as mentioned in the programme, for increasing morphine availability would be addressed by Department of Revenue in coordination with Central Drug Standards Control Organization. Cooperation of international and national agencies in the field of palliative care would be taken for successful implementation of the programme.

The major strategies proposed are provision of funds for establishing state palliative care cell and palliative care services at the district hospital.

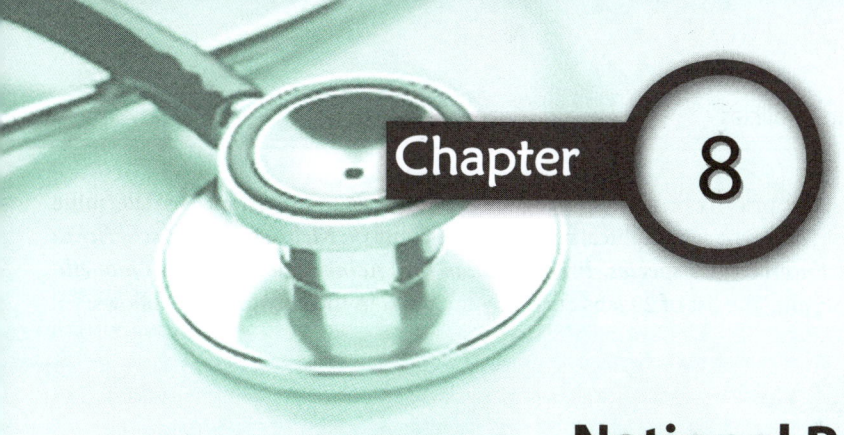

Chapter 8

National Programme on Containment of Antimicrobial Resistance

INTRODUCTION

Antimicrobial resistance (AMR) in pathogens causing important communicable diseases has become a matter of great public health concern globally including our country. Resistance has emerged even to newer and more potent antimicrobial agents like Carbapenems.

The rapid spread of multi-resistant bacteria and the lack of new antibiotics to treat infections caused by these organisms pose a rapidly increasing threat to public and animal health and needs to be tackled if we are to contain the problem and prevent untreatable illnesses.

India has given due cognizance to the problem of antimicrobial resistance and to tackle this issue, Government of India has launched a "National Programme on Containment of Antimicrobial Resistance" under the 12th five-year plan (2012–2017).

OBJECTIVES

The main objectives of this programme are:
- To establish a laboratory-based AMR surveillance system of 30 network labs in the country and to generate quality data on antimicrobial resistance for pathogens of public health importance.
- To strengthen infection control guidelines and practices and promote rational use of antibiotics.
- To generate awareness among healthcare providers and in the community about rational use of antibiotics.

Activities to be carried out under the programme:
- Surveillance for Containment of Antimicrobial Resistance in various geographical regions.
- Rational use of antibiotics.
- Development and implementation of national infection control guidelines.
- Training and capacity building of professionals in relevant sectors.
- IEC for dissemination of information about rational use of antibiotics.
- Development of National Repository of Bacterial strains/cultures.

CURRENT STATUS OF AMR PROGRAMME (AS OF OCTOBER 2018)

AMR Surveillance

National Center for Disease Control (NCDC) is the focal point for implementation of the programme. Currently the network of labs includes 20 state medical colleges from 18 states. These labs are required to submit AMR surveillance data of seven priority bacterial pathogens of public health importance to determine the magnitude and trends of AMR in different geographical regions of the country: *Klebsiella spp., Escherichia coli, Staphylococcus aureus,* **and** *Enterococcus species, Pseudomonas spp, Acinetobacter spp., Salmonella enterica serotypes* Typhi and Paratyphi. The list of 20 labs currently included in the network is as follows:

- BJMC Pune, Maharashtra
- BJMC Ahmedabad, Gujarat
- GSVM Medical College Kanpur, UP
- GMCH Chandigarh
- SMS Medical College Jaipur, Rajasthan
- LHMC, Delhi
- VMMC and Safdarjung Hospital, Delhi
- MMC and RI Mysore, Karnataka
- KAPV Government Medical College, Trichy, Tamil Nadu
- Government Medical College, Thiruvananthapuram, Kerala
- Guwahati Medical College, Guwahati, Assam
- Mahatma Gandhi Memorial Medical College, Indore, Madhya Pradesh
- NEIGRIHMs, Shillong, Meghalaya
- IGMC, Shimla, HP
- Medical College, Jammu
- Medical College, Aurangabad, Maharashtra
- Osmania General Hospital and Osmania Medical College, Hyderabad, Telangana
- SCB Medical College and Hospital, Cuttack, Odisha
- Agartala Govt. Medical College and GBP Hospital
- Guntur Medical College and Govt. General Hospital, Andhra Pradesh

Under the programme, AMR surveillance data is to be submitted in the WHONET format on a quarterly basis and feedback is provided to the labs by NCDC regarding completeness of data, etc. The data is analyzed was at NCDC on an annual basis. In 2019-20, this network was expanded to another 5 state medical colleges, representing states which are not yet included under the network.

For the year 2017, AMR surveillance data was submitted by 10 network labs (first 10 in the list above). The data has been analyzed and analyzed data has been uploaded on NCDC website. As per trends obtained from the 10 network laboratories for the year 2017, resistance rates to most of the antimicrobials are high in these common pathogens including fluoroquinolones, third generation cephalosporins and carbapenems. However, no resistance has been reported for reserve drugs such as for vancomycin in *S. aureus* and for colistin in Gram-negative bacteria.

NATIONAL TREATMENT GUIDELINES

A common unified National Treatment Guidelines for antimicrobial use in infectious diseases has been released and uploaded on the website. It can serve as a guide to all the hospitals to formulate their own guidelines on basis of which physicians will be trained.

Infection prevention and control guidelines and surveillance of healthcare associated infections:
- An interim concise guideline on infection control has been uploaded on NCDC website as a ready reference for the hospitals to start implementing infection control practices in their settings.

- National Infection Control Guidelines have been drafted with support from WHO India and is in the process of finalization.
- NCDC sites in a phased manner are joining the ICMR-AIIMS HAI surveillance network.

IEC ACTIVITIES

Various IEC activities are conducted round the year including quiz competition in schools, public lectures in academic institutions and radio programmes, participation in health fairs, etc.

Review Meetings, Trainings and Workshops

The network labs are provided training on WHONET software and onsite support through site visits. All the labs have been trained for micro broth dilution testing for colistin and vancomycin. Annual meetings are conducted to review the working of the network labs under the programme.

Strengthening Laboratory Capacity for AMR Detection

During onsite visits, the lab capacity is assessed and hand holding is done for strengthening Internal Quality Control and Proficiency Testing in these labs. 1% resistant strains are to be submitted every quarter by the sites for confirmation to National Center for Disease Control (NCDC). Most labs under the programme are enrolled into the External Quality Assessment System Programme under the banner of Indian Association of Medical Microbiologist (IAMM - EQAS) Programme.

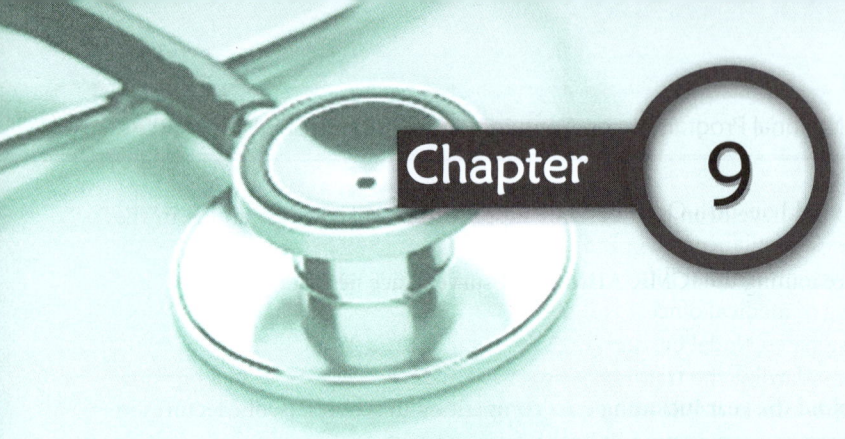

Chapter 9

National Rabies Control Programme

INTRODUCTION

Rabies is responsible for extensive morbidity and mortality in India. The disease is endemic throughout the country. With the exception of Andaman and Nicobar and Lakshadweep Islands, human cases of rabies are reported from all over the country. The cases occur throughout the year. About 96% of the mortality and morbidity is associated with dog bites. Cats, wolf, jackal, mongoose and monkeys are other important reservoirs of rabies in India. Bat rabies has not been conclusively reported from the country.

To address the issue of rabies in the country, National Rabies Control Programme was approved during 12th FYP by Standing Finance Committee meeting held on 3 October 2013 as Central Sector Scheme to be implemented under the Umbrella of NHM.

The Programme had two components – Human and Animal Components in 12th FYP.

Human Component for roll out in all States and UTs through nodal agency NCDC with total budget of ₹20 Crores and Animal Health Component for pilot testing in Haryana and Chennai through nodal agency Animal Welfare Board of India (AWBI) under the aegis of the Ministry of Environment and Forests (MoEF) under Government of India MoEF and CC, GOI with total budget of ₹30 Crores for the plan period. The Human Health Component has been rolled out in 26 States and UTs (Pilot Project for **Animal Health Component by Animal Welfare Board of India (AWBI) has been ended with closure of last FY of 12th FYP, i.e. with effect from 31.3.2017)**

OBJECTIVES

- Training of Health Care professionals on appropriate Animal Bite Management and Rabies Post-exposure Prophylaxis.
- Advocacy for states to adopt and implement intradermal route of post exposure prophylaxis for Animal Bite Victims and Pre-exposure Prophylaxis for high risk categories.
- Strengthen Human Rabies Surveillance System.
- Strengthening of Regional Laboratories under NRCP for Rabies Diagnosis.
- Creating awareness in the community through Advocacy and Communication and Social Mobilization.

Activities Undertaken in Last One Year (2018–19) Under NRCP

- **Training and capacity building:** Under the programme to review the activities undertaken by the states, Review Meeting of State Nodal Officers (SNOs) and Training of Master Trainers and under National Rabies

Control Programme (NRCP) was held on 11th October and 12th October 2018. States advocated in the meeting to put emphasis on rabies surveillance and ensuring the availability of ARV and ARS for animal bit victims. State level training plans on Animal Bite Management and Rabies Prophylaxes, Surveillance received from 6 States and training of medical officers and health workers are being conducted across the states. All states and UTs have designated Nodal Officers for NRCP and District Nodal Officers, which are being appointed in 7 states. To standardize the trainings under NRCP, Technical Committee of experts has been formed for developing modules and following training modules are being prepared.

- Training module for the Medical Officers
- Training module for the Health workers
- Manual for Rabies diagnostics.
- **Guidelines and technical support to states:** To review the recent WHO recommendation on Rabies Post Exposure Prophylaxis (2017), expert group meeting on Revision of National Guidelines for Rabies Prophylaxis was held at NCDC on 8th January, 2019 and minutes were circulated to stakeholders Review of Rabies Control in the state of Goa under the Mission Rabies in Oct. 2018.
- **Rabies and animal bite surveillance:** The standard case definition on suspected, probable and confirmed cases has been finalized in the expert group meeting held at NCDC. The probable case definition for suspected human rabies has been included under Integrated Disease Surveillance Project (IDSP). Apart from this, programme is also mapping and networking tertiary care hospital (Infectious disease hospitals/ Medical College, District Hospital, etc.) in the States and Districts. Reporting formats on animal bite, rabies, laboratory surveillance are being finalized to standardize the reporting process for rabies as a notifiable disease initiated.
- **Laboratory strengthening for rabies diagnosis**: Four regional laboratories have been supported under the programme to Strengthen Rabies Diagnostics (National Institute of Mental Health and Neurosciences [NIMHANS], Disease Investigation Unit Lab, Directorate of Animal Husbandry and Veterinary Services, Government of Goa, Panaji, Goa, AIIMS Jodhpur, National Center for Disease Control [NCDC], Delhi. Review meeting of above labs was conducted on 12th Oct, 2018 for further labs. Strengthening in the country of regional workshops is planned for Medical and Vet Microbiologists. NIMHANS Bengaluru organized the workshop in March, 2019 and more 30 microbiologists were trained during the workshop from 4-5 states.
- **IEC activities:** Under the Programme, Prototype IEC material was developed and disseminated to the States. World Rabies Day is observed on 28th September each year at NCDC and States were advocated to observe it at State/District level as per the theme of audio and recommended video. Spots were created and mass media campaign was conducted for 10 days for generating community awareness on rabies from 25 Sept to 4 Oct, 2018.
- **Intersectoral coordination for Rabies Control:** To institutionalize the "ONE HEALTH" approach at National level, collaboration with Department of Animal Husbandry, Dairying and Fisheries (DADF), Ministry of Agriculture and Farmer Welfare (MoA and FW), for development of technical guidelines for animal component of rabies control has been done. MoU is proposed to be signed between DADF, MoA and FW, MoH and FW, Wildlife Institute of India for prevention and control of Zoonotic Diseases in India including rabies. 14 States constituted State Level Zoonosis Committee (SLZC) for intersectoral coordination for prevention and control of zoonosis including Rabies. SOPs for institutionalizing "One Health" approach for Rabies is under process.
- **Operational research:** Preliminary meeting on study on assessment of rabies burden in the country was held with stakeholders, National Institute of Epidemiology (NIE) Chennai, Association for Prevention and Control of Rabies in India (APCRI) at ICMR on 28th December, 2018.

Chapter 10

National Submission to Provide Safe Drinking Water

INTRODUCTION

The National Submission to Provide Safe Drinking Water is to be completed on mission mode before March 2020. The urgency of implementation of the mission is due to:

- Criticality and urgency of the matter.
- Requirement of significant increase in operational efficiency.
- Requirement of additional funds, robust monitoring and surveillance of those.
- Requirement of special technology, manpower and strategy to achieve the goal.

GOAL

To cover all the arsenic and fluoride affected habitations with safe and perennial surface water based piped water supply schemes as the permanent and sustainable solution.

SUBMISSION PHASES

The submission have three phases namely:

1. **Diagnostic phase:** To correctly determine the action plan based on most recent and authentic data.
2. **Implementation phase:** Roll-out of area specific schemes as per guidelines.
3. **Sustain phase:** To ensure that schemes are running successfully with adequate monitoring and surveillance.

STANDARD DRINKING WATER QUALITY

Bureau of Indian Standards has set specifications in IS-10500-2012 standards for drinking water. However, this standard is only voluntary in nature and not legally supported for enforcement. This standard has two limits:

1. Desirable limits
2. Maximum permissible or cause for rejection limits

If any parameter exceeds the cause for rejection limit, that water is considered as contaminated. Broadly speaking, water is defined as contaminated if it is biologically contaminated (presence of microscopic organisms such as algae, Zoo-plankton, flagellates, *E. coli*, etc.) or chemical contamination exceeds permissible limits (e.g., excess fluoride D 1.5 mg/L), salinity, i.e.,

- Total Dissolved Solids (TDS >2,000 mg/L)

- Dissolved iron (>0.3 mg/L)
- Arsenic (>0.01 mg/L)
- Nitrates (>45 mg/L)

In rural areas, more than 85% of drinking water sources are ground water based and in the short term, chemical constituents in groundwater do not change much, therefore testing once in a year for chemical contaminants is adequate. Testing for bacteriological contamination is recommended 4 times a year, once in every season. However, every year it should be carried out at least twice, i.e., during pre-monsoon and post-monsoon seasons.

STEPS TO ROLL OUT THE PROJECTS

- The action plan will contain unambiguous timelines, proposed schemes and corresponding village coverage, scheme wise funding requirements, potential sources of funding and tasks to be executed over the course of next four years to ensure that the state is Arsenic/Fluoride free.
- Identification of habitations: Identify the habitations, affected by water contaminated by Arsenic and Fluoride. The habitations will be geo-tagged for all future uses. The geo-tagged location will be accessible on the 'Mobile Application', Integrated Management Information System (IMIS) for real time monitoring.
- Priorities may be as follows:
  - Habitations not covered by any other existing long term programme of central or state government.
  - Habitations having higher degree of contamination according to IMIS data.
- Identification of source: State has to identify, geo-tag and select the source on the basis of following parameters.
  - Source/Aquifer must be contaminant free
    - ❖ Source must be perennial in nature.
    - ❖ Source must be the most economically feasible (least lifecycle cost) option which has the ability to provide clean drinking water in perpetuity.
  - **Quality testing of source:** States have to follow the Uniform Drinking Water Quality Monitoring Protocol published and widely distributed by the Ministry of Drinking Water and Sanitation.
- **Preparation of schemes:** On the basis of identification of habitation and source, State has to prepare a proposal.

Mandatory Requirements

- Per capita cost of supply of safe and adequate drinking water to the end user.
- Operation and maintenance cost.
- Cost of implementation for all en-route non-arsenic/non-fluoride affected habitations, towns, industries, and cities should be borne fully by the concerned State Government, also clear break up of capital costs for rural, en-route nonarsenic/nonfluoride affected habitations, urban town/city and industries must be provided.
- Detailed phase wise and time bound plan.
- The State should firmly commit in providing, State matching share corresponding to release of Central Share for Arsenic and Fluoride affected habitations and entire share corresponding to en-route non-arsenic/nonfluoride affected habitations.
- Ground Level Service Reservoir (GLSR)/Over Head Tanks (OHT/ESR) should not be far away from the source to minimize raising mains.

- Ground Level Service Reservoir (GLSR)/Over Head Tanks (OHT/ESR) should be located so as to give adequate distribution by gravity to cover maximum number of habitations.
- The schemes should have recycling/reuse of filter bed washed water in Water Treatment Plants (WTP).
- The schemes should have sufficient capacity of chlorination plants including online booster chlorination plants, so that end user should get purified/safe water.
- All the mega water supply schemes shall have dedicated Three Phase Electrical Power Supply.
- All Water Treatment Plants (WTP's) shall necessarily have a basic level water quality testing laboratory with adequate manpower.
- It is up to the State Government to decide the service level of water supply delivery, however, in no case the service level shall not be less than 40 liters per capita per day (LPCD) based on current population.
- All mega schemes shall be commissioned within a span of 24 months from the date of award of work.
- The schemes should have the provision for bulk water meter before the entry point of Gram Panchayat/ Habitation.

Advisory

- It is advised to use renewable energy like solar power/solar panels/solar light wherever necessary and it is required to minimize the O and M cost and to save the electricity.
- For all mega schemes utility of Supervisory Control and Data Acquisition (SCADA) system for real time monitoring may be exploded.
- It is advised to have sufficient number of flow meters in the scheme.
- It is advisable that, the schemes should be designed so that it makes minimum energy consumption.
- It is advised to have necessary provision for extension, in future.
- It is advised to have a suitable water tariff plan, if not existing already.

Chapter 11

National Tuberculosis Elimination Programme

RNTCP RENAMED

At the start of 2020, the central government renamed the RNTCP as the National Tuberculosis Elimination Programme (NTEP). In a letter to all the State Chief Secretaries of states and UTs, the commitment is emphasized by the Union Government to achieve the sustainable development goals of ending TB by 2025, five years ahead of the global targets (Fig. 1).

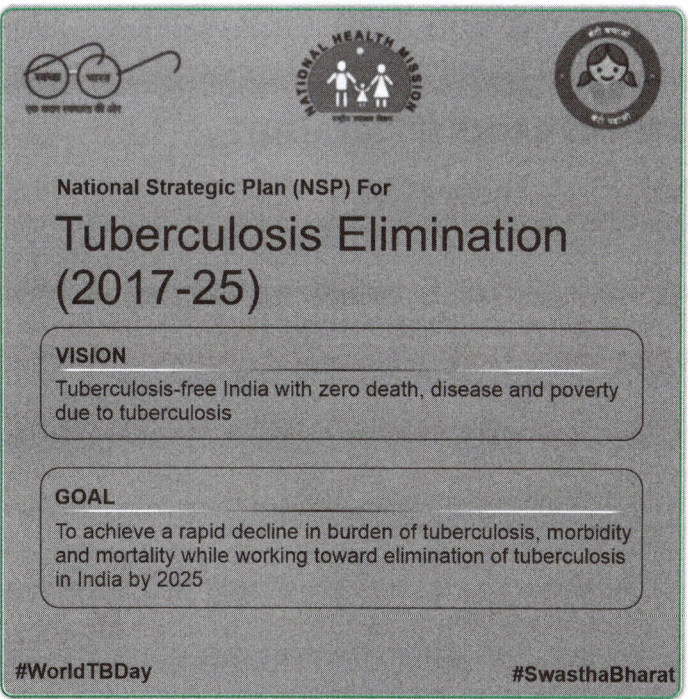

Figure 1: Tuberculosis elimination

The RNTCP in India

The large scale implementation of the Indian Government's Revised National TB Control Programme (RNTCP) (sometimes known as RNTCP 1) was started in 1997. The RNTCP was then expanded across India until the entire nation was covered by the RNTCP in March 2006. At this time the RNTCP also became known as RNTCP II. RNTCP II was designed to consolidate the gains achieved in RNTCP I, and to initiate services to address TB/HIV, MDR-TB and to extend RNTCP to the private sector.

RNTCP uses the World Health Organization (WHO) recommended Directly Observed Treatment Short Course (DOTS) strategy and reaches over a billion people in 632 districts/reporting units. The RNTCP is responsible for carrying out the Government of India Five-Year TB National Strategic Plans.

With the RNTCP both diagnosis and treatment of TB are free. There is also, at least in theory, no waiting period for patients seeking treatment and TB drugs.

The initial objectives of the RNTCP in India were:

- To achieve and maintain a TB treatment success rate of at least 85% among new sputum positive (NSP) patients.
- To achieve and maintain detection of at least 70% of the estimated new sputum positive people in the community.

New sputum positive patients are those people who have never received TB treatment before, or who have taken TB drugs for less than a month. They have also had a positive result to a sputum test, which diagnoses them as having TB.

There is more information about the current provision of TB treatment in India and the Testing and Diagnosis of TB in India.

NATIONAL STRATEGIC PLAN (NSP) 2012–2017

There has been a number of five year National Strategic Plans (NSP) since the start of the RNTCP. The NSP 2012–2017 had the aim of achieving universal access to quality diagnosis and treatment. Before this there was little treatment available through the RNTCP for the treatment of drug resistant TB.

A number of significant improvements were made during the five years of the plan. These included:

- **Complete geographical coverage:** Complete geographical coverage for diagnostic and treatment services for multi-drug resistant TB was achieved in 2013. A total of 93,000 people with MDR TB were diagnosed and had been given treatment for drug resistant TB by 2015. Also, the National AIDS Control Organization (NACO) had collaborated with the RNTCP and had made HIV-TB collaboration effective. Most TB patients registered by the RNTCP were receiving HIV screening and 90% of HIV positive TB patients were receiving antiretroviral treatment.
- **Notification by the private sector:** A government order in May 2012 made it compulsory for health care providers to notify every TB case diagnosed. This was done with the aim of improving the collection of patient care information. It meant that in future all private doctors, caregivers and clinics treating a TB patient had to report every case of TB to the government.

   There was also concern about that when people are referred to the RNTCP from the private sector there would be a good enough service, and TB treatment would be available in practice.
- **Banning of serodiagnostic tests:** In June 2012, the GoI prohibited the import and sale of serodiagnostic tests for TB. It is now believed that this has saved countless people from having inaccurate results.

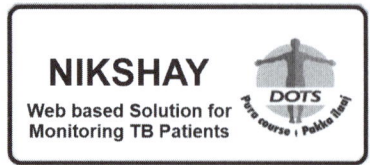

DEVELOPMENT OF NIKSHAY

The Central TB Division developed a case-based and web-based system called "Nikshay". This helped with the reporting of all TB cases. It was scaled up nationally (Fig. 2).

Standards for TB Care in India

The Standards for TB Care in India were also developed and published in 2014. The standards described what should be done, and the TB treatment and care that should be provided throughout India, including what should be provided in the private sector.

- **Vision:** TB-Free India with zero deaths, disease and poverty due to tuberculosis.
- **Goal:** To achieve a rapid decline in burden of TB, morbidity and mortality while working towards elimination of TB in India by 2025.

Continuation of prior efforts have yielded inadequate declines, and will not accelerate the progress toward ending TB. New, comprehensively-deployed interventions are required to hasten the rate of decline of incidence of TB many fold, to more than 10-15% annually.

The requirements for moving toward TB elimination have been integrated into the four strategic pillars of **"Detect – Treat – Prevent – Build" (DTPB)**.

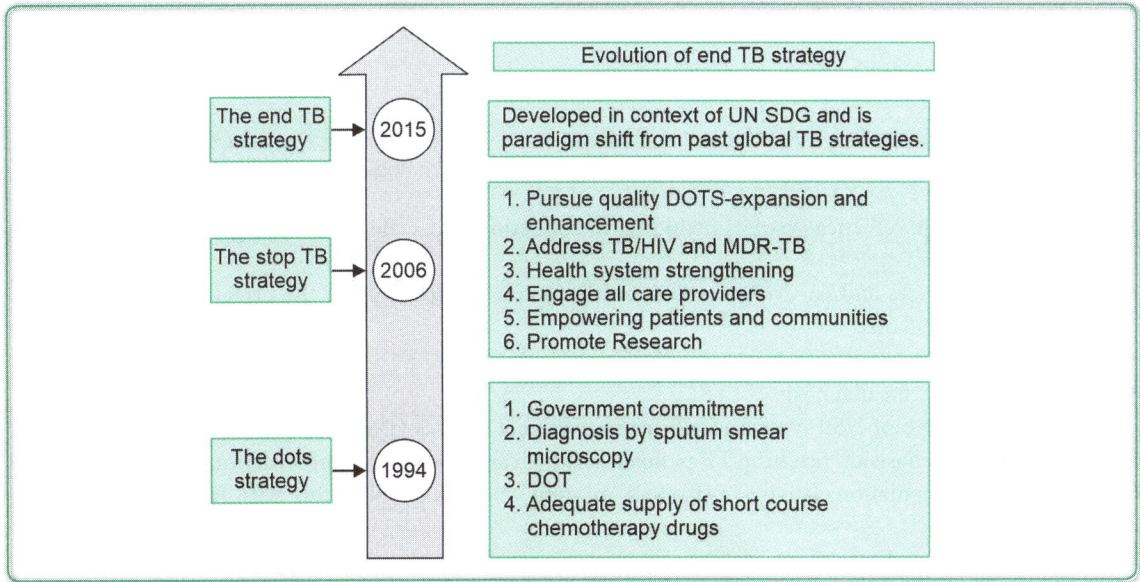

Figure 2: Development of Nikshay

NATIONAL STRATEGIC PLAN FOR TUBERCULOSIS ELIMINATION 2017–2025

RNTCP has released a 'National strategic plan for tuberculosis elimination 2017–2025' (NSP) for the control and elimination of TB in India by 2025 (Fig. 3). According to the NSP, TB elimination has been integrated into the four strategic pillars of **"Detect – Treat – Prevent – Build" (DTPB)**.

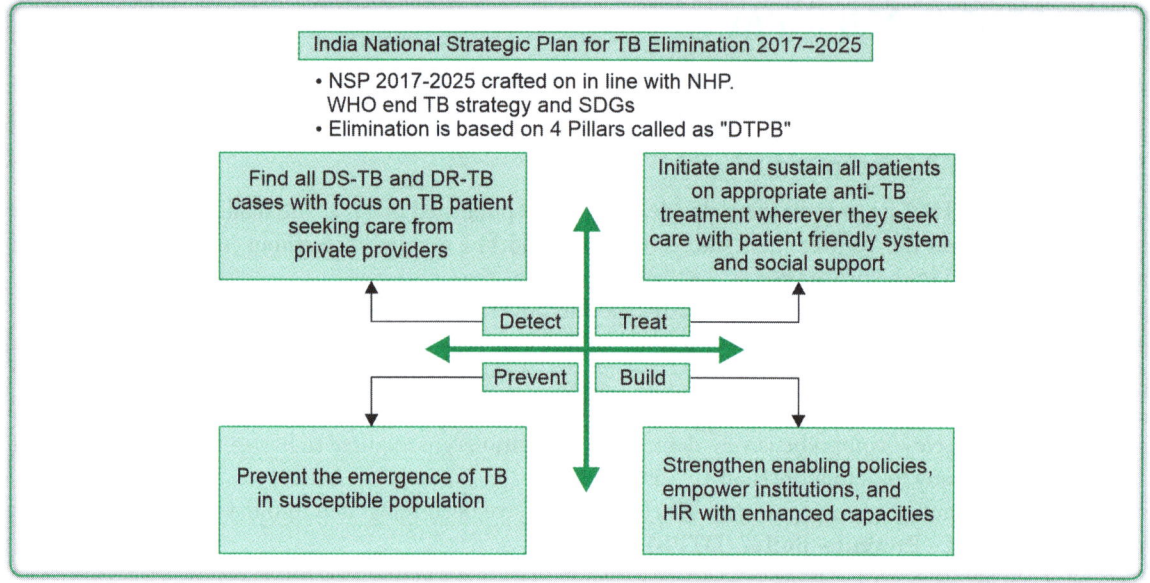

Figure 3: National strategic plan for tuberculosis elimination

Detect

What does it entail?

- To use high efficiency diagnostic tools for early and accurate diagnosis linked treatment across the country.
- To strengthen surveillance systems including introduction and scale up of next generation sequencing platforms.
- Purchasing services and ensuring notification through laboratories from the private sector and link to laboratory surveillance.
- To promote and foster research for new diagnostic tools.
- To build capacity for diagnosis of LTBI.

The first objective of NSP is to find all drug sensitive TB cases (DS-TB) and drug resistant TB cases (DRTB) with an emphasis on reaching TB patients seeking care from private providers and undiagnosed TB cases in high-risk populations (such as prisoners, migrant workers, people living with HIV/AIDS, contacts, etc.).

Early diagnosis and treatment of TB cases in the community is an important step in TB elimination, which will help in decreasing the risk of transmission of disease to others, poor health outcomes, and social and economic hardships of the patient and their family.

Notification of TB Cases

Notification of all TB patients from all health care providers is made mandatory by Ministry of Health and Family Welfare, Government of India since 2012. All health care providers (clinical establishments run or managed by government (including local authorities), private, or NGO sectors, and/or individual practitioners) should notify every TB case to local health authorities (district health officer, chief medical officer of a district, and municipal health officer of a municipal corporation/municipality) every month. With its amendment in 2015, all laboratories are also included to notify TB cases.

Till now, only medical practitioners, hospitals and laboratories were notifying TB patients to government health system, now according to 'Mandatory TB notification Gazette for private practitioners, chemists and public health staff' March 2018, all chemists will also inform about TB patients for whom they have dispensed the TB drugs. TB patients themselves are also encouraged to notify themselves. Every TB patient will be attempted to reach out by the local public health authority, namely, District Health Officer or Chief Medical Officer of a District and Municipal Health Officer of urban local bodies, so that the incentives and support to patients, families and communities can be properly extended.

Nikshay

To facilitate TB notification, RNTCP has developed a case-based, web-based, TB surveillance system called 'NIKSHAY' (https://nikshay.gov.in) for both government and private health care facilities. Future enhancements under NIKSHAY are for patients support, logistics management, direct data transfers, adherence support and to support interface agencies which are supporting programme to expand the reach.

Public Private Partnership

For promotion of public-private mix (PPM) in TB prevention and care, private providers are provided incentives for TB case notification, and for ensuring treatment adherence and treatment completion. The incentives are provided through direct beneficiary transfer.

The incentives to the Private Sector TB Care Provider are as follows:
- ₹250/- on notification of a TB case diagnosed as per Standards for TB Care in India (STCI).
- ₹250/- on completion of every month of treatment.
- ₹500/- on completion of entire course of TB treatment.
- ₹2750/- for notification and management of a drug-sensitive patient over 6–9 months as per STCI.
- ₹6750/- for notification and correct management of a drug-resistant case over 24 months as per STCI.

Free Drugs and Diagnostic Tests to TB Patients in Private Sector

Free drugs and diagnostic tests are provided to TB patients seeking treatment from private health sector. There are two approaches for ensuring access to free drugs and diagnostic tests to TB patients in private sector.
- First is access to programme- provided drugs and diagnostics through attractive linkages
- Second is reimbursement of market - available drugs and diagnostics.

Significant cost reduction of select diagnostics is achieved by 'Initiative for Promoting Affordable and Quality TB Tests' (IPAQT). One hundred and thirty-one private sector labs networked to provide four quality tests for TB at or below the ceiling prices.

For TB diagnosis, more than 14,000 designated microscopy centers are spread across the country. Cartridge Based Nucleic Acid Amplification Tests (CBNAAT)/Line Probe Assay (LPA) have been established at district levels for decentralized molecular testing for drug resistant TB. Reference laboratories have been established at state and national levels which provide culture and drug sensitivity test (DST) services as well as molecular diagnosis.

Treat

What does it entail?
- Providing daily regimen using FDCs to all TB patients.
- DST guided treatment for DR TB.

- Patient centric approach to treatment.
- Prevent loss at cascade of TB care

Next step under the programme is initiation and sustaining all TB patients on appropriate anti-TB treatment wherever they seek care, with patient friendly system and social support. Provision of free TB drugs in the form of daily Fixed Dose Combinations (FDCs) for all TB cases is advised with the support of Directly Observed Treatment (DOT).

(DOT is a specific strategy to improve adherence by any person observing the patient taking medications in real time. The treatment observer does not need to be a healthcare worker, but could be a friend, a relative or a lay person who works as a treatment supervisor or supporter. If treatment is incomplete, patients may not be cured and drug resistance may develop).

Screening of all patients for rifampicin resistance (and for additional drugs wherever indicated) is done. For drug sensitive TB, daily fixed dose combinations (FDCs) of first-line anti-tuberculosis drugs in appropriate weight bands for all forms of TB and in all ages should be given. First line treatment of drug-sensitive TB consists of two-months (8 weeks) intensive phase with four drug FDCs followed by a continuation phase of four months (16 weeks) with three drug FDCs.

- **For new TB cases**, the treatment in intensive phase (IP) consists of eight weeks of Isoniazid (INH), Rifampicin, Pyrazinamide and Ethambutol (HRZE) in daily doses as per four weight band categories and in continuation phase three drug FDCs—Rifampicin, Isoniazid, and Ethambutol (HRE) are continued for 16 weeks.
- **For previously treated cases of TB**, the Intensive Phase is of 12 weeks, where injection streptomycin is given for 8 weeks along with four drugs (INH, Rifampicin, Pyrazinamide and Ethambutol) and after 8 weeks the four drugs (INH, Rifampicin, Pyrazinamide and Ethambutol) in daily doses as per weight bands are continued for another four weeks. In continuation phase Rifampicin, INH, and Ethambutol are continued for another 20 weeks as daily doses.

  The continuation phase in both new and previously treated cases may be extended by 12–24 weeks in certain forms of TB like skeletal, disseminated TB based on clinical decision of the treating physician.

  Patients eligible for retreatment should be referred for a rapid molecular test or drug susceptibility testing to determine at least rifampicin resistance, and preferably also isoniazid resistance status. On the basis of the drug susceptibility profile, a standard first-line treatment regimen (2HRZE/4HR) can be repeated if no resistance is documented; and if rifampicin resistance is present, shorter regimen for MDR-TB (multidrug resistant TB) regimen should be prescribed according to WHO's recent drug resistant TB treatment guidelines.

  RNTCP has introduced Bedaquiline CAP for MDR-TB under conditional access programme in 2016 across six sites, with a country wide scale up plan in 2017–2020.

- **Nikshay Poshan Yojana:** It is centrally sponsored scheme under National Health Mission (NHM), financial incentive of ₹500/- per month is provided for nutritional support to each notified TB patient for duration for which the patient is on anti-TB treatment. Incentives are delivered through Direct benefit transfer (DBT) scheme to bank accounts of beneficiary.

Expending options for ICT based treatment adherence support mechanisms:
- Mobile based "Pill-in-Hand" adherence monitoring tool.
- Interactive Voice Response (IVR), SMS reminders.
- Specially designed electronic pill boxes or strips with GSM connection and pressure sensor.
- **Patient compliance toolkit:** A mobile app for patients to report treatment compliance using video, audio or text message.

- Automated pill loading system.
- Innovatively designed ICT enabled smart cards SMS gateway.

Intensifying TB control activities in following key populations is addressed in NSP:
- TB-HIV.
- Diabetics, Tobacco use and Alcohol dependence.
- Poor, undernourished, economically and socially backward communities.
- TB control in hilly and difficult terrains.
- Substance dependence and sexual minorities.
- TB and pregnancy.
- Pediatric population.
- Prison inmates and staff of prisons/jails.
- Management of extra pulmonary TB.

Prevent

What does it entail?
- Scale up airborne infection control measures at health care facilities.
- Treatment for latent TB infection in contacts of bacteriologically-confirmed cases.
- Addressing social determinants of TB through intersectoral approach.

With the objective to prevent emergence of TB in susceptible population various measures are indicated as:
- Scale up airborne infection control measures at health care facilities.
- Treatment for latent TB infection in contacts of bacteriologically-confirmed cases.
- Address social determinants of TB through intersectoral approach.

a.   Airborne infection control measures: TB infection control is a combination of measures aimed at minimizing the risk of TB transmission within population and hospital and other settings. The foundation of such infection control lies in:
- Early diagnosis, and proper management of TB patients.
- Health education about cough etiquettes and proper disposal of sputum by patient. Cough etiquette means covering nose and mouth when coughing or sneezing. This can be done with a tissue, or if the person doesn't have a tissue they can cough or sneeze into their upper sleeve or elbow, but they should not cough or sneeze into their hands. The tissue should then be safely disposed of.
- Houses should be adequately ventilated.
- Proper use of air borne infection control measures in health care facilities and other settings.

b.   Contact tracing: Since transmission can occur from index case to the contact any time (before diagnosis or during treatment. Contacts of TB patients must be evaluated. These groups include:
- All close contacts, especially household contacts.
- In case of pediatric TB patients, reverse contact tracing for search of any active TB case in the household of the child must be undertaken.
- Particular attention will be paid to contacts with the highest susceptibility to TB infection.

c.   Isoniazid preventive therapy (IPT): Preventive therapy is recommended to Children <6 years of age, who are close contacts of a TB patient. Children will be evaluated for active TB by a medical officer/ pediatrician and after excluding active TB he/she will be given INH preventive therapy. In addition to above, INH preventive therapy will be considered in following situation:

- For all HIV infected children who either had a known exposure to an infectious TB case or are Tuberculin skin test (TST) positive (≥5 mm induration) but have no active TB disease.
- All TST positive children who are receiving immunosuppressive therapy (e.g., children with nephrotic syndrome, acute leukemia, etc.).
- A child born to mother who was diagnosed to have TB in pregnancy will receive prophylaxis for 6 months, provided congenital TB has been ruled out. BCG vaccination can be given at birth even if INH preventive therapy is planned.

Close contacts of index cases with proven DR-TB (drug resistant-TB) will be monitored closely for signs and symptoms of active TB as isoniazid may not be prophylactic in these cases.

d.   BCG vaccination: It is provided at birth or as early as possible till one year of age. BCG vaccine has a protective effect against meningitis and disseminated TB in children.

e.   Addressing social determinants of TB like poverty, malnutrition, urbanization, indoor air pollution, etc. require inter departmental/ministerial coordinated activities and the programme is proactively facilitating this coordination.

Build

What does it entail?
- Build synergies with existing health service delivery mechanism under Urban Health Mission and plan for integration of services.
- Reform and restructure HR in TB programme to align with the enhanced programme needs for surveillance, participation of private sector and community participation.
- Strengthen RNTCP's regulatory capacity to control TB drugs through appropriate laws, regulations, and policies.
- Position TB high on the health and development agenda of the nation to ensure adequate resources, greater demand for and universal access to TB care services.

Health system strengthening for TB control under the National Strategic Plan 2017–2025 is recommended in the form of building and strengthening enabled policies, empowering institutions and human resources with enhanced capacities.

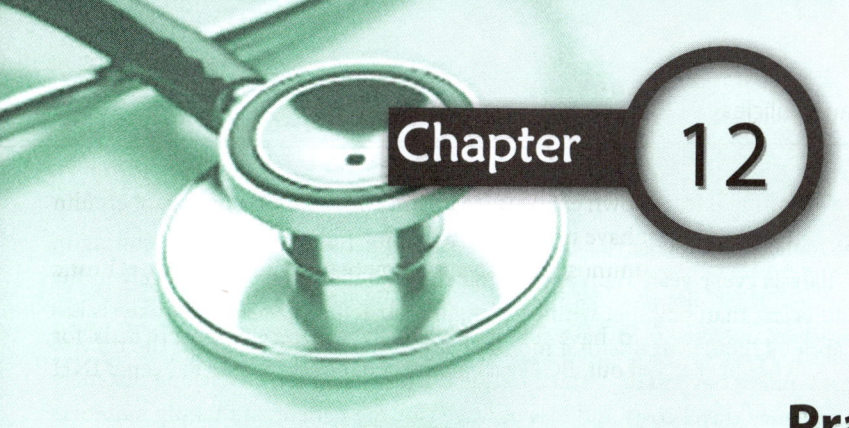

Chapter 12

Pradhan Mantri National Dialysis Programme

INTRODUCTION

The Pradhan Mantri National Dialysis Programme was rolled out in 2016 as part of the National Health Mission (NHM) for provision of free dialysis services to the poor.

The Guidelines for Pradhan Mantri National Dialysis Programme envisage provision of dialysis services under NHM in Public Private Partnership (PPP) mode (Fig. 1).

- It aims to provide free dialysis services to the poor.
- The first phase of the programme envisaged setting up of hemodialysis centers in all districts of the country.

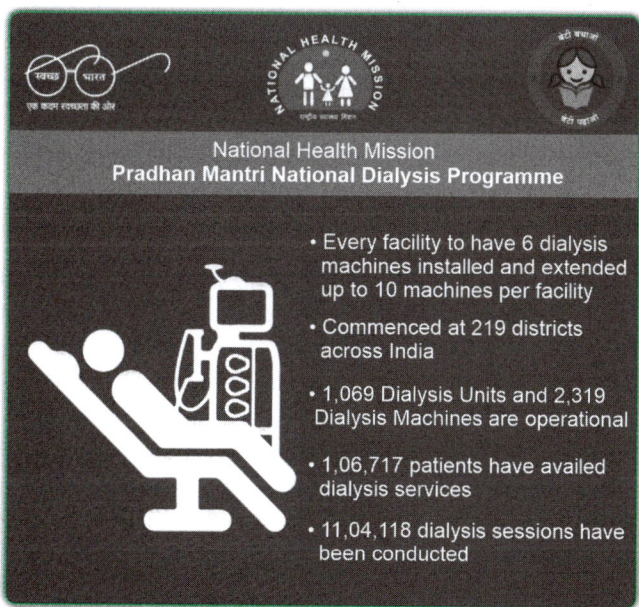

National Health Mission
Pradhan Mantri National Dialysis Programme

- Every facility to have 6 dialysis machines installed and extended up to 10 machines per facility
- Commenced at 219 districts across India
- 1,069 Dialysis Units and 2,319 Dialysis Machines are operational
- 1,06,717 patients have availed dialysis services
- 11,04,118 dialysis sessions have been conducted

Figure 1: Pradhan Mantri National Dialysis Programme

Rationale

Every year about 2.2 lakh new patients of End Stage Renal Disease (ESRD) get added in India resulting in additional demand for 3.4 Crore dialysis every year. With approximately 4950 dialysis centers, largely in the private sector in India, the demand is less than half met with existing infrastructure. Since every dialysis has an additional expenditure tag of about ₹2000, it results in a monthly expenditure for patients to the tune of ₹3–4 lakhs annually. Besides, most families have to undertake frequent trips, and often cover long distances to access dialysis services incurring heavy travel costs and loss of wages for the patient and family members accompanying the patient. Therefore, this leads to financial catastrophe for practically all families with such patients. With substantial gain in quality of life and extension of progression free survival for patients, families continue to stretch financially to make large out of pocket spends. It has been felt that both in terms of provision of this important lifesaving procedure and also for reducing impoverishment on account of out of pocket expenditure for patients, a Dialysis Programme is required.

SOLUTION STRATEGY

There are two main types of dialysis, which are hemodialysis and peritoneal dialysis.

- **Hemodialysis (HD, commonly known as blood dialysis)**: In HD, the blood is filtered through a machine that acts like an artificial kidney and is returned back into the body. HD needs to be performed in a designated dialysis center. It is usually needed about three times per week, with each episode taking about 3–4 hours.
- **Peritoneal dialysis (PD, commonly known as water dialysis)**: In PD, the blood is cleaned without being removed from the body. The abdomen sac (lining) acts as a natural filter. A solution (mainly made up of salts and sugars) is injected into the abdomen that encourages filtration such that the waste is transferred from the blood to the solution. There are two types of PD—continuous ambulatory peritoneal dialysis (CAPD) and automated peritoneal dialysis (APD). CAPD needs to be done 3–5 times every day, but does not require a machine. APD uses an automated cycler machine to perform 3–5 exchanges during the night while the patient is asleep.

Close medical supervision is not required for most PD cases, thus making it a feasible option for patients who may want to undergo dialysis in the home setting. Each treatment option has its advantages and disadvantages, which vary with the condition of the patient and presence of underlying diseases. It is, therefore, important for every patient with ESRD to discuss various treatment options in detail with his doctor before starting treatment.

The majority of patients in India receive renal replacement therapy in hemodialysis center. The number of patients on Hemodialysis and the number of hospital-based and free standing units is steadily growing. A dialysis unit delivers patient care, and has specific requirements of treated water, electricity, medical gases and waste disposal. It additionally requires accommodating all the workers involved in patient care, allow emergency procedures, permit adequate hygiene and maintenance of specialized equipment. The design and layout of a unit must take into account all the above features in order to function smoothly and prevent development of complications. Proper planning of a dialysis unit is therefore essential.

Public Private Partnership for Hemodialysis Services

As per the guidelines, the private partner is to provide medical human resource, dialysis machine along with Reverse Osmosis (RO) water plant infrastructure, dialyzer and consumables, while the space, power, and water supply within District Hospitals is to be provided by the State Government.

Based on consultation with experts and discussion with some of the states implementing the Dialysis Programme in the PPP mode, the following was considered as the ideal and cost-effective approach.

- It is desirable to roll out dialysis services in the states, beginning with the District Hospitals in a PPP mode. Direct provisioning by the state governments would be time consuming and likely to be costly and risky.
- Service Provider should provide medical human resource, dialysis machine along with RO water plant infrastructure, dialyzer and consumables.
- Payer Government should provide space in District Hospitals, Drugs, Power and water supply and pay for the cost of dialysis for the poor patients.

Financial Support

Currently, under NHM, 100% of the service procedure fees for patients below poverty line (BPL) economic group is covered. However, non BPL patients would have the benefit of accessing the services close to the community at the district hospitals at same rates as paid by the Government for the BPL patient.

While there exist health schemes such as Rashtriya Swasthya Bima Yojana (RSBY) funded by Govt. of India which covers hemodialysis procedure, it is evident that due to high cost and recurring sessions required over the life time, the total cost for providing dialysis cannot be adequately covered. However, for BPL families registered under RSBY, the cost of dialysis care shall be catered through RSBY funding up to its maximum coverage. The additional resources required would be provided to the state under the National Health Mission.

Financing

- For below poverty line (BPL) economic group: 100% expenses are directly covered under NHM by the government.
- For non-BPL patients: They can get treated at the district hospitals by paying the same rates as paid by the government for the BPL patient.

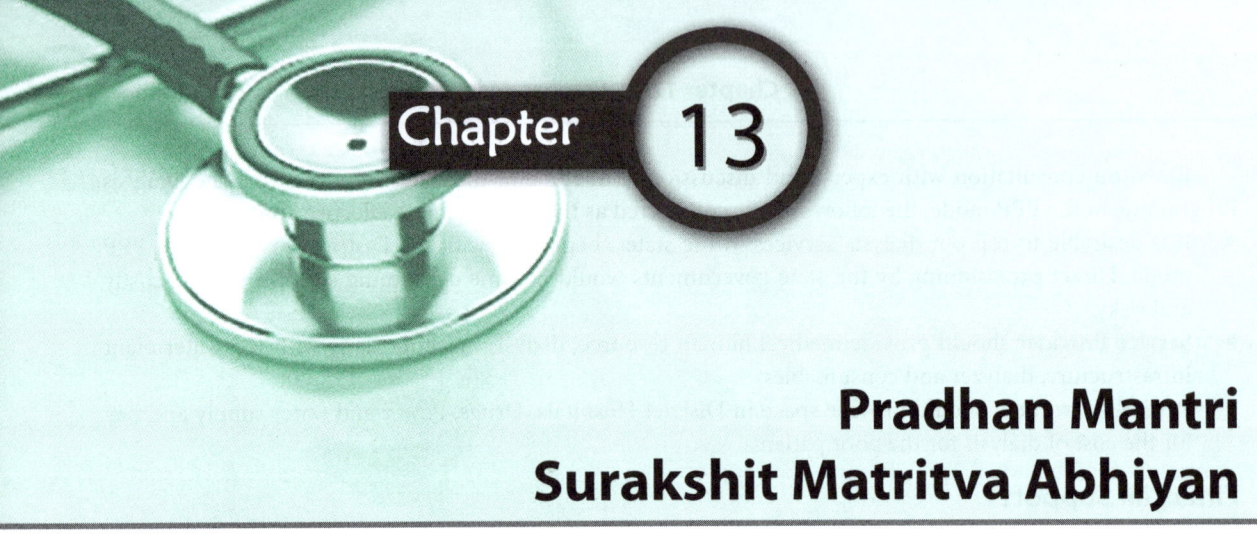

Chapter 13

Pradhan Mantri Surakshit Matritva Abhiyan

INTRODUCTION

Pradhan Mantri Surakshit Matritva Abhiyan (PMSMA) is a fixed day strategy, every month across the country during which a range of quality maternal health services are envisaged to be provided as part of antenatal care.

Under the campaign, a minimum package of antenatal care services is to be provided to the beneficiaries on the 9th day of every month at the Pradhan Mantri Surakshit Matritva Clinics to ensure that every pregnant woman receives at least one checkup in the 2nd/3rd trimester of pregnancy. If the 9th day of the month is a Sunday/a holiday, then the clinic should be organized on the next working day.

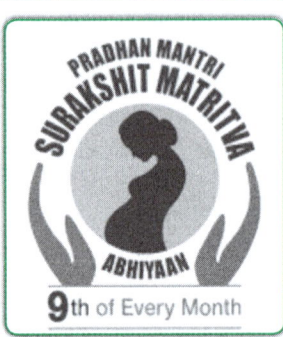

GOAL OF PRADHAN MANTRI SURAKSHIT MATRITVA ABHIYAN

The PMSMA envisages improvement in the quality and coverage of antenatal care (ANC) including diagnostics and counseling services as part of the Reproductive Maternal Neonatal Child and Adolescent Health (RMNCH+A) Strategy.

OBJECTIVES

- Ensure at least one antenatal checkup for all pregnant women in their second or third trimester by an OBGYN specialist/physician.
- Improve the quality of care during antenatal visits. This includes ensuring provision of the following services:
  - All applicable diagnostic services.
  - Screening for applicable clinical conditions.
  - Appropriate management of any existing clinical condition such as anemia, pregnancy-induced hypertension, gestational diabetes, etc.
  - Appropriate counseling services and proper documentation of services rendered.
  - Additional service opportunity to pregnant women who have missed antenatal visits.
  - Identification and line-listing of high-risk pregnancies based on obstetric/medical history and existing clinical conditions.

- Appropriate birth planning and complication readiness for each pregnant woman especially those identified with a risk factor or a co-morbid condition.
- Special emphasis on early diagnosis, adequate and appropriate management of women with malnutrition.

KEY FEATURES

The PMSMA is based on the premise—that if every pregnant woman in India is examined by a physician and appropriately investigated at least once during the PMSMA and then appropriately followed up—the process can result in reduction in the number of maternal and neonatal deaths in our country.

Antenatal checkup services would be provided by OBGYN specialists/Radiologist/Physicians with support from private sector doctors to supplement the efforts of the government sector.

- A minimum package of antenatal care services (including investigations and drugs) would be provided to the beneficiaries on the 9th day of every month at identified public health facilities (PHCs/ CHCs, DHs/ urban health facilities, etc.) in both urban and rural areas in addition to the routine ANC at the health facility/outreach.
- Using the principles of a single window system, it is envisaged that a minimum package of investigations (including one ultrasound during the 2nd trimester of pregnancy) and medicines such as IFA supplements, calcium supplements, etc. would be provided to all pregnant women attending the PMSMA clinics.
- While the target would reach out to all pregnant women, special efforts would be made to reach out to women who have not registered for ANC (left out/missed ANC) and also those who have registered but not availed ANC services (dropout) as well as high-risk pregnant women.
- OBGYN specialists/Radiologist/physicians from private sector would be encouraged to provide voluntary services at public health facilities where government sector practitioners are not available or inadequate.
- Pregnant women would be given Mother and Child Protection Cards and safe motherhood booklets.
- One of the critical components of the Abhiyan is identification and follow up of high-risk pregnancies. A sticker indicating the condition and risk factor of the pregnant women would be added onto MCP card for each visit:
  - **Green sticker**—for women with no risk factor detected.
  - **Red sticker**—for women with high-risk pregnancy.
- A National Portal for PMSMA and a Mobile application have been developed to facilitate the engagement of private/ voluntary sector.
- 'IPledgeFor9' Achievers Awards have been devised to celebrate individual and team achievements and acknowledge voluntary contributions for PMSMA in states and districts across India.

TARGET BENEFICIARIES

The programme aims to reach out to all pregnant women who are in the 2nd and 3rd trimesters of pregnancy.

PUBLIC HEALTH FACILITIES TO ACCESS SERVICES UNDER PMSMA

- **Rural areas:** Primary Health Centers, Community Health Centers, Rural Hospitals, Sub-District Hospital, District Hospital, Medical College Hospital
- **Urban areas:** Urban Dispensaries, Urban Health Posts, Maternity Homes

PROVISION OF SERVICES

- All the beneficiaries visiting the facility are first registered in a separate register for PMSMA.
- After registration, ANM and SN ensures that all basic laboratory investigations are done before the beneficiary is examined by the OBGYN Medical Officer. The report of the investigations should ideally be handed over within an hour and before the beneficiaries are meeting the doctors for further checkups. This will ensure identification of high-risk status (like anemia, gestational diabetes, hypertension, infection, etc.) at the time of examination and further advice. In certain cases, where additional investigations are required, beneficiaries are to be advised to get those investigations done and share the report during next PMSMA or during her routine ANC check-up visit.
- Lab investigations—USG, and all basic investigations–Hb, Urine Albumin, RBS (Dip stick), rapid Malaria test, rapid VDRL test, Blood Grouping, CBC ESR, USG.

SERVICES

- A detailed history of all the beneficiaries needs to be taken and then examined and assessed for any danger signs, complications or any high-risk status.
- Blood Pressure, per abdominal examination and examination for fetal heart sounds should be done for all the beneficiaries coming for ANC check-up.
- If a woman visiting a public health facility requires a specific investigation, sample should be collected at the facility itself and transported to the appropriate center for testing. ANM/MPW should be responsible for transporting the collected sample, conveying the results to the pregnant women and appropriate follow-up.
- After examination by ANM/Staff Nurse, Medical Officer to also examine and attend to every beneficiary attending PMSMA.
- All identified high-risk pregnancies should be referred to higher facilities and JSSK help desks that have been set up at these facilities should be responsible for guiding the referred women once they reach the facilities. MCP cards to be issued to all beneficiaries.
- All identified high-risk women including those with complications to be managed and treated by OBGYN/Comprehensive Emergency Obstetric Care (CEmOC)/Basic Emergency Obstetric Care (BEmOC) specialist. If needed, such cases should be referred to higher level facilities and a referral slip with probable diagnosis and treatment given should be mentioned on the slip.
- One ultrasound is recommended for all pregnant women during the 2nd/3rd trimester of pregnancy. If required, USG services may be made available in a PPP mode and expenditure booked under JSSK.
- Before leaving the facility every pregnant woman to be counseled, may be individually or in groups, on nutrition, rest, safe sex, safety, birth preparedness, identification of danger signs, institutional delivery and Postpartum Family Planning (PPFP).
- Filling out the MCP cards at these clinics should be mandatory and a sticker indicating the condition and risk factor of the pregnant women should be added onto MCP card for each visit:
  - Green sticker—for women with no risk factor detected.
  - Red sticker—for women with high-risk pregnancy.
  - Blue—for women with pregnancy induced hypertension.
  - Yellow—pregnancy with comorbid conditions such as diabetes, hypothyroidism, STIs.

- Counseling session to focus on the following topics:
  - Care during pregnancy.
  - Danger signs during pregnancy.
  - Birth preparedness and complication readiness, contact details to be used in case of need.
  - Family Planning
  - Importance of nutrition including iron, folic acid consumption and calcium supplementation.
  - Rest
  - Safe sex
  - Institutional delivery.
  - Identification of referral transport.
  - Entitlements under Janani Suraksha Yojana (JSY).
  - Entitlements and service guarantee under Janani Shishu Suraksha Karyakram (JSSK).
  - Postnatal care.
  - Breastfeeding and complementary feeding.

Those pregnant women with unwanted pregnancies need to be provided with safe abortion care services after proper counseling.

Referral transport mechanism for high-risk women: During PMSMA, 108/102/State owned ambulances/ Private empanelled ambulances can also be used for referring those cases identified as high-risk.

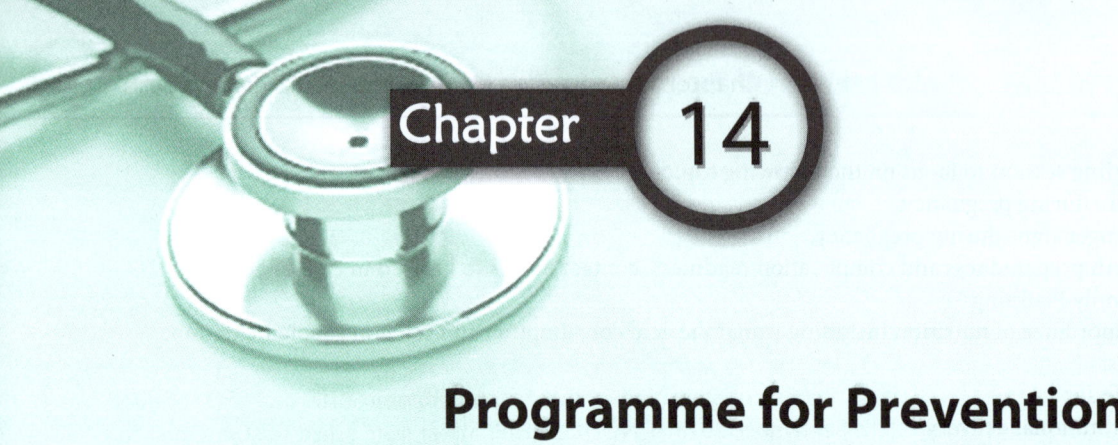

Chapter 14

Programme for Prevention and Control of Leptospirosis

INTRODUCTION

Leptospirosis is a public health problem in Gujarat, Kerala, Karnataka, Tamil Nadu, Maharashtra and Andaman and Nicobar Islands. Frequent outbreaks of leptospirosis are being reported, predominantly affecting young adult males. The disease is easily treatable and the mortality is preventable if detected and treated early. Under XII plan, Programme for Prevention and Control of Leptospirosis has been approved and is being implemented in five endemic states and one union territory as mentioned above. The strategy includes:

- Strengthening of diagnostics laboratories for early diagnosis.
- Strengthening of patient management facilities.
- Trained manpower development.
- Strengthening of inter sectoral coordination.
- Create awareness in general community.

Background: Leptospirosis is a significant public health problem in India and the outbreaks of Leptospirosis are increasingly being reported from States such as Kerala, Gujarat, Tamil Nadu, Maharashtra and Karnataka. Leptospirosis is also being reported from nonendemic states wherever facility for diagnosis of such cases exists. Early case detection, accurate diagnosis, appropriate and timely treatment reduce the morbidity and mortality due to the disease.

To address the rising burden of the disease, the Government of India initially launched a Pilot project on Prevention and Control of Leptospirosis as a "New Initiative" under XIth Five-Year Plan. Following the success of the pilot project, the Government of India then launched the Programme for Prevention and Control of Leptospirosis (PPCL) during 12th Five-Year Plan in the endemic states viz. Gujarat, Kerala, Tamil Nadu, Maharashtra, Karnataka and UT of Andaman and Nicobar Islands. National Center for Disease Control (NCDC) has been designated as the nodal agency for implementation of Programme.

OBJECTIVE

To reduce the morbidity and mortality due to leptospirosis in humans.
The strategies of programme for prevention and control of leptospirosis include:

- Developing of trained manpower.
- Strengthening the surveillance of leptospirosis in humans.
- Strengthening diagnostic laboratory in programme states.

- Creating awareness regarding timely detection and appropriate treatment of patients.
- Strengthening patient management facilities in programme states.
- Strengthening intersectoral coordination at state and district level for outbreak detection, prevention and control of leptospirosis.

ACTIVITIES UNDERTAKEN BY NCDC IN 2018–19

- **Monitoring and review:** Review meeting of State Nodal officers of programme states and SSOs of flood affected states was held on 28th September 2018 at NCDC, Delhi. States were asked to strengthen the activities under programme including leptospirosis surveillance, improving case management facility for patients and expediting the financial expenditure under the programme. State of Kerala, Gujarat and UT of Andaman and Nicobar have submitted the activity report, action plan and fund utilization.
- **Surveillance**: Regular surveillance of presumptive and laboratory confirmed cases of leptospirosis is undertaken through IDSP and monitored under the programme.
- **Technical support to states:** Advisory was issued in July 2018 under the programme from Director, NCDC to all flood affected states on preventive and control measures to be undertaken for Leptospirosis. In this regard, visits to Mumbai, Maharashtra and Karnataka in August and September 2018 were paid to review leptospirosis control activities.
- **IEC activities:** IEC material (Radio spots and Radio Jingle) under Programme for Prevention and Control of Leptospirosis (PPCL) was prepared through NFDC.
- **Intersectoral coordination:** Follow-up is done with states to constitute and operationalize state and district level zoonotic committees for One Health for Prevention and Control of Zoonotic Diseases including leptospirosis.
- **Financial support to states:** Approval from Ministry and IFD for fund transfer amounting to 52 lakhs to states (Kerala and Gujarat) is obtained, however, the fund transfer could not be completed in FY 2018–19.

IMPACT OF THE PROGRAMME

Although the programme is still in its nascent stage but it has been able to sensitize the State Governments about the significant public health impact of the disease. The surveillance of the disease has been strengthened and cases and outbreaks are regularly reported through IDSP portal.

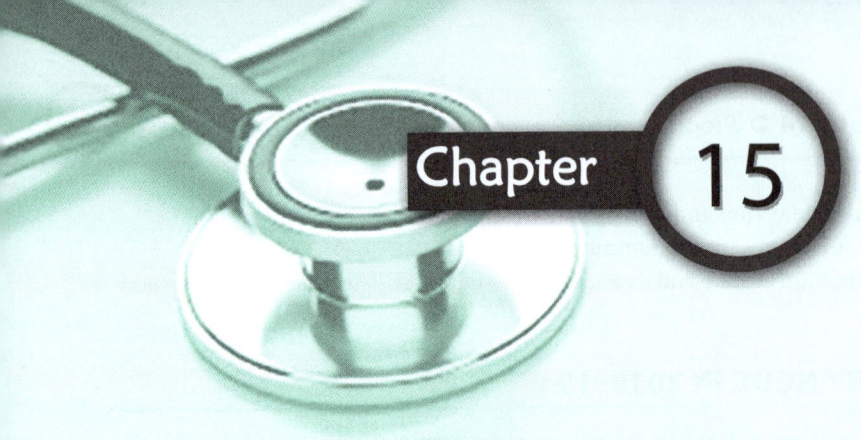

Chapter 15

National Oral Health Programme

INTRODUCTION

India has a high prevalence of oro-dental disease and it is well established that oral diseases are public health problems and have a great impact on systemic health. Poor oral health can cause poor aesthetics, affects mastication adversely, causes agonizing pain and can lead to loss of productivity due to loss of man-hours.

Oral health is important for overall health and good quality of life. Oral diseases affect all the age groups. Some common oral diseases are dental caries, periodontal diseases, malocclusion, oral sub-mucous fibrosis, oral cancer, cleft lip, cleft palate, etc.

According to the World Health Organization (WHO), oral health is a state of being free from chronic mouth and facial pain, oral and throat cancer, oral sores, birth defects such as cleft lip and palate, periodontal (gum) disease, tooth decay and tooth loss, and other diseases and disorders that affect the oral cavity.

Dental caries and gum diseases affect nearly 60% and 80%, of the Indian population, respectively. Oral diseases have also been linked to bacterial endocarditis, atherosclerosis, chronic obstructive lung diseases and preterm low birth weight. Periodontal health has been directly linked with diabetes.

National Oral Health Programme (NOHP) was launched during 2014–15 to strengthen the public health facilities of the country for an accessible, affordable and quality oral healthcare delivery.

Routine dental check-ups and early intervention can prevent the most common dental problems. To our dismay, oral health has been neglected over the years, due to lack of awareness among general population and even the care providers, especially in the underprivileged areas. According to the data from Dental Council of India, 72% of the population live in villages which remain deprived of dental care.

Though some states have made progress in providing comprehensive oral healthcare through its primary care system, a lot still remains to be achieved in the whole country. Therefore, oral healthcare delivery of the country needs to be strengthened for efficient oral healthcare delivery and improvement of oral health indicators and overall health of the population of the country.

Ministry of Health and Family Welfare, Government of India has envisaged the National Oral Health Programme (NOHP) for an affordable, accessible and equitable oral healthcare delivery in a well-coordinated manner for bringing about 'optimal oral health' for all by 2020.

OBJECTIVES

- To improve the determinants of oral health.
- To reduce morbidity from oral diseases.
- To integrate oral health promotion and preventive services with general healthcare system.
- To encourage promotion of Public Private Partnerships (PPP) model for achieving better oral health.

- To achieve these objectives, Government of India has decided to assist the State Governments in initiating provision of dental care along with other ongoing health programmes implemented at various levels of the primary healthcare system under the umbrella of National Health Mission.

Through NOHP, states are provided necessary funds by the government of India to establish dental units equipped with necessary trained manpower, equipment including dental chair and consumable dental materials.

Government of India also helps in developing prototype Information, Education and Communication (IEC) materials/Behavior Change Communication (BCC) materials for dissemination of information and to raise awareness about Oral Health across the country.

Monitoring of programme implementation and progress of NOHP is carried out by the National Oral Health Cell (NOHC) at central level and at state level, programme is monitored by state nodal officer. Organizational structure of NOHP includes:

- National Oral Health Cell (NOHC)
- State Oral Health Cell (SOHC)
- District Oral Health Cell (DOHC)
- Improvement in the determinants of oral health, e.g., healthy diet, oral hygiene improvement, etc. and to reduce disparity in oral health accessibility in rural and urban population.
- Reduce morbidity from oral diseases by strengthening oral health services at Sub district/district hospital to start with.
- Integrate oral health promotion and preventive services with general healthcare system and other sectors that influence oral health; namely various National Health Programmes.
- Promotion of Public Private Partnerships (PPP) for achieving public health goals.

COMPONENTS

The programme has two components as under:
1. **National health mission component:** Support is provided to States to set up Dental Care Units at District Hospitals or below. Support is provided for the following components:
   - Manpower support (Dentist, Dental Hygienist, Dental Assistant)
   - Equipment including dental chair
   - Consumables for dental procedures
2. **Tertiary component:** For central level activities such as:
   - Designing IEC materials like Posters, TV, Radio Spots, Training Modules.
   - Organizing national, regional nodal officers training programme to enhance the programme management skills, review the status of the programme.
   - Preparing State/District level trainers by conducting national and regional workshops to train the paramedical health functionaries associated to healthcare delivery.

IVRS Oral Health Helpline

The Ministry of Health and Family Welfare launched an Interactive Voice Response System (IVRS) Helpline for Oral Health Programme on the occasion of World Oral Health Day on 20 March 2017. It can be accessed through a toll free number by any individual by dialing 1800-11-2032.

The aim is to:
- Provide information regarding common oral health concerns.
- Create awareness regarding the importance of oral health.
- Dispel common myths regarding oral diseases.
- Provide emergency instructions in case of common oral health diseases.

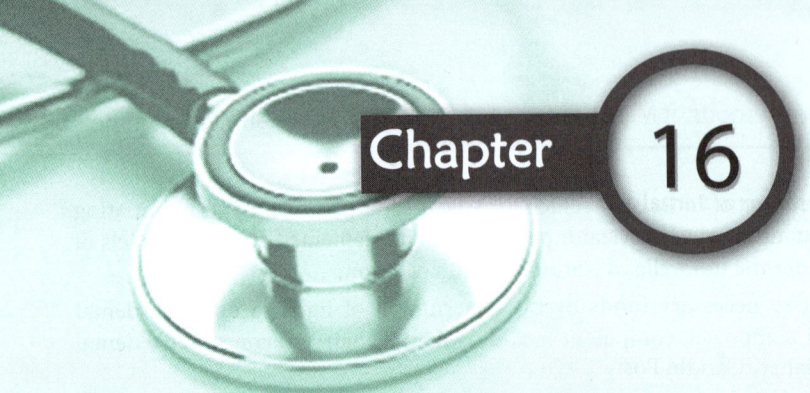

Chapter 16

Unique Methods of Management and Treatment of Inherited Disorders

INTRODUCTION

- Training and diagnostic services under UMMID
- List of Training Centers
- List of NIDAN Kendras
- List of aspirational districts covered under the programme
- Expected outcomes of UMMID

UMMID is a Department of Biotechnology (DBT), Ministry of Science and Technology initiative to create awareness about genetic disorders amongst clinicians and establish molecular diagnostics in hospitals for the benefit of patients in India.

The plan of the UMMID initiative is to link the well-established centers of Medical Genetics in India to upcoming centers and to establish clinical genetics facilities in district hospitals. This will improve patient care services for genetic disorders and impart latest medical genetics education to medical students to prepare them for the era of molecular medicine.

TRAINING AND DIAGNOSTIC SERVICES UNDER UMMID

UMMID plans to work at three levels of medical care which will work in close collaboration with a close link between training and establishment of diagnostic services. The three components of UMMID are given below:

1. **Fellowship in genetic diagnostics:** Hands-on training for 6 months will be provided to doctors working in government hospitals by eight departments with state-of-the-art DNA-based diagnostic services for genetic disorders. Each center will train four fellows per year thus providing 96 trained doctors in genetic diagnostics during the period of 3 years.

2. **NIDAN Kendras (diagnostic centers):** Hospitals with interested doctors, committed administrators and basic infrastructure have been selected and funded to establish genetic laboratories. The financial support and twinning with established Medical Genetics centers will help them to develop state-of-the-art facilities in molecular diagnostics.

3. **Prevention of genetic disorders in aspirational districts:** Each of the seven centers providing genetic training have adopted one aspirational district and will establish a programme for prevention of genetic disorders including beta thalassemia and newborn screening for treatable disorders. This will be a prototype of an outreach programme which will take latest genetic diagnostics to the population and lead

the way to incorporate genetic services in maternal and child care. This will provide onsite training to the doctors in these district hospitals in addition to creating awareness about genetic disorders amongst the general population.

List of Training Centers

- Department of Medical Genetics, Sanjay Gandhi Postgraduate Institute of Medical Sciences (SGPGIMS), Raebareli Road, Lucknow, Uttar Pradesh.
- Division of Genetics, Department of Pediatrics, All India Institute of Medical Sciences (AIIMS), New Delhi.
- Genetics Unit, Department of Pediatrics, Maulana Azad Medical College (MAMC), New Delhi.
- Department of Clinical Genetics, Christian Medical College (CMC), Vellore, Tamil Nadu.
- Center for Genetic Studies and Research, The Madras Medical Mission, Chennai, Tamil Nadu.
- Diagnostics Division, Center for DNA Fingerprinting and Diagnostics (CDFD), Hyderabad, Telangana.
- Department of Hematology, Christian Medical College (CMC), Vellore, Tamil Nadu.
- ICMR National Institute of Immunohematology (NIIH), KEM Hospital, Parel, Mumbai, Maharashtra.

List of NIDAN Kendras

- Lady Hardinge Medical College (LHMC), New Delhi.
- Nizam's Institute of Medical Sciences (NIMS), Hyderabad, Telangana.
- All India Institute of Medical Sciences (AIIMS), Jodhpur, Rajasthan
- Army Hospital Research and Referral, New Delhi.
- Nil Ratan Sircar (NRS) Medical College and Hospital, Kolkata, West Bengal.

List of Aspirational Districts Covered under the Programme

Expected outcomes of UMMID

- Contribute to patient care services for genetic disorders which account for 80% of rare disorders, by developing trained manpower in the cutting-edge area of genomic technologies.
- Establish genetic diagnostic centers in different parts of the country which will not only provide patient care services but improve the component of medical genetics training in medical education and equip medical doctors of the twenty-first century for the era of molecular medicine.
- Create awareness about genetic disorders amongst clinicians and laypersons, so that the patients and families get appropriate diagnosis, management and preventive services through government (Beneficiaries—70,000 pregnant women and 35,000 newborn babies per year).
- UMMID will spread the reach of diagnostic facilities for rare genetic disorders, pharmacogenetics, prenatal diagnosis and population-based screening for prevention.
- Establishment of genomic techniques will contribute to research into genetic aspects of rare and common genetic disorders.

Chapter 17

Rajiv Gandhi National Drinking Water Mission

INTRODUCTION

The Accelerated Rural Water Supply Programme (ARWSP) was introduced in 1972–73 by the Government of India to assist the States and Union Territories to accelerate the pace of coverage of drinking water supply. The programme was given a missionary approach with the launch of the Technology Mission of Drinking Water and Related Water Management, also called the National Drinking Water Mission (NDWM) in 1986. The NDWM was renamed as the Rajiv Gandhi National Drinking Water Mission (RGNDWM) in 1991.

Rural water supplies being a state subject, the state governments have been implementing the rural water supply programme under the Minimum Needs Programme (MNP). The central government through RGNDWM supplements the efforts of the state governments by providing assistance under the Accelerated Rural Water Supply Programme.

SALIENT FEATURES

The salient features of the revised policy for implementation of Accelerated Rural Water Supply Programme during the Ninth Plan period are as follows:

- The present allocation criteria of funds under ARWSP to the states based on normative criteria should be replaced with a need-based approach. The states having large number of 'Not Covered' and quality affected habitations in drought-prone, desert regions and hard rock areas would get more allocation than the states well-endowed with water resources.
- Decentralization of powers to the states for implementation of sub-mission programmes.
- Enhancing ceiling for operation and maintenance from the present level of 10–15% of annual plan allocation.
- Providing 100% funds for the nascent programmes such as HRD, R&D, IEC and Management Information System.
- Institutionalizing community-based, demand-driven rural water supply programme with cost-sharing instruments by communities, gradually replacing the current supply-driven, centrally maintained non-people participating rural water supply programme.
- Institutionalizing water quality monitoring and surveillance systems. Out of 1.43 million rural habitations in the country, 1.40 million habitations have access to safe drinking water. Special efforts are being made for ensuring sustainability of the facilities provided under the Accelerated Rural Water Supply Programme, by initiating action to institutionalize community-based rural water supply programme. Special emphasis is being given to areas affected with quality problems due to excess fluoride, arsenic, iron and other pollutants.

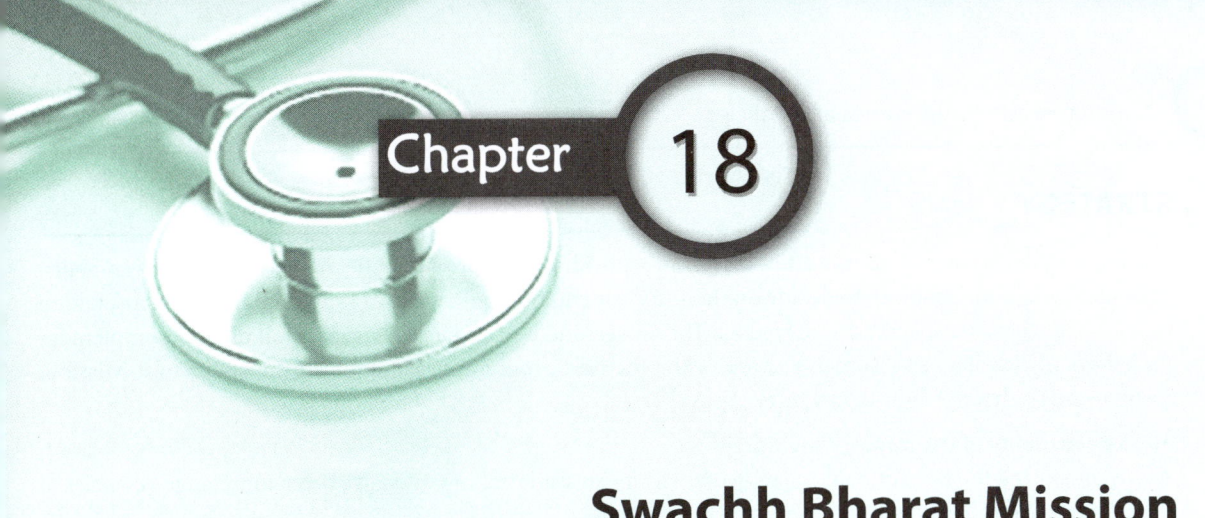

Chapter 18

Swachh Bharat Mission

INTRODUCTION

To accelerate the efforts to achieve universal sanitation coverage and to put focus on sanitation, the Prime Minister of India had launched the Swachh Bharat Mission on 2nd October 2014. The mission was implemented as nation-wide campaign/Janandolan which aimed at eliminating open defecation in rural areas during the period 2014 to 2019 through mass scale behavior change, construction of household-owned and community-owned toilets and establishing mechanisms for monitoring toilet construction and usage.

Under the mission, all villages, Gram Panchayats, Districts, States and Union Territories in India declared themselves "open-defecation free" (ODF) by 2nd October 2019, the 150th birth anniversary of Mahatma Gandhi, by constructing over 100 million toilets in rural India.

To ensure that the open defecation free behaviors are sustained, no one is left behind, and that solid and liquid waste management facilities are accessible, the Mission is moving towards the next Phase II of SBMG, i.e., ODF-Plus. ODF Plus activities under Phase II of Swachh Bharat Mission (Grameen) will reinforce ODF behaviors and focus on providing interventions for safe management of solid and liquid waste in villages.

VISION

The aim of Swachh Bharat Mission (Gramin) phase II is to ensure the open defecation free behaviors are sustained.

OBJECTIVES

- Open defecation free behaviors are sustained and no one is left behind.
- Solid and liquid waste management facilities are accessible and reinforcing ODF behaviors and focus on providing interventions for safe management of solid and liquid waste in villages.
- To encourage cost-effective and appropriate technologies for ecologically safe and sustainable sanitation.
- To develop, wherever required, community managed sanitation systems focusing on scientific Solid and Liquid Waste Management systems for overall cleanliness in the rural areas.
- To create significant positive impact on gender and promote social inclusion by improving sanitation especially in marginalized communities.

STRATEGY

The focus of the strategy is to move towards a 'Swachh Bharat' by providing flexibility to State governments, as sanitation is a State subject, to decide on their implementation policy, use of funds and mechanisms, taking into account the state specific requirements. The Government of India's role is essential only to complement the efforts of the State governments through the focused programme being given the status of a Mission, recognizing its dire need for the country.

The key elements of the strategy include:

- Augmenting the institutional capacity of districts for undertaking intensive behavior change activities at the grassroots level.
- Strengthening the capacities of implementing agencies to roll out the programme in a time-bound manner and to measure collective outcomes.
- Incentivizing the performance of State-level institutions to implement behavioral change activities in communities.

Focus on Behavior Change

Behavior change has been the key differentiator of Swachh Bharat Mission and therefore emphasis is placed on Behavior Change Communication (BCC). BCC is not a 'stand-alone' separate activity to be done as a 'component' of SBM-G, but about nudging communities into adopting safe and sustainable sanitation practices through effective BCC.

Emphasis is placed on awareness generation, triggering mindsets leading to community behavior change and demand generation for sanitary facilities in houses, schools, Anganwadis, places of community congregation, and for Solid and Liquid Waste Management activities. Since Open Defecation Free villages cannot be achieved without all the households and individuals conforming to the desired behavior of toilet use every day and every time, community action and generation of peer pressure on the outliers are key.

Flexibility to States

States have flexibility regarding the utilization of the IHHL incentive. The provision of incentives for IHHLs for rural households is available to States (from the IHHL component) in addition to extensive motivational and behavioral change interventions (from the IEC component). This is also used to maximize coverage so as to attain community outcomes.

Foot Soldiers of Swachh Bharat

There is a need for a dedicated, trained and properly incentivized sanitation workforce at the GP level. An army of 'foot soldiers' or 'Swachhagrahis', earlier known as 'Swachhata Doots' is developed and engaged through existing arrangements like Panchayati Raj Institutions, Cooperatives, ASHAs, Anganwadi workers, Women Groups, Community-based Organizations, Self-help Groups, water linemen/pump operators, etc. who are already working in the GPs, or through engaging Swachhagrahis specifically for the purpose. In case existing employees of line departments are utilized, their original line departments are in clear agreement to the expansion of their roles to include activities under the Swachh Bharat Mission.

Sanitation Technologies

Appropriate participation of the beneficiary/communities, financially or otherwise in the setting up of the toilets is advised to promote ownership and sustained use, both at the household and community levels.

The built-in flexibility in the menu of options is to give the poor and the disadvantaged families' opportunity for subsequent upgrading of their toilets depending upon their requirements and financial position and to ensure that sanitary toilets are constructed for safe confinement and disposal of feces. An illustrative list of technology options, with cost implications is provided to meet the user preferences and location-specific needs. While the Government provides flexibility in choosing the toilet technology considering area's topography, soil conditions, etc., properly constructed Twin-Pit is considered the most preferred technology.

Monitoring Mechanisms

A robust monitoring arrangement has been put in place to monitor Open Defecation Free status of a village, the implementation of Solid and Liquid Waste Management projects as well as the construction and use of household toilets, school and Anganwadi toilets, and Community Sanitary Complexes. The monitoring also uses a robust community led system, like Social Audit. Community-based monitoring and vigilance committees will help in creating peer pressure. States decide the delivery mechanisms to be adopted to meet the community needs.

Verification of ODF Communities

The term 'ODF' has been defined by GoI and indicators for the same have been developed. To institute credible process to verify villages against these indicators, an effective verification mechanism is a must. As sanitation is a State subject, and States are the key entities in implementation of the programme, the mechanism for ODF verification is best evolved by the States themselves. The role of the Center is to cross-share processes adopted by different States and evolve a mechanism to validate a small percentage of GPs/villages declared ODF by the States and further facilitate and guide the States where there is large difference in evaluation of Center/State.

Sustaining ODF Communities

The achievement of ODF involves working on behavior change to a great extent, sustenance of which requires concerted efforts by the community. Many districts and States have evolved parameters to maintain sustainability of ODF.

SWACHH BHARAT MISSION FOR URBAN AREAS

The programme includes elimination of open defecation, conversion of unsanitary toilets to pour flush toilets, eradication of manual scavenging, municipal solid waste management and bringing about a behavioral change in people regarding healthy sanitation practices.

The mission aims to cover 1.04 crore households, provide 2.5 lakh community toilets, 2.6 lakh public toilets, and a solid waste management facility in each town. Under the programme, community toilets will be built in residential areas where it is difficult to construct individual household toilets. Public toilets will also be constructed in designated locations such as tourist places, markets, bus stations, railway stations, etc. The programme will be implemented over a five-year period in 4,401 towns.

The total assistance available for construction of an individual toilet is ₹4000/- from the Central Government and an amount of ₹1333/- at least from the State Government. In the case of the North East States, the states are required to contribute only ₹400/- per individual toilet. However, there is no bar on releasing any extra funds at any stage by the ULB/State Government through additional resources.

The expected assistance for construction of community toilets - Central Government will contribute up to 40% of the cost of construction of community toilet as a VGF/outright grant. As per SBM guidelines, the States/UTs shall provide an additional 13.33% for the said component. The NE and special category states shall be required to contribute 4% only. The balance shall have to be arranged through innovative mechanisms by the urban local body. The approximate cost per seat for a community toilet is ₹65,000/-.

₹62,009 crore is likely to be spent on the programme. Of this, the Center will pitch in ₹14,623 crore. Of the Center's share of ₹14,623 crore, ₹7,366 crore will be spent on solid waste management, ₹4,165 crore on individual household toilets, ₹1,828 crore on public awareness and ₹655 crore on community toilets.

SWACHH BHARAT MISSION (GRAMIN)

Phase I

The Nirmal Bharat Abhiyan has been restructured into the Swachh Bharat Mission (Gramin). The SBM(G) was launched on 2nd October 2014 to ensure cleanliness in India and make it Open Defecation Free (ODF) in Five Years. It seeks to improve the levels of cleanliness in rural areas through Solid and Liquid Waste Management activities and making Gram Panchayats Open Defecation Free (ODF), clean and sanitized.

Incentive as provided under the Mission for the construction of Individual Household Latrines (IHHL) was available for all Below Poverty Line (BPL) households and Above Poverty Line (APL) households restricted to SCs/STs, small and marginal farmers, landless laborers with homestead, physically handicapped and women-headed households. The Incentive amount provided under SBM(G) to Below Poverty Line (BPL) /identified APLs households was up to ₹12,000 for construction of one unit of IHHL and for water availability, including for storing for hand-washing and cleaning of the toilet. Central share of this Incentive for IHHLs was ₹9,000/- (75%) from Swachh Bharat Mission (Gramin). The State share was ₹3,000/-(25%). For North Eastern States, and Special Category States, the Central share was ₹10,800/- and the State share was ₹1,200/- (90% : 10%). The beneficiary was encouraged to additionally contribute in the construction of his/her IHHL to promote ownership.

Said to be the world's largest behavior change programme, it achieved the seemingly impossible task by generating a people's movement at the grassroots. All stakeholders worked together from 2014 to 2019 and in a time bound manner ensured that, as on 2nd October 2019 all districts across India, declared themselves as ODF.

Phase II

Having achieved the milestone of an ODF India in a time bound manner in the last five years from 2014 to 2019, the work on sanitation and the behavior change campaign has to continue to sustain the gains made under the programme and also to ensure no one is left behind and the overall cleanliness (Sampoorn Swachhata) in villages as well.

In February 2020, the Phase-II of the SBM(G) with a total outlay of ₹1,40,881 crores was approved with a focus on the sustainability of ODF status and Solid and Liquid Waste Management (SLWM). SBM(G) Phase-II is planned to be a novel model of convergence between different verticals of financing and various schemes of Central and State Governments. The programme will be implemented in mission mode from 2020–21 to 2024–25.

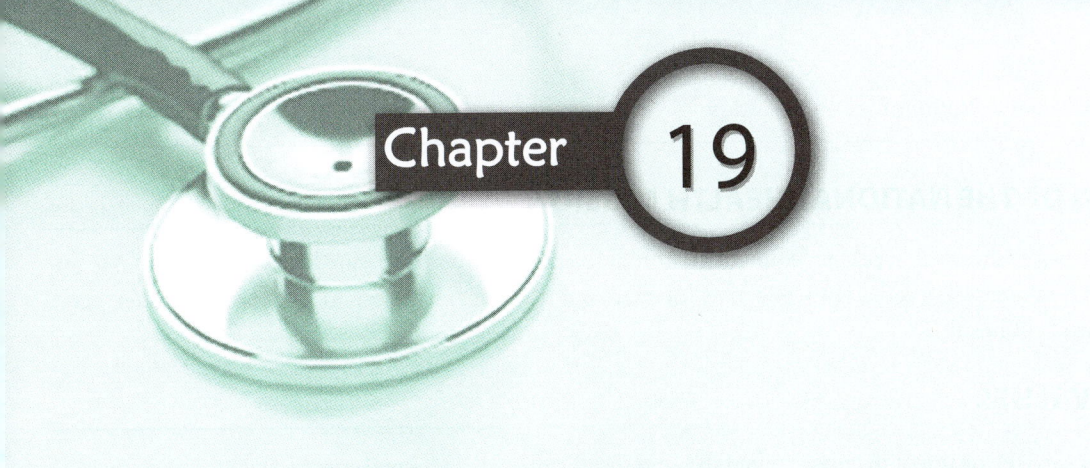

Chapter 19

National Health Mission

INTRODUCTION

The National Health Mission (NHM) encompasses its two submissions, NRHM and NUHM. The Union Cabinet vide its decision dated 1st May 2013 has approved the launch of National Urban Health Mission (NUHM) as a submission of an over-arching National Health Mission (NHM), with National Rural Health Mission (NRHM) being the other submission of NHM.

The NHM envisages achievement of universal access to equitable, affordable and quality health care services that are accountable and responsive to people's needs.

GOALS

The key goals of this phase of NHM will be towards enabling and achieving the stated vision, making the system responsive to the needs of citizens, building a broad based inclusive partnership for realizing National health goals, focusing on the survival and well-being of women and children, reducing existing disease burden and ensuring financial protection for households.

HEALTH INDICATORS TO BE ACHIEVED BY NATIONAL HEALTH MISSION

- Reduce maternal mortality rate (MMR) to 1/1000 live births.
- Reduce infant mortality rate (IMR) to 25/1000 live births.
- Reduce total fertility rate (TFR) to 2.1.
- Prevention and reduction of anemia in women aged 15–49 years.
- Prevent and reduce mortality and morbidity from communicable, non-communicable, injuries and emerging diseases.
- Reduce household out-of-pocket expenditure on total health care expenditure.
- Reduce annual incidence and mortality from tuberculosis by half.
- Reduce prevalence of leprosy to <1/10000 population and incidence to zero in all districts.
- Annual malaria incidence to be <1/1000.
- Less than 1% microfilaria prevalence in all districts.
- Kala-azar elimination by 2015, <1 case per 10,000 population in all blocks.

VISION OF THE NATIONAL HEALTH MISSION

"Attainment of universal access to equitable, affordable and quality health care services, accountable and responsive to people's needs, with effective intersectoral convergent action to address the wider social determinants of health."

CORE VALUES

- Safeguard the health of the poor, vulnerable and disadvantaged, and move toward a right-based approach to health through entitlements and service guarantees.
- Strengthen public health systems as a basis for universal access and social protection against the rising costs of health care.
- Build environment of trust between people and providers of health services.
- Empower community to become active participants in the process of attainment of highest possible levels of health.
- Institutionalize transparency and accountability in all processes and mechanisms.
- Improve efficiency to optimize the use of available resources.

GUIDING PRINCIPLES

- Build an integrated network of all primary, secondary, and a substantial part of tertiary care, providing a continuum from community level to the district hospital, with robust referral linkages to tertiary care and a particular focus on strengthening the primary health care system including outreach services in both rural areas and urban slums.
- Ensure coordinated intersectoral action to address issues of food security and nutrition, access to safe drinking water and sanitation, education particularly girls' education, occupational and environmental health determinants, women's rights and empowerment and different forms of marginalization and vulnerability.
- Incentivize states and UTs to undertake health sector reforms that lead to greater efficiency and equity in health care delivery.
- Ensure prioritization of services that address the health of women and children and the prevention and control of communicable and non-communicable diseases, including locally endemic diseases.
- Reduce out of pocket expenditure on health care, eliminate catastrophic health expenditures and provide social protection to the poor against the rising costs of health care, through cashless services delivered by public health care facilities, supplemented by contracted in private sector facilities wherever necessary.
- Ensure that all public health care facilities or publicly financed private care facilities provide assured quality of health care services.
- Ensure increased access and utilization of quality health services to minimize disparity on account of gender, poverty, caste, other forms of social exclusion and geographical barriers.
- Plan for differential financial investments and technical support to cities, districts and states with higher proportions of vulnerable population groups, urban poor and destitute, and with difficult geographical terrain that face special challenges to meeting health goals.

- Strengthen state level implementation capacity to progress towards achievement of universal health care through flexible and responsive resource allocation, the creation of efficient institutional mechanisms, rules, regulations and processes to enable effective decentralized health planning and management.
- Incentivize good performance of both facilities and providers.
- Address shortages of skilled workers in remote, rural areas, and other underserved pockets through appropriate monetary and nonmonetary incentives.
- Promote partnerships with private, for profit, and not for profit agencies including civil society organizations to achieve health outcomes.
- Facilitate knowledge networks and create effective public health institutions.
- Encourage and enable the involvement of representatives of Panchayati Raj Institutions (PRIs)/Urban Local Bodies (ULBs) in the governance and in the health services, and undertake proactive efforts for convergence and concerted action on social determinants of health such as food and nutrition, safe drinking water, sanitation and hygiene, housing, environment and waste management, education, child marriage, gender and social inequity.
- Establish an accountability and governance framework that would include social audits through people's bodies, community-based monitoring and an effective mechanism of concurrent evaluation.
- Mainstream AYUSH, so as to enhance choice of services for users and to learn from and revitalize local health care traditions.
- Expand focus beyond maternal and child survival to ensuring quality of life for women, children and adolescents.

STRATEGIES

- Support and supplement state efforts to undertake sector wide health system strengthening through the provision of financial and technical assistance.
- Build state, district and city capacity for decentralized outcome-based planning and implementation, based on varying diseases burden scenarios, and using a differential financing approach. There will be a focus on results and performance-based funding including linkage to caseloads.
- Enable integrated facility development planning which would include infrastructure, human resources, drugs and supplies, quality assurance, and effective Rogi Kalyan Samitis (RKS).
- Create a district level knowledge center within each district hospital to serve as the hub for a range of tasks including inter alia, provision of secondary care and selected elements of tertiary care, and the site for skill-based training for all cadres of health workers, collating and analyzing data and coordinating district planning.
- Improve delivery of outreach services through a mix of static facilities and mobile medical units with a team of health service providers with the skill mix and capacity to address primary health care needs.
- Strengthen the sub-center/Urban Primary Health Center (UPHC) with additional human resources and supplies to deliver a much larger range of preventive, promotive and curative care services—so that it becomes the first port of call for each family to access a full range of primary care services.
- Prioritize achievement of universal coverage for Reproductive Maternal, Newborn, Child Health + Adolescent (RMNCH+A), National Communicable Disease Control and Non-Communicable Diseases programmes.
- Expand focus from child survival to child development of all children 0–18 years through a mix of community, *anganwadi*, and school-based health services. The focus of such services will be on prevention and early identification of diseases through periodic screening, health education and promotion of good

health practices and values during these formative years and timely management including assured referral for secondary and tertiary level care as appropriate.

- Achieve the goals of safe motherhood and transition to addressing the broader reproductive health needs of women.
- Focus on adolescents and their health needs.
- Ensure the control of communicable diseases which includes prompt response to epidemics and effective surveillance.
- Use primary health care delivery platforms to address the rising burden of non-communicable diseases.
- Converge with Ministry of Women and Child Development and other related Ministries for effective prevention and reduction of under-nutrition in children aged 0–3 years and anemia among children, adolescents and women.
- Empower the ASHA to serve as a facilitator, mobilizer and provider of community level care.
- Strengthen people's organizations such as the Village Health Sanitation and Nutrition Committees (VHSNC) and Mahila Arogya Samitis (MAS) for convergent intersectoral planning to address social determinants of health and increasing utilization of health and related public services at the community level.
- Create mechanisms to strengthen behavior change communication efforts for preventive and promotive health functions, action on social determinants and to reach the most marginalized.
- Enable social protection function of public hospitals through the universal provision of free consultations, free drugs and diagnostics, free emergency response and patient transport systems. Develop effective partnerships with the not-for-profit, nongovernmental organizations and with the for-profit, private sector to bring in additional capacity where needed to close gaps or improve quality of services.
- Improve public health management by encouraging states to create public health cadre, and strengthening/ creating effective institutions for programme management, providing incentives for improved performance and building high quality research and knowledge management structures. Support states to develop a comprehensive strategy for human resources in health, through policies to support improved recruitment, retention and motivation of health workers in rural, remote and underserved areas, improved workforce management, required staff to help achieve IPHS norms of human resource deployment, development of mid-level care providers and creation of new cadres with appropriate skill sets, and in-service training.
- Enhance use of Information and Communication Technology to improve health care and health systems performance.
- Strengthen Health Management Information Systems as an effective instrument for programme planning and monitoring, supplemented by regular district level surveys and a strong disease surveillance system.
- Ensure universal registration of births and deaths with adequate information on cause of death, to assist in health outcome measurements and health planning.
- Establish accountability frameworks at all levels for improved oversight of programme implementation and achievement of goals. Mechanisms for accountability shall range from participatory community processes like *Jan Sunwais/Samwads*, Social Audit through Gram Sabhas to professional independent concurrent evaluation.
- Implement pilots for Universal Health Coverage (UHC) in selected districts in both EAG and non EAG States to test approaches and innovations before scaling up.

INSTITUTIONAL MECHANISMS

National Level

- At the National level, the Mission Steering Group (MSG) and the Empowered Programme Committee (EPC) are in place. The MSG provides policy direction to the Mission. The Union Minister of Health and Family Welfare chairs the MSG. The convener is the Secretary, Department of Health and Family Welfare and the co-convener is the Additional Secretary and Mission Director. Financial proposals brought before the MSG are first placed before and examined by the EPC, which is headed by the Union Secretary of Health and Family Welfare. The composition, role and powers of the MSG and EPC are in accordance with the Cabinet approval of May 1, 2013.
- The Mission is headed by a Mission Director, of the rank of Additional Secretary, supported by a team of Joint Secretaries. The Mission handles not just the day-to-day administrative affairs of the Mission but is responsible for planning, implementing and monitoring Mission activities. Up to 0.5% of NHM outlay is earmarked for programme management and activities for policy support at the national level through a National Programme Management Unit (NPMU).
- The National Health Systems Resource Center (NHSRC) serve as the apex body for technical support to the center and states. Technical support focuses on problem identification, analysis and problem solving in the process of implementation. It also includes capacity building for district/city planning, and organization of community processes and over all dimensions of institutional capacity, of which skills is only a part. NHSRC also undertake implementation research and evaluation and support the development of State Health Systems Resource Centers (SHSRC) and knowledge networks and partnerships in the states. NHSRC also provide support for policy and strategy development, through collating evidence and knowledge from published work, from experiences in implementation and serve as institutional memory.
- The National Institute of Health and Family Welfare (NIHFW) is the country's apex body for training. Its main focus is on public health education, development of skills in public health management and all training needs of the health care providers. Training is focused on skill-based training of service providers and includes selected aspects of health management training. Its primary accountability is to see that along with its state counterparts, necessary skills for public health management and service provision are in place. One of the major roles of the NIHFW is to revitalize and strengthen the State Institutes of Health and Family Welfare (SIHFW). Another role is to develop into a center of e-learning. The NIHFW also play a leading role in public health research and support to health and family welfare programmes.
- The huge need of institutional capacity development across the nation can be met only by coordinated efforts between planned networks of a large number of public health institutions. Knowledge resources for the National Disease Control Programmes are supported by the National Center for Communicable Diseases. Additional knowledge resources can be harnessed from a number of emerging public health institutions, such as the public health divisions of centrally sponsored institutes namely, All India Institutes of Medical Sciences (AIIMS), and Postgraduate Medical Education and Research (PGIMER), others, such as, the Public Health Foundation of India (PHFI), the Indian Institutes of Health Management and Research (IIHMR), and institutes and schools of public health in states.

State Level

- At the state level, the mission functions under the overall guidance of the State Health Mission (SHM) headed by the State Chief Minister. The State Health Society (SHS) would carry the functions under the Mission and would be headed by the Chief Secretary.

- The District Health Mission (DHM)/City Health Mission (CHM) would be headed by the head of the local self-government, i.e., Chairperson Zila Parishad/Mayor as decided by the state depending upon whether the district is predominantly rural or urban. Every district will have a District Health Society (DHS), which will be headed by the District Collector. At the city level, the Mission or Society may be established based on local context. Existing vertical societies for various national and state health programmes will be merged in the DHS.
- The management of NUHM activities may be coordinated by a city level Urban Health Committee headed by the Municipal Commissioner/District Magistrate/Deputy Commissioner/District Collector/ Sub-Divisional Magistrate/Assistant Commissioner based on whether the city is the district headquarter or a sub-divisional headquarter as may be decided by the State. This would facilitate coordination with other related departments like Women and Child Development, Water Supply and Sanitation especially in times of response to disease outbreaks/epidemics in the cities.
- For the seven mega cities of Delhi, Mumbai, Chennai, Kolkata, Bengaluru, Hyderabad and Ahmedabad, NHM will be implemented by the City Health Mission.
- The State Programme Management Unit (SPMU), State Health System Resource Centers (SHSRC) and the State Institutes of Health and Family Welfare (SIHFW) will continue to play similar roles for the State as do their national counterparts for the Center. The SPMU acts as the main secretariat of the SHS. The constitution and functioning of the SPMU and Executive Committee of the SHS shall be such that there is no hiatus between the Directorate of Health and Family Welfare services and the SPMU.
- SIHFWs and SHSRCs will be strengthened with the necessary infrastructure and human resources to enable provision of quality trainings and skill development programmes. Linkages with research institutes, schools of public health and medical colleges at state and national level would be supported.
- The District Programme Management Unit (DPMU) would be linked to a District Health Knowledge Center (DHKC) and its partners for the requisite technical assistance. The District Training Center (DTC) would be the nodal agency for training requirements of the District Health Society (DHS).

Strengthening State Health Systems

The NHM shall be a major instrument of financing and support to the states to strengthen public health systems and health care delivery. This financing to the state will be based on the state's Programme Implementation Plan (PIP). The PIP shall have following parts:

Part I: NRHM RCH Flexipool
Part II: NUHM Flexipool
Part III: Flexible Pool for Communicable Diseases
Part IV: Flexible Pool for Non-communicable Diseases, Injury and Trauma
Part V: Infrastructure Maintenance

Critical Areas for Concerted Action Toward Health Systems Strengthening

- Decentralized health planning.
- Facility-based service delivery.
- The District Hospital and Knowledge Center.
- Outreach services.
- Community Processes, Behavior Change Communication, and Addressing Social Determinants.
- Social Protection Function of Public Health Services.
- Partnerships with the NGOs, Civil Society, and Profit Private Sector.
- Human Resource Development.

- Public Health Management.
- Health of Tribals and People in Left Wing Extremist (LWE) affected areas.
- Health of the Urban Poor.
- Pilots for Universal Health Coverage.
- Health Management Information Systems.
- Governance and Accountability Framework.

SERVICE DELIVERY STRATEGIES

- Reproductive, Maternal, Newborn, Child Health and Adolescent (RMNCH+A) Services.
- Control of communicable diseases.
- Non-communicable diseases.

Primary Care List of Assured Services

The assured services provided by a primary care team (includes staff of PHC, sub-centers and CHWs) is as follows:

Reproductive and Child Health

- Care in pregnancy—all care including identification of complications, but excluding management of complications requiring surgery or blood transfusion.
- All aspects of Essential Newborn Care.
- Care for common illnesses of newborn and of children—identify, stabilize and refer life threatening conditions beyond the approved skill sets of the mid-level care provider, immunization.
- Universal use of iodized salt.
- All aspects of prevention and management of malnutrition, excepting those that require institutional care.
- All family planning services except female sterilization. Provision of safe abortion services—medical and surgical.
- Identification and management of anemia, common sexual and urogenital problems which can be treated syndromically, or diagnosed with point of care diagnostics, and identification of those which need referral.
- All public health measures that lead to improved maternal and child survival and lower RCH morbidity.
- All health education and individual counseling measures needed for promotion of desirable health behaviors and health care practices and change from inappropriate health care practices and behaviors, related to RCH.
- All activities under the Rashtriya Bal Suraksha Karyakram—at *anganwadi* and school level.
- All laboratory support needed for the same.
- Patient transport systems that can bring and drop back patients, for example, sick infants up to one year of age, institutional delivery, for disability, and address problems of access due to lack of transport.

Emergency and Trauma Care

- Prevention and appropriate management for bites and stings—snakes, scorpions, wild animals. Management of poisoning, including food poisoning.
- Complete first aid including management of minor injuries.
- Stabilization care in poisoning and major injuries and ensuring referral through emergency response systems.

Control of Communicable Disease

- Screening for leprosy, referral on suspicion, and follow-up of cases with confirmed diagnosis and prescribed treatment.
- Referral of suspect tuberculosis, family level screening of known patients, and follow-up of cases with confirmed diagnosis and prescribed treatment.
- HIV testing, appropriate referral and follow-up of specialist-initiated treatment.
- All measures for the prevention of Vector Borne Diseases; early and prompt treatment for these diseases, with referral of complicated cases.
- Control of helminthiasis.
- Reduction in burden of water borne disease, especially diarrhea and dysentery, typhoid and water borne hepatitis, prompt and appropriate care leading to reduction of mortality and morbidity due to these diseases.
- Reduction of infectious hepatitis B and identification and referral for the same.
- Primary care for other infectious diseases, presenting as fever especially ARI, UTI with referral where institutional care is required or where diagnosis is not ascertained.

Control of Non-communicable Disease

- Screening for breast and cervical cancers in all women over the age of 30.
- Screening for mental disorders, counseling, and follow-up to specialist initiated care.
- Detection of epilepsy and stroke and follow-up to specialist initiated drugs and rehabilitative measures.
- Screening for visual impairments, correction of refractive errors and referrals for the rest.
- Screening for diabetes and hypertension in all population above 30 annually.
- Ensuring follow-up on doctor initiated drugs in diabetes and hypertension—and secondary prevention—so that no complications develop.
- Prevention—primary, secondary and tertiary preventive care in rheumatic heart disease. (Prevention of rheumatic disease, prevention of rheumatic heart disease, and prevention of mortality and excess morbidity in rheumatic heart disease).
- Primary and secondary prevention in COPD and bronchial asthma, with provision of follow-up care in patients put on treatment by specialists.
- Counseling and support to victims of violence.
- Preventive measures against all harmful addictive substances—tobacco in the main, but also alcohol and addictive drugs.
- Community based geriatric care support.
- Preventive and promotive measures to address musculoskeletal disorders—mainly osteoporosis, arthritis of different types and referral or follow-up as indicated.
- Community based rehabilitative and disability care support.

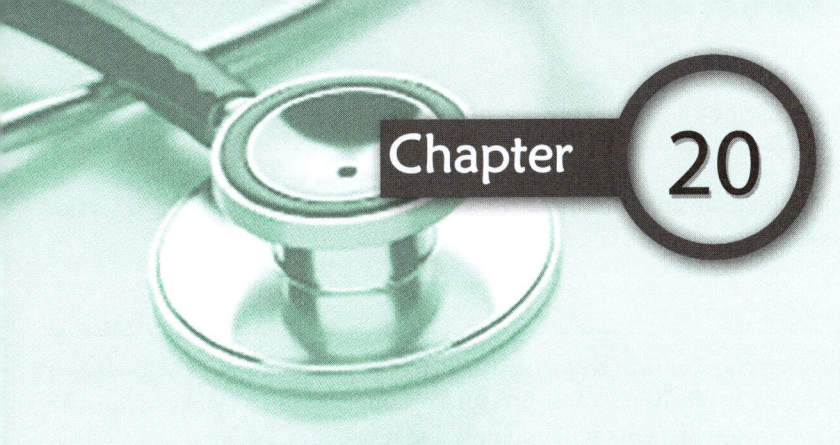

Chapter 20

National Urban Health Mission

INTRODUCTION

In order to effectively address the health concerns of the urban poor population, the Ministry propose to launch a National Urban Health Mission (NUHM). The Mission Steering Group of the National Rural Health Mission (NRHM) will be expanded to work as the apex body for NUHM also. Every Municipal Corporation, Municipality, Notified Area Committee, and Town Panchayat will become a unit of planning with its own approved broad norms for setting up of health facilities. The separate plans for Notified Area Committees, Town Panchayats and Municipalities will be part of the District Health Action Plan drawn up for NUHM. The Municipal Corporations will have a separate plan of action as per broad norms for urban areas. The existing structures and mechanisms of governance under NRHM will be suitably adapted to fulfill the needs of NUHM also. NUHM is a new sub-mission under the over-arching National Health Mission (NHM). Under the scheme, the following proposals have been approved:

- One Urban Primary Health Center (U-PHC) for every population.
- One Urban Community Health Center (U-CHC) for five to six U-PHCs in big cities.
- One Auxiliary Nursing Midwive (ANM) for a population of 10,000.
- One Accredited Social Health Activist (ASHA) (community link worker) for 200–500 households.

FOCUS

NUHM focuses on:
- Urban poor population living in listed and unlisted slums.
- All other vulnerable population such as homeless, rag-pickers, street children, rickshaw pullers, construction and brick and lime kiln workers, sex workers, and other temporary migrants.
- Public health thrust on sanitation, clean drinking water, vector control.

NUHM would endeavor to achieve its goal through:
- Need-based city specific urban health care system to meet the diverse health care needs of the urban poor and other vulnerable sections.
- Institutional mechanism and management systems to meet the health-related challenges of a rapidly growing urban population.
- Partnership with community and local bodies for a more proactive involvement in planning, implementation and monitoring of health activities.
- Availability of resources for providing essential primary health care to urban poor.

- Partnerships with Non-Governmental Organization (NGO) for profit and not for profit health service providers and other stakeholders.

AIMS

To improve the health status of the urban population in general, particularly the poor and other disadvantaged sections by facilitating equitable access to quality health care, through a revamped primary public health care system, targeted outreach services and involvement of the community and urban local bodies.

The scheme will focus on primary health care needs of the urban poor. This mission will be implemented in 779 cities and towns with more than 50,000 population and cover about 7.75 crore people. The interventions under the sub-mission will result in:

- Reduction in Infant Mortality Rate (IMR).
- Reduction in Maternal Mortality Ratio (MMR).
- Universal access to reproductive health care.
- Convergence of all health related interventions.

The existing institutional mechanism and management systems created and functioning under NRHM will be strengthened to meet the needs of NUHM.

City wise implementation plans will be prepared based on baseline survey and felt need. Urban local bodies will be fully involved in implementation of the scheme.

GOAL

The NUHM would aim to improve the health status of the urban population in general, but particularly of the poor and other disadvantaged sections, by facilitating equitable access to quality health care through a revamped public health system, partnerships, community-based mechanism with the active involvement of the urban local bodies.

CORE STRATEGIES

- Improving the efficiency of public health system in the cities by strengthening, revamping and rationalizing existing government primary urban health structure and designated referral facilities.
- Promotion of access to improved health care at household level through community-based groups—Mahila Arogya Samitis.
- Strengthening public health through innovative, preventive and promotive action.
- Increased access to health care through creation of revolving fund.
- IT enabled services (ITES) and E-governance for improving access to surveillance and monitoring.
- Capacity building of stakeholders.
- Prioritizing the most vulnerable amongst the poor.
- Ensuring quality health care services.

OUTCOMES

The NUHM would strive to put in place a sustainable urban health delivery system for addressing the health concerns of the urban poor. The NUHM proposes to measure results at different levels with a long-term as well as intermediate term view.

Process/Throughput Level Indicators

- Number of cities/population where mission has been initiated
- Number of city specific urban health plans developed and operationalized
- Number of U-PHCs with outreach made operational
- Number of cities/population with all slums and facilities mapped
- Number of slum/cluster level health and sanitation per day
- Number of MAS formed
- Number of U-PHCs with programme managers
- Number of ASHAs trained and functioning

Output Level Indicators

- Increase in outpatient department (OPD) attendance
- Increase in below poverty line (BPL) referrals from U-PHCs/referral availed
- Increase in institutional deliveries as percentage of total deliveries
- Increase in complete immunization among children <12 months
- Increase in case detection of malaria through blood examination
- Increase in case detection of tuberculosis (TB) through chest symptoms
- Increase in referral for sputum microscopy examination for TB
- Increase in number of cases screened and treated for dental ailments
- Increase in antenatal check-up (ANC) of pregnant women
- Increased tetanus toxoid (2nd dose) coverage among pregnant women
- Strengthened civil registration system to achieve 100% registration of births and deaths.

Impact Level Focus on Urban Poor

- Reduce IMR by 40% (in urban areas)—National Urban IMR down to 20 per 1000 live births by 2017.
  - 40% reduction in under-five mortality rate (U5MR) and IMR.
  - Achieve universal immunization in all urban areas.
- Reduce MMR by 50%.
  - 50% reduction in MMR (among urban population of the state/country).
  - 100% ANC coverage (in urban areas).
- Achieve universal access to reproductive health including 100% institutional delivery.
- Achieve replacement level fertility (Total fertility rate 2.1).
- Achieve all targets of Disease Control Programmes.

INSTITUTIONAL ARRANGEMENT FOR IMPLEMENTATION

- The NUHM would leverage the institutional structures of the NRHM at the National, State and District level for operationalization of the NUHM. However, in order to provide dedicated focus to issues relating to Urban Health, the institutional mechanism under the NRHM at various levels would be strengthened for NUHM implementation.
- At the central level, the Mission Steering Group under the Union Health Minister, the Empowered Programme Committee under the Secretary (Health and Family Welfare), and the National Programme Coordination Committee under the Mission Director will be responsible for providing overall guidance and taking important decisions.

- For effective implementation and monitoring of NUHM, a National Programme Management Unit (NPMU) will be set up at the central level. The NPMU will also be expected to provide technical assistance to the Urban Health Division of the Ministry.
- At the State level, for improving the Programme Management under NUHM, a State Programme Management Unit (SPMU) will be set up, which would essentially be an extension of the NRHM SPMU, with a separate Urban Health Cell, reporting to the State Mission Director. The staff at the SPMU- Urban Health Cell may be proposed:
  - State Urban Health Programme Manager
  - State Urban Health MIS Manager
  - State Urban Health Finance Manager
  - State Urban Health Consultant (M and E and Community Participation).
- In addition to the above, at the city level, the States may either decide to constitute a separate City Urban Health Mission/City Urban Health Society or use the existing structure of the District Health Society/Mission under NRHM with additional stakeholder members.
- At the city level, the management of NUHM activities may be coordinated by a city level Urban Health Committee headed by the District Magistrate/Additional District Magistrate/Sub-division Magistrate based on whether the city is a district headquarter or a sub-division headquarter. This would help ensure better coordination with municipal departments like sanitation, water, waste management, especially in times of response to disease outbreaks/epidemics in the city.
- Further for enhancing the Programme Management, a City Programme Management Unit (CPMU) may be established. The staff at the City PMU level may be as proposed:
  - Urban Health Data Manager
  - Urban Health Accounts Manager
  - Consultant (Epidemiologist)

The NUHM would promote participation of the urban local bodies in the planning and management of the urban health programmes.

- For the seven mega cities, namely Delhi, Mumbai, Kolkata, Chennai, Bengaluru, Hyderabad and Ahmedabad, the NUHM may be implemented through the respective ULBs. For the remaining cities, health department would be the primary implementation agency for NUHM. However, for cities/towns where capacity exists with the ULBs, the states may decide to hand over the management of the NUHM to them.
- A generic institutional model for a National/State/District/City level Urban Health Mission and Society is illustrated, notwithstanding the flexibilities provided to the states.
- The National Urban Health service delivery model would make a concerted effort to rationalize and strengthen the existing public health care system in urban areas and promote effective engagement with the non-governmental sector (profit/not for profit) for expanding reach to urban poor, along with strengthening the participation of the community in planning and management of the health care service delivery (Fig. 1).

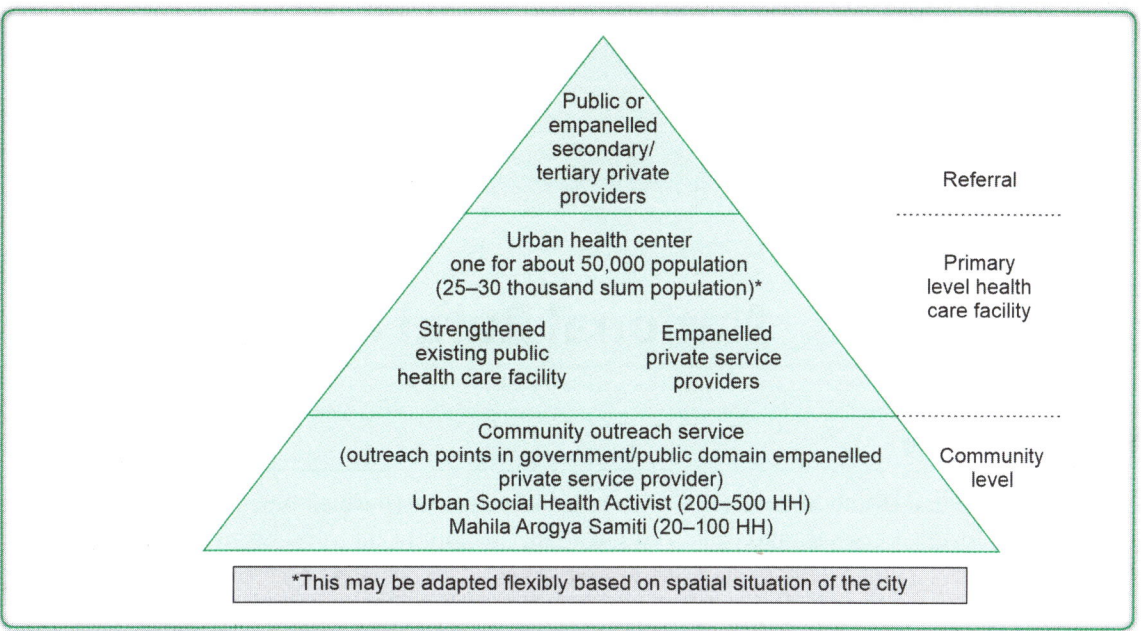

Figure 1: Urban health care delivery model

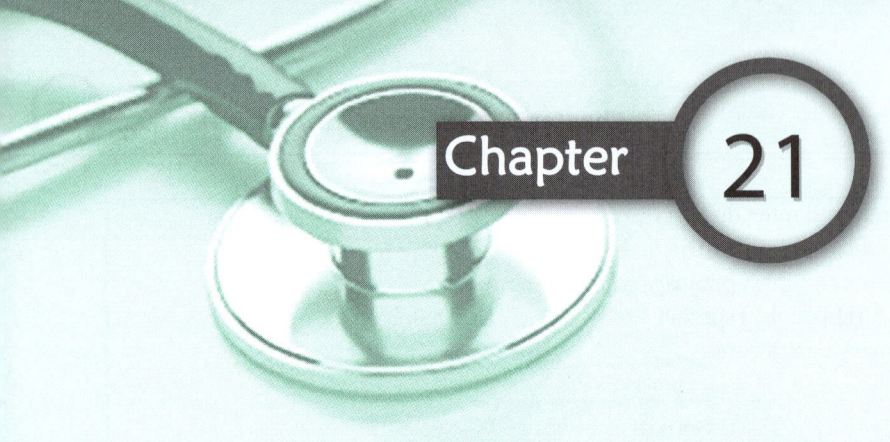

Chapter 21

National Rural Health Mission

INTRODUCTION

The National Rural Health Mission (NRHM) was launched by the Hon'ble Prime Minister on 12th April 2005, to provide accessible, affordable and quality health care to the rural population, especially the vulnerable groups.

The NRHM seeks to provide equitable, affordable and quality health care to the rural population, especially the vulnerable groups. Under the NRHM, the Empowered Action Group (EAG) States as well as North Eastern States, Jammu and Kashmir and Himachal Pradesh have been given special focus. The thrust of the mission is on establishing a fully functional, community-owned, decentralized health delivery system with intersectoral convergence at all levels, to ensure simultaneous action on a wide range of determinants of health such as water, sanitation, education, nutrition, social and gender equality. Institutional integration within the fragmented health sector was expected to provide a focus on outcomes, measured against Indian Public Health Standards for all health facilities.

VISION

- The NRHM (2005–12) seeks to provide effective health care to rural population throughout the country.
- The mission is an articulation of the commitment of the Government to raise public spending on health from 0.9% of GDP to 2–3% of GDP.
- It aims to undertake architectural correction of the health system to enable it to effectively handle increased allocations as promised under the National Common Minimum Programme and promote policies that strengthen public health management and service delivery in the country.
- **Key Components**
    - Provision of a female health activist in each village.
    - A village health plan prepared through a local team headed by the Health and Sanitation Committee of the Panchayat; strengthening of the rural hospital for effective curative care and made measurable and accountable to the community through Indian Public Health Standards (IPHS).
    - Integration of Vertical Health and Family Welfare Programmes and Funds for optimal utilization of funds and infrastructure and strengthening delivery of primary health care.
- It seeks to revitalize local health traditions and mainstream AYUSH into the public health system.
- It aims at effective integration of health concerns with determinants of health like sanitation and hygiene, nutrition, and safe drinking water through a District Plan for Health.
- It seeks decentralization of programmes for district management of health.

- It seeks to address the inter-state and inter-district disparities, especially among the 18 high focus States, including unmet needs for public health infrastructure.
- It shall define time-bound goals and report publicly on their progress.
- It seeks to improve access of rural people, especially poor women and children, to equitable, affordable, accountable and effective primary health care.

GOALS

- Reduction in Infant Mortality Rate (IMR) and Maternal Mortality Ratio (MMR).
- Universal access to public health services such as womens health, child health, water, sanitation and hygiene, immunization, and nutrition.
- Prevention and control of communicable and non-communicable diseases, including locally endemic diseases.
- Access to integrated comprehensive primary health care.
- Population stabilization, gender and demographic balance.
- Revitalize local health traditions and mainstream AYUSH.
- Promotion of healthy lifestyle.

OBJECTIVES

- Facilitating increased access and utilization of quality health services by all.
- Reducing child and maternal mortality.
- Universalizing access to public services for food and nutrition, sanitation and hygiene and universalizing access to public health services with emphasis on services addressing women's and children's health and universal immunization.
- Preventing and controlling communicable and non-communicable diseases, including locally endemic diseases.
- Improving access to integrated comprehensive primary health care.
- Stabilizing population, gender and demographic balance.
- Raising public expenditure on health along with giving flexibility to states and communities to pool risks through local initiatives.
- Seeing a concomitant reduction in IMR, MMR and total fertility rate (TFR).
- Revitalizing local health traditions.
- Promoting healthy lifestyles.

STRATEGIES

- To fulfill these ends, the mission has the following core and supplementary strategies.
- Training and capacity enhancement of Panchayati Raj Institutions to own, control and manage public health services.
- Promoting access to improved health care at the household level through the female health activists (the Accredited Social Health Activist or ASHA).
- Improving facilities for institutional childbirths through provision of referral transport, escort and improved hospital care subsidized under the Janani Suraksha Yojana (JSY) for the below poverty line families.

- Creating and upgrading sub-centers, primary health centers (PHCs) and community health centers (CHCs) using untied, flexi-pool grant and maintenance funding.
- Initiating Village Health and Nutrition Days (VHNDs), to educate and mobilize the community.
- Setting up Hospital Development Societies (HDS) or Rogi Kalyan Samitis (RKS) and Village Health and Sanitation Committees (VHSCs), for encouraging the involvement of the community at decentralized levels.
- Generating health plans for each village through the Village Health Committee of the Panchayat.
- Implementing intersectoral District Health Plans (DHPs) prepared by the District Health Mission, which converge health, nutrition, water, sanitation and hygiene activities.
- Integrating Health and Family Welfare Programmes at the National, State, District and Block levels.
- Providing technical support to National, State and District Health Missions, for public health management.
- Strengthening capacities for data collection, assessment and review for evidence-based planning, monitoring and supervision.
- Formulating transparent policies for deployment and career development of human resource for health.
- Developing capacities for preventive health care at all levels for promoting healthy lifestyles and reducing consumption of tobacco and alcohol.
- Promoting non-profit organizations particularly in underserved areas.
- Revitalizing and mainstreaming other forms of medicine particularly Ayurveda, Yoga and Naturopathy, Unani, Siddha and Homeopathy (or AYUSH).
- Fostering public-private partnerships while regulating the private sector including the informal Rural Medical Practitioners (RMPs) to ensure availability of quality service to citizens at reasonable cost; and
- Instituting Indian Public Health Standards (IPHS).

Core Strategies

- Train and enhance capacity of Panchayati Raj Institutions (PRIs) to own, control and manage public health services.
- Promote access to improved health care at household level through the female health activist (ASHA).
- Health plan for each village through Village Health Committee of the Panchayat.
- Strengthening sub-center through an untied fund to enable local planning and action and more Multi-purpose Workers (MPWs).
- Strengthening existing PHCs and CHCs, and provision of 30–50 bedded CHC per lakh population for improved curative care to a normative standard (Indian Public Health Standards defining personnel, equipment and management standards).
- Preparation and implementation of an intersectoral District Health Plan prepared by the District Health Mission, including drinking water, sanitation and hygiene and nutrition.
- Integrating vertical Health and Family Welfare Programmes at National, State, Block, and District levels.
- Technical support to National, State and District Health Missions for Public Health Management.
- Strengthening capacities for data collection, assessment and review for evidence-based planning, monitoring and supervision.
- Formulation of transparent policies for deployment and career development of human resources for health.
- Developing capacities for preventive health care at all levels for promoting healthy lifestyles, reduction in consumption of tobacco and alcohol, etc.
- Promoting non-profit sector particularly in underserved areas.

Supplementary Strategies

- Regulation of private sector including the informal rural practitioners to ensure availability of quality service to citizens at reasonable cost.
- Promotion of public private partnerships for achieving public health goals.
- Mainstreaming AYUSH—revitalizing local health traditions.
- Reorienting medical education to support rural health issues including regulation of medical care and medical ethics.
- Effective and viable risk pooling and social health insurance to provide health security to the poor by ensuring accessible, affordable, accountable and good quality hospital care.

Mission Outcomes

The mission outcomes are expected to follow a phased approach and are at two levels.

National Level

- Infant mortality rate to be reduced to 30/1000 live births.
- Maternal mortality ratio to be reduced to 100/100,000.
- Total fertility rate to be brought to 2.1.
- Malaria mortality reduction rate –50% up to 2010, additional 10% by 2012.
- Kala-azar to be eliminated by 2010.
- Filaria/Microfilaria reduction rate 70% by 2010, 80% by 2012 and elimination by 2015.
- Dengue mortality reduction rate 50% by 2010 and sustaining at that level until 2012.
- Japanese encephalitis mortality reduction rate: 50% by 2010 and sustaining at that level until 2012.
- Cataract operation increasing to 46 lakhs per year until 2012.
- Leprosy prevalence rate to be brought to less than 1/10,000.
- Tuberculosis DOTS services from the current rate of 1.8/1000, 85% cure rate to be maintained through the entire mission period.
- 2000 Community Health Centers to be upgraded to Indian Public Health Standards.
- Utilization of First Referral Units to be increased from less than 20–75%.
- 250,000 women to be engaged in 18 States as Accredited Social Health Activists (ASHA).

Community Level

- Availability of trained community level workers at village level, with a drug kit for generic ailments.
- Health Day at *Anganwadi* level on a fixed day/month for provision of immunization, ante/post-natal checkups and services related to mother and child health care, including nutrition.
- Availability of generic drugs for common ailments at sub-center and hospital level.
- Good hospital care through assured availability of doctors, drugs and quality services at PHC/CHC level.
- Improved access to universal immunization through induction of auto-disabled syringes, alternate vaccine delivery and improved mobilization services under the programme.
- Improved facilities for institutional delivery through provision of referral, transport, escort and improved hospital care subsidized under the Janani Suraksha Yojana (JSY) for the Below Poverty Line families.
- Availability of assured health care at reduced financial risk through pilots of Community Health Insurance under the mission.
- Provision of household toilets.
- Improved outreach services through mobile medical unit at district level.

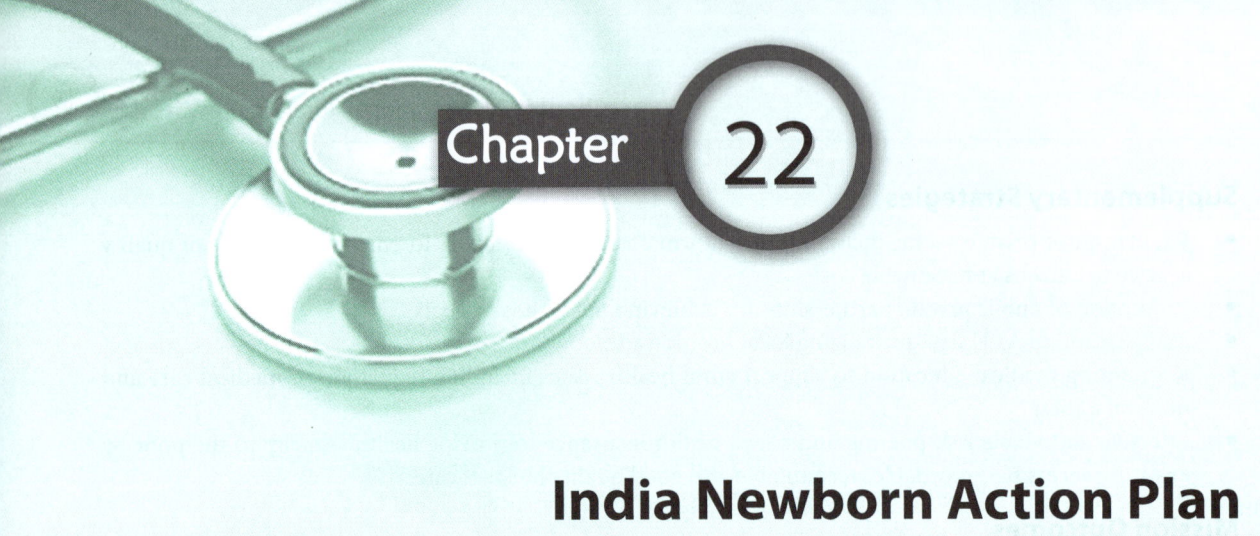

Chapter 22

India Newborn Action Plan

INTRODUCTION

The India Newborn Action Plan (INAP) is India's committed response to the Global Every Newborn Action Plan (ENAP), launched in June 2014 at the 67th World Health Assembly, to advance the global strategy for women's and children's health. The ENAP sets forth a vision of a world that has eliminated preventable newborn deaths and stillbirths. INAP lays out a vision and a plan for India to end preventable newborn deaths, accelerate progress, and scale up high-impact yet cost-effective interventions. INAP has a clear vision supported by goals, strategic intervention packages, priority actions, and a monitoring framework. For the first time, INAP also articulates the Government of India's specific attention on preventing stillbirths. INAP was launched in September 2014, for accelerating the reduction of preventable newborn deaths and stillbirths in the country with the goal of attaining 'Single Digit Neonatal Mortality Rate (NMR) by 2030' and 'Single Digit Still Birth Rate (SBR) by 2030'. Currently, there are estimated 7.47 lakh neonatal deaths annually. The neonatal deaths are expected to reduce to below 2.28 lakh annually by 2030, once the goal is achieved. The INAP is a concerted effort towards translating commitments into meaningful change for newborns. INAP will serve as a framework for the states to develop their area-specific action plans.

MILESTONES IN CHILD SURVIVAL PROGRAMMES IN INDIA

- 1992 – Child Survival and Safe Motherhood Programme (CSSM)
- 1997 – RCH I
- 2005 – RCH II
- 2005 – National Rural Health Mission
- 2013 – RMNCH+A Strategy
- 2013 – National Health Mission
- 2014 – INAP

OBJECTIVES

- Builds on existing commitments under the National Health Mission and 'Call to Action' for child survival and development.
- Aligns with the ENAP; defines commitments based on specific contextual needs of the country.
- Aims at attaining single digit NMR by 2030, five years ahead of the global plan.

- Emphasizes strengthened surveillance mechanism for tracking stillbirths.
- Focuses on ending preventable newborn deaths, improving quality of care and care beyond survival.
- Prioritizes those babies that are born too soon, too small, or sick—as they account for majority of all newborn deaths.
- Aspires towards ensuring equitable progress for girls and boys, rural and urban, rich and poor, and between districts and states.
- Identifies major guiding principles under the overarching principle of integration: equity, gender, quality of care, convergence, accountability, and partnerships.
- Defines six pillars of interventions: pre-conception and antenatal care; care during labor and childbirth; immediate newborn care; care of healthy newborn; care of small and sick newborn; and care beyond newborn survival.
- Serves as a framework for states/districts to develop their own action plan with measurable indicators.

GOALS

The two specific goals of INAP are as follows:
- **Goal 1:** Ending preventable newborn deaths to achieve "Single Digit NMR" by 2030, with all the states to individually achieve this target by 2035.
- **Goal 2:** Ending preventable stillbirths to achieve "Single Digit SBR" by 2030, with all the states to individually achieve this target by 2035.

Under INAP, the newborn care/postnatal care component of the RMNCH+A continuum (for high impact interventions and commodities) has been further delineated into four distinct categories: immediate newborn care, care of healthy newborn, care of small and sick newborn, and care of newborn beyond survival. Further, pre-conception and antenatal care and care during labor and childbirth—the two stages impacting newborn outcomes including stillbirths have been included.

As a result, six pillars of intervention packages have been identified. The interventions under each of the six pillars have been described below in detail including the strategic/priority actions required to deliver high-impact interventions for achieving effective coverage. As such, the interventions have been categorized as:
- Essential [E], to be implemented universally.
- Situational [S], implementation dependent on epidemiological context.
- Advanced [A], implementation based on health-system capacity of the state/district.

ACTION PLAN BASED ON SIX PACKAGES

The states are urged to develop their action plan based on the **Six Packages** described in Table 1.

Table 1: Action plan based on six packages develop by state

Package 1	Preconception and antenatal care
Package 2	Care during labor and childbirth
Package 3	Immediate newborn care
Package 4	Care of healthy newborn
Package 5	Care of small and sick newborn
Package 6	Care beyond newborn survival

Package 1: Preconception and Antenatal Care

Priority Actions

- Prioritize actions for delaying age at 1st pregnancy in convergence with stakeholders and other departments with special focus on teenage pregnancy.
- Train an adequate number of service providers for Family Planning Services and ensure availability of commodities, as per FP 2020.
- Saturate high case-load facilities to provide Postpartum Intrauterine Contraceptive Device (PPIUCD).
- Train an adequate numbers of ANMs in SBA (including ANC component).

Scale up nutritional interventions of periconceptional folic acid, maternal calcium supplementation, and iron folic acid supplementation National Iron Plus Initiative/Weekly Iron and Folic Acid Supplementation (NIPI/WIFS).

- Strengthen convergence with related departments for nutrition counseling.
- Screening of high-risk pregnancies and their management as per protocols.
- Accelerate implementation of preventive measures against malaria for pregnant women in endemic area
- Promote counseling and birth preparedness.

Package 2: Care during Labor and Childbirth

Priority Actions

- Prioritize and strengthen public health facilities at all levels (L1, L2, L3) for conducting safe delivery, including provision of emergency obstetric care as per the norms of Maternal and Newborn Health (MNH) Toolkit.
- Provision of dedicated MCH wings in facilities with high caseload, including functional WASH facilities.
- All delivery points to be saturated with adequately trained health workers: Ensure trained and skilled staff at all designated delivery points: L1 delivery point should have Skilled Birth Attendants (SBA) trained ANMs/SNs, L2 delivery point to have at least one Basic Emergency Obstetric Care (BEmOC) trained MO, and L3 delivery point must have at least four obstetricians and gynecologists/Comprehensive Emergency Obstetric Care (CEmOC) trained Medical Officers (MOs) and four Anesthetist/Life Saving Anesthesia Skills (LSAS) trained MOs.
- Expand the availability of SBA-trained birth attendants. In addition to ANM, SBA training to be rolled out for AYUSH doctors (as per state-specific need).
- Establish Quality Assurance mechanism at each level, like—use of safe birth checklist and regular quality audits including perinatal death audits.
- Institutionalize referral mechanism to ensure to-and-fro referral, including inter-facility referral, as and where required.
- Accelerate scale-up of new policy decisions on management of preterm labor through use of antenatal corticosteroids and antibiotics for premature rupture of membranes.
- Develop a mechanism of supportive supervision through existing systems or through partnerships (with professional organizations, medical colleges, and private hospitals) at the regional and state level.
- Generate awareness on JSSK entitlements, promote community participation, and demand for safe institutional delivery.
- Establish a sound surveillance system for tracking stillbirths.

Package 3: Immediate Newborn Care

Priority Actions

- Establish fully functional Newborn Care Corners (NBCCs) at all facilities conducting deliveries, according to the norms prescribed in the MNH toolkit.
- Saturate all facilities conducting deliveries with NSSK-trained staff.
- Implement standardized clinical protocols for essential newborn care, including resuscitation.
- Develop quality assurance mechanisms/cells to monitor training quality and adherence to standard protocols.
- Regular quality audits of facilities, including death audits.
- Ensure availability of injection vitamin K at all delivery points and its inclusion in the State's Essential Drugs List.
- Develop a mechanism of ongoing supportive supervision at the facility level.
- Strengthen counseling for breastfeeding, postnatal care, and community and home care practices.
- Focus on community strategies to promote demand for essential newborn care.

Package 4: Care of Healthy Newborn

Priority Actions

- Recruitment and rational deployment of ASHAs as per the population norm capacity-building of ASHAs to provide newborn care at the community level.
- Ensure uninterrupted supply of ASHA HBNC kits and replenishment thereof, from PHC inventory.
- Ensure timely payments of HBNC incentives for ASHAs.
- Set up mechanisms for monitoring of HBNC visits, with regards to quality and coverage.
- Ensure implementation of standardized training norms and uniform mechanism (formats, checklist) for quality of home visits.
- Strengthen and revitalize the role of ANM as supervisor cum mentor to ASHA.
- Institutionalize a framework for supportive supervision and mentoring of ASHAs (ARC, DRC, DCM, BCM, Supervisor/Facilitator).
- Build responsive referral system—easy access and availability of referral transport and medical care at the health facilities for all sick/high-risk newborns referred by ASHAs.
- Strengthen counseling for breastfeeding, postnatal care, entitlements, and home care practices using counselors and audiovisuals.
- Ensure availability of vaccines and logistic support for immunization at all delivery points.

Package 5: Care of Small and Sick Newborn

Priority Actions

- Ensure dissemination of guidelines at all levels of facilities with priority to high caseload facilities and High Priority Districts (HPDs).
- Establish fully functional NBSUs, SNCUs with the requisite HR in blocks/districts with priority to High Priority Districts (HPDs) and scale up KMC unit/wards on the existing FBNC system.
- Saturate all districts in the state with fully functional SNCUs followed by all facilities with >3000 deliveries/year.
- Upgrade NICUs at the medical colleges/tertiary care facilities to provide referral services for advanced newborn care support (ventilation, surgery) at regional level, and to strengthen linkages with SNCUs and NBSUs.

- Operationalize SNCU monitoring software across all SNCUs/NICUs.
- Institutionalize network of Regional/State FBNC collaborating centers and Medical Colleges to:
  - Accelerate capacity building of MOs/Staff Nurses/ANMs posted in NBSUs, SNCUs and KMC units, and of ANMs for IMNCI.
  - Develop an integrated framework for supportive supervision.
- Ensure mechanisms for timely procurement and supply chain management of equipment, drugs, and laboratory reagents as per the defined norms and technical specifications.
- Regularly monitor quality of trainings.
- Develop Quality Assurance mechanisms/cells to ensure compliance with norms for quality of care for small and sick newborns, including tools for adherence to admission and discharge criteria, SOPs for clinical management, infection prevention and control.
- Conduct regular quality audits of facilities including death audits.
- Scale up new operational guidelines, allowing ANMs to administer injectable antibiotics for neonatal sepsis.

Package 6: Care Beyond Newborn Survival

Priority Actions
- Train all levels of service providers engaged in screening of birth defects and developmental delays.
- Deploy trained mobile health teams for screening.
- Establish fully functional District Early Intervention Centers (DEICs).
- Institutionalize a robust referral mechanism between screening points and District Early Intervention Centers (DEICs).
- Establish centers of excellence at tertiary care hospitals for management of conditions, especially the birth defects requiring surgical correction.
- Screen birth defects by the service providers at the facility and in community by ASHAs during home visits.
- Facility-based follow-up of small and sick babies for developmental delay and appropriate management.
- Follow-up of all sick/high-risk newborns discharged from the SNCU for a period of one year by ASHAs.
- Develop resource network, including private practitioners, to provide specialized care for identified cases.

NATIONAL TARGETS

The national targets of INAP are given in Table 2.

Table 2: INAP—National targets

Targets	Current	2017	2020	2025	2030
Impact targets					
NMR (per 1000 live births)	29	24	21	15	<10
SBR (per 1000 live births)	22	19	17	13	<10
Coverage targets					
Safe delivery (institutional + home delivery by SBA (%)	76	90	95	95	95

Contd...

Targets	Current	2017	2020	2025	2030
Initiation of breastfeeding within one hour of birth (%)	—	75	90	90	90
Women with preterm labor receiving at least one dose of antenatal corticosteroids (%)	—	75	90	95	95
Babies born in health facilities with birth asphyxia received resuscitation (%)	—	75	90	95	95
Babies received complete schedule of home visits under HBNC by ASHA (%)	—	50	75	95	95
Newborn with sepsis in the community received Gentamicin by ANM (%)	—	50	75	75	75
Newborn discharged from SNCU followed until age one (%)	—	35	50	75	75
Newborn with low birth weight/ Prematurity managed with KMC at facility (%)	—	35	50	75	90

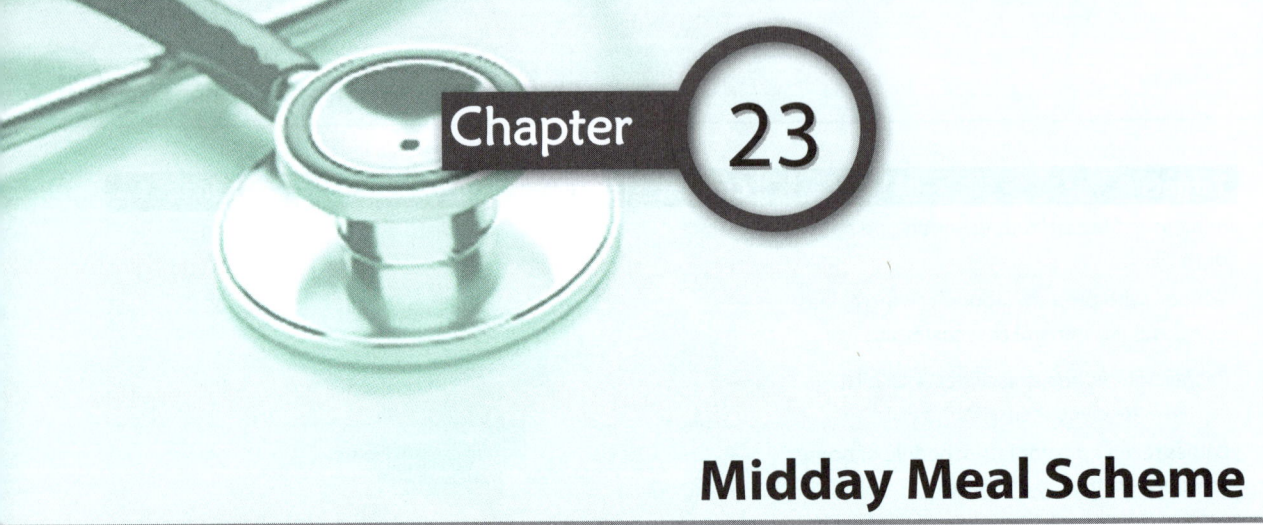

Chapter 23

Midday Meal Scheme

INTRODUCTION

With a view to enhancing enrolment, retention and attendance and simultaneously improving nutritional levels among children, the National Programme of Nutritional Support to Primary Education (NP-NSPE) was launched as a Centrally Sponsored Scheme on 15th August 1995.

In 2001, MDMS became a cooked Midday Meal Scheme under which every child in every Government and Government-aided primary school was to be served a prepared midday meal with a minimum content of 300 calories of energy and 8–12 g protein per day for a minimum of 200 days. The scheme was further extended in 2002 to cover not only children studying in Government, Government-aided and local body schools, but also children studying in Education Guarantee Scheme (EGS) and Alternative and Innovative Education (AIE) centers.

In September 2004, the Scheme was revised to provide for Central Assistance for Cooking cost @ ₹1 per child per school day to cover cost of pulses, vegetables, cooking oil, condiments, fuel and wages and remuneration payable to personnel or amount payable to agency responsible for cooking. Transport subsidy was also raised from the earlier maximum of ₹50 per quintal to ₹100 per quintal for special category states and ₹75 per quintal for other states. Central assistance was provided for the first time for management, monitoring and evaluation of the scheme @ 2% of the cost of food grains, transport subsidy and cooking assistance. A provision for serving midday meal during summer vacation in drought affected areas was also made.

In July 2006, the scheme was further revised to enhance the cooking cost to ₹1.80 per child/school day for States in the North Eastern Region and ₹1.50 per child/school day for other States and UTs. The nutritional norm was revised to 450 calories and 12 g of protein. In order to facilitate construction of kitchen-cum-store and procurement of kitchen devices in schools, provision for central assistance @ ₹60,000 per unit and @ ₹5,000 per school in phased manner were made.

In October 2007, the scheme was extended to cover children of upper primary classes (i.e. class VI to VIII) studying in 3,479 Educationally Backwards Blocks (EBBs) and the name of the scheme was changed from 'National Programme of Nutritional Support to Primary Education' to 'National Programme of Midday Meal in Schools'. The nutritional norm for upper primary stage was fixed at 700 calories and 20 g of protein. The scheme was extended to all areas across the country from April 1, 2008.

The scheme was further revised in April 2008 to extend the scheme to recognized as well as unrecognized *Madarsas/Maqtabs* supported under SSA.

OBJECTIVES

The objectives of the midday meal scheme are as follows:

- Improving the nutritional status of children in classes I–VIII in government, local body and government-aided schools, and EGS and AIE centers.
- Encouraging poor children, belonging to disadvantaged sections, to attend school more regularly and help them concentrate on classroom activities.
- Providing nutritional support to children of primary stage in drought-affected areas.

From the year 2009 onwards, the following changes have been made to improve the implementation of the scheme:

- Food norms have been revised to ensure balanced and nutritious diet to children of upper primary group by increasing the quantity of pulses from 25 g to 30 g, vegetables from 65 g to 75 g and by decreasing the quantity of oil and fat from 10 g to 7.5 g.
- Cooking cost (excluding the labor and administrative charges) has been revised from ₹1.68 to ₹2.50 for primary and from ₹2.20 to ₹3.75 for upper primary children from 1.12.2009 to facilitate serving meal to eligible children in prescribed quantity and of good quality. The cooking cost for primary is ₹2.69 per child per day and ₹4.03 for upper primary children from April 1, 2010. The cooking cost will be revised prior approval of competent authority by 7.5% every financial year from April 1, 2011.
- The honorarium for cooks and helpers was paid from the labor and other administrative charges of ₹0.40 per child per day provided under the cooking cost. In many cases the honorarium was so little that it became very difficult to engage manpower for cooking the meal. A separate component for payment of honorarium @ ₹1000 per month per cook-cum-helper was introduced from December 1, 2009. Honorarium at the above prescribed rate is being paid to cook-cum-helper. However, in some of the states the honorarium to cook-cum-helpers are being paid more than ₹1000/- through their state fund. Following norms for engagement of cook-cum-helper have been made:
  - One cook-cum-helper for schools up to 25 students.
  - Two cooks-cum-helpers for schools with 26–100 students.
  - One additional cook-cum-helper for every addition of up to 100 students.
    More than 25.70 lakhs cook-cum-helper are engaged by the State/UTs during 2013–14 for preparation and serving of midday meal to children in elementary classes.
- A common unit cost of construction of kitchen shed @ ₹60,000 for the whole country was impractical and also inadequate. Now the cost of construction of kitchen-cum-store will be determined on the basis of plinth area norm and State Schedule of Rates. The Department of School Education and Literacy vide letter No.1-1/2009-Desk (MDM) dated December 31, 2009 had prescribed 20 sq.m plinth area for schools having up to 100 children. For every additional up to 100 children, additional 4 sq.m plinth area will be added. States/UTs have the flexibility to modify the slab of 100 children depending upon the local condition.
- Due to difficult geographical terrain of the Special Category States, the transportation cost @ ₹1.25 per quintal was not adequate to meet the actual cost of transportation of food grains from the FCI godowns to schools in these States. On the request of the North Eastern States the transportation assistance in the 11 Special Category States (Northern Eastern States, Himachal Pradesh, Jammu and Kashmir and Uttarakhand) have been made at par with the public distribution system (PDS) rates prevalent in these States with effect from December 1, 2009.

- The existing system of payment of cost of food grains to FCI from the Government of India is prone to delays and risk. Decentralization of payment of cost of food grains to the FCI at the district level from 1.4.2010 allowed officers at State and National levels to focus on detailed monitoring of the scheme.

REVISION IN SCHEME

Since its inspection, the scheme has been revised from time to time and the present provisions are as given below:
- Free supply of food grains @ 100 g per child per school day at Primary and @ 150 g per child per school day at upper primary.
- Subsidy for transportation of food grains is provided to 11 special category states at PDS rate prevalent in these states and up to a maximum of ₹75.00 per quintal for other than special categories States/UTs.
- In addition to food grains, a midday meal involves major input, viz., cost of cooking, which is explained below.

Cost of cooking includes cost of ingredients, e.g. pulses, vegetables, cooking oil and condiments as given in Table.

Table: Food norm with effect from December 1, 2009

| Sl. no. | Items | Quantity/day/child | |
		Primary	Upper primary
1.	Food grains	100 g	150 g
2.	Pulses	20 g	30 g
3.	Vegetables (leafy also)	50 g	75 g
4.	Oil and fat	5 g	7.5 g
5.	Salt and condiments	As per need	As per need

- **Engagement of cook-cum-helpers**
  - A separate provision for payment of honorarium to cook-cum-helper @ ₹1000/- per month has been made. One cook-cum-helper may be engaged in a school having up to 25 students, two cooks-cum-helpers for schools having 26–100 students and one additional cook-cum-helper for every addition of up to 100 students.
  - The expenditure towards the honorarium of cook-cum-helper is shared between the Center and the NER States and 3 Himalayan States (Himachal Pradesh, Jammu and Kashmir and Uttarakhand) on 90:10 basis, 100% for UTs and with other States on 60:40 basis vide order dt. 8-12-2015.
- **Management, monitoring and evaluation**
  Provide assistance to States/UTs for Management, Monitoring and Evaluation (MME) at the rate of 1.8% of total assistance on:
  (a) free food grains, (b) transport cost (c) cooking cost and (d) Honorarium to cook-cum-helpers. Another 0.2% of the above amount will be utilized at the Central Government for management, monitoring and evaluation. The detailed guidelines issued by the Ministry vide letter No. F.1-15/2009-Desk (MDM) dated 21st June, 2010.
- Provision of midday meal during summer vacation in drought affected areas.
- **Provision of essential infrastructures:**
  - Kitchen-cum-stores
  - Kitchen devices.

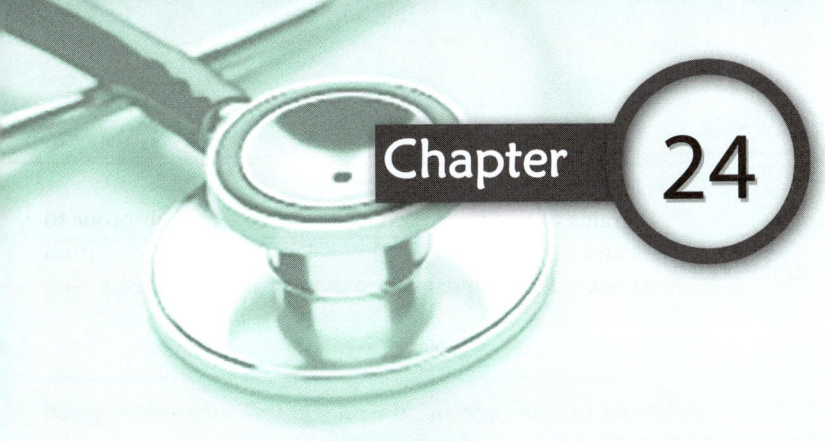

Chapter 24

Janani Suraksha Yojana

INTRODUCTION

Janani Suraksha Yojana (JSY) is a safe motherhood intervention under the National Rural Health Mission (NRHM). It is being implemented with the objective of reducing maternal and neonatal mortality by promoting institutional delivery among poor pregnant women. The scheme is under implementation in all States and Union Territories (UTs), with a special focus on low performing states (LPS). JSY was launched in April 2005 by modifying the National Maternity Benefit Scheme (NMBS). The NMBS came into effect in August 1995 as one of the components of the National Social Assistance Programme (NSAP). The scheme was transferred from the Ministry of Rural Development to the Department of Health and Family Welfare during the year 2001–02. The NMBS provides for financial assistance of ₹500/- per birth up to two live births to the pregnant women who have attained 19 years of age and belong to the below poverty line (BPL) households. When JSY was launched the financial assistance of ₹500/-, which was available uniformly throughout the country to BPL pregnant women under NMBS, was replaced by graded scale of assistance based on the categorization of States as well as whether beneficiary was from rural/urban area. States were classified into low performing states (LPS) and high performing states (HPS) on the basis of institutional delivery rate, i.e. states having institutional delivery 25% or less were termed as LPS and those which have institutional delivery rate more than 25% were classified as HPS. Accordingly, eight erstwhile EAG States namely Uttar Pradesh, Uttarakhand, Madhya Pradesh, Chhattisgarh, Bihar, Jharkhand, Rajasthan, Odisha and the States of Assam and Jammu and Kashmir were classified as Low Performing States. The remaining States were grouped into High Performing States.

GOALS

To reduce maternal and infant mortality through increasing institutional delivery
- Access to quality antenatal and postpartum health care the programme provides a continuum of care package that includes ANC, institutional delivery, postpartum care, and family planning coordinated by the ASHA.

VISION

- To promote institutional deliveries
- To reduce overall maternal mortality ratio and infant mortality rate.

BENEFICIARIES

- Pregnant women of all section of the society.
- No age bar.
- Irrespective of birth order.
- In rural and urban areas.

IMPORTANT FEATURES OF JANANI SURAKSHA YOJANA

- The scheme focuses on the poor pregnant woman with special dispensation for states having low institutional delivery rates namely the States of Uttar Pradesh, Uttaranchal, Bihar, Jharkhand, Madhya Pradesh, Chhattisgarh, Assam, Rajasthan, Odisha and Jammu and Kashmir. While these states have been named as Low Performing States (LPS), the remaining states have been named as High Performing States (HPS).
- **Tracking Each Pregnancy:** Each beneficiary registered under this yojana should have a JSY card along with a MCH card. ASHA/AWW/any other identified link worker under the overall supervision of the ANM and the MO, PHC should mandatorily prepare a micro-birth plan. This will effectively help in monitoring antenatal check-up, and the post-delivery care.
- **Eligibility for Cash Assistance:** BPL Certification—This is required in all HPS. However, where BPL cards have not yet been issued or have not been updated, States/UTs would formulate a simple criterion for certification of poor and needy status of the expectant mother's family by empowering the gram pradhan or ward member (Table 1).

Table 1: Cash assistance for institutional delivery (in ₹)

Category	Rural Area		Urban Area	
	Mother's package	ASHA's package*	Mother's package	ASHA's package**
LPS	1400	600	1000	400
HPS	700	600	600	400

* ASHA package of ₹600 in rural areas include ₹300 for ANC component and ₹300 for facilitating institutional delivery
**ASHA package of ₹400 in urban areas include ₹200 for ANC component and ₹200 for facilitating institutional delivery

- **Cash assistance for home delivery:** The BPL pregnant women, who prefer to deliver at home, are entitled to a cash assistance of ₹500 per delivery regardless of the age of pregnant women and number of children.
- **Direct benefit transfer under Janani Suraksha Yojana:** Direct benefit transfer (DBT) mode of payment has been rolled out in 43 districts with effect from January 1, 2013 and in 78 districts from July 1, 2013. Recently, instructions have been issued to all States/UTs regarding extension of DBT mode of payment throughout the country in all districts. Under this initiative, eligible pregnant women are entitled to get JSY benefit directly into their bank accounts.

JANANI SHISHU SURAKSHA KARYAKARAM (JSSK)

INTRODUCTION

In view of the difficulty being faced by the pregnant women and parents of sick newborn along-with high expenditure on delivery and treatment of sick-newborn, Ministry of Health and Family Welfare (MoHFW) has taken a major initiative to ensure better facilities for women and child health services. It is an initiative to provide completely free and cashless services to pregnant women including normal deliveries and cesarean operations and sick newborn (up to 30 days after birth) in Government Health Institutions in both rural and urban areas.

Government of India launched Janani Shishu Suraksha Karyakaram (JSSK) on June 1, 2011. The scheme is estimated to benefit more than 12 million pregnant women who access Government health facilities for their delivery. Moreover, it will motivate those who still choose to deliver at their homes to opt for institutional deliveries. It is an initiative with a hope that states would come forward and ensure that benefits under JSSK would reach every needy pregnant woman coming to government institutional facility. All the States and UTs have initiated implementation of the scheme.

The following are the free entitlements for pregnant women:

- Free and cashless delivery
- Free C-Section
- Free drugs and consumables
- Free diagnostics
- Free diet during stay in the health institutions
- Free provision of blood
- Exemption from user charges
- Free transport from home to health institutions
- Free transport between facilities in case of referral
- Free drop back from institutions to home after 48 hours stay.

The following are the free entitlements for sick newborns till 30 days after birth:

This has now been expanded to cover sick infants:

- Free treatment
- Free drugs and consumables
- Free diagnostics
- Free provision of blood
- Exemption from user charges
- Free transport from home to health institutions
- Free transport between facilities in case of referral
- Free drop back from institutions to home.

KEY FEATURES

- The initiative entitles all pregnant women delivering in public health institutions to absolutely free and no expense delivery, including cesarean section.
- The entitlements include free drugs and consumables, free diet up to 3 days during normal delivery and up to 7 days for C-section, free diagnostics, and free blood wherever required. This initiative also provides for free transport from home to institution, between facilities in case of a referral and drop back home. Similar entitlements have been put in place for all sick newborns accessing public health institutions for treatment till 30 days after birth. This has now been expanded to cover sick infants.
- The scheme aims to eliminate out of pocket expenses incurred by the pregnant women and sick newborne while accessing services at Government health facilities.
- The scheme is estimated to benefit more than 12 million pregnant women who access Government health facilities for their delivery. Moreover, it will motivate those who still choose to deliver at their homes to opt for institutional deliveries.
- All the States and UTs have initiated implementation of the scheme.

BENEFITS

Drugs and Consumables

Drugs and consumables including supplements such as iron folic acid shall be given free of cost to the pregnant women: During ANC, INC, PNC up to 6 weeks which includes management of normal delivery, C-section and any complications during the pregnancy and childbirth. The same is also to be provided when a neonate is sick and needs urgent and priority treatment.

Diagnostics

During pregnancy, childbirth and in postnatal period, investigations are essential for timely diagnosis of complications and likely problems which the women can face during the process of child birth. Both essential and desirable investigations shall be conducted free of cost for the pregnant women: During ANC, INC, PNC up to 6 weeks. Investigations required prior to both normal delivery and C-section. The same are also to be provided when a neonate is sick and needs urgent and priority treatment for conditions like infection, pneumonia, etc.

Diet

The first 48 hours after delivery are vital for detecting any complications and its immediate management. Care of the mother and baby (including immunization) are essential immediately after delivery and at least up to 48 hours. During this period, mother is guided for initiating breastfeeding and advised for extra calories, fluids and adequate rest which are needed for the well-being of the baby and herself. Non-availability of diet at the health facilities demotivates the delivered mothers from staying at the health facilities and most of the mothers prefer returning home immediately after delivery. This hampers adequate care of the pregnant women and neonates, which is important for quality PNC services. The diet shall be provided to the pregnant women as per following norms: Up to maximum of 3 days in case of normal delivery. Up to maximum of 7 days in case of C-section. Up to maximum of 5 days for the mother of sick newborn child. The unit cost of the diet should not exceed ₹100 per day.

Provision of Blood

Blood transfusion may be required to tackle emergencies and complication of deliveries such as management of severe anemia, PPH and C-sections, etc. The provision of blood will be free of any cost and without any user charges; however, the relatives and attendants accompanying the pregnant women shall be encouraged to donate blood for replacement.

Referral Transport

It is well proven that a significant number of maternal and neonatal deaths could be saved by providing timely referral transport facility to the pregnant women for normal delivery or C-section. This also needs to be provided to a neonate up to 30 days, when the baby is sick and needs urgent and priority treatment particularly for conditions like infection, pneumonia, etc. A drop back facility alleviates the pressure to leave the health facility earlier than desirable and obviates out of pocket expenses. The free referral transport entitlements for pregnant women and sick neonates up to 30 days and therefore are as under:
- Transport from home to the health facility.
- Referral to the higher facility in case of need (reasons for referral needs to be recorded).
- Drop back from the facility to home the referral transport between home to facility, drop back, refer to higher facility must be provided to pregnant woman/sick neonate. No cash to be paid to beneficiary. Ambulances will be utilized and in case of non-availability of Ambulance PPP mode/Hired vehicle can be used in case of dire emergencies.

Exemption from User Charges

User charges are levied in Government health institutions of the State for OPD, admissions, diagnostic tests, blood, etc. These add up to the out of pocket expenses.

IMPLEMENTATION OF THE NEW INITIATIVE

Action at State Level

- State Nodal Officer nominated for JSSK.
- Institute a grievance redressal mechanism for ensuring that the commitments are fulfilled in letter and spirit.
- Provide required finances and necessary administrative steps/GOs for the above activities.
- Regularly monitor and report on designated formats at specified periodicity.
- Review the implementation status during District CMOs meetings.

Action at District Level

The District Health Societies are required to take following actions:
- Deputy Chief Medical Officer (CMO) has been nominated as the District Nodal Officer.
- Widely publicize free entitlements in public domain.
- Institute a grievance redressal mechanism for ensuring that the commitments are fulfilled in letter and spirit and furnish copy of the grievance cell constituted to the State Health Society.
- Regularly review the stocks of drugs and consumables for ensuring availability at the public health institutions.

- Ensure lab facilities and diagnostic services are functional at all designated facilities, particularly at District Health (DH), Sub District Hospital (SDH), First Referral Units (FRU), Community Health Center (CHC) and 24 × 7 Primary Health Center System (PHCs).
- Prepare time bound action plans for establishing and operationalizing Blood Bank at District level and Blood Storage Centers at identified FRUs.
- Review referral linkages and their utilization by beneficiaries.
- Provide required finances/empowerment for utilization of funds to the Block MOs and facility in-charges for the above activities, particularly in emergency situations/stock outs.
- Regularly monitor and report on designated formats at specified periodicity.
- Review the implementation status during Block MOs/MOs meetings.

DISSEMINATION OF THE ENTITLEMENTS IN THE PUBLIC DOMAIN

- Widely publicize these entitlements through print and electronic media.
- Display them prominently on adequate size hoardings and boards, which are clearly visible from distance in all Government health facilities, e.g., SCs, PHCs, CHCs, SDHs and DHs/FRUs.
- IEC budget sanctioned in the Project Implementation Plan (PIP) under RCH/NRHM can be utilized for this.

Ensure Drugs and Consumable

- Notify the essential drug list for RCH services to be notified at all the service delivery points.
- Ensure regular procurement, uninterrupted supply and availability of drugs and consumables at all public health institutions.
- The daily availability of the drugs should be displayed at the health facility.
- Empower the head of the district/health facility to procure drugs and consumables to prevent stock outs.
- Ensure the quality and shelf life of drugs supplied.
- Ensure a proper inventory of drugs and consumables at each health facility for timely reporting on stock outs and expiry.
- In-charge pharmacist of the facility to ensure availability of drugs at dispensing points, i.e. labor room, OT, indoors, casualty, etc. after the routine hours.
- Ensure that first expiry drugs and consumables are used first. "FIRST in and FIRST out" protocol.
- Ensure proper storage of drugs and consumables by keeping drug stores clean and tidy with adequate ventilation and cooling.

Strengthen Diagnostics

- Ensure lab and diagnostic services at DH, SDH, FRU, CHC, and 24 × 7 PHCs.
- Ensure availability of basic routine investigations like pregnancy test, Hb and routine urine at sub-center level, particularly those designated as delivery points.
- Ensure rational posting of lab technicians for integrated and comprehensive utilization in the entire programme.
- Make emergency investigations available round-the-clock, at least at DH, SDH and FRU level.
- Ensure uninterrupted supply of reagents, consumables and other essentials required for lab investigations.
- Empower the head of the District/health facility to procure reagents, consumables and other essentials to prevent their shortage/stock out.

- In case in-house lab and diagnostic services are not available, free investigations can be provided through PPP/outsourcing.

Ensure Provision of Diet

- Ensure provision of diet (cooked food) at all delivery points from District Hospital up to 24 × 7 PHC.
- If proper kitchen and adequate manpower is not available, then this service can be outsourced.
- Local seasonal foods, vegetables, fruits, milk and eggs can be given to her for a proper nutritious diet.
- MO in-charge should monitor the quality of food being served at the health facility.
- Diet is to be provided up to three days for normal delivery and up to seven days stay for cesarean section (C-section) and up to maximum of 5 days for the mother of sick newborn child.
- The health facility should receive the funds in advance for ensuring provision of free diet for the pregnant women and the mothers who have delivered.

Ensure Availability of Blood in Case of Need

- Prepare time bound action plans for establishing and operationalizing blood bank at district level and blood storage centers at identified FRUs.
- Maintain adequate stocks for each blood group.
- Ensure availability of reagents and consumables for blood grouping, cross-matching and blood transfusion.
- Blood banks to ensure mandatory screening of blood before storage, and organize periodic voluntary blood donation camps for maintaining adequate number of blood units.
- Provide adequate funds to blood banks for electric backup and POL, and alternate source of power backup for blood bag refrigerators for blood storage units.
- Medical officer in-charge/lab technician of the blood bank to periodically visit blood storage units for monitoring and supervision.

Exemption from All Kinds of User Charges

- Government order issued for exemption from any user charges for pregnant women and sick newborns up to 30 days, at public health facilities.

Referral Transport

- Ensure universal reach of the referral transport (no area left uncovered), with 24 × 7 referral services.
- State is free to use any suitable model of transportation, e.g. government ambulances, EMRI, referral transport PPP model, etc.
- Establish linkages for the inaccessible areas (hilly terrain, flooded or tribal areas, etc.) to the road head/pick up points.
- Widely publicize the free and assured referral transport through print and electronic media.
- Monitor and supervise services at all levels, including utilization of each vehicle and number of cases transported.

Grievance Redressal

- Prominently display the names, addresses, emails, telephones, mobiles and fax numbers of grievance redressal authorities at health facility level, district level and state level, and disseminate them widely in the public domain (i.e., Chief Medical Officer, Deputy Chief Medical Officer, Medical Superintendent, Block Medical Officer).
- Set up help desks and suggestion/complaint boxes at government health facilities.

- Keep fixed hours (at least 1 hour) on any two working days per week in all the health facilities for meeting the complainants and redressing their grievances related to free entitlements.
- Take action on the grievances within a suitable timeframe, and communicate to the complainants.
- Maintain proper records of actions taken.
- The State Health Society should be kept informed of action taken with respect to all the above (on monthly basis).

MONITORING AND FOLLOW-UP

- At National level, the scheme will be monitored by National Health Systems Resource Center (NHSRC) under guidance and support from Maternal Health Division, Ministry of Health and Family Welfare, Government of India.
- At State level, the State Nodal Officer (JSSK) and District Monitors will follow-up the progress in implementation of the scheme. In CMOs meeting at State level, the Mission Director, NRHM/Director Health Services will review the progress of the scheme.
- At District level, the CMOs/District Nodal Officers (Dy. CMOs) will monitor and follow-up the progress with regard to implementation of the scheme at the facility level. During monthly meetings of in-charges of Health Institutions, CMO will review the progress of the scheme wherein the deputy CMOs will also be present to give their feedback/inputs.

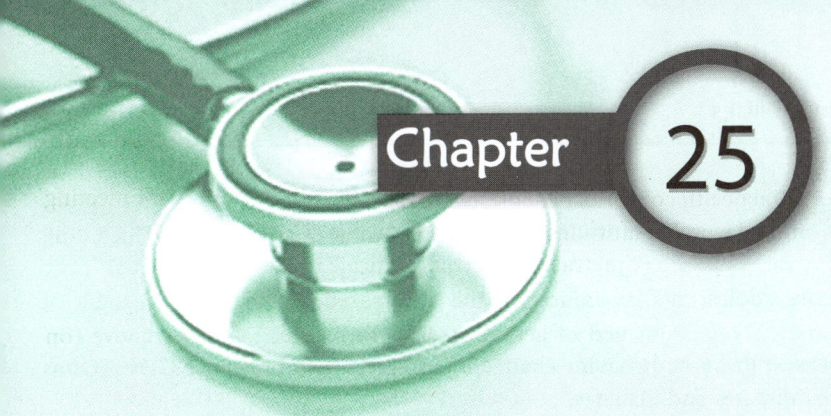

Chapter 25

Rashtriya Kishor Swasthya Karyakram

INTRODUCTION

The Ministry of Health and Family Welfare has launched a health programme for adolescents, the age group of 10–19 years, which would target their nutrition, reproductive health and substance abuse, among other issues.

The Rashtriya Kishor Swasthya Karyakram (RKSK) was launched on 7th January, 2014. The key principles of this programme are adolescent participation and leadership, equity and inclusion, gender equity and strategic partnerships with other sectors and stakeholders.

The programme envisions enabling all adolescents in India to realize their full potential by making informed and responsible decisions related to their health and well-being and by accessing the services and support they need to do so.

- **Purpose:** Guidance on preparation of the adolescent health (AH) related components of state and district NHM PIPs including budgets and reporting on progress/indicators.

To guide the implementation of this programme, MoHFW, in collaboration with UNFPA, has developed a National Adolescent Health Strategy. It realigns the existing clinic-based curative approach to focus on a more holistic model based on a continuum of care for adolescent health and developmental needs.

The RKSK (National Adolescent Health Programme) will comprehensively address the health needs of the 243 million adolescents. It introduces community-based interventions through peer educators, and is underpinned by collaborations with other ministries and state governments.

OBJECTIVES

Improve nutrition:
- Reduce the prevalence of malnutrition among adolescent girls and boys
- Reduce the prevalence of iron-deficiency anemia (IDA) among adolescent girls and boys.

Improve sexual and reproductive health:
- Improve knowledge, attitude and behavior, in relation to SRH
- Reduce teenage pregnancies
- Improve birth preparedness, complication readiness and provide early parenting support for adolescent parents.

Enhance mental health: Address mental health concerns of adolescents.

Prevent injuries and violence: Promote favorable attitudes for preventing injuries and violence (including GBV) among adolescents.

Prevent substance misuse: Increase adolescents' awareness of the adverse effects and consequences of substance misuse.

Address non-communicable diseases: Promote behavior change in adolescents to prevent NCDs such as hypertension, stroke, cardiovascular diseases and diabetes.

TARGET GROUPS

The new adolescent health (AH) strategy focuses on age groups 10–14 years and 15–19 years with universal coverage, i.e., males and females; urban and rural; in school and out of school; married and unmarried; and vulnerable and under-served.

STRATEGIES

Strategies/interventions to achieve objectives can be broadly grouped as:
- Community-based interventions.
- Peer Education (PE).
- Quarterly Adolescent Health Day (AHD).
- Weekly Iron and Folic Acid Supplementation Programme (WIFS).
- Menstrual Hygiene Scheme (MHS).

Facility-based Interventions

Strengthening of Adolescent Friendly Health Clinics (AFHC).

Convergence

- **Within health and family welfare:** FP, MH (including VHND), RBSK, NACP, National Tobacco Control Programme, National Mental Health Programme, NCDs and IEC.
- **With other departments/schemes:** WCD (ICDS, KSY, BSY, SABLA), HRD (AEP, MDM), Youth Affairs and Sports (Adolescent Empowerment Scheme, National Service Scheme, NYKS, NPYAD).

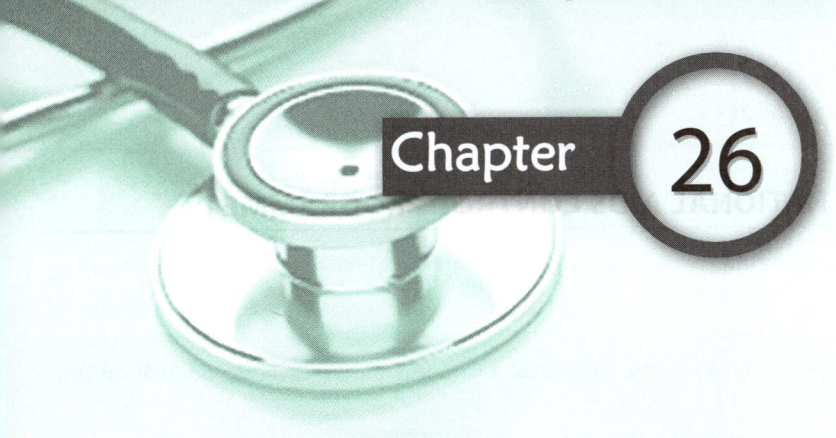

Chapter 26

National AIDS Control Programme

INTRODUCTION

India's AIDS Control Programme is globally acclaimed as a success story. The **National AIDS Control Programme (NACP)**, launched in 1992, is being implemented as a comprehensive programme for prevention and control of HIV/AIDS in India. Over time, the focus has shifted from raising awareness to behavior change, from a national response to a more decentralized response and to increasing involvement of NGOs and networks of PLHIV.

In 1992, the Government launched the first National AIDS Control Programme (NACP I) with an IDA Credit of USD 84 million and demonstrated its commitment to combat the disease. NACP I was implemented with an objective of slowing down the spread of HIV infections so as to reduce morbidity, mortality and impact of AIDS in the country. National AIDS Control Board (NACB) was constituted and an autonomous National AIDS Control Organization (NACO) was set up to implement the project. The first phase focused on awareness generation, setting up surveillance system for monitoring HIV epidemic, measures to ensure access to safe blood and preventive services for high risk group populations.

In November 1999, the second National AIDS Control Project (NACP II) was launched with World Bank credit support of USD 191 million. The policy and strategic shift was reflected in the two key objectives of NACP II: (i) to reduce the spread of HIV infection in India, and (ii) to increase India's capacity to respond to HIV/AIDS on a long-term basis. Key policy initiatives taken during NACP II included: adoption of National AIDS Prevention and Control Policy (2002); Scale up of Targeted Interventions for high risk groups in high prevalence states; Adoption of National Blood Policy; a strategy for greater involvement of people with HIV/AIDS (GIPA); launch of National Adolescent Education Programme (NAEP); introduction of counseling, testing and PPTCT programmes; launch of National Anti-Retroviral Treatment (ART) programme; formation of an inter-ministerial group for mainstreaming; and setting up of the National Council on AIDS, chaired by the Prime Minister; and setting up of State AIDS Control Societies in all States.

In response to the evolving epidemic, the third phase of the National Programme (NACP III) was launched in July 2007 with the goal of Halting and Reversing the Epidemic by the end of project period. NACP was a scientifically well-evolved programme, grounded on a strong structure of policies, programmes, schemes, operational guidelines, rules and norms. NACP-III aimed at halting and reversing the HIV epidemic in India over its five-year period by scaling up prevention efforts among high risk groups (HRG) and general population and integrating them with care, support and treatment services. Thus, prevention and care, support and treatment (CST) form the two key pillars of all the AIDS control efforts in India. Strategic information management and institutional strengthening activities provide the required technical, managerial and administrative support for implementing the core activities under NACP III at National, State and District levels.

KEY PRIORITIES UNDER NATIONAL AIDS CONTROL PROGRAMME IV

- Preventing new infections by sustaining the reach of current interventions and effectively addressing emerging epidemics.
- Prevention of parent to child transmission.
- Focusing on IEC strategies for behavior change in HRG, awareness among general population and demand generation for HIV services.
- Providing comprehensive care, support and treatment to eligible PLHIV.
- Reducing stigma and discrimination through greater involvement of PLHA (GIPA).
- Decentralizing rollout of services including technical support.
- Ensuring effective use of strategic information at all levels of programme.
- Building capacities of NGO and civil society partners especially in states with emerging epidemics.
- Integrating HIV services with health systems in a phased manner.
- Mainstreaming of HIV/AIDS activities with all key central/state level Ministries/departments will be given a high priority and resources of the respective departments will be leveraged. Social protection and insurance mechanisms for PLHIV will be strengthened.

NATIONAL AIDS CONTROL PROGRAMME IV COMPONENTS

Component 1

Intensifying and Consolidating Prevention Services with a Focus on HRG and Vulnerable Populations

This component will support the scaling up of Targeted interventions with the aim of reaching out to the hard-to-reach population groups who do not yet access and use the prevention services of the programme, and saturate coverage among the HRGs. In addition, this component will support the bridge population, i.e. migrants and truckers. Component 1 includes the following two subcomponents:

Scaling up Coverage of TIs among HRG

The interventions under this sub-component will include:
- The provision of behavior change interventions to increase safe practices, testing and counseling, and adherence to treatment, and demand for other services.
- The promotion and provision of condoms to HRG to promote their use in each sexual encounter.
- Provision or referral for STI services including counseling at service provision centers to increase compliance of patients with treatment, risk reduction counseling with focus on partner referral and management.
- Needle and syringe exchange for IDUs as well as scaling up of Opioid Substitution Therapy (OST) provision. This sub-component also includes the financing of operating costs for about 25 State Training Resource Centers as well as participant training costs over a period of 5 years.

Scaling up of Interventions among other Vulnerable Populations

The activities under this subcomponent will include:
- Risk assessment and size estimation of migrant population groups and truckers at transit points and at workplaces.

- Behavior change communications (BCC) for creating awareness about risk and vulnerability, prevention methods, availability and location of services, increase safe behavior and demand for services as well as reduce stigma.
- Promotion and provisioning of condoms through different channels including social marketing.
- Development of linkages with local institutions, both public and NGO owned, for testing, counseling and STI treatment services.
- Creation of "peer support groups" and "safe spaces" for migrants at destination.
- Establishment of need-based and gender-sensitive services for partners of IDUs.
- Strengthening networks of vulnerable populations with enhanced linkages to service centers and risk reduction interventions, specifically condom use.

Component 2

Expanding IEC Services

- General population, and
- High risk groups with a focus on behavior change and demand generation.

The IEC has been an important component of the NACP. With the expansion of services for counseling and testing, ART, STI treatment and condom promotion, the demand generation campaigns will continue to be the focus of the NACP-IV communication strategy. IEC will remain an important component of all prevention efforts and will include:

- Behavior change communication strategies for HRGs, vulnerable groups and hard-to-reach populations.
- Increasing awareness among general population, particularly women and youth.

Component 3

Comprehensive Care, Support and Treatment

The NACP IV will implement comprehensive HIV care for all those who are in need of such services and facilitate additional support systems for women and children affected and infected with HIV/AIDS. It is envisaged that greater adherence and compliance would be possible with wide network of treatment facilities and collaborative support from PLHIV and civil society groups. Additional Centers of Excellence (CoEs) and upgraded ART Plus centers will be established to provide high-quality treatment and follow-up services, positive prevention and better linkages with health care providers in the periphery.

With increasing maturity of the epidemic, it is very likely that there will be greater demand for second-line ART, OI management. NACP IV will address these needs adequately. It is proposed that the comprehensive care, support and treatment of HIV/AIDS will inter alia include:

- Anti-retroviral treatment (ART) including second line.
- Management of opportunistic infections, and
- Facilitating social protection through linkages with concerned departments/ministries. The programme will explore avenues of public-private partnerships. The programme will enhance activities to reduce stigma and discrimination at all levels particularly at health care settings.

Component 4

Strengthening Institutional Capacities

The objective of NACP IV will be to consolidate the trend of reversal of the epidemic seen at the national level to all the key districts in India. Programme, planning, and management responsibilities will be strengthened at state and district levels to ensure high quality, timely and effective implementation of field level activities and desired programmatic outcomes.

The planning processes and systems will be further strengthened to ensure that the annual action plans are based on evidence, local priorities and in alignment with NACP IV objectives. Sustaining the epidemic response through increased collaboration and convergence, where feasible, with other departments will be given a high priority during NACP IV. This will involve phased integration of the HIV services with the routine public sector health delivery systems, streamlining the supply chain mechanisms and quality control mechanisms and building capacities of governmental and non-governmental institutions and networks.

Component 5

Strategic Information Management Systems (SIMS)

The roll-out of SIMS is ongoing and will be firmly established at all levels to support evidence-based planning, programme monitoring and measuring of programmatic impacts. The surveillance system will be further strengthened with focus on tracking the epidemic, incidence analysis, identifying pockets of infection and estimating the burden of infection. Research priorities will also be customized to the emerging needs of the programme. NACP IV will also document, manage and disseminate evidence and effective utilization of programmatic and research data. The relevant, measurable and verifiable indicators will be identified and used appropriately.

SERVICES FOR PREVENTION AT DIFFERENT LEVELS

Core Services at District Level

In packaging of services, care is taken for the special needs of the region and availability of complementary health care system. In high prevalence districts, the full spectrum of preventive, supportive and curative services are available in medical colleges or district hospitals. These hospitals provide HIV/AIDS prevention services including treatment and cure for sexually transmitted infections, psycho-social counseling and support for people infected or affected by HIV, management of opportunistic infections and anti-retroviral therapy for people living with HIV/AIDS, counseling and testing facility for prevention of parent to child transmission of HIV infection, specialized pediatric HIV care and treatment as well as referral for specialist needs such as surgery, ENT and ophthalmology, etc.

Community Health Centers Give Basic Services

Community health centers (CHCs) and primary health centers are integrated in the programme and facilitate prevention through promotion of condoms, counseling and testing for HIV (ICT centers), prevention of parent to child transmission (PPTCT), treatment and cure for sexually transmitted diseases and management of opportunistic infections.

CBOs for Better Service Outreach

Hospitals providing HIV services are linked to NGOs/CBOs which play a significant role in providing peer support services and home-based care for people living with HIV/AIDS. CBOs also facilitate follow-up with children born to HIV-positive women, support at the community level and outreach to services at the district level.

PREVENTIVE SERVICES

Awareness Raising

The HIV infection is entirely preventable through awareness raising. Therefore, awareness raising about its occurrence and spread is very significant in protecting the people from the epidemic. It is for this reason that the National AIDS Control Programme lays maximum emphasis on the widespread reach of information, education and communication on HIV/AIDS prevention. Changing knowledge, attitude and behavior as a prevention strategy of HIV/AIDS thus is a key thrust area of the National AIDS Control Programme.

Addressing the Vulnerable

Awareness raising brings behavior change. Through this route the programme promotes prevention, and aims to reach out to 80% of the high risk groups and 95% of the young people. In fact, the awareness campaign of NACP has received a big boost with the formation of National Council on AIDS that has mainstreamed HIV prevention activities in various government institutions and programmes.

The programme focuses on saturating an estimated four million high risk groups (commercial sex workers, injecting drug users, men-who-have-sex-with-men), twelve million highly vulnerable population—migrants and truckers, and a large number of young women and men in the general community, who constitute almost 40% of the country's population, with information on various aspects of vulnerability to HIV infection.

MANAGEMENT OF STI/RTI

Sexually transmitted diseases are one of the determinants of HIV transmission. An estimated 5% adult population affected by STDs, also has HIV infection. HIV vulnerability from STDs is furthermore increased as access to treatment or medical care for these diseases is very low, especially among the high risk groups. Limited diagnostic facilities to manage complicated STDs and drug resistance to major STDs are the other issues of concern that NACP III addresses.

Making STD Services Common

Under NACP III, a demand for STD services is generated through its awareness on one hand and on the other STD services are expanded through its integration with the reproductive and child health programme. The programme supports increased demand for the services through capacity building among the medical practitioners of primary health care centers and community health care centers, and the private regional medical practitioners providing STD services. The programme also supports not-for-profit private practitioners and NGOs in the management of STDs among the high risk groups.

Checking Drug Resistance and Improving Surveillance

Apart from expanding the network providing STD services, NACP III plans routine screening of HRGs for drug resistance to certain STDs. Regional centers are planned to be set up for this during the programme period to monitor drug resistance in syndromic oral/anal STDs, and develop guidelines for their treatment.

Integrated Counseling and Testing Center

The HIV counseling and testing services were started in India in 1997. As on 31st August 2016 in India, there were 20,756 integrated counseling and testing centers (ICTC), mainly located in government hospitals. An ICTC is a place where a person is counseled and tested for HIV, of his own free will or as advised by a medical provider. The main functions of an ICTC are:

- Conducting HIV diagnostic tests.

- Providing basic information on the modes of HIV transmission, and promoting behavioral change to reduce vulnerability.
- Link people with other HIV prevention, care and treatment services.

Ideally, a health facility should have one ICTC for all groups of people. However, an ICTC is located in facilities that serve specific categories such as high risk group, pregnant women, STI cases, TB patients, HIV/AIDS symptomatic patients. Accordingly, an ICTC is located in the general OPD or obstetrics and gynecology department of a medical college or a district hospital or in a maternity home where the majority of clients can access counseling and testing services.

The HIV counseling and testing service is a key entry point to prevention of HIV infection and to treatment and care of people who are infected with HIV. When availing counseling and testing services, people can access accurate information about HIV prevention and care and undergo HIV test in a supportive and confidential environment. People who are found HIV negative are supported with information and counseling to reduce risks and remain HIV negative. People who are found HIV positive are provided psycho-social support and linked to treatment and care.

Prevention of Parent to Child Transmission

The Prevention of Parent to Child Transmission (PPTCT) of HIV/AIDS programme was launched in the country in the year 2002 following a feasibility study in 11 major hospitals in the five high HIV prevalence states. As on August 31, 2016 in India there are 20,756 ICTC, most of these in government hospitals, which offer PPTCT services to pregnant women.

The HIV exposed baby is initiated on Cotrimoxazole prophylaxis at 6 weeks and is tested for HIV DNA PCR at 6 weeks by dry blood spot (DB) collection. If the DBS sample is positive for HIV DNA PCR, then a repeat DBS sample is tested for HIV DNA PCR. The HIV exposed baby is then initiated on lifelong ART at the earliest if confirmed HIV positive through 2 DNA PCR test.

The PPTCT services cover about 47% annual estimated pregnancies in the country. In the year 2015–16, 12.7 million pregnant women accessed this service. Of these, 11,918 pregnant women were HIV positive. In order to provide universal access to these services, further scale up is planned up to the level of Community Health Center and the Primary Health Center through NHM integration, as well as private sector by forging public-private partnerships.

Post-exposure Prophylaxis (PEP)

Occupational Exposure

Occupational exposure refers to exposure to potential blood-borne infections (HIV, HBV and HCV) that may occur in health care settings during performance of job duties. Post-exposure prophylaxis (PEP) refers to comprehensive medical management to minimize the risk of infection among health care personnel (HCP) following potential exposure to blood-borne pathogens (HIV, HBV, HCV). This includes counseling, risk assessment, relevant laboratory investigations based on informed consent of the source and exposed person, first aid and depending on the risk assessment, the provision of short term (four weeks) of antiretroviral drugs, with follow-up and support.

Condom Promotion Programme

Consistent condom use has been one of the most critical aspects of NACO's prevention strategy for HIV/AIDS control. To this effect, NACO started its condom promotion programme under National AIDS Control Programme (NACP) phase III and continued expanding in Phase IV also. The specific condom promotion objectives are:

- Increase demand for condoms among high risk, bridge and general population.
- Expanding social marketing programme to saturate coverage in high HIV prevalence and/or high fertility districts and to increase.
- The demand for condoms among high risk, bridge and general population.
- Maximize access of free condoms with most vulnerable groups—while minimizing wastage.
- Increase sales in rural areas and expand availability through condom sales through non-traditional outlets (stores not previously). Selling/that do not usually sell condoms.
- Introduce brand management innovations and demand generation activities to promote consistent condom use.
- Increase the accessibility of condoms to make it available within 15 minutes of walking distance from any location.

Access to Safe Blood

Access to safe blood is mandated by law, and is the primary responsibility of NACO. The specific objective of the blood safety programme is to ensure reduction in the transfusion associated with HIV transmission to 0.5%, while making available safe and quality blood within one hour of requirement in a health facility.

However, there is a serious mismatch between demand and availability of blood in the country: against 8.5 million units/year requirement, the availability is only 4.4 million units/year. Another concern is that voluntary blood donation is only 52%. NACO is committed to bridge the gap in the availability and improve quality of blood under NACP III. To achieve these objectives, NACO plans to:

- Raise voluntary blood donation to 90%.
- Establish blood storage centers in community health centers.
- Expand external quality assessment services for blood screening.
- Quality management in blood transfusion services.
- Sensitize clinicians on optimum use of blood, blood components and products.
- Add 39 blood banks in districts that do not have blood transfusion facility.
- Establish blood storage centers in 3222 community care centers.
- Provide refrigerated vans in 500 districts for networking with blood storage centers.
- Establish additional model blood banks in 22 states; 10 are functional already.
- Set up additional blood component separation units (BCSU) in 80 tertiary care hospitals and separate at least 50% of the collection at all BCSUs (162) into components.
- Promote autologous blood donation.
- Liaise with Indian Red Cross Society and Ministry of Youth Affairs and Sports to promote voluntary blood donation among the youth.
- Set up 32 model blood banks in various states.
- Liaise with the Indian Medical Council (IMC) to mandate the requirement of a department of transfusion medicine in all medical colleges and appropriate transfusion practices in the syllabus of MD/MS clinical subjects.
- Establish one additional plasma fractionation facility in the country.
- Establish four centers of excellence in blood transfusion services in the four metros in order to cater to any region of the country at the time of a crisis.
- Introduce accreditation of blood banks.

The activities and functioning of a large network of blood banks and blood component separation facilities in the country are supervised at district, state and national level.

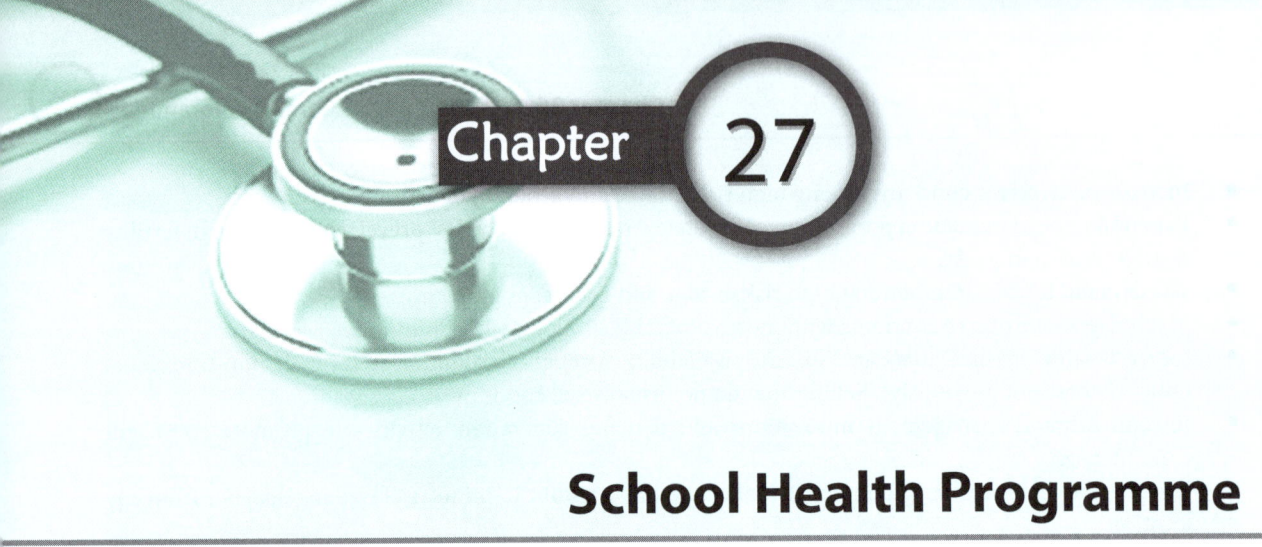

Chapter 27

School Health Programme

INTRODUCTION

National Rural Health Mission (NRHM) has taken cognizance of the potential impact of the school health programme on the health of the students, their families and the generations to come and brought this initiative to forefront within the context of the Reproductive and Child Health (RCH) Programme.

Providing easy access to health, nutrition and hygiene, education and services to children in schools is a simple and a cost effective tool which can go a long way in the prevention and control of communicable and non-communicable diseases. It also enables revitalization of local health traditions and the mainstreaming of AYUSH and promotion of healthy lifestyles in the health curriculum programme in schools.

As NRHM promotes flexibility in the states, under the school health programme, the states have been given an option to implement the programme comprehensively. According to the needs of the children, institutional capacity and available service delivery options, 26 States have provisioned for the School Health Programme in their programme implementation plans. It is expected that all the states that have taken up this challenge and introduced a school health programme from the year 2008 will continue with this initiative, expanding it as per the need so that ultimately it has a universal coverage. It is also expected that the other states will start providing school health services in the near future. It is envisaged that all schools, both rural and urban, will be covered under various aspects of the school health programme in all parts of the country.

OBJECTIVES

The main objectives of this service is the prevention of illness as well as the promotion of health and well-being of the students through:
- Early detection and care of students with health problems.
- Development of healthy attitudes and healthy behaviors by students.
- Ensure a healthy environment for children at school.
- Prevention of communicable diseases at school.

ESSENTIAL ELEMENTS

Essential elements of school health are:
- **Health-related school policies** that include children of all communities, encourage healthy lifestyles, address priority public health problems and promote collaboration among teachers. It also enables students and their parents on one side and departments like health, education, women and child development on the other side to bring about convergence.

- **Provision of safe (physically and psychosocially) and supportive environment** to ensure healthy development of students and provide a healthy learning environment. Provision of nutrition relieves the hunger of the child coming from deprived circumstances and provision of safe water and adequate sanitation reinforces hygienic behavior. It is especially important to provide privacy (functional women toilets and support for menstrual management) and safety to promote participation of adolescent girls in education. Keeping the school free of violence and various forms of discrimination is also an important dimension.
- **Health, hygiene and nutrition education** that focuses upon the development of age appropriate knowledge, attitudes, values and life skills needed to establish lifelong healthy practices. Additionally, the school environment must provide opportunities to practice the acquired healthy behavior in order to reduce the vulnerability of youth and teachers to common health risks. For example, midday, meal programmes cooked and served hygienically, sanitary toilets/latrines with running water, soap and water for handwashing, adequate supply of potable water, provision of sanitary napkins for girls and kitchen garden to demonstrate feasibility of growing healthy food.
- **School-based health and nutrition services** that are equitable, simple, sustainable, safe and familiar and address problems that are prevalent and recognized as important within the community, e.g., Midday meal scheme, midday school meals.

Operational Framework

School age population is extremely vulnerable to health risks and illness. Illnesses and behavior formed during this period can have a detrimental effect on health during the adult years of an individual's life.

Services

Health Screening and Referral Linkage with Health Services for Remedial and Preventive Measures

Screening helps in early detection and the timely institution of treatment for the most-common causes of morbidity.

Ophthalmic and dental conditions, skin lesions and nutritional problems in particular are conditions where early identification can affect cure and prevent further progress and complications. By attending to some health determinants like anemia and malnutrition, it could play a preventive role in addressing these critical problems.

It also helps identify children with refractive errors and hearing deficits, which are a major source of learning difficulties and by arranging to correct them, can dramatically improve school performance. Identification and support to children with disabilities is another major role that screening can play.

It is, therefore, recommended to carry out health checkups of all students at least once in a year, but preferably twice a year. Much of the success of school health screening programmes lies in constructing effective post screening referral arrangements. This is needed to ensure that the roughly 1% of children who are identified during the screening process as having serious but correctable ailments receive the higher level of clinical care that they need.

Health Education

This ensures the provision of age appropriate information on health, hygiene and nutrition, and to put it simply, education about the physical and mental aspects of growing up. It has great potential on promotion of healthy development and preventing risk behavior. There are four broad activity groups that constitute school health education.

1. **Promote health and hygiene practices within schools:** Understanding of health issues in the formal curriculum. The second is the construct of a series of informal sessions for students on specific necessary health issues which are not part of the formal learning system. This form of communication inculcates interest and enhances retention. It is effective for issues which require interpersonal dialogue, like life skills, education and menstrual hygiene or for issues which require demonstrations, for instance, first aid education.

   The third is the use of the school for behavior change and communication to disseminate health information and mold health related behaviors through extracurricular activities like poster making, plays, competitions, quiz contests. Finally, it is also the health and hygiene related practices that the school consciously inculcates in its students; for example, the use of toilets, handwashing before meals, the disposal of waste and the cleanliness of class-rooms and school campus.

2. **Addressing nutritional issues, particularly anemia and malnutrition:** Health department can assist in providing specific interventions in the school setting for the priority areas or micro- and macronutrients deficiency. This includes identification and correction of anemia, periodic treatment for worm infestation, the promotion of use of iodized salt, organizing talks on relevant nutrition issues and a linkage with the school midday meal programme to ensure that this acts as the critical supplement to correct macro-nutritional deficiency, rather than being a substitute for food intake at home. School health programme offers a unique opportunity to reach students and through them, their families at home. The nutrition counseling given herein has the potential to last through to the next generation as these students are the parents of tomorrow.

3. **Providing safe and supportive environment in schools:** It is a given pre-requisite that schools need to provide the basic amenities like potable drinking water, separate sanitary toilets for boys and girls and clean classrooms.

   It is also necessary that schools strive to ensure safety of their students and staff from physical injuries, stress, corporal punishment and abuse. The school environment needs to be supportive of its teachers and students and also to be sensitive and alert to manifest signs and symptoms of these conditions and provide the opportunity to seek appropriate help in effective and confidential management.

4. **Service provision:** Services for minor ailments like headache, fever, cuts can be provided by the trained teachers while all other services can be offered through health care providers. **Following activities need to be ensured to provide these services.**

   - **Capacity Building:** This is needed to ensure that both school teachers as well as the health staff and their supervisors comprehend the school health programme and are equipped with the knowledge, skills and system support needed to implement this programme optimally.

     As teachers are required to participate actively, nodal teachers need to be identified by principal or headmistress and their training is planned and organized. Each school has to have at least one designated nodal teacher for the school health programme and in large schools there has to be one nodal teacher per 250 students, with a school level coordinator. Based on these norms, the number of teachers from each school who act as nodal officers are identified. Ongoing refresher training of those trained before is essential as also is the continuous enrolment and training of new teachers to ensure adequate replacement of those staff members who are transferred or retire in their service tenure.

- **Monitoring and Evaluation:** It is essential that the school health programme put in place is implemented with the requisite quality and scale needed to reach all students and make a significant impact. This system would not only measure the functioning of the programme but is an essential tool for further fine tuning and improvement. For monitoring and evaluation to become operational, a system needs to be developed and incorporated in the routine health monitoring system.
- **Core Management Group:** A core management group responsible for overseeing the implementation of school health programme needs to be constituted at state, district, block and village levels with representatives from various departments and stakeholders like:
  - ❖ Department of health, including the AIDS control division.
  - ❖ Department of education.
  - ❖ Department of women and child development (WCD).
  - ❖ Principal and teachers.
  - ❖ Parents' representative.
  - ❖ Students' representative.

At the state and district levels, overall oversight may be provided by the NRHM Mission Director/District Magistrate/local body and at the village level by Village Health and Sanitation Committee.

COMPONENTS OF THE SCHOOL HEALTH PROGRAMME

Health Screening and Remedial Measures

The students would be screened at least annually by medical and paramedical personnel assisted by school teachers trained for this purpose. Ideally screening should be done twice a year. Since the number of students to be screened is massive the critical limitation is the availability of skilled human resource for this task.

Health Conditions to be Screened

Under this programme, all students would be screened for a minimum set of pre-defined conditions, which would include:

- **General health and personal hygiene:** Weight and height recording would be done with computation of BMI and identification of underweight or overweight children. Such children need to be managed by counseling along with their caregivers. In the underweight child, support is needed to ensure that adequate food is being accessed and medical examination rules out secondary causes of malnutrition.
- **Clinical/laboratory assessment of anemia:** Over 70% of children could be anemic. In case of children with anemia of mild and moderate severity, we also need to note response to treatment and those who fail to respond should be referred since they need to be explored for non-dietary causes of anemia. Most cases, however, are due to dietary gaps and worm infestation and could be treated in the school setting itself. Case of severe anemia must be urgently referred to hospital.
- **Eye examination:**
  - Eyes should be checked for refractory errors, night blindness, trachoma, conjunctivitis.
  - Refractory errors are a major treatable cause of learning problems.
- **Ear discharge and hearing problems:** Repeated ear discharge can lead to deafness. Many times deafness remains unnoticed but contributes to poor scholastic performance. Screening proformas designed under the national programme would be used for those students who have any such suspicion during health screening.

- **Common dental conditions:** Dental caries and periodontal disease are common ailments and detected early, further progression can be prevented.
- **Common skin diseases and infestations:** Scabies, pyoderma and lice are some of the most common diseases. These are contagious and simultaneous treatment of all those affected is the easiest and the surest way to cut down the spread.
- **Heart defects—rheumatic and congenital:** There have been successful incidences where these have been detected and managed appropriately through school health programmes in our country.
- **Disabilities: Visual, hearing, locomotor, others:** Children with disabilities have special needs to be able to keep up with the class. Equipment, as well as support and guidance could help them. It is crucial for school health programmes to detect these as well as to create awareness about the special needs of people with disabilities.

Learning Disorders/Problem Behaviors/Stress/Anxiety

Teachers need to be sensitized to identify children with such problems at an early stage and send them to appropriate referral centers. These conditions may not be detected during health screening, but a trained teacher would notice it during the regular course of school.

Planning the Screening and the Referral

A school-wise schedule of visits of the health personnel needs to be drawn up and communicated to the school authorities, students, parents and local government well in advance so that all preparations can be made. The students would be examined, screened and treated/referred/counseled as necessary on the prescribed dates.

A resource manual would be prepared and distributed to all the providers (health staff and teachers) so that they are aware of the interventions, methodology and responsibilities. After screening, the students found to be suffering from any disease/abnormality would be referred to the designated health facilities for each type of illness. A list of such referral facilities would be drawn up. The list will include adolescent's health clinics that may have been established in nearby health facilities under RCH-II ARSH strategy. The minimum that states would need to do is to provide referral slips to the students with information to them and their parents as to which center to go to and when.

Planning for Remedial Action at the School Itself

There is also considerable remedial action that would be taken at the school level itself. Appropriate first-line treatment for small cuts and injuries and certain common illnesses like skin ailments, which would otherwise become septic. For this a first aid kit should be put in place. This is useful irrespective of screening.

Immunization with DT at 6 years and with tetanus toxoid at 10 and 16 years is also another action but this would need the nurse and could be combined with the health screening.

Documentation and Health Records

Teachers would maintain the health record of each student in the school on a child health card and a school health register that ensures that each child who has been screened gets the follow-up required.

It is also valuable for every school after the screening to provide information of common illnesses detected. The very presentation of this record indicates the seriousness with which the screening was carried out. It also tells us what was screened for and what was not. Tamil Nadu is one State that regularly compiles such statistics and it is an example that is worth emulating.

Equipment and Supplies for Health Screening

Health department would provide the equipment and supplies required for health screening. This would include a functional weighing scale and height measurement equipment (Stadiometer or a wall mounted one). Health department would also provide a Snellen's Chart for testing visual acuity. For smaller schools, health team would carry these equipment during the screening visits to schools. For bigger schools, the health department could supply these equipment to schools who would ensure safe keeping of the equipment.

Health department would supply first-aid kits containing common medicines like paracetamol for mild pain, headache, fever and Dysmenorrhea, ORS packets for diarrhea; dressing material and antiseptic solution and antibiotic cream for managing minor wounds.

School health register is a record kept by the school on the results of the screening and helps in organizing the follow-up.

Transport for Screening and Referrals

Adequate provision for funds would be ensured to provide appropriate transport (including provision for hiring vehicle, if necessary) to health staff to visit the schools and more important, to take children for referrals.

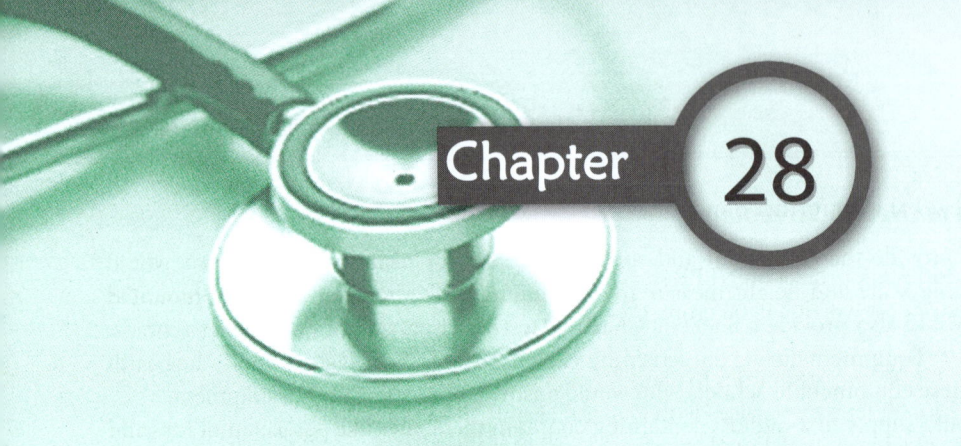

Chapter 28

National Leprosy Eradication Programme

INTRODUCTION

The National Leprosy Control Programme (NLCP) was launched by the Government of India in 1955. Multidrug Therapy (MDT) came into wide use from 1982 and the National Leprosy Eradication Programme (NLEP) was introduced in 1983.

Since then, remarkable progress has been achieved in reducing the disease burden.

The NLEP is 100% centrally sponsored scheme. MDT is supplied free of cost by WHO.

It was only in 1970s that a definite cure was identified in the form of MDT. The MDT came into wide use from 1982, following the recommendation by the WHO Study Group, Geneva in October 1981. Government of India (GoI) established a high power committee under chairmanship of Dr. MS Swaminathan in 1981 for dealing with the problem of leprosy. Based on its recommendations the NLEP was launched in 1983 with the objective to arrest the disease activity in all the known cases of leprosy. However, coverage remained limited due to a range of organizational issues and fear of the disease and the associated stigma. Districts were covered in a phased manner and all the districts in the country could be covered only by the year 1996. At this stage in view of substantial progress achieved with MDT, in 1991, the World Health Assembly resolved to eliminate leprosy at a global level by the year 2000. In order to strengthen the process of elimination in the country, the first World Bank supported project was introduced in 1993.

MILESTONES IN NATIONAL LEPROSY CONTROL PROGRAMME

- 1955 - National Leprosy Control Programme (NLCP) launched
- 1983 - National Leprosy Eradication Programme launched
- 1983 - Introduction of Multidrug Therapy (MDT) in Phases
- 2005 - Elimination of Leprosy at National Level
- 2012 - Special action plan for 209 high endemic districts in 16 States/UTs

PHASES OF NLCP

- The first phase of the World Bank supported project started from 1993–94 where the project supported the vertical programme structure formulated by GoI for the high endemic districts, while in the moderate and low endemic districts, Mobile Leprosy Treatment Units (MLTU) were established. The project was completed on 31 March 2020 with further 6 months, extension to complete the preparation of proposal for second phase project.

- The second phase of World Bank project on NLEP started for a period of 3 years from 2000–02, WHO to provide MDT drugs free of cost worth ₹48.00 crore.

  Objectives of second phase

  - Decentralization of NLEP responsibilities to States/UTs through State/District Leprosy Societies.
  - Accomplish integration of leprosy services with General Health Care System (GHS) and
  - Achieve elimination of leprosy at National level by the end of the project.

This second phase of NLEP also aimed to detect 11.0 lakh new leprosy cases and cure 11.5 lakh leprosy cases with MDT while reducing the disability rate to 2% among new leprosy cases. Well-planned activities were efficiently implemented in close association of various NLEP partners viz. State and UTs Governments, World Bank, WHO, ILEP, DANLEP, NGOs and Community, Pvt. Medical Practitioners and various concerned Government Ministries/Departments such as Information and Broadcasting, Social Justice and Empowerment, Education, Railways, Defense/paramilitary, Labor and Industries, etc. The second National Leprosy Elimination Project successfully ended on 31 December 2004.

The National Leprosy Eradication Programme is being continued with GoI funds from January 2005 onwards. Additional support for the programme is continued to be received from the WHO and ILEP organizations. MDT is to be supplied free of cost as of now by NOVARTIS through WHO.

In the year 2001, after the global elimination was achieved, a target was reset for the remaining 14 countries to achieve elimination on national basis by December, 2005. India was one of these countries.

The National Health Policy, GoI sets the goal of elimination of leprosy, i.e. to reduce the number of cases to <1/10,000 population by the year 2005.

The National Leprosy Eradication Programme took up the challenge with the active support of the State/UT Governments and dedicated partners in the World Health Organization, the International Federation of Anti Leprosy Associations (ILEP), the Sasakawa Memorial Health Foundation and the Nippon Foundation, NOVARTIS, DANLEP (1986–2003) and the World Bank (1993–2004).

As a result of the hard work and meticulously planned and executed activities, the country achieved the goal of elimination of leprosy as a public health problem, defined as less than 1 case per 10,000 population, at the National Level in the month of December, 2005. As on December 31, 2005, Prevalence Rate recorded in the country was 0.95/10,000 population.

Following are the programme components:

- Decentralized integrated leprosy services through General Health Care System.
- Training in leprosy to all General Health Services functionaries.
- Intensified Information, Education and Communication (IEC).
- Renewed emphasis on Prevention of Disability and Medical Rehabilitation and
- Monitoring and supervision.

STRATEGY

Leprosy Elimination in India

- Decentralized integrated leprosy services through general health care system.
- Early detection and complete treatment of new leprosy cases.
- Carrying out house hold contact survey in detection of multibacillary (MB) and child cases.

Contd…

- Early diagnosis and prompt MDT, through routine and special efforts.
- Involvement of Accredited Social Health Activists (ASHAs) in the detection and complete treatment of leprosy cases for leprosy work.
- Strengthening of Disability Prevention and Medical Rehabilitation (DPMR) services.
- Information, Education and Communication (IEC) activities in the community to improve self-reporting to primary health center (PHC) and reduction of stigma.
- Intensive monitoring and supervision at Primary Health Center/Community Health Center.

Results (Objectives) achieved during 12th plan period, i.e., 2012–2017 were as follows:

- Improved early case detection.
- Improved case management.
- Stigma reduced.
- Development of leprosy expertise sustained.
- Research supported evidence based programme practices.
- Monitoring supervision and evaluation system improved.
- Increased participation of persons affected by leprosy in society.
- Programme management ensured.

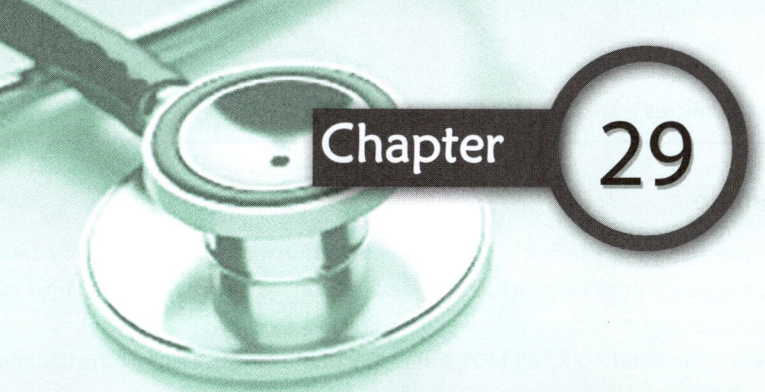

Chapter 29

National Programme for Prevention and Control of Deafness

INTRODUCTION

Hearing loss is the most common sensory deficit in humans today. As per WHO estimates in India, there are approximately 63 million people, who are suffering from significant auditory impairment; this places the estimated prevalence at 6.3% in Indian population.

As per National Sample Survey Office (NSSO) survey, currently there are 291 persons per one lakh population who are suffering from severe to profound hearing loss (NSSO, 2001). Of these, a large percentage is of children between the ages of 0–14 years. With such a large number of hearing impaired young Indians, it amounts to a severe loss of productivity, both physical and economic. An even larger percentage of our population suffers from milder degrees of hearing loss and unilateral (one-sided) hearing loss.

OBJECTIVES

- To prevent the avoidable hearing loss on account of disease or injury.
- Early identification, diagnosis and treatment of ear problems responsible for hearing loss and deafness.
- To medically rehabilitate persons of all age groups, suffering with deafness.
- To strengthen the existing intersectoral linkages for continuity of the rehabilitation programme, for persons with deafness.
- To develop institutional capacity for ear care services by providing support for equipment and material and training personnel.

Long-term objective: To prevent and control major causes of hearing impairment and deafness, so as to reduce the total disease burden by 25% of the existing burden by the end of 12th Five-Year Plan.

STRATEGIES

- To strengthen the service delivery including rehabilitation.
- To develop human resource for ear care.
- To promote outreach activities and public awareness through appropriate and effective IEC strategies with special emphasis on prevention of deafness.
- To develop institutional capacity of the district hospitals, community health centers and primary health centers, selected under the project.

Components of the Programme

- **Manpower training and development:** For prevention, early identification and management of hearing impaired and deafness cases, training would be provided by medical college level specialists (ENT and Audiology) to grassroot level workers.
- **Capacity building:** For the district hospital, CHC and PHC in respect of ENT/Audiology infrastructure.
- **Service provision including rehabilitation:** Screening camps for early detection of hearing impairment and deafness, management of hearing and speech impaired cases and rehabilitation (including provision of hearing aids), at different levels of health care delivery system.
- **Awareness generation through IEC/BCC activities:** For early identification of hearing impaired, especially children so that timely management of such cases is possible aid to remove the stigma attached to deafness.

Service Components

Early Detection

The detection would be by sensitized personnel at grassroot level including family members/parents, selected school teachers, MPWs at subcenter level, public health nurses and medical officers in PHCs and CHCs and district level personnel. Personnel at all levels would be assigned a specific task in order to ensure that the right guidance is provided at the appropriate time to the affected persons. House to house surveys will be conducted by the AWWs and ASHAs, under the supervision of the male and female MPWs for detection of cases of hearing impairment and deafness. The deafness cases will be noted in the disability column of ANM's village register. The MPWs will maintain records of each family based on a family proforma provided to them. The district level pediatricians and gynecologists will be responsible for referring any child born of a high risk pregnancy or delivery, as well as other children who are exposed to a high risk factor in infancy and who show features suggestive of hearing impairment. These children will be screened by the district level ENT doctor/ Audiologist with OAE and then subjected to diagnostic tests. School teachers will undertake to screen the children in the school with the help of pre-prepared proformas. These will help to identify children with any ear or hearing problem. They will then be referred to the school health doctor for evaluation, diagnosis and guidance regarding treatment.

Ear Screening Camps

Functions
- Screening camps will be organized in collaboration with NRHM (RBSK)/ M/o SJ and E at the PHC/CHC and district level for screening the general population in respect of ear problems, hearing impairment and deafness.
- Detection and treatment of common ear problems.
- Spreading awareness regarding ear problems, early detection of deafness, available treatment and health care facilities for referral of such cases.
- Education of community, especially the parents of young children regarding importance of right feeding practices, various common ear problems, early detection of deafness in young children and available treatment for hearing impairment/deafness.
- Education of *panchayat* members, members of *mahila mandals* and *youth leaders.*

Conducting Camps

Ear screening camps will be conducted by the PHC/CHC doctors and district level ENT specialists, trained under the programme.

- The screening camps will be facilitated in collaboration with NRHM (RBSK) or by the NGOs, identified by the M/o SJ and E/District Health Society. These NGOs will require adequate infrastructure to carry out screening camps and experience of work at the community level.
- One screening camp will be organized per month at any PHC or CHC or district hospital by rotation.

Treatment: Medical and Surgical

Treatment of all affected persons would be undertaken at the following levels:

- **Public Health Nurses and MPWs:** Would provide treatment of common ear ailments such as Wax, Acute Suppurative Otitis Media, etc. under the guidance of the PHC doctor. The Public Health Nurses and MPWs will have the capacity to distribute relevant ear drops and medicines under the guidance of the PHC doctor.
- Trained PHC/CHC doctors will provide early diagnosis of ear diseases and treatment of all common ear ailments. All persons requiring special diagnostic facilities, complicated cases and those needing surgical intervention will be referred to the district hospital.
- **District hospital:** The district level ENT doctors and audiologists will provide comprehensive preventive, promotive and curative and medical rehabilitative services. Wherever feasible, suitable linkages would be developed with the comprehensive rehabilitation centers (CRC) and DDRC in coordination with the Ministry of Social Justice and Empowerment, for provision of rehabilitative services.
- The district level pediatricians will also be responsible for treating ear diseases such as acute otitis media, so that progress to deafness can be prevented.

Appropriate Referral

Effective linkages would be developed from peripheral level to district level with the help of functionaries and personnel from grass-roots level (AWW, ASHA and sensitized parents and PRIs), subcenter level (Male and female MPWs), PHC level medical officers, public health nurses, school teachers and school health doctors, ENT private practitioners and district level officers.

Rehabilitation of Hearing and Speech disorders and Hearing-Aid Provision

- All patients who are identified as having an ear problem and either require surgery, hearing aid fitting or rehabilitative therapy will be referred to the ENT doctor and audiologist at the district level.
- Those who need surgery will be given the appropriate treatment at the district hospital.
- Complicated cases that cannot be adequately handled at the district hospital will be further referred to the State Medical College for expert treatment.
- Patients who suffer with sensorineural hearing loss that is not amenable to medical or surgical correction and which requires hearing aid, will be fitted with the same at the district level provided by Ministry of Social Justice and Empowerment. This will include children who are suffering with bilateral sensorineural hearing loss.
- The hearing aids will be issued as per existing rules. It is proposed that collaboration with the Ministry of Social Justice and Empowerment will be established for this purpose.
- The requirement for speech therapy and hearing therapy will be met with by the audiologist at the district level.

Awareness Creation in the Community

- Community level health workers and doctors will undertake this activity on a continuous basis. This will also form a part of the IEC activities at various levels.
- Sensitization will be done regarding various aspects relating to early detection of hearing loss. They will be educated about the various ill effects of hearing loss on the speech, mental and social development of the child.
- Information regarding various treatment modalities as well as techniques of rehabilitation.
- Sensitization to ill effects of hearing loss in the elderly so that they may refer the aged and hearing-impaired persons for suitable management/rehabilitation.

Expected Benefits of the Programme

The programme is expected to generate the following benefits in the short as well as in the long run:

- Large scale direct benefit of various services like prevention, early identification, treatment, referral, rehabilitation, etc. for hearing impairment and deafness as the primary health center/community health centers/district hospitals largely cater to their need.
- Decrease in the magnitude of hearing impaired persons.
- Decrease in the severity/extent of ear morbidity or hearing impairment in large number of cases.
- Improved service network for the persons with ear morbidity/hearing impairment in the states and districts covered under the project.
- Awareness creation among the health workers/grass-roots level workers through the primary health center medical officers and district officers which will percolate to the lowest level as the lower level health workers function within the community.
- Larger community participation to prevent hearing loss through panchayati raj institutions, mahila mandals, village bodies and also creation of a collective responsibility framework in the broad spectrum of the society.
- Leadership building in the primary health center medical officers to help create better sensitization in the grassroots level which will ultimately ensure better implementation of the programme.
- Capacity building at the district hospitals to ensure better care.
- State of the art department of ENT at the medical colleges in the state/union territory under the project.

Programme Execrates and Expansion

The programme was a 100% centrally-sponsored scheme during 11th five-year plan. However, as per the 12th five-year plan, the center and the states will have to pool in resources financial norms of NRHM. The programme was initiated in year 2007 on pilot more in 25 Districts of 11 States UTs. The programme has been expanded to 192 Districts of 20 States and UTs. Additional 200 Districts in a phase hammer probably carding all the States and UTs by March 2017.

Chapter 30

National Programme for Prevention and Control of Cancer, Diabetes, Cardiovascular Diseases and Stroke

INTRODUCTION

Pilot phase of the National Programme for Prevention and Control of Cancer, Diabetes, Cardiovascular Diseases and Stroke (NPCDCS) launched on January 4, 2008 by Deputy Chairman, Planning Commission in the presence of Hon'ble Minister for Health and Family Welfare and Hon'ble Minister of State.

Objectives of the Pilot Phase

- Risk reduction for prevention of NCDs (Diabetes, CVD and Stroke).
- Early diagnosis and appropriate management of diabetes, cardiovascular diseases and stroke strategies.
- Health promotion for the general population.
- Disease prevention for the high risk groups.

Objectives of NPCDCS

- Prevent and control common NCDs through behavior and lifestyle changes.
- Provide early diagnosis and management of common NCDs.
- Build capacity at various levels of health care for prevention, diagnosis and treatment of common NCDs.
- Train human resource within the public health setup viz. doctors, paramedics and nursing staff to cope with the increasing burden of NCDs.
- Establish and develop capacity for palliative and rehabilitative care.

STRATEGIES

The strategies to achieve above objectives are as follows:
- Prevention through behavior change.
- Early diagnosis.
- Treatment.
- Capacity building of human resource.
- Surveillance, monitoring and evaluation.

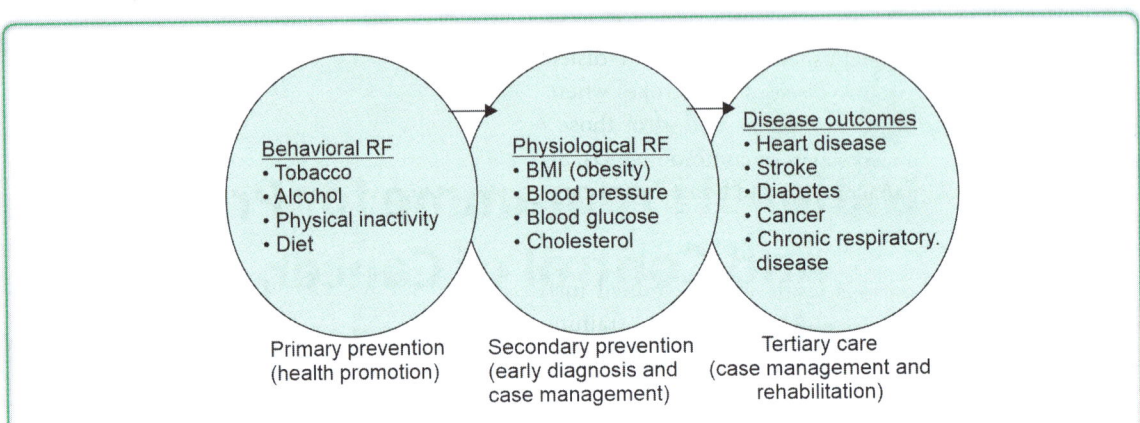

Figure 1: Risk factors (RF) and level of NCD prevention and management

Prevention through Behavior Change

The major risk factors to cancer, hypertension, obesity, diabetes and cardiovascular diseases are unhealthy diet, physical inactivity, stress and consumption of tobacco and alcohol. Attempts will be made to prevent these risk factors by creating general awareness about the non-communicable diseases (NCD) and promotion of healthy lifestyle habits among the community (Fig. 1). Such interventions will be done through the peripheral health functionaries and NGOs.

The various approaches such as mass media, community education and interpersonal communication will be used for behavior change focusing on the following five messages:

1.   Increased intake of healthy foods.
2.   Increased physical activity through sports, exercise, etc.
3.   Avoidance of tobacco and alcohol.
4.   Stress management.
5.   Warning signs of cancer.

Interpersonal communication will be carried out through ASHAs/AWWs/SHGs/ Youth clubs, Panchayat members etc. For which education material will be developed at central/state level to facilitate IEC/BCC activities. These workers/groups will also help in social mobilization for diagnostic camps. Targeted intervention programmes will be designed to bring awareness in schools and workplaces.

Early Diagnosis

Strategy for early diagnosis of chronic non-communicable diseases will consist of opportunistic screening of persons above the age of 30 years at the point of primary contact with any health care facility, be it the village, CHC, district hospital, tertiary care hospital, etc. Opportunistic screening will have in-built components of mass awareness creation, self screening and trained health care providers.

Such screening involves simple clinical examination comprising relevant questions and easily conducted physical measurements (such as history of tobacco consumption and measurement of blood pressure etc.) to identify those individuals who are at a high risk of developing diabetes and CVD, warranting further investigation/action. The investigations which may not be carried out in the health facilities can be outsourced.

Treatment

"NCD clinic" will be established at CHC and district hospital (NCD here refers to cancer, diabetes, hypertension, cardiovascular diseases and stroke) where comprehensive examination of patients referred by lower health facility/health worker as well as of those reporting directly will be conducted for ruling out complications or advanced stages of common NCDs. Screening, diagnosis and management (including diet counseling, lifestyle management) and home-based care will be the key functions.

Capacity Building of Human Resource

Health personnel at various levels will be trained for health promotion, prevention, early detection and management by a team of trainers at identified training institutes/centers. These training institutes/centers will be identified by the state in consultation with the center.

Surveillance, Monitoring and Evaluation

Regular monitoring and review of the scheme will be conducted at the district, state and central level through monitoring formats and periodic visits and review meetings. For the purpose, NCD cell at different levels is envisaged to supervise and monitor the programme and also other NCD programmes. The evaluation is the integral part of the programme and will be carried out concurrently and periodically, as and when required.

The strategies proposed will be implemented in 20,000 sub-centers and 700 community health centers, in 100 districts across 21 States during 2010–12. The guidelines on operational aspects and financial norms of the programme have been given in details to facilitate the effective implementation of the programme (Table 1).

Table 1: Packages of services to be made available at different levels under NPCDCS

Health facility	Packages of services
Sub center	• Health promotion for behavior change • 'Opportunistic' Screening using BP measurement and blood glucose by strip method • Referral of suspected cases to CHC
CHC	• Prevention and health promotion including counseling • Early diagnosis through clinical and laboratory investigations (Common lab investigations: Blood sugar, lipid profile, ECG, ultrasound, X-ray, etc.) • Management of common CVD, diabetes and stroke cases (outpatient and in patients.) • Home-based care for bed ridden chronic cases • Referral of difficult cases to district hospital/higher health care facility
District hospital	• Early diagnosis of diabetes, CVDs, stroke and cancer • Investigations: Blood sugar, lipid profile, kidney function test (KFT), liver function test (LFT), ECG, Ultrasound, X-ray, colposcopy, mammography etc. (if not available, will be outsourced) • Medical management of cases (outpatient, inpatient and intensive care) • Follow-up and care of bed-ridden cases • Day care facility • Referral of difficult cases to higher health care facility • Health promotion for behavior change
Tertiary cancer center	Comprehensive cancer care including prevention, early detection, diagnosis, treatment, minimal access surgery after care, palliative care and rehabilitation

MANAGEMENT STRUCTURE

National Non-communicable Disease Cell (National NCD Cell)

Organization structure and services available are given in Table 2 and Figure 2.

National NCD cell will be responsible for overall planning, implementation, monitoring and evaluation of the different activities and achievement of physical and financial targets planned under the programme. The National NCD cell shall function under the guidance of programme in-charge from the Ministry of Health and Family Welfare and will be supported by the identified officers/officials from the Directorate General of Health Services.

Table 2: Organization structure of national NCD cell

Technical wing	Administrative wing
Deputy Director General	Additional Secretary/Joint Secretary
CMO (Cancer)	Director (NCD)
CMO (Diabetes and CVD)	Under Secretary (NCD)
CMO (Geriatric care)	Under Secretary (NCD)
Consultants	Section officer

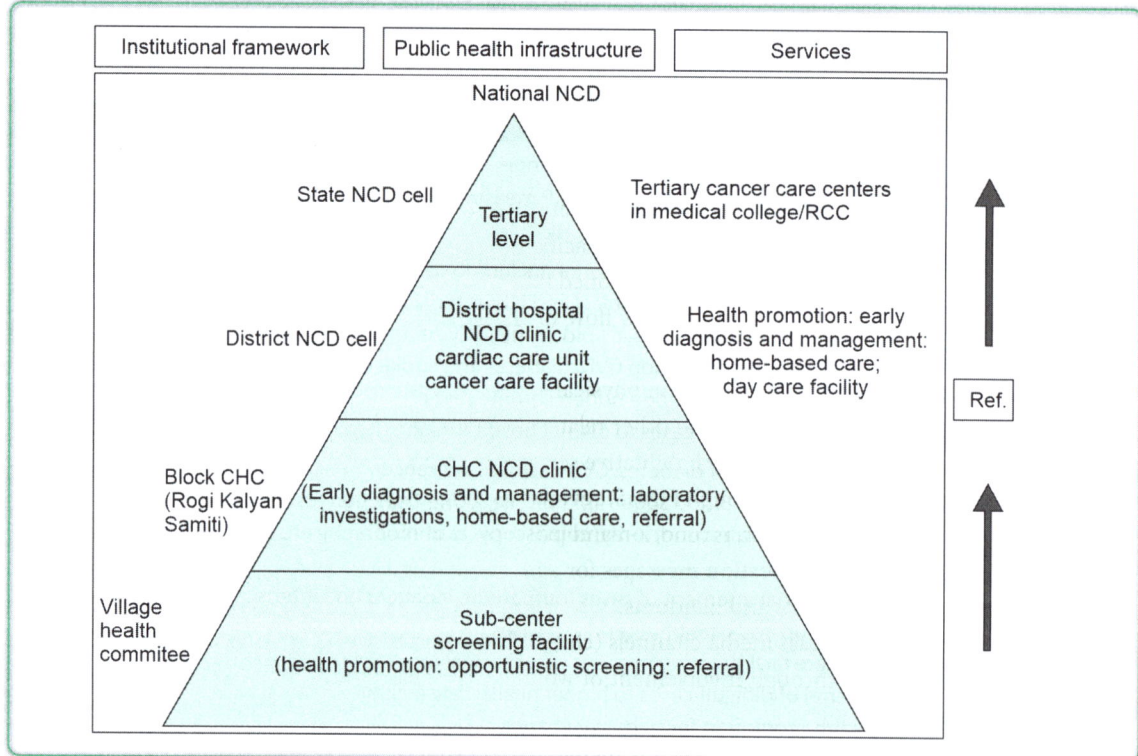

Figure 2: Services available under NPCDCS at different levels

Roles and Responsibilities of the National NCD Cell

- Nodal body to roll out NPCDCS in the country.
- Plan, coordinate, and monitor all the activities at National and State level.
- Develop operational guidelines, standard operating procedures (SOP), training modules, quality benchmarks, monitoring and reporting systems and tools.
- Monitoring and evaluation of the programme through HMIS, review meetings, field observations, surveillance, operational research and evaluation studies.
- Prepare National Training Plan: Curriculum, training resource centers, training modules and organize national level training programmes.
- Procurement of equipment and supplies for items to be provided as commodity assistance.
- Release of funds and monitoring of expenditure.

State NCD Cell

State NCD cell will be established preferably in the Directorate of Health Services or any other space provided by the State Government. The NCD cell will be responsible for overall planning, implementation, monitoring and evaluation of the different activities, and S. No. The cell shall function under the guidance of State Programme Officer (SPO NCD) and will be supported by the identified officers/officials from the Directorate/Director General of Health Services. SPO (NCD) will be a state level health official identified by the State Government.

Roles and Responsibilities of the State NCD Cell

- Preparation of state action plan for implementation of NPCDCS strategies.
- Develop district wise information of NCD diseases including cancer, diabetes, cardiovascular disease and stroke through health facilities including sentinel sites.
- Organize state and district level trainings for capacity building.
- Ensure appointment of contractual staff sanctioned for various facilities.
- Release of funds to districts for continuous flow of funds and submit statement of expenditure and utilization certificates.
- Maintaining state and district level data on physical, financial, epidemiological profile.
- Convergence with NRHM activities and other related departments in the State/District.
- Ensure availability of palliative and rehabilitative services including oral morphine.
- Monitoring of the programme through HMIS, review meetings, field observations.
- Public awareness regarding health promotion and prevention of NCDs through following approaches:
  - Development of communication messages for audio-visual and print media.
  - Distribution of pamphlets and handouts.
  - Campaigns through mass media channels (electronic and print media).
  - Social mobilization through involvement of women's self-help groups, community leaders, NGOs, etc.
- Advocacy and public awareness through mid-media (Street Plays, folk methods, wall paintings, hoardings, etc.)
- Flip charts to ground level workers for health education in the community.

District NCD Cell

District NCD cell will be established preferably in the Directorate of Health Services or any other space provided by district headquarter. The NCD cell will be responsible for overall planning, implementation, monitoring and evaluation of the different activities and achievement of physical and financial targets planned under the programme in the district. The cell shall function under the guidance of district programme officer (DPO NCD) and will be supported by the identified officers/officials from the district health system. DPO NCD shall be a district level health official and be identified by the State Government.

Roles and Responsibilities of the District NCD Cell

- Preparation of district action plan for implementation of NPCDCS strategies.
- Maintain and update district database of NCD diseases including cancer, diabetes, cardiovascular disease and stroke.
- Conduct sub-district/CHC level trainings for capacity building.
- Engage contractual personnel sanctioned for various facilities in the district.
- Maintain fund flow and submit utilization certificates.
- Maintaining district level data on physical, financial, epidemiological progress.
- Convergence with NRHM activities.
- Convergence with the other related departments in the states/district.
- Ensure availability of palliative and rehabilitative services including oral morphine.

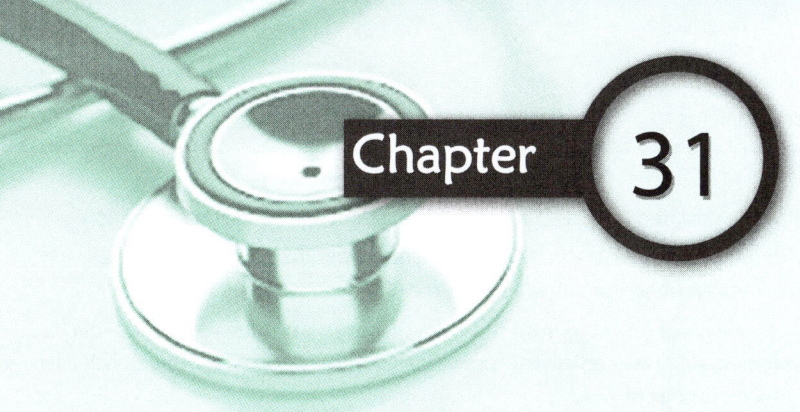

Chapter 31

Universal Immunization Programme

BACKGROUND OF IMMUNIZATION PROGRAMME IN INDIA

The success of smallpox eradication in the 70s brought attention to the immunization programme globally as well as in India. The Expanded Programme on Immunization (EPI), a programme for immunizing all children during the first year of life with DPT, OPV, BCG and typhoid–paratyphoid fever vaccines, was launched in 1978. In 1985, the name of EPI was changed to the Universal Immunization Programme (UIP). The stated objectives of UIP are to:

- Rapidly increase immunization coverage.
- Improve the quality of services.
- Establish a reliable cold chain system to the health facility level.
- Introduce a district-wise system for monitoring of performance.
- Achieve self-sufficiency in vaccine production.

Evolution of the programme over the years is listed in Table.

Table: Evolution of the programme

1978	Expanded Programme of Immunization (EPI) • Limited reach - mostly urban
1985	Universal Immunization Programme (UIP) • For reduction of mortality and morbidity due to 6 VPDs • Indigenous vaccine production capacity enhanced • Cold chain established • Phased implementation • All districts covered by 1989–90 • Monitoring and evaluation system implemented
1986	Technology mission on immunization • Monitoring under PMO's 20-point programme • Coverage in infants (0–12 months) monitored
1992	Child survival and safe motherhood (CSSM) • Included both UIP and safe motherhood programme
1997	Reproductive child health (RCH 1)
2005	National rural health mission (NRHM)

Contd…

2012	Government of India declared 2012 as "Year of Intensification of Routine Immunization"
2013	India, along with other South-East Asia Region, declared commitment towards measles elimination and rubella/congenital rubella syndrome (CRS) control by 2020
2013	No wild Polio virus case was reported from the country for the last three years and India had a historic achievement and was certified as "polio free country" along with other South East Asia Region (SEAR) countries of WHO

The goal of the current comprehensive multiyear plan for 2013–2017 was to reduce mortality and morbidity due to vaccine preventable diseases with the help of high quality immunization programmes. Its key objectives are to:

- Improve programme service delivery for equitable and efficient immunization services in all districts.
- Increase demand and reduce barriers for people to access immunization services through improved advocacy at all levels and social mobilization.
- Strengthen and maintain robust surveillance system for vaccine preventable diseases (VPDs) and adverse events following immunization (AEFI).
- Introduce and expand the use of new and underutilized vaccines and technology in UIP.
- Strengthen health system for the immunization programme.
- Contribute to global polio eradication and the elimination of measles, maternal and neonatal tetanus.

VACCINES UNDER UIP

- **Under UIP, following vaccines are provided:**
  - Bacillus Calmette Guerin (BCG)
  - Diphtheria, Pertussis and Tetanus Toxoid (DPT)
  - Oral Polio Vaccine (OPV)
  - Measles
  - Hepatitis B
  - Tetanus Toxoid (TT)
  - JE vaccination (in selected high disease burden districts)
  - Hib containing pentavalent vaccine (DPT+HepB+Hib) (In selected states).
- **Diseases protected by vaccination under UIP**
  - Diphtheria
  - Pertussis
  - Tetanus
  - Polio
  - Tuberculosis
  - Measles
  - Hepatitis B
  - Japanese encephalitis (commonly known as brain fever).
  - Meningitis and pneumonia caused by Haemophilus influenzae type VPD surveillance.
- Vaccine preventable diseases (VPD) surveillance system is needed to create evidence base to enable planning and deployment of effective interventions.
- India has different surveillance models. Integrated Disease Surveillance Project (IDSP) is one of those surveillance systems.
- IDSP is a case-based surveillance system for detection of early warning signals of outbreaks. There are other sentinel surveillance systems which fall under different vertical National Health Programmes for diseases targeted for control, elimination or eradication.

- Another source is the National Polio Surveillance Project (NPSP), which has done extremely well in acute flaccid paralysis (AFP) and measles surveillance in India.
- WHO/NPSP provides needed technical and training support for AFP and measles surveillance.
  New vaccines to be introduced as per National Technical Advisory Group on Immunization (NTAGI) recommendation.
- Injectable polio vaccine (IPV): National Technical Advisory Group on Immunization (NTAGI) recommended injectable polio vaccine (IPV) introduction as an additional dose along with third dose of DPT in the entire country in the first quarter of 2016.
- Rota virus vaccine: NTAGI recommended the introduction of rota virus vaccine in Universal Immunization Programme in a phased manner.
- Rubella vaccine is to be introduced as MR vaccine replacing the measles containing vaccine first dose (MCV1) at 9 months and second dose (MCV2) at 16–24 months.

IMPLEMENTATION OF ROUTINE IMMUNIZATION

- Routine immunization targets to vaccinate 27 million newborns each year with all primary doses and ~100 million children of 1–5 years' age with booster doses of UIP vaccines. In addition, 30 million pregnant mothers are targeted for TT vaccination each year.
- To vaccinate this cohort of 157 million beneficiaries, ~10 million immunization sessions are conducted, majority of these are at village level.
- As per Coverage Evaluation Survey (2009), 89.8% of vaccination in India is provided through public sector [(53% from outreach session held at *Anganwadi* center (25.6%), subcenter (18.9%) etc.)] while private sector contributed to only 8.7%.
- ASHA and AWW support ANM by mobilizing eligible children to session site thus try to ensure that no child is missed. ASHA is also provided an incentive of ₹150/–session for this activity.
- To ensure potent and safe vaccines are delivered to children, a network of ~27,000 cold chain points have been created across the country where vaccines are stored at recommended temperatures.

COMPONENTS

Strategy and Policy

National Health Policy (2002) is directed towards achieving an acceptable, affordable and sustainable standard of health through an appropriate health system. Provision of universal immunization of children against vaccine preventable diseases is one of the major goals under this policy. Country's five-year plan also puts emphasis on reduction in maternal and infant mortality rates as major maternal and child health indicators. Country developed a comprehensive Multi-Year Strategic Plan for immunization in 2005, which has been revised in 2013. This document is a national strategy document to guide development of UIP plans at national and state levels. Ministry of Health and Family Welfare also revised the National Vaccine Policy in 2011. The goal of this vaccine policy is to guide decision making in order to develop a long term plan to strengthen the UIP. This policy addresses issues of vaccine security, management, regulation guidelines, vaccine research and development and product development. To ensure informed decision making for any modification in UIP. Schedule or inclusion of new vaccines, there is a National Technical Advisory Group on Immunization (NTAGI) which comprises a number of technical experts, national programme leaders and managers, representatives from development partners and professional bodies. All issues related to the programme and vaccines are presented to this group for review and discussions and final recommendations.

Cold Chain System, Vaccines and Logistics

Cold chain is a system of storing and transporting vaccine at the recommended temperature range from the point of manufacture to point of use. India has built a vast cold chain infrastructure to ensure that only potent and effective vaccines reach millions of beneficiaries across the country. The vaccines are supplied by manufacturers directly to four Government Medical Store Depots (at Karnal, Mumbai, Chennai and Kolkata) and state and regional vaccine stores. The GMSDs supply to the states and regional vaccine stores; state and regional vaccine stores supply vaccines to divisional vaccine stores and district. The vaccines are further supplied to last cold chain points which are usually situated in primary health centers (PHCs) and community health centers. Transportation of vaccines from states/regional stores to divisions and districts is done in cold boxes using insulated vaccine vans. Vaccine carriers with icepacks are used to transport vaccines from PHCs to the outreach sessions in the village. The performance and efficiency of the cold chain system at different levels is monitored continuously, through supervisory visits, review meetings.

Injection Safety and Waste Disposal

A large number of injection procedures are undertaken in lakhs of vaccination sessions across the country every year. Unsafe injection practices can harm the recipient of the injection, the health worker and the community resulting in potentially life-threatening infections such as HIV/AIDS, Hepatitis B and C, etc. To ensure safe injection practices, Government of India endeavors to ensure continuous supply of injection safety equipment (AD syringes, reconstitution syringes, hub cutters and waste disposal bags). Trainings are conducted and supported by job-aids, on job training (supportive supervision). Disposal of immunization waste is strictly as per central pollution control board (CPCB) guidelines for biomedical waste disposal. The principles followed are segregation of waste at source (at the session site), transportation to the PHC or CHC, treatment of sharps and potentially biohazardous plastic waste, disposal of sharps in sharp pits and treated plastic waste through proper recycling. The states are provided funds to procure hub cutters, black and red plastic bags and construction of sharp pits in PHCs and CHCs.

ADVERSE EVENT FOLLOWING IMMUNIZATION (AEFI) SURVEILLANCE SYSTEM IN INDIA

History

- 1988: AEFI surveillance started in India.
- 2005: National AEFI guidelines developed and disseminated.
- 2007 onwards: State and District Level AEFI Committees formed.
- 2008: National AEFI Committee constituted.
- 2010: Guidelines revised, printed and widely circulated.
- 2011: SOPs printed and disseminated.
- 2012: AEFI Secretariat establishment.
- Over the years: Improved trends of reporting.
- The WHO defines AEFI as "a medical incident that takes place after an immunization, causes concern, and believed to be caused by immunization".
- AEFI surveillance in country monitors immunization safety, detects and responds to adverse events following immunization; corrects unsafe immunization practices, reduces the negative impact of the event on health and contributes to the quality of immunization activities.

- Special focus is being provided by Government of India to strengthen the system for reporting and responding to any adverse event following immunization (AEFI).
- Operational Guidelines for AEFI surveillance and response were first published in 2005 and revised in 2010. These have been disseminated to medical officers all over the country. Subsequent revision of these guidelines is under process.
- An AEFI secretariat has been established under immunization technical support unit (ITSU) to strengthen and coordinate all issues related to AEFI.
- India National Regulatory Authority (NRA) assessment has passed successfully in December 2012.
- The National AEFI committee has been revised in 2013 and broader range of expertise has been added to the National AEFI committee such as pharmacology, forensic medicine, pathology, immunology, epidemiology, communication, etc. besides pediatrics and immunization programme related experts.
- Workshops have been conducted at national level and for the pentavalent using States (Gujarat, Goa, Jammu and Kashmir, Haryana, Tamil Nadu, Kerala, Karnataka and Puducherry) for capacity building through latest WHO AEFI causality assessment guidelines and developing an effective AEFI monitoring system.
- To strengthen collaboration between stakeholders of vaccine pharmacovigilance programme at state level, participants from the regulator (DCGI) and in charges from the network of ADR monitoring centers of the Pharmacovigilance Programme of India (PvPI) have also been included from each state in these trainings.
- The National AEFI guidelines are being currently revised to include the new WHO causality assessment methodology and add verbal autopsy and forensic autopsy protocols for investigating AEFI deaths along with SOPs for AEFI case-related sample collections.

STRATEGIC COMMUNICATION

Strategic communication refers to policy-making and guidance for consistent information activity through coherent messaging. The issue of media advocacy, proactive planning and effective media response is emerging as one of the key elements of strategic communication support to achieving full routine immunization coverage in the country. Demand generation gains critical importance in raising immunization coverage in the country, especially when India is poised to sustain polio eradication, increase visibility and coverage of routine immunization (RI) by motivating people to demand immunization services, sustain and report vaccine related features, timely completion of routine immunization schedules of their children, and build grounds for new vaccines.

Development of Routine Immunization Logo

The new logo of the baby holding the syringe, indicating routine immunization (RI) as his right, has been developed in purple color. This will give RI a distinct identity. Deliberate efforts have been made to stay away from the polio brand colors of yellow and pink.

Immunization Trainings

The immunization programme runs due to the coordinated efforts of different cadres of health staff working in the states at different levels (states, districts, PHCs and CHCs).

In the year of intensification of routine immunization (2012–13), the Government of India has supported the training of approximately 12,50,000 frontline workers (ANMs, LHVs, *Anganwadi* workers and ASHAs) in 9 high priority States—UP, MP, Rajasthan, Bihar, Chhattisgarh, Jharkhand, Haryana, Gujarat and West Bengal. The objective is to motivate and strengthen the capacity of frontline workers to reduce dropouts and left outs and improve the quality of services. The process followed is a cascade model.

Monitoring and Evaluation

Universal immunization programme has a set of indicators to monitor progress under different components of the programme and evaluate the coverage of immunization amongst the target population. In the country, UIP performs monitoring and evaluation at three levels.

1. There is a regular reporting system from the health sub-center to PHC, district, state and national level. This reporting has been computerized in the country as a part of health management information system (HMIS), and the data is available from health facility level and above every month. Recently MoHFW has also implemented mother and child tracking system (MCTS) to track every pregnant woman, mother and child up to 5 years of age to ensure delivery of health services.

2. To evaluate immunization coverage, country conducts period population-based surveys. These include National Family Health Survey (NFHS), District Level Health Survey (DLHS), Annual Health Survey (AHS) and UNICEF Coverage Evaluation Survey (CES).

3. In between periodic surveys and administrative reporting, country also plans targeted studies and surveys to evaluate the performance of various components under UIP. Some of the examples are VMAT/EVSM, PIE, MCTS field assessment, etc.

SCHEMES

Routine Immunization

Objectives

- The stated objectives of UIP are:
    - To rapidly increase immunization coverage.
    - To improve the quality of services.
    - To establish a reliable cold chain system to the health facility level.
    - Monitoring of performance.
    - To achieve self-sufficiency in vaccine production.

Immunization Campaigns

Japanese Encephalitis (JE) Vaccination

- JE vaccination has been expanded from 113 districts in 15 states to 179 districts in 20 states. Two doses of JE vaccine have been introduced under the routine immunization in 2013 to further protect children from JE.
- JE vaccination campaign covered 154 endemic districts out of 179 identified districts and has covered 108 million children. Remaining districts were covered by March 2015.

Measles Supplementary Immunization Activity (SIA)

- Based on National Technical Group on Immunization (NTAGI) recommendation, Government of India introduced second dose of measles under the Universal Immunization Programme (UIP) in 2010 through a two-pronged strategy.
- 21 states with first dose of measles coverage of >80% introduced 2nd dose directly in their routine immunization.

Polio Eradication Programme in India
- There is a remarkable achievement, particularly considering the fact that in 2009, India accounted for nearly half of the total number of polio cases globally and there were an estimated 2 lakh cases of polio every year in the country in the year 1978.
- India reported its last case of polio on 13th January 2011.

Chapter 32

Mission Indradhanush

INTRODUCTION

Mission Indradhanush was launched by Ministry of Health and Family Welfare (MoHFW) Government of India on 25th December, 2014. It ensures that all children under the age of two years as well as pregnant women are fully immunized with seven vaccine preventable diseases.

The Mission Indradhanush, depicting seven colors of the rainbow, targets to immunize all children against seven vaccine preventable diseases, namely:

1. Diphtheria
2. Pertussis (Whooping cough)
3. Tetanus
4. Tuberculosis
5. Polio
6. Hepatitis B
7. Measles.

In addition to this, vaccines for Japanese Encephalitis (JE) and *Haemophilus influenzae* type B (HIB) are also being provided in selected states.

PHASES OF MISSION

First Phase of Mission Indradhanush

For the first phase, 201 high focus districts across 28 states in the country that have the peak number of partially immunized and unimmunized children were identified by the Government. There were total four rounds in the first phase of the mission. The first round of the first phase was started on 7th April, 2015 and continued for more than a week. Further, second, third and fourth rounds were held for more than a week in the month of May, June and July starting from 7th of each month. The first phase of this mission was very successful.

The main highlights of the first phase of Mission Indradhanush are as given below:

- Total 9.4 lakh sessions were organized during these four rounds of Mission Indradhanush.
- About 2 crore vaccines were given to the children as well as pregnant women.
- Tetanus toxoid vaccine was given to more than 20 lakh pregnant women, 75.5 lakh children were vaccinated and about 20 lakh children were fully vaccinated.
- More than 57 lakh zinc tablets and 16 lakh ORS packets were freely distributed to all the children to protect them against diarrhea.

Second Phase of Mission Indradhanush

Union Health Minister launched phase-2 of Mission Indradhanush in 352 districts targeting full immunization. The second phase of Mission Indradhanush was started on 7th October, 2015.

The second, third and fourth rounds of this phase started on 7th November and 7th December, 2015 and 7th January, 2016 respectively.

AIM

To achieve full immunization in 352 districts which includes 279 mid priority districts, 33 districts from the North East states and 40 districts from phase one where huge number of missed out children were detected.

OBJECTIVES

General Objective

The objective of Mission Indradhanush is to ensure high coverage of children and pregnant women with all available vaccines throughout the country, with emphasis on the identified 201 high focus districts.

Specific Objectives

With the launch of Mission Indradhanush, the government aims at:

- Generating high demand for immunization services by addressing communication challenges;
- Enhancing political, administrative and financial commitment through advocacy with key stakeholders; and
- Ensuring that the partially immunized and unimmunized children are fully immunized as per national immunization schedule.

FOCUS AREAS

Mission Indradhanush will be a nationwide drive, with focus on 201 identified high focus districts. Key areas reached through Mission Indradhanush will be:

- Areas with vacant sub-centers: No auxiliary nurse midwife (ANM) posted for more than three months.
- Villages/areas with three or more consecutive missed routine immunization (RI) sessions: ANMs on long leave or other similar reasons.
- High risk areas (HRAs) identified by the polio eradication programme. These include populations living in areas such as:
  - Urban slums with migration
  - Nomadic sites
  - Brick kilns
  - Construction sites
  - Other migrant settlements (fisherman villages, riverine areas with shifting populations)
  - Underserved and hard to reach populations (forested and tribal populations, hilly areas, etc.).
- Areas with low RI coverage, identified through measles outbreaks, cases of diphtheria and neonatal tetanus in last two years.
- Small villages, hamlets, dhanis, purbas, basas (field huts), etc., clubbed with another village for RI sessions and not having independent RI sessions.

STRATEGY FOR MISSION INDRADHANUSH

Mission Indradhanush was a nationwide intensified RI drive for ensuring high coverage throughout the country and was conducted between March and June 2015 in the country, with focus on 201 high focus districts. The two main components of this mission will be:

- Operational planning
- Communication planning

Implementation of Mission Indradhanush

- All ANMs will plan activities for seven days of each drive. This will include 1–2 days of activities in the ANM's own sub-center area and remaining days in same/adjoining blocks or urban areas of her district.
- All identified areas that require RI strengthening but have no/infrequent RI sessions must be reached through Mission Indradhanush sessions.
- Mission Indradhanush will be implemented according to a roster prepared during the microplanning meetings at block and district levels for each ANM in the district. Once these rosters have been prepared for each ANM in the district for the duration of the Indradhanush week, the DIO must assess the requirement of any hired vaccinators, which if required, should be identified, hired as per NHM financial norms (Annexure 8) and trained by the DIO.

Operational Planning

The following two operational mechanisms will be utilized to reach out to the unreached or poorly reached beneficiaries:

- **Fixed and Outreach Sessions:** Medical officer in charge for the block/urban planning unit will conduct a detailed planning for the additional sessions to be conducted in the planning unit. Provision for vaccination should be made at health posts, primary health centers (PHCs) and district hospital.
- **Sites for Vaccination:** In urban areas, urban health posts, post-partum (PP) centers, family welfare centers or local leaders' premises in urban slums can also be used as immunization sites. For other areas, primary schools, *anganwadi* centers, private dispensaries, nongovernmental organization (NGO) sites or any other locations that are easily accessible and acceptable to community can be used as immunization sites. Efforts have to be made to provide regular immunization services from these sites even after the Indradhanush weeks are over.
- **Availability of Human Resources:** In addition to health staff available from the same or neighboring community health center (CHC)/Block PHC, NGOs (LIONS, Rotary etc.), it is necessary to utilize retired health workers, and staff available from other government agencies such as Employee's State Insurance Corporation, Central Government Health Scheme, armed forces, railways, District Urban Development Agency (DUDA)/State Urban Development Agency (SUDA) and community based organizations to reach large number of children.
- **Timing:** The activity will be conducted from 9 am to 4 pm. However, sessions should be planned and based on the availability of the targeted population to maximize the benefits achieved.
- **Team:** A team will comprise one vaccinator and up to two mobilizers (at least one should be from local mohallas/locality). An additional vaccinator will be included in the team if the estimated injection load is more than 60–70.
- **Mobile Sessions:** Mobile sessions should be planned at places where routine immunization coverage is weak and the small number of beneficiaries does not warrant an independent session. These areas include

periurban areas, scattered slums, brick kilns and construction sites. For these sessions, alternate means such as mobile vans should be planned in the attached format.

It is important to ensure that the vials of BCG, measles and JE vaccines that are reconstituted at one site should not be used at the next site. The integrated child development services (ICDS) department may support these mobile clinics through supplementary nutrition services that may be provided to beneficiaries in these difficult-to reach areas.

Planning Considerations

Based on evidence and best practices from the polio eradication programme, following activities will be critical for the successful implementation of Mission Indradhanush:

- **Meticulous planning of immunization sessions at all levels:** Plan sessions for identified areas with inadequate reach of immunization programme. Ensure availability of sufficient vaccinators and all vaccines during routine immunization sessions.
- **Effective communication and social mobilization efforts:** Generate awareness and demand for immunization services through need-based communication and social mobilization activities (mass media, mid media, interpersonal communication, school and youth networks and corporates).
- **Intensive training of health officials and frontline workers:** Build capacity of health officials and workers for routine immunization activities to ensure the highest quality of immunization services delivery to beneficiaries.
- **Establish accountability framework through task forces:** Enhance involvement and accountability/ ownership of state and district administrative and health officials through state and district task forces for immunization. It is important to use concurrent session monitoring data to plug gaps in implementation.

Communication Planning

Need-based communication and social mobilization activities should be planned to achieve the following objectives:

- Demand generation through increased visibility;
- Advocacy through media, professional bodies and political leadership;
- Capacity building of immunization workforce on communication;
- Social mobilization through interpersonal communication, school and youth networks and corporates; and
- Monitoring of communication interventions.

STEPS FOR ROLLOUT OF MISSION INDRADHANUSH

The rollout of Mission Indradhanush requires meticulous planning at all levels. The special sessions under Mission Indradhanush should be conducted in areas that are unreached or poorly reached for routine immunization services to ensure maximum improvement in full immunization coverage of states. Prior to conducting these sessions, headcount must be done in such areas for enlisting beneficiaries and preparing due lists.

Chapter 33

National Programme for Control of Blindness

INTRODUCTION

National Programme for Control of Blindness (NPCB) was launched in the year 1976 as a 100% centrally sponsored scheme with the goal to reduce the prevalence of blindness from 1.4% to 0.3%. As per survey in 2001–02, prevalence of blindness is estimated to be 1.1%.

Rapid survey on avoidable blindness conducted under NPCB during 2006–07 showed reduction in the prevalence of blindness from 1.1% (2001–02) to 1% (2006–07). Various activities/initiatives undertaken during the five-year plans under NPCB are targeted towards achieving the goal of reducing the prevalence of blindness to 0.3% by the year 2020.

Main causes of blindness are given in Table.

Table: Main causes of blindness

Cataract	62.6%
Refractive error	19.70%
Corneal blindness	0.90%
Surgical complication	1.20%
Posterior capsular opacification	0.90%
Glaucoma	5.80%
Posterior segment disorder	4.70%
Others	4.19%

Estimated National Prevalence of Childhood Blindness/low vision is 0.80 per thousand.

GOALS AND OBJECTIVES OF NPCB IN THE XII FIVE-YEAR PLAN

- To reduce the backlog of blindness through identification and treatment of blind at primary, secondary and tertiary levels based on assessment of the overall burden of visual impairment in the country.
- Develop and strengthen the strategy of NPCB for—Eye Health II and prevention of visual impairment; through provision of comprehensive eye care services and quality service delivery.

- Strengthening and upgradation of RIOs to become center of excellence in various sub-specialities of ophthalmology.
- Strengthening the existing and developing additional human resources and infrastructure facilities for providing high quality comprehensive eye care in all districts of the country.
- To enhance community awareness on eye care and lay stress on preventive measures.
- Increase and expand research for prevention of blindness and visual impairment.
- To secure participation of voluntary organizations/private practitioners in eye care.

STRATEGIES TO ACHIEVE THE OBJECTIVES

- Decentralized implementation of the scheme through District Health Societies (NPCB).
- Reduction in the backlog of blind persons by active screening of population above 50 years, organizing screening eye camps and transporting operable cases to eye care facilities.
- Development of eye care services and improvement in quality of eye care by training of personnel, supply of high-tech ophthalmic equipment, strengthening follow-up services and regular monitoring of services.
- Screening of school age group (primary and secondary) children for identification and treatment of refractive errors, with special attention in under-served areas.
- Public awareness about prevention and timely treatment of eye ailments.
- Special focus on illiterate women in rural areas. For this purpose, there should be convergence with various ongoing schemes for development of women and children.
- To make eye care comprehensive, besides cataract surgery, provision of assistance for other eye diseases like diabetic retinopathy, glaucoma management, laser techniques, corneal transplantation, vitreoretinal surgery, treatment of childhood blindness, etc.
- Construction of dedicated eye wards and eye OTs in district hospitals in NE States and few other States as per need.
- Development of Mobile Ophthalmic Units [renamed as Multipurpose District Mobile Ophthalmic Units (MDMOU)] in the district level for patient screening and transportation of patients.
- Continuing emphasis on primary health care (eye care) by establishing vision centers in all PHCs with a PMOA in position.
- Participation of community and Panchayati Raj Institutions in organizing services in rural areas.
- Involvement of private practitioners in the programme.

REVISED STRATEGIES

Based upon the finding of the survey conducted during 1998–99 and 1999–2000:
- To make the NPCB more comprehensive by:
  - Strengthening services for other blindnesses like corneal blindness.
  - Refractive errors in school going children.
  - Improved follow-up service of cataract operated persons.
  - Treating other causes of blindness like glaucoma.
- To shift:
  - From eye camp approach to a fixed facility.
  - From conventional surgery to IOL implantation for better quality post-operative vision.
- To expand the World Bank project activities like constructions of eye OTs, eye wards at district level, training of eye surgeons, modern cataract surgery and supply of eye equipment.

- To strengthen participation of voluntary organizations in the programme and to earmark geographic areas to NGOs and government hospital and improve the performance of government units.
- To enhance coverage of eye care services in tribal and underserved areas through identification of bilateral blind patients, preparation of village wise blind register and giving preference to bilateral blind patients for cataract surgery.

New Initiatives

- Dedicated eye wards and eye OTs in DH and SDH as per demand.
- Appointment of ophthalmic surgeons and O.A. in new DHs and SDHs.
- Appointment of OA in PHCs.
- Appointment of eye donation counselors in eye banks.
- Grant-in-aid for NGOs for management of various eye diseases.
- PPP.
- Special attention to NE States.
- Telemedicine in ophthalmology.
- Vitamin A supplement and MMR vaccination through DBCS funds.

World Bank assisted cataract blindness control project (1994–2002):

- Implemented in 8 States.
- 15.35 million operations had been done against 11 million target.
- IOL implantation had been increased from 3% in 1993 to 75% in 2002.

Danish assistance to NPCB (1998–2003):

- Funds were utilized for the training, development of MIS, supply of equipment.

VISION 2020

Vision 2020 is a global initiative that aims to eliminate avoidable blindness by the year 2020. It was launched on 18 February 1999 by the World Health Organization together with more than 20 international non-governmental organizations involved in eye care and prevention and management of blindness that comprise the International Agency for the Prevention of Blindness (IAPB).

Vision 2020 is a partnership that provides guidance, technical and resource support to countries that have formally adopted its agenda.

Mission

The mission of the vision 2020 global initiative is to eliminate the main causes of all preventable and treatable blindness as a public health issue by the year 2020.

Objectives

Vision 2020: The Right to Sight accomplishes its mission as it attains the three major objectives:

1. Raise the profile, among the key audiences, of the causes of avoidable blindness and the solutions that will help to eliminate the problem.
2. Identify and secure the necessary resources around the world in order to provide an increased level of prevention and treatment programmes.

3. Facilitate the planning, development and implementation of the three core Vision 2020 strategies by National Programmes.

Strategies and Activities

Over two decades, it is hoped that Vision 2020 will prevent 100 million people from becoming blind.

Vision 2020, through WHO, IAPB and its member organizations, provides technical support and advocacy to prevention of blindness activities worldwide. At the national level, a strong partnership between Ministry of Health, national and international NGOs, professional organizations, and civil society groups—brought together in a national prevention of blindness or vision 2020 committee—should facilitate the development and implementation of effective and sustainable national eye care plans.

Vision 2020 seeks to eliminate the main causes of avoidable blindness in the world: The goal is to eliminate avoidable blindness. In the long term, the initiative seeks to ensure the best possible vision for all people, thereby improving their quality of life. This goal should be achieved through the establishment of a sustainable, comprehensive eye care system as an integral part of every national health system.

Core Strategies

*   **Disease control:** Facilitate the implementation of specific programmes to control and treat the major causes of blindness.
*   **Human resource development:** Support training of ophthalmologists and other eye care personnel to provide eye care.
*   **Infrastructure and appropriate technology development:** Assist to improve infrastructure and technology to make eye care more available and accessible.

Essential Components

*   Cost-effective disease control interventions
*   Human resource development (training and motivation)
*   Infrastructure development (facilities, appropriate technology, consumables, funds).

Principles are Summarized in the Acronym ISEE
*   Integrated into existing health care systems
*   Sustainable in terms of money and other resources
*   Equitable care and services available to all, not just the wealthy
*   Excellence—a high standard of care throughout.

Structure of vision 2020 is illustrated in Figure 1.

Fifty-sixth World Health Assembly resolution WHA 56.26, elimination of avoidable blindness
Global political commitment to vision 2020 was reaffirmed in 2003 by the adoption of this resolution that urged each Member State to:
*   Support the global initiative for the elimination of avoidable blindness by setting up, not later than 2005, a national vision 2020 plan, in partnership with WHO and in collaboration with nongovernmental organizations and the private sector.
*   Commence implementation of such plans by 2007 at the latest; and
*   Include in such plans effective information systems with standardized indicators and periodic monitoring and evaluation, with the aim of showing a reduction in the magnitude of avoidable blindness by 2010.

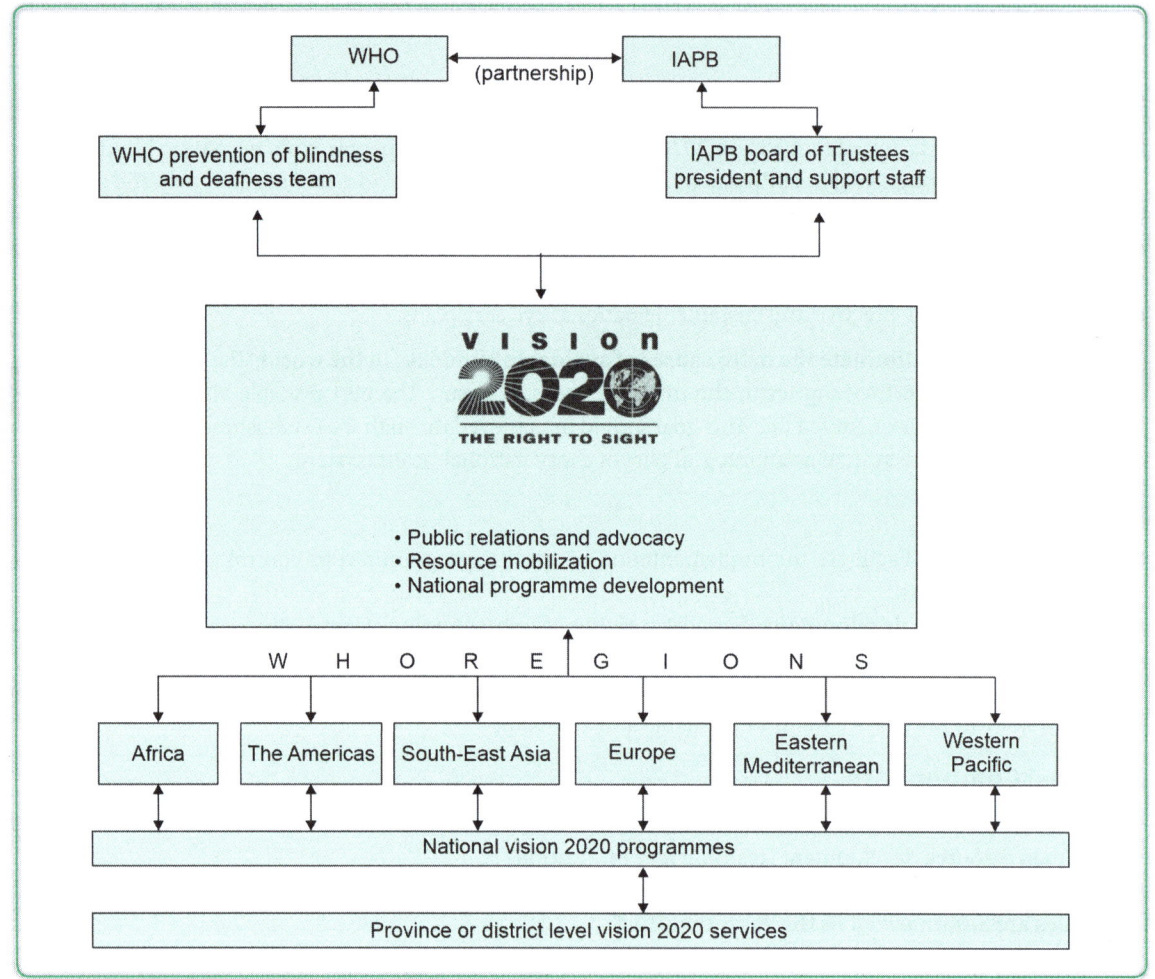

Figure 1: The Vision 2020 structure

*(*Source: World Health Organization, Prevention of Blindness Programme (WHO/PBD), 2005.)*

The resolution also requested the Director-General of WHO to:

- Maintain and strengthen WHO's collaboration with Member States and the partners of the global initiative for the elimination of avoidable blindness; and
- Ensure coordination of the implementation of the global initiative, in particular by setting up a monitoring committee grouping all those involved.

VISION 2020 INDIA

India is a national forum for eliminating avoidable blindness by year 2020. It is a key driver of the World Health Organization (WHO) and International Agency for the Prevention of Blindness (IAPB) joint global initiative for eliminating avoidable blindness.

- **Vision 2020:** The Right to Sight—India was launched in 2004. It is a collaborative effort of INGOs, NGOs, eye care organizations in India and the Government to coordinate and advocate for improved eye care programmes; gaining and sharing knowledge and think solutions together to achieve quality, comprehensive and equitable eye care.
- **Vision 2020:** The Right to Sight—India's programmes and action plans are aligned with government's programme of National Programme for Control of Blindness. Our programmes are focused on developing all the departments in our member organizations' eye hospitals.
- Key strengths are our leadership, passion, knowledge, skills, experience and commitment brought together by like-minded member organizations to fulfill our vision and mission.

    80% of blindness in India is because of cataract and uncorrected refractive errors. History has provided us (VISION 2020 INDIA Forum) with a unique privilege and opportunity to work as a team in mission mode with a laser sharp focus—to eliminate avoidable blindness to a level that it ceases to be a public health problem for our citizens residing in our 626 districts in India.

Six key strategic areas to produce an impact are:

1. Advocacy for eye health
2. Policy and programme development
3. Quality in eye care
4. Resource mobilization and sustainability
5. Resource center
6. Organizational development

Vision

An India free of avoidable blindness, where every citizen enjoys the gift of sight and the visually challenged have enhanced quality of life as a right.

Mission

To work with eye care organizations in India for the elimination of avoidable blindness by provision of equitable and affordable services as well as rehabilitation of visually challenged persons through development of appropriate policies, quality standards, advocacy, training, and promotion of best practices with a special emphasis on the poor and marginalized sections of society and underserved areas.

Core Values

India is committed to being a transparent, accountable, inclusive and sustainable organization that respects all its members and stakeholders whose participation is actively sought in democratic decision-making and organizational learning. We promote quality and equity in eye care, with the highest ethical standards.

Key Result Areas

- Advocacy
- Coordination
- Government liaison
- Best practices
- Capacity building
- Human resource development

- Monitoring
- Information
- Sustainability

GLOBAL ACTION PLAN 2014–2019

(*'Universal Eye Health' - the WHO Global Action Plan*)

"Universal Eye Health: A global action plan 2014–2019" (GAP) was unanimously adopted by Member States at the World Health Assembly in 2013 as part of WHA resolution 66.4 (also read: What is universal eye health?).

GAP has a global target—the reduction in prevalence of avoidable blindness and visual impairment by 25% by 2019 from the baseline of 2010.

The Vision of the GAP is:

"A world in which nobody is needlessly visually impaired, where those with unavoidable vision loss can achieve their full potential and where there is universal access to comprehensive eye care services."

Goals of the GAP

- To reduce visual impairment as a global public health problem
- To secure access to rehabilitation for visually impaired services

Objectives of GAP

- To generate evidence on magnitude and causes of VI and use it in advocacy;
- To develop and implement integrated national eye health policies and plans;
- To ensure multi-sectoral engagement and effective partnerships.

The GAP sets itself a global target of a "Reduction in prevalence of avoidable visual impairment by 25% by 2019" (from the baseline prevalence in 2010).

Key Indicators

To monitor progress
- Prevalence and causes of visual impairment.
- Numbers of ophthalmologists, optometrists and allied ophthalmic personnel.
- Cataract surgical rate and cataract surgical coverage.

The GAP is built upon VISION 2020: The right to sight, the global initiative for the elimination of avoidable blindness, a joint programme of the World Health Organization (WHO) and the International Agency for the Prevention of Blindness (IAPB).

Strategies

National Eye Health Plans must be geared to:
- **Collect evidence:**
  - Collect data on prevalence of visual impairment through RAAB (Rapid Assessment of Avoidable Blindness).
  - Assess a country's eye health system using ECSA (Eye Care Service Assessment).

- **Train more eye care professionals:**
  - Address acute shortage in every cadre of eye health—nurses, optometrists, ophthalmologists, etc.
  - Ensure equitable access to eye health personnel.
- **Provide comprehensive eye care:**
  - Eye care is well-funded and integrated into health care.
  - Covers all major causes of visual impairment and rehabilitation.
  - Increase cataract surgical rate and coverage.
- **Eliminate social and economic obstacles:**
  - Point-of-care payment should not prevent access and should be free for the poorest.
  - Gender disaggregated data should be collected at all levels.

The action plan provides us with 'indicators' to measure progress at the national level:
- The prevalence and causes of visual impairment.
- The number of eye care personnel.
- Cataract surgical rate and coverage.

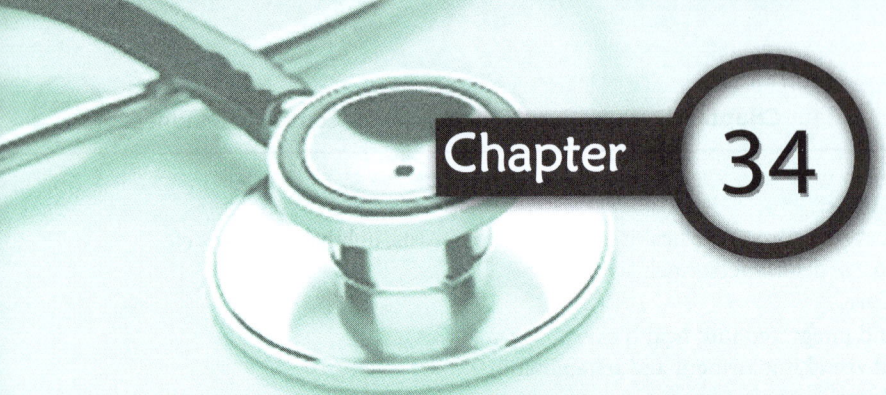

Chapter 34

Revised National Tuberculosis Control Programme, Evolution of TB Control

INTRODUCTION

Tuberculosis is a major public health problem in India. India accounts for one-fifth of the global TB incidence and is estimated to have the highest number of active TB cases amongst all the countries of the entire World. Every year there are approximately 18 lakh new cases in the country of which approximately 8 lakhs are new smear-positive and therefore infectious. Each sputum positive case if not treated, on an average, infects 10–15 persons in a year. Two persons die from TB in India every three minutes, i.e., more than 1,000 people every day.

To control TB, National Tuberculosis Control Programme (NTCP) has been in operation in the country since 1962. This could not achieve the desired results. Therefore, it was reviewed by an expert committee in 1992 and based on its recommendations, Revised National TB Control Programme (RNTCP). It was formed is an application to India of WHO and which recommended strategy of Directly Observed Treatment Short course (DOTS), was launched in the country on 26 March 1997. The objectives of RNTCP are:

- To achieve and maintain a cure rate of at least 85% among newly detected infectious TB cases
- Achieve and maintain detection of at least 70% of such cases in the population.

The RNTCP was implemented in the country in a phased manner and by March 23, 2006 the entire country has been covered under RNTCP. The programme is being implemented with assistance from World Bank, DFID, USAID, GDF and GFATM.

1950s–60's Important TB research at TRC and NTI	
1962 National TB Programme (NTP)	
1992	Programme review • Only 30% of patients diagnosed; • Of these, only 30% treated successfully
1993	RNTCP pilot began
1997–2006	RNTCP I
2006–2011	RNTCP II
2012–17	National Strategic Policy

REVISED NATIONAL TB CONTROL PROGRAMME

The large scale implementation of the Indian government's Revised National TB Control Programme (RNTCP) (sometimes known as RNTCP 1) was started in 1997. The RNTCP was then expanded across India until the entire nation was covered by the RNTCP in March 2006. At this time, the RNTCP also became known as RNTCP II. RNTCP II was designed to consolidate the gains achieved in RNTCP I, and to initiate services to address TB/HIV, MDR-TB and to extend RNTCP to the private sector. RNTCP uses the World Health Organization (WHO) recommended Directly Observed Treatment Short Course (DOTS) strategy and reaches over a billion people in 632 districts/reporting units.

With the RNTCP, both diagnosis and treatment of TB are free. There is also, at least in theory, no waiting period for patients seeking treatment and TB drugs.

The initial objectives of the RNTCP in India were:

- To achieve and maintain a TB treatment success rate of at least 85% among new sputum positive (NSP) patients.
- To achieve and maintain detection of at least 70% of the estimated new sputum positive people in the community.

Objectives of RNTCP

General Objectives

- To reduce morbidity and mortality due to tuberculosis.
- To break the chain of transmission.

Operational Objectives

- To provide SCC to all detected TB patients for the recommended duration of treatment till they are cured.
- To treat annually on an average about 750 sputum positive cases per million population as against the existing rate of 375 per million population.
- To administer antituberculous drugs under direct observation during the intensive phase and maintaining good quality supervision of drug administration during the continuation phase. Treatment services will be made most accessible to the patients through the involvement of the peripheral health functionaries with a view to achieve a cure rate of at least 85% amongst all newly detected sputum positive cases.
- To detect at least 70% of the estimated incidence of smear positive pulmonary tuberculosis patients. Efforts at case detection to be made only after achieving 85% cure rate.

Strategy

Strategies Relating to Case-finding

Case-finding will be passive. Emphasis will be laid on diagnosis through sputum examination. The quality of diagnosis will be improved by:

- Provision of binocular microscopes.
- Uninterrupted supply of good quality reagents, slides and sputum cups.
- Training and supervision of microscopist.
- Three sputum smears for diagnosis.
- Establishing quality control with a cross checking mechanism at sub-district, state and national level through networking of laboratories; and
- Monitoring the proportion of cases diagnosed without bacteriological confirmation.

Strategies Related to Treatment and Case-holding

All identified TB patients will be given SCC as per treatment regimens for different categories of patients.

The intensive phase will be directly observed through responsible peripheral functionaries and continuation phase appropriately supervised by observing the intake of the first dose of the medicine during the weekly drug collections and checking of empty foils of combi packs at the time of collection of next dosages and by random check by health workers.

Strategies Related to Operational Management

Strengthening at the Central, State and District levels will be done by providing necessary manpower, equipment and training to facilitate monitoring, supervision and training. A tuberculosis unit (TU) will be established at the sub-district in an existing CHC/Block PHC/Taluk hospital which will function as the managerial unit of the programme for 0.3 to 0.5 million population and comprise a senior treatment supervisor (STS) and a senior TB laboratory supervisor (STLS). This team will be responsible for implementation and supervision of all facets of the programme in their areas of jurisdiction, maintenance of the records and preparation of progress reports. The team will be under supervision of one of the medical officers in position at the TB unit who shall be designated.

Strategy for Other Key Areas

For regular monitoring and evaluation of programme activities, a health information network will be established. NGOs and private practitioners will be appropriately involved to support the RNTCR. An effective IEC strategy will be developed involving professional organizations and communication experts. Emphasis will be laid on awareness of community with regard to symptoms and signs of TB and availability of diagnostic and treatment centers.

Activities

Case-finding

In the rural areas, the existing laboratories at the PHCs/CHCs level up to maximum of one per lakh population strengthening to function as a microscopic center.

Treatment and Case-holding

DOTs three days a week will be given throughout the intensive phase. Facility of treatment will be made available at sub-centers/treatment centers close to patients' residence/village, to enhance patient compliance.

Information, Education and Communication (IEC)

For programme success, it is of paramount importance to enhance the knowledge and awareness of providers, users and community at large about different aspects of tuberculosis and its control measures.

Training of Staff

The training institutes at Central, State and District levels will be appropriately strengthed in terms of staff, equipment, vehicles and civil works. It is proposed to train the key trainers at Central and State levels and these in turn will train District trainers who will be responsible for giving training to all categories of staff within the district.

Management Information System (MIS)

Cohort analysis of treatment results as per specially designed RNTCP formats would be the main indications of programme effectiveness.

NATIONAL STRATEGIC PLAN FOR TUBERCULOSIS CONTROL 2012–17

Objectives

- To ensure early and improved diagnosis of all TB patients including drug resistant and HIV-associated tuberculosis.
- To provide access to high-quality treatment for all diagnosed cases of TB.
- To scale-up access to effective treatment for drug-resistant TB.
- To decrease the morbidity and mortality of HIV-associated TB.
- To extend RNTCP services to patients diagnosed and treated in the private sector.

Strategies

- Strengthening and improving the quality of basic DOTS services.
- Further strengthening and aligning with health system under NRHM.
- Deploying improved rapid diagnostics to the field level.
- Expanding efforts to engage all care providers.
- Strengthening urban TB control.
- Expanding diagnosis and treatment of drug resistant TB.
- Improving communication, outreach, and social mobilization.
- Promoting research for development and implementation of improved tools and strategies.

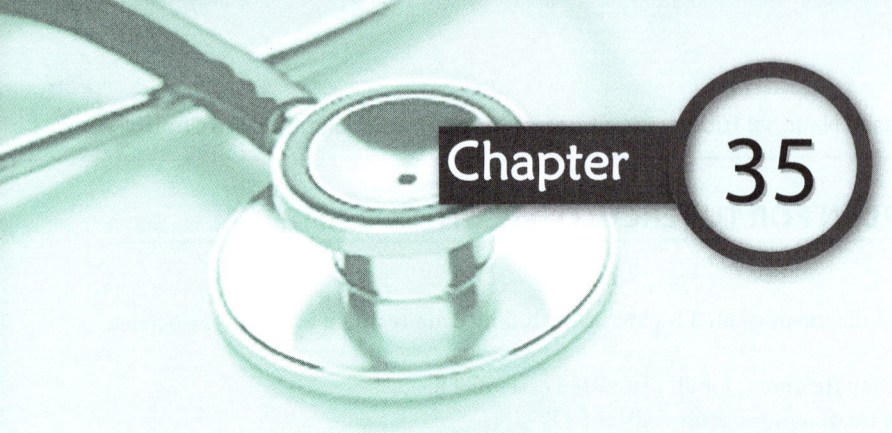

Chapter 35

National Malaria Control Programme

INTRODUCTION

National Malaria Control Programme (NMCP) was launched in 1953. Spectacular success of NMCP enthused health planner to convert it into Eradication Programme (NMEP) in 1958. The success achieved by NMEP was short-lived; due to various constraints like financial, logistic, administrative and technical. Resurgence of malaria after 1964, reached its peak in 1975, when state recorded 712 thousand malaria cases. To overcome this situation, modified plan of operation was introduced in 1977.

This led to significant reduction in malaria incidence which was maintained up to 1986. Since then, there was gradual increase in incidence along with increase in mortality. During 1975, 0.7 million cases of malaria were reported in the state. State responded this challenge by adopting modified plan of operation in 1977 and malaria was once again controlled in the state, which is revealed by the fact that during the year 1986 only 47 thousand malaria cases were reported. This achievement did not last longer. During 1995–96 malaria outbreaks and deaths due to malaria were reported from tribal parts of the state. In this year, there were about 380 thousand malaria cases and 242 deaths due to malaria.

Evolution of malaria control programme

1953	National Malaria Control Programme (NMCP)
1958	National Malaria Eradication Programme (NMEP)
1977	Modified Plan of Operation (MPO)
1979	Multipurpose Worker Scheme (MPW Scheme)
1995	Implementation of Malaria Action Plan–1995 (MAP – 95)
1997	Launching of World Bank Assisted Enhanced Malaria Control Project in tribal districts of the state (EMCP)
2000	National Antimalaria Programme (NAMP)
2004	National Vector Borne Disease Control Programme (NVBDCP)

OBJECTIVES

- To reduce morbidity due to malaria.
- To prevent deaths due to malaria.

- Industrial and agricultural development activities should not be affected due to malaria.
- The gains achieved so far should be maintained.

ACTIVITIES

Early Detection and Prompt Treatment

Identification of High Risk Areas

During the year 1995, the state experienced major malaria outbreaks especially in tribal districts of the state more prominently in Thane, Dhule, Nasik, Yeotmal, Chandrapur and Gadchiroli. Every year, high risk PHCs and sub centers were being identified as per guidelines given by Government of India (GoI). Following are the epidemiological parameters for identification of high risk areas.

- Recorded deaths due to malaria with *Plasmodium falciparum* (Pf) infection during transmission season with evidence of local infection in an endemic area in any of the last 3 years.
- Doubling of slide positivity rate (SPR) during last three years provided the SPR of 2nd and 3rd year reached 4% or more.

Surveillance

Active Surveillance

Blood smear collection of fever cases through regular house to house visits by multipurpose workers.

Passive Surveillance

Blood smear collection of fever cases coming at primary health centers, rural and cottage hospitals, district hospitals, and all government medical institutions, etc.

Contact Mass Nomad (CMN)–Contact

Blood smear collection irrespective of fever of all family members of malaria positive case.

Mass

Blood smear collection irrespective of fever of all families around malaria positive case.

Nomad

Blood smear collection irrespective of fever of all persons of nomadic tribes.

- **Through drug distribution centers (DDCs):**
  - About 66000 drug distribution centers are established in *Grampanchayats, Aanganwadi* and primary schools at village level. Chloroquine 150 mg tablets were being distributed to fever cases coming to them without obtaining blood smears through these depot holders.
- **Through fever treatment depots (FTDs):**
  - 1500 fever treatment depots were established only in tribal districts of the state. Chloroquine 150 mg tablets were being distributed to fever cases coming to them with obtaining blood smears through these depot holders.
- **Through malaria clinics:**
  - Malaria clinics were established in the state in hospitals and primary health centers where laboratory technicians were posted. At present, 1028 malaria clinics are functioning in the state at various level.

Vector Control Measures

Since 1999, the use of DDT has been stopped in indoor residual spraying due to development of resistance in vector species. Synthetic pyrethroid has been introduced for IRS since 1995–96 in Maharashtra State.

- Indoor residual spraying (IRS) is being carried out in identified high risk villages, i.e., in rural area.
- Two regular rounds of IRS are being carried out every year during transmission season.
- Focal spraying is also being carried out in outbreak areas.
- **Antilarval spraying:** Weekly spraying of larvicides (Temephos, Fenthion, MLO, BTI, etc.) on mosquito breeding places is being carried out in urban areas.

Mosquito Control—Source Reduction

Source reduction involves preventing development of mosquito larvae. The female anopheles mosquito lays eggs in collections of clean water. Each female anopheles mosquito lays millions of eggs in its lifetime of 4–8 weeks. The eggs hatch into larvae which then develop into pupae and adults in a span of 7–10 days. The best method of mosquito control is preventing the development of the eggs into adult mosquitoes. These anti-larval measures are not only simple and cost effective, but also environment-friendly.

STRATEGIES

Implementation Strategies

Major components of implementation strategies are:
- **Early detection and prompt treatment:**
  - Identification of high risk area.
  - Strengthening of surveillance activities.
  - Decentralization of laboratory services.
  - Availability of anti-malarial drugs up to the village level.
- **Selective vector control:**
  - Indoor residual spraying.
  - Anti-larval measures.
  - Use of biocides.
  - Personal protection methods mainly use of impregnated bednets.
  - Biological control measures.
- **Capacity Building:** Training to field staff and Nongovernmental Organizations (NGOs).
- **World Bank assisted enhanced malaria control project to intensify malaria control activities in tribal belt of the state.**

Celebration of Anti-Malaria Month–June up to village level every year. Activities carried out during Anti-Malaria Month—June are as under:
- Organization of state level press conference on 1st June.
- Organization of district level press conference.
- Special edition of Arogya Patrika on malaria.
- Broadcasting of speech on Aakashwani/Doordarshan by state level officers.
- Broadcasting of TV spots on Doordarshan.
- Broadcasting of radio jingles.
- Advertises in different local newspapers.
- Organization of Malariology workshops for NGOs.

SPECIAL FEATURES

Early Detection and Prompt Treatment

- Identification of High Risk areas on the basis of parameters like slide positivity rate (SPR), Annual Parasite Incidence (API), Pf proportion, deaths due to malaria.
- Strengthening of surveillance activities.
- Decentralization and strengthening of laboratory services.
- One-day condensed radical treatment, presumptive treatment to all fever cases and suspected malaria cases at referral institutions.
- Chemoprophylaxis to pregnant women.
- Establishment of drug distribution centers, fever treatment depots in tribal districts and malaria clinics in every village.
- Treatment of malaria cases at every sub-center, PHC, RH totally free of cost.
- Introduction of Twin Blister Pack containing Chloroquine 600 mg and Primaquine 45 mg for easy consumption of tablets and to reduce parasitic load in community.
- Appointment of pada workers and malaria link volunteers (MLVs) in tribal and remote areas.
- P–falciparum infection is known to lower blood glucose level causing death due to hypoglycemia in complicated cases. To avert these death, Glucometers are provided at all community health centers.

Vector Control

- IRS—Insecticidal residual spraying with synthetic pyrethroid in selected high risk population.
- Use of larvivorous Guppy fish under biological control.
- Distribution of medicated mosquito bednets in selected villages. Totally free of cost to families below poverty line, and ₹20/– for families above poverty line.
- Reimpregnation of distributed bednets is made every six months' interval. Re-impregnation of bed nets of other users will also be made if required by villagers.
- Use of biocides in towns under urban malaria scheme.
- Routine entomological studies.
- To intensify malaria control activities, establishment of district malaria control societies in 16 tribal districts under World Bank assisted enhanced malaria control project.
- Intersectoral coordination with nonhealth departments such as building and constructions, irrigation, railway, urban development, fisheries, tribal development, education, forest etc.
- Training of various health personnel and peripheral staff throughout the year.
- Involvement of non-government organizations in malaria control activities.
- Implementation of bye laws for mosquito prevention.
- Emphasis on IEC for active community participation.

WORLD BANK ASSISTED ENHANCED MALARIA CONTROL PROJECT (EMCP)

The anti-malaria activities are being carried out in the state as recommended by the Expert Committee in Malaria Action Plan–1995.

To intensify malaria control activities, World Bank assisted EMCP started in October 1997 in 7 States; one of them is Maharashtra.

Project activities under EMCP are as follows:
- Early detection and prompt treatment
- Selective vector control
- Personal protection method
- Early detection and containment of epidemics
- Intersectoral coordination
- Institutional and management capacity building

URBAN MALARIA SCHEME

Urban malaria scheme (UMS) was sanctioned in 1971 after the recommendations of Madhok Committee in 1969. Initially, 23 towns were selected for programme implementation. Subsequently, the scheme was extended to 131 towns in 19 states/UTs covering a population of 116 million.

Objectives

- To control malaria by reducing the vector population in the urban areas
- To reduce morbidity and mortality.

The norms for establishment of Urban Malaria Scheme (UMS) are as follows:
- The towns should have a minimum population of 40,000 (now 50,000).
- The API should be 2 or above.
- The towns should promulgate and strictly implement the civic byelaws to prevent.
- Eliminate domestic and peridomestic breeding places.

Control Strategies

- Anti-larval measures on weekly intervals.
- Source reduction, i.e. land filling/drainage through minor engineering methods.
- Biological control by introduction of larvivorous fish.
- Anti-parasitic measures through passive surveillance for detection of cases and complete treatment.
- Legislative measures (Enactment of byelaws).

NATIONAL VECTOR BORNE DISEASE CONTROL PROGRAMME (NVBDCP)

Introduction

The National Vector Borne Disease Control Programme (NVBDCP) is an umbrella programme for prevention and control of Vector Borne Diseases. Earlier the Vector Borne Diseases were managed under separate National Health Programmes, but now NVBDCP covers all 6 Vector borne diseases namely: (1) Malaria, (2) Dengue, (3) Chikungunya, (4) Japanese Encephalitis, (5) Kala-Azar, (6) Filaria (*Lymphatic filariasis*). At the time of independence, there were an estimated 75 million cases of malaria and 0.8 million deaths due to malaria were being reported annually. Government of India launched National Malaria Control Programme (NMCP) in 1953. Under this programme, indoor residual spray was being done with DDT twice a year. As a result, incidence of malaria cases came down from 75 million cases in 1953 to 2 million cases in 1958 in India. In 1958, this control programme was switched over to National Malaria Eradication Programme (NMEP), under which initially every house in the state was to be sprayed with DDT twice a year. Later on, spraying was withdrawn but surveillance activities were carried out vigorously.

This went on but gradually malaria incidence began to rise. In Punjab State, the number of malaria cases went from 321 in 1966 to 5 lac in 1977. Due to this setback to the programme, a revised strategy was started called "Modified Plan of Operation" (MPO) w.e.f. 1.4.1977. Under this, all the rural population and towns having less than 40,000 populations were under active surveillance. Every dwelling unit was visited by health worker fortnightly to detect fever cases and to give presumptive treatment to them against malaria. Radical treatment was administered to declared positive cases.

The main features of this programme are:
* Surveillance
* Malaria clinics
* Drug distribution centers (DDCs)
* Fever treatment depots (FTDs)
* Spray operations
* Urban malaria scheme (UMS)

Surveillance

Active Surveillance

Under this, the fortnightly domiciliary visits are made by MPHW (M) under primary health care system and by this fortnightly visit large number of secondary cases can be avoided where malaria transmission is seasonal.

The components of active surveillance are:
* Search for fever cases
* Collection of blood smears from fever cases
* Administration of appropriate presumptive treatment.

Malaria surveillance includes maintenance of ongoing watch over the status of malaria in a group or community. It provides a basis for measuring effectiveness of anti-malaria programme and helps control measures. Malaria surveillance presumes that every malaria case presents itself with symptoms of fever at some point of time during the course of infection. These all fever cases are examined for blood smears to know the malaria parasite load.

Malaria surveillance includes:
* Laboratory confirmation of presumptive diagnosis
* To find out the source of the infection
* Identification of cases and susceptible contacts in order to prevent further spread of disease.

The timely collection and examination of blood smears are the key elements in the National Malaria Control strategy. By giving early radical treatment to detected cases, the human reservoir of malaria parasite is reduced.

Passive Surveillance

All the health institutions screen the fever cases visiting the hospital for malaria by blood slides collection.

Malaria Clinic

Malaria clinics are working in the state in medical institutions where the blood slides are examined same day and radical treatment is also given to positive cases on the spot.

Drug Distribution Center (DDCs)

Antimalaria drugs are distributed to fever cases through drug distribution centers (DDC) in the village; free of cost.

The DDC's do not collect blood slides but administer presumptive treatment to fever cases.

As per revised National Malaria Drug Policy 2008, DDCs are being phased out and instead establishment of FTDs is being promoted.

NATIONAL FRAMEWORK FOR MALARIA ELIMINATION

India 2016–2030

Overview

Overview encouraged by the success achieved in malaria control in recent years, the vision of India's malaria control programme has been now shifted to sustained malaria elimination to contribute more effectively to improved health and quality of life of the people. The National framework for malaria elimination in India 2016–2030 was launched in February 2016.

Vision

- Eliminate malaria nationally and contribute to improved health, quality of life and alleviation of poverty.

Goals

- In line with the WHO Global Technical Strategy (GTS) for Malaria 2016–2030 and the Asia Pacific Leaders Malaria Alliance Malaria Elimination Roadmap, the goals of the National framework for malaria elimination in India 2016–2030 are:
  - Eliminate malaria (zero indigenous cases) throughout the entire country by 2030; and
  - Maintain malaria–free status in areas where malaria transmission has been interrupted and prevent reintroduction of malaria.

Objectives

The National framework for malaria elimination in India has formulated the following objectives:

- By 2022, transmission of malaria interrupted and zero indigenous cases attained in all 26 States/UTs that were under categories 1 and 2 in 2014;
- By 2024, incidence of malaria reduced to less than 1 case per 1000 population in all States and UTs, and their districts;
- By 2027, indigenous transmission of malaria interrupted in all States and UTs of India; and
- By 2030, malaria eliminated throughout the entire country, and re-establishment of transmission prevented.

Phases of Programme

Targets set for malaria elimination in India are as follows:

- **By the end of 2016**
  - All States and UTs have included malaria elimination in their broader health policies and planning framework.

- **By 2020**
  - All 15 States/UTs that were under category 1 (elimination phase) in 2014 have completely interrupted malaria transmission and achieved zero indigenous cases and deaths due to malaria;
  - All 11 States/UTs under category 2 (pre-elimination phase) in 2014 have entered into category 1 (elimination phase);
  - 5 States/UTs under category 3 (intensified control phase) in 2014 have entered into category 2 (pre-elimination phase);
  - 5 States/UTs under category 3 (intensified control phase) in 2014 have reduced disease burden but continue to remain in category 3; and
  - Estimated malaria burden at national level has reduced by 15–20% as compared to 2014.
  - Additionally, states with stronger health systems such as Gujarat, Maharashtra and Karnataka may implement accelerated malaria elimination programmes to achieve interruption of transmission and demonstrate early elimination followed by sustenance of zero indigenous cases.
- **By 2022**
  - All 26 States/UTs that were under categories 1 and 2 in 2014 have interrupted malaria transmission and achieved zero indigenous cases and deaths due to malaria;
  - 5 States/UTs which were under category 3 (intensified control phase) in 2014 have entered into category 1 (elimination phase);
  - 5 States/UTs which were under category 3 (intensified control phase) in 2014 have entered into category 2 (pre-elimination phase); and
  - Estimated malaria burden at national level has reduced by 30–35% as compared to 2014.
- **By 2024**
  - All States and UTs and their districts have reduced API to less than 1 case per 1000 population at risk, sustain zero deaths due to malaria and establish fully functional malaria surveillance to track, investigate and respond to each case.
  - 31 States/UTs have interrupted transmission of malaria and zero indigenous cases and deaths attained.
  - 5 States/UTs which were under category 3 (intensified control phase) in 2014 have entered into elimination phase.
- **By 2027**
  - Indigenous transmission of malaria interrupted, and the entire country has no indigenous cases and no deaths due to malaria.
- **By 2030**
  - The entire country sustained status of zero indigenous cases and deaths due to malaria for 3 consecutive years; and India has initiated the processes for certification of malaria elimination status.

Chapter 36

National Nutritional Anemia Prophylaxis Programme

INTRODUCTION

The Ministry of Health and Family Welfare has revised the guidelines on iron folic acid (IFA) supplementation related to the National nutritional anemia prophylaxis programme (NNAPP).

This is the outcome of a long process, initiated with different consultations on anemia in adolescent girls. The National Consultation on Micronutrients in the end of 2003 with ICMR/MoHFW, worked with the committee (chaired by DG ICMR) constituted subsequently with NRHM and different groups on the 11th plan.

OBJECTIVES

The specific objectives of the programme are:
- To assess the baseline prevalence of nutritional anemia in mothers and young children through estimation of hemoglobin (Hb) levels.
- To put the mothers and children with low Hb levels (<10 g and <8 g respectively) on anti-anemia treatment.
- To put the mother with Hb level >10 g/dL and children with Hb >8 g/dL on the prophylaxis programme.
- To monitor continuously the quality of the tablets, distribution and consumption of the supplements.
- To assess periodically the Hb levels of the beneficiaries.
- To motivate the mothers to consume the tablets through relevant nutrition education (and to give to their children also).

BENEFICIARIES

The scheme beneficiaries are children in 1–5 years of age, pregnant and nursing mothers, female acceptor of terminal methods of family planning and IUDs.

The target beneficiaries of the scheme are 50% of total pregnant and nursing mothers and 25% of total women acceptors of terminal methods and IUDs. The target child population is 50% of total population in the age group of 1–5 years.

ACTIVITIES

The programme focuses on the following activities:
- Promotion of regular consumption of foods rich in iron.

- Supply of iron and folate supplements in the form of tablets (folifer tablets) to the target group.
- Identification and treatment of severely anemic cases. The recommended daily dosages of iron and folic acid (IFA) tablets are as follows:
  - **Adult women:** 60 mg elemental iron + 0.5 mg folic acid.
  - **Children (1–5 years):** 20 mg elemental iron + 0.1 mg folic acid.
    - ❖ For young children, who cannot swallow, liquid syrup containing the same amount of IFA was given (2 mL at a time). This has been discontinued since 1991.

ORGANIZATION

The programme is implemented through the primary health centers and its sub-centers. The multipurpose worker female and other para-medics in the PHC's are responsible for the distribution of IFA tablets (adult and pediatric doses) to beneficiaries. The functionaries of ICDS scheme assist in implementation of programme.

HIGHLIGHTS

- The infants between 6 months and 12 months should also be included in the programme as there is sufficient evidence that iron deficiency affects this age also.
- Children between 6 months and 60 months should be given 20 mg elemental iron and 100 mcg folic acid per day per child as this regimen is considered safe and effective.
- National IMNCI guidelines for this supplementation to be followed.
- For children (6–60 months), ferrous sulfate and folic acid should be provided in a liquid formulation containing 20 mg elemental iron and 100 mcg folic acid per mL of the liquid formulation. For safety reason, the liquid formulation should be dispensed in bottles so designed that only 1 mL can be dispensed each time.
- Dispersible tablets have an advantage over liquid formulations in programmatic conditions. These have been used effectively in other parts of the world and in large scale Indian studies. The logistics of introducing dispersible formulation of iron and folic acid should be expedited under the programme.
- The current programme recommendations for pregnant and lactating women should be continued.
- School children, 6–10 years old, and adolescents, 11–18 years old, should also be included in the National nutritional anemia prophylaxis programme (NNAPP).
- Children 6–10 years old will be provided 30 mg elemental iron and 250 mcg folic acid per child per day for 100 days in a year.
- Adolescents, 11–18 years will be supplemented at the same doses and duration as adults. The adolescent girls will be given priority.

Multiple channels and strategies are required to address the problem of iron deficiency anemia. The newer products such as double fortified salts/sprinkles/ultra rice and other micronutrient candidates or fortified candidates should be explored as an adjunct or alternate supplementation strategy.

WEEKLY IRON FOLIC SUPPLEMENTATION

Weekly iron folic supplementation (WIFS) is an approach that can be effective for ensuring adequate iron status of women, particularly before pregnancy and during the first trimester in communities where food-based strategies are not yet fully implemented or effective.

Short- and medium-term WIFS has been effective in reducing the prevalence of anemia among women of reproductive age in several community settings where the necessary support, social marketing and interpersonal advocacy ensured adequate compliance.

Although the proven method for decreasing the risk for neural tube defects (NTDs) is through daily dosing with folic acid before pregnancy through the first trimester of pregnancy. WIFS provides an additional opportunity for ensuring adequate folate status before pregnancy and in the very early stages of pregnancy particularly for those who may become pregnant or do not know that they are already pregnant and are not covered by other programmes. The impact of weekly supplementation with 60 mg of iron was similar to daily supplementation except in severely anemic women.

CONSULTATION RECOMMENDATIONS

- Strategies to combat both iron deficiency and anemia, and to improve iron reserves and folate status in women of reproductive age should be integrated. Deworming, measures to prevent hookworm infections, the promotion of improved bioavailable iron intake, as well as interventions to control other prevalent causes of anemia, particularly malaria and other infections, and vitamin A deficiency need to be considered.

- In population groups where the prevalence of anemia is above 20% among women of reproductive age and mass fortification programmes of staple foods with iron and folic acid are unlikely to be implemented within 1–2 years, WIFS should be considered as a strategy for the prevention of iron deficiency, the improvement of pre-pregnancy iron reserves and the improvement of folate status in some women. If data on anemia prevalence in women of reproductive age is not available, anemia prevalence in other groups such as pregnant women (>40% anemia prevalence) or children under 5 years of age may be used as a proxy. In the absence of such information, criteria such as dietary patterns and socioeconomic status may be considered. Women from low income groups who may not have access to processed iron-fortified food products and other sources of highly bioavailable iron could be considered a priority group for this intervention.

The weekly supplement should contain 60 mg iron in the form of ferrous sulfate ($FeSO_4.7H_2O$) and 2800 μg folic acid, although evidence for the effective dose of folic acid for weekly supplementation is very limited. Daily folic acid supplementation is effective for reducing the risk of NTDs (Botto LD et al., 1999). The recommendation for the weekly folic acid dosage is based on the participants' rationale of providing 7 times the recommended daily dose to prevent NTDs and the limited experimental evidence demonstrating that this dose can improve red blood cell folate concentrations to levels that have been associated with a reduced risk for NTDs. The iron dose recommended for WIFS may cause short-term gastrointestinal discomfort and black stool, but there is no reported risk of long-term toxicity. The participants also agreed that the recommended weekly folic acid dose has no known toxicity, although evidence for this was limited. Two published studies evaluating weekly folic acid supplementation were considered. In Mexico, women received 5.0 mg folic acid for 3 months, and their red blood cell folate levels were still in the range associated with a 50% lower risk of NTDs one week after the last tablet was consumed (Martinez-de Villarreal LE et al., 2001). They also showed a 50% decrease in the incidence of anencephaly and spina bifida cases, and a significant reduction in infant mortality and disability after two years (Martinez-de Villarreal LE et al., 2002). In New Zealand, once a week supplement of 2.8 mg of folic acid taken for 12 weeks increased women's red blood cell folic acid levels to concentrations associated with a reduced risk of bearing a child with a NTD (Norsworthy B et al., 2004).

Two situations may necessitate supplementation with iron alone. Fortification of staple foods with folic acid has been shown to be very effective and is being widely implemented. Iron alone should be used in weekly supplementation programmes where mandatory folic acid fortification has been introduced and shown to be effective if fortification with iron has not been implemented or is ineffective. Antifolate antimalarial treatment is employed in some malaria endemic regions. There is some evidence to suggest that the efficacy of these drugs may be reduced by folic acid supplementation. In these settings, it is considered prudent to provide iron only weekly supplements.

Upon confirmation of pregnancy, women should receive standard antenatal care. The current WHO recommendation is to provide daily supplementation with 60 mg iron and 400 µg folic acid to women during pregnancy and the first 3 months postpartum.

The WIFS programmes must be integrated with other efforts to control iron deficiency and anemia and should be planned as long-term self-sustained interventions that women of reproductive age will utilize during their childbearing years.

Successful implementation of WIFS programmes will require motivation and creation of demand by women of reproductive age as the starting point for promoting this new approach, establishing adequate mechanisms to start and sustain programmes, including adequate funding, community level support and public-private partnerships including nongovernmental organizations, an uninterrupted supply of good quality iron and folic acid supplements, the development and implementation of effective communication strategies with the media and other information channels, establishment of methods for promoting compliance by women of reproductive age, especially when consumption is not supervised, and integration with effective existing delivery systems in health, education and the private sector (e.g. in factories, markets, and local shops) as well as through community organizations.

Baseline data are needed before launching WIFS interventions; programmes must be monitored closely with regard to both processes and outcomes, during the first year, and then annually for the first 5 years. Monitoring and evaluation systems should be implemented to determine if the intended outcomes are being achieved.

WIFS PROGRAMME IN INDIA

- Government of India decided to implement the WIFS programme for the adolescents from financial year 2013–14.
- Evidence-based programmatic response to the prevailing anemia situation.
- Based on the weekly supplementation of WIFS.
- Provided free of cost iron and folic acid and deworming tablet, along with testing and counseling.
- Cover approximately 13 crore beneficiaries.

Goals

- **Long-term goal:** Break the inter-generational cycle of anemia.
- **Short-term goal:** Nutritionally improved human capital.

Objectives

To reduce the prevalence and severity of nutritional anemia in adolescent population (10–19 years).

Target Group: Implemented in both rural and urban areas and focus on:
- School-based (boys and girls): Three fourth school going adolescent girls and boys in government-aided/municipal schools from 6th to 12th class (10–19 years).

- Community-based through *Anganwadi* center (girls only): Three fourth adolescent girls who are out of school/married/pregnant and lactating adolescent girls.

Strategies

- Screening of target groups for moderate/severe anemia and referring these cases to health facility.
- Administration of weekly iron and folic acid supplementation (WIFS). Each IFA tablet containing 100 mg elemental iron and 500 μg folic acid for 52 weeks in a year.
- Biannual de-worming (Albendazole 400 mg), 6 months apart, for control of worm infestation.
- Information and counseling for improving dietary intake and for taking actions for prevention of intestinal worm infestation.

Benefits

- WIFS may be a more efficient preventive approach because:
  - Three fourth fewer side effects.
  - Three fourth easier to manage at the community level.
  - Three fourth more sustainable.
- Daily dosing of iron and folic acid reduce the risk for
  - Three fourth neural tube defects (NTDs).
  - Three fourth neonatal mortality.
  - Three fourth enhance maternal and infant health.
- Weekly versus daily supplementation with 60 mg of iron had similar impact, except in severity.

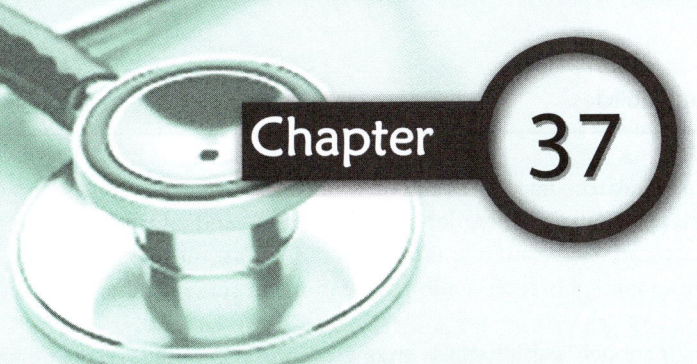

Chapter 37

National Programme for Control and Treatment of Occupational Diseases

INTRODUCTION

Occupational health was one of the components of the National Health Policy 1983 and now also included in National Health Policy 2002 but very little attention has been paid to mitigate the effect of occupational disease through proper programme. Ministry of Health and Family Welfare, Government of India has launched a scheme entitled "National Programme for Control and Treatment of Occupational Diseases" in 1998–99. The National Institute of Occupational Health, Ahmedabad (ICMR) has been identified as the nodal agency for the same.

Major occupational diseases can be divided in following categories:
- Occupational injuries
- Occupational lung diseases
- Occupational cancers
- Occupational dermatosis
- Occupational infections
- Occupation toxicology
- Occupational mental disorders
- Others

Occupational disorders can be grouped according to the etiological factors:
- Occupational injuries: Ergonomic related.
- Chemical occupational factors: Dust, gases, acid, alkali, metals, etc.
- Physical occupational factors: Noise, heat, radiation.
- Biological occupational factors.
- Behavioral occupational factors.
- Social occupational factors.

In India, prevalence of silicosis was 6.2–34% in mica miners, 4.1% in manganese miners, 30.4% in lead and zinc miners, 9.3% in deep and surface coal miners, 27.2% in iron foundry workers, and 54.6% in slate-pencil workers. Prevalence of asbestosis was extended from 3% in asbestos miners to 21% in mill workers. In textile workers, the byssinosis was as common as 28–47%. Nutritional status in terms of body mass indices (BMI) of the workers is also significantly low.

Research projects have been proposed to initiate by the Government:
- Prevention, control and treatment of silicosis and silicotuberculosis in agate industry.

- Occupational health problems of tobacco harvesters and their prevention.
- Hazardous process and chemicals, database generation, documentation, and information dissemination.
- Capacity building to promote research, education, training at National Institute of Occupational Disease.
- Health risk assessment and development of intervention programme in cottage industries with high risk of silicosis.
- Prevention and control of occupational health hazards among salt workers in the remote desert areas of Gujarat and Western Rajasthan.

GLOBAL STRATEGY FOR OCCUPATIONAL HEALTH

The global strategy for achieving occupational health for all [World Health Organization-South-East Asia Regional Office (WHO-SEARO 1999)] includes the following 10 major areas for action:

1. Strengthening of International and National policies for health at work and development of policy tools.
2. Developing healthy work environments.
3. Developing healthy work practices and promoting health at work.
4. Strengthening occupational health services.
5. Establishing support services for occupational health.
6. Developing occupational health standards based on scientific risk assessment.
7. Developing human resources for occupational health.
8. Establishing registration and data system including development of information services for experts, effective transmission of data, and raising public awareness through strengthened public information system.
9. Strengthening research.
10. Developing collaboration in occupational health services and organizations.

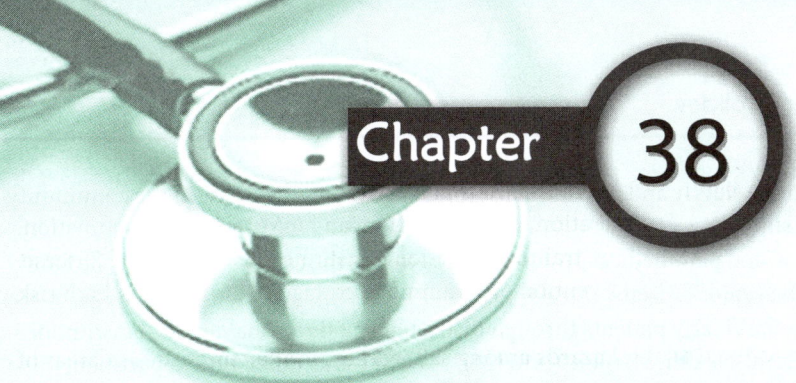

Chapter 38

National Programme for Health Care of the Elderly

INTRODUCTION

The National Programme for Health Care of the Elderly (NPHCE) is an articulation of the International and National commitments of the Government as envisaged under the UN Convention on the Rights of Persons with Disabilities (UNCRPD), National Policy on Older Persons (NPOP) adopted by the Government of India in 1999 and Section 20 of "The Maintenance and Welfare of Parents and Senior Citizens Act, 2007" dealing with provisions for medical care of senior citizen.

The programme has envisaged to provide promotional, preventive, curative and rehabilitative services in an integrated manner for the elderly in various Government health facilities. The range of services will include health promotion, preventive services, diagnosis and management of geriatric medical problems (out and in-patient), day care services, rehabilitative services and home-based care as needed. Districts will be linked to regional geriatric centers for providing tertiary level care.

VISION

The visions of the NPHCE are:
- To provide accessible, affordable, and high-quality long-term, comprehensive and dedicated care services to an aging population.
- To create a new "architecture" for aging.
- To build a framework to create an enabling environment for "a society for all ages".
- To promote the concept of active and healthy aging.

OBJECTIVES

- Main objective of the programme is to provide preventive, curative and rehabilitative services to the elderly persons at various levels of health care delivery system of the country.
- Other objectives are to strengthen referral system, to develop specialized manpower and to promote research in the field of diseases related to old age.

Specific Objectives

- To provide an easy access to promotional, preventive, curative and rehabilitative services through community-based primary health care (PHC) approach.

- To identify health problems in the elderly and provide appropriate health interventions in the community with a strong referral backup support.
- To build capacity of the medical and paramedical professionals as well as the care-takers within the family for providing health-care to the senior citizen.
- To provide referral services to the elderly patients through district hospital regional medical institutions.
- To converge with National Rural Health Mission (NRHM), AYUSH and other line departments like Ministry of Social Justice and Empowerment.

STRATEGIES

Core Strategies

- Community-based PHC approach including domiciliary visits by trained health-care workers.
- Dedicated services at PHC/Community Health Center (CHC) level including provision of machinery, equipment, training, additional human resources, information, education and communication (IEC), etc.
- Dedicated facilities at the district hospital with 10-bedded wards, additional human resources, machinery and equipment, consumables and drugs, training and Information, Eduction and Communication (IEC).
- Strengthening of eight regional medical institutions to provide dedicated tertiary level medical facilities for the elderly, introducing PG courses in geriatric medicine, and in-service training of health personnel at all levels.
- IEC using mass media, folk media and other communication channels to reach out to the target community.
- Continuous monitoring and independent evaluation of the programme and research in geriatrics and implementation of NPHCE.

Supplementary Strategies

- Promotion of public private partnerships in geriatric health care.
- Mainstreaming AYUSH—revitalizing local health traditions and convergence with programmes of Ministry of Social Justice and Empowerment in the field of geriatrics.
- Reorienting medical education to support geriatric issues.

EXPECTED OUTCOMES

- Regional geriatric centers (RGC) in eight regional medical institutions by setting up RGCs with a dedicated geriatric out-patient department (OPD) and 30-bedded geriatric ward for management of specific diseases of the elderly, training of health personnel in geriatric health care and conducting research.
- Postgraduates in geriatric medicine (16) from the eight regional medical institutions.
- Video conferencing units in the eight regional medical institutions to be utilized for capacity building and mentoring.
- District geriatric units with dedicated geriatric OPD and 10-bedded geriatric ward in 80–100 district hospitals.

- Geriatric clinics/rehabilitation units set up for domiciliary visits in community/primary health centers in the selected districts.
- Sub-centers provided with equipment for community outreach services.
- Training of Human Resources in the Public Health-Care System in geriatric care.

PACKAGE OF SERVICES UNDER NPHCE

The programme has envisaged to providing promotional, preventive, curative and rehabilitative services in an integrated manner for the elderly in various Government health facilities. The package of services would depend on the level of health facility and may vary from facility to facility. The range of services will include health promotion, preventive services, diagnosis and management of geriatric medical problems (out- and in-patient), day care services, rehabilitative services and home-based care as needed. Districts will be linked to RGCs for providing tertiary level care. The services under the programme would be integrated below district level and will be an integral part of existing PHC delivery system and vertical at district and above as more specialized health care are needed for the elderly (Table 1).

Table 1: Packages of services to be made available at different levels under NPHCE

Health facility	Packages of services
Sub-center	• Health education related to healthy aging • Domiciliary visits for attention and care to home bound/bedridden elderly persons and provide training to the family care providers in looking after the disabled elderly persons • Arrange for suitable calipers and supportive devices from the PHC to the elderly disabled persons to make them ambulatory • Linkage with other support groups and day care centers, etc. operational in the area Institutional framework for the implementation of NPHCE
Primary health center	• Weekly geriatric clinic run by a trained Medical Officer • Maintain record of the elderly using standard format during their first visit • Conducting a routine health assessment of the elderly person based on simple clinical examination relating to eye, BP, blood sugar, etc. • Provision of medicines and proper advice on chronic ailments • Public awareness on promotional, preventive and rehabilitative aspects of geriatrics during health and village sanitation day/camps • Referral for diseases needing further investigation and treatment, to community health center or the district hospital as per need
Community health center	• First referral unit (FRU) for the elderly from PHCs and below • Geriatric clinic for the elderly persons twice a week • Rehabilitation unit for physiotherapy and counseling • Domiciliary visits by the rehabilitation worker for bed-ridden and elderly patients and counseling of the family members on their home-based care • Health promotion and prevention • Referral of difficult cases to district hospital/higher health care facility

Contd…

Health facility	Packages of services
District hospital	• Geriatric clinic for regular dedicated OPD services to the elderly. • Facilities for laboratory investigations for diagnosis and provision of medicines for geriatric medical and health problems • 10-bedded geriatric ward for in-patient care of the elderly • Existing specialties like general medicine; orthopedics, ophthalmology; ENT services, etc. will provide services needed by elderly patients • Provide services for the elderly patients referred by the CHCs/PHCs, etc. • Conducting camps for geriatric services in PHCs/CHCs and other sites • Referral services for severe cases to tertiary level hospitals
Regional geriatric center	• Geriatric clinic (specialized OPD for the elderly) • 30-bedded geriatric ward for in-patient care and dedicated beds for the elderly patients in the various specialties viz. surgery, orthopedics, psychiatry, urology, ophthalmology, neurology, etc. • Laboratory investigation required for elderly with a special sample collection center in the OPD block • Tertiary health care to the cases referred from medical colleges, district hospitals and below

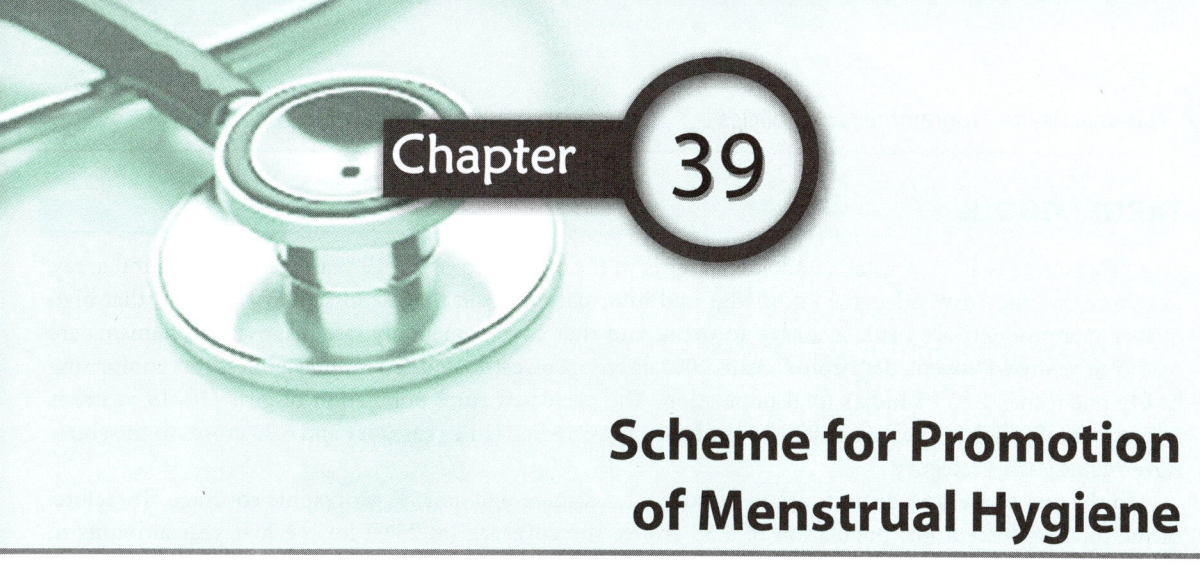

Chapter 39

Scheme for Promotion of Menstrual Hygiene

INTRODUCTION

The Ministry of Health and Family Welfare has introduced a scheme for promotion of menstrual hygiene among adolescent girls in the age group of 10–19 years in rural areas.

The scheme for promotion of menstrual hygiene aims at ensuring that adolescent girls in the target group have adequate knowledge and information about menstrual hygiene and the use of sanitary napkins, that high quality, safe products are made available to them, and that environmentally safe disposal mechanisms are readily accessible. The scheme has been launched as part of the adolescent reproductive and sexual health (ARSH) component under RCH II.

OBJECTIVES

The major objectives of the scheme are:
- To increase awareness among adolescent girls on menstrual hygiene.
- To increase access to and use of high quality sanitary napkins to adolescent girls in rural areas.
- To ensure safe disposal of sanitary napkins in an environment-friendly manner.

Under the scheme, a pack of six sanitary napkins is provided under the NHM's brand 'Freedays'.

In the first phase, the scheme is expected to cover approximately 25% of the country's adolescent girl population (aged 10–19 years), i.e. 1.5 crore girls in 152 districts across 20 states. Out of these, supply of sanitary napkins in 107 districts was envisaged initially in a central supply mode, wherein sanitary napkins were to be supplied by the Government of India. The supply of sanitary napkins in the remaining 45 districts was envisaged in a self-help group (SHG) mode, wherein SHGs were to manufacture the sanitary napkins that are to be sold to adolescent girls. Procurement of sanitary napkins, whether through central supply by the Government of India, or through SHGs, has to be done at a fixed price of ₹7.50/- per pack of six sanitary napkins. The sanitary napkins are provided under NHM's brand, 'Freedays'. These napkins are being sold to adolescents girls at the rate of ₹6 per pack of six napkins by accredited social health activists (ASHAs). From out of the sale proceeds, the ASHA gets an incentive amount of Re. 1 per pack, besides getting a free pack of sanitary napkins per month and the balance ₹5 is to be deposited in the state/district treasury. The scheme has taken off in 107 districts in the 17 States that are being supplied sanitary napkins through central procurement.

TARGET GROUP

This programme will be targeted at adolescent girls in the age group of 10–19 years, residing in rural areas, to ensure that they have adequate knowledge and information about the use of sanitary napkins, that high quality safe products are made available to them, and that environmentally safe disposal mechanisms are readily accessible. Based on data from Census 2001, there are an estimated 225 million adolescents comprising nearly one-fifth (22%) of India's total population. The projected rural population of girls (10–19 years) is 8.55 crores, of which 2.42 crores belong to the below poverty line (BPL) category and 6.13 crores to the above poverty line (APL) category.

In the first phase, 150 districts are to be covered, i.e. there will be 25% geographic coverage. Therefore, of the total adolescent girl population of 8.55 crores, the coverage (at 25%) for the first year amounts to 2.14 crore girls in the target group. Assuming that approximately 70% of population of 2.14 crores of adolescent girls is to be reached, and given varying ages of onset of menarche between 10–12 years, the calculation in this programme is based upon a target population of 1.5 crore girls in the age group of 10–19 years. Out of these 1.5 crore girls, the approximate proportion of APL girls is about 70% (105 lakhs) and that of BPL girls is 30% (45 lakhs).

OVERALL STRATEGY

The scheme adopts two key strategies. Demand generation through ASHA and other community mechanisms such as Women's Groups/Kishori Mandals. An additional mechanism for in-school youth would be that of the AEP through the life skills courses for Classes IX and XI. Supply side intervention through ensuring a supply of a product (sanitary napkin) which is reasonably priced and of high quality.

SELECTION OF DISTRICTS

The initiative will be rolled out in phases, with 25% of the country being covered in the first phase, i.e., 150 districts in selected states. The following criteria are suggested to the states for selection of districts where these interventions may be taken up:
- Existing adolescent health programme.
- Strong AEP intervention.
- Active Self-help Group (SHG) federations.
- Effective ASHA training and support systems.

In the selected districts, the states would cover approximately 70% of the adolescent girl population because of the varying ages of onset of menarche between 10 and 12 years.

COMPONENTS OF THE PROGRAMME

- Community-based health education and outreach in the target population to promote menstrual health.
  - Outreach through ASHA/other community mechanisms.
  - Outreach through schools.
- Ensuring regular availability of sanitary napkins to the adolescents.
  - In the community.
  - In the school.
- Sourcing and procurement of sanitary napkins.
  - Training of ASHA in menstrual hygiene.

- Behavior change communication.
- Safe disposal of sanitary napkins.

The roles and responsibilities at various service delivery levels are given in Table 1.

Table 1: Service delivery framework: Roles and responsibilities at various service delivery levels

Level of care	Service provider	Service package
Village	ASHA/CBOs/SHGs	1. Mobilize adolescent girls. Conduct monthly meetings. Provide health education to adolescent girls 2. Conduct women's group meetings 3. Distribute sanitary napkins to adolescent girls 4. Ensure regular refill and supply of sanitary napkins to the village from the sub-center. Sell sanitary napkins and maintain accounts 5. Track supplies and estimate requirement for the following month 6. Submit progress report on key indicators
Sub-center	ANMs	1. Train ASHA on menstrual hygiene booklet, and conduct periodic refreshers 2. Monitor the monthly meetings periodically 3. Transport the sanitary napkin stock from block PHC to sub-center 4. Ensure safe storage of the sanitary napkin stock 5. Supply requisite number of sanitary napkin packs to ASHA in her sub-center area 6. Provide imprest funds and transportation costs to ASHA 7. Conduct spot checks during regular field visits and village health and nutrition day (VHND) 8. Review and validate ASHA tracking system and accounts register 9. Maintain inventory, tracking and accounts register
PHC	Medical officer/Block account officer	1. Ensures that ASHA training on menstrual hygiene takes place. 2. Ensures safe storage of sanitary napkins. 3. Conducts spot checks during regular field visits. 4. Maintains inventory, tracking and accounts register.
District	CMHO/CS/DPM	1. Serves as the nodal point for the programme. 2. Engages the services of a bookkeeper on a contractual basis to train MO/Block accounts officer and ANM in all blocks on maintaining inventory and accounts for the scheme. 3. Ensures remittance of funds obtained to district health society through the block. 4. Ensures safe storage of sanitary napkins. 5. Monitors the programme on a regular basis. 6. Organizes monthly programme and financial review of the scheme along with other health programmes. 7. Manages convergence of various departments
State	Mission director, NRHM	1. Organizes sourcing of sanitary napkins from SHGs/bidding process 2. Sets up quality cell to ensure conformity with prescribed standards 3. Ensures sound logistics systems for smooth supply to district and below

The operationalization of the programme at the district and sub-district levels is given in Table 2.

Table 2: Operationalization of the programme at the district and sub-district levels

Step 1	Sanitary napkins are supplied to the block warehouse. Storage will need to be organized by states at the block level. Such storage needs to be clean, dry, rodent-free and secure
Step 2	The ANM will collect the sanitary napkins from the block during her monthly meeting visits and transport it to the sub-center. Even when packaged for delivery at the level of the PHC, the commodity is lightweight but bulky, needing adequate space which is free of moisture and pests/rodents. It will be stored at the sub-center or at a place rented for this particular purpose, if the space in the sub-center is insufficient. Such storage will need to be organized by states
Step 3	The ANM will provide the ASHA with a one-time imprest fund of ₹300 (or more if decided by the state steering committee) which she will take from the untied funds pool of the sub-center
Step 4	The ASHA will use the imprest funds to purchase sanitary napkins from the ANM. ASHA will also get a pack of sanitary napkins free every month for her own use to be able to become an effective change agent
Step 5	The ASHA will sell sanitary napkins to the adolescent girls at a price decided by the Government
Step 6	In case ASHA is selling the sanitary napkin packs, she will retain an incentive for every pack sold, the incentive amount being decided by the state steering committee
Step 7	The ASHA will retain the amount recovered from the sale to replenish the imprest amount which the ASHA will use for subsequent purchase
Step 8	The ANM will deposit the funds obtained from the sale of napkins to the ASHA in the united funds of the sub-center
Step 9	These funds will be used for meeting the costs of transportation from Block to sub-center and then to the village and rental to store the sanitary napkins at the Sub-Center level if required
Step 10	The balance fund, if any, after meeting the above costs will be returned to the district health society through the block. The district health society should use these funds for programmes for adolescents

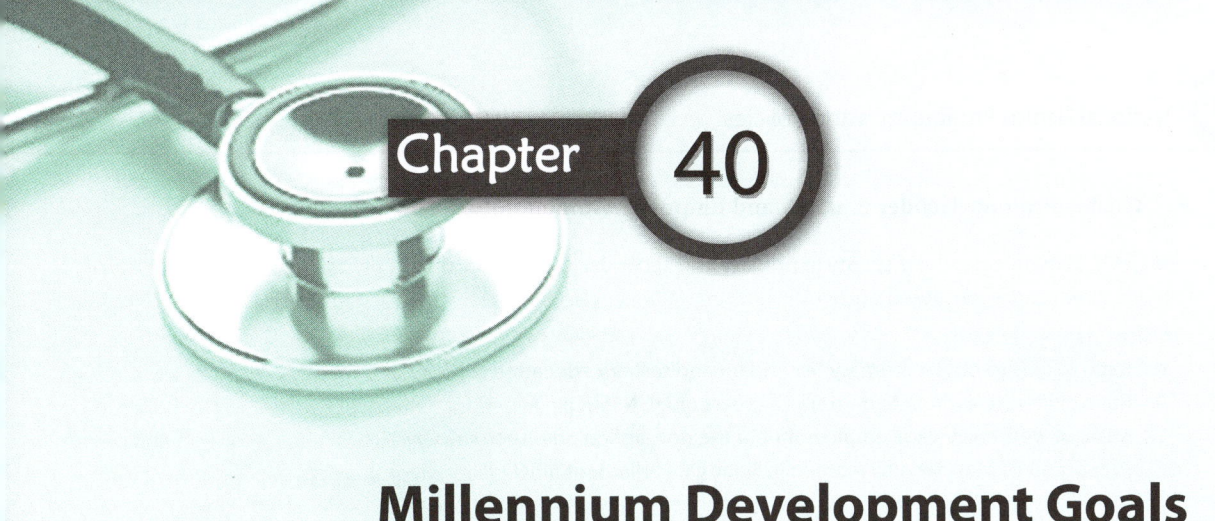

Millennium Development Goals

INTRODUCTION

In September 2000, building upon a decade of major United Nations conferences and summits, world leaders came together at the United Nations Headquarters in New York to adopt the United Nations Millennium Declaration.

The declaration committed nations to a new global partnership to reduce extreme poverty, and set out a series of eight time-bound targets—with a deadline of 2015—that have become known as the **millennium development goals** (MDGs).

The MDGs have helped in bringing out a much needed focus and pressure on basic development issues, which in turn led the governments at national and sub national levels to do better planning and implement more intensive policies and programmes. The MDGs originated from the millennium declaration adopted by the general assembly of the United Nations in September 2000. The MDGs consist of eight goals, and these eight goals address myriad development issues.

MILLENNIUM DEVELOPMENT GOALS

- **Goal 1: Eradicate Extreme Poverty and Hunger**

Target 1. Halve, between 1990 and 2015, the proportion of people whose income is less than $1 a day

Indicators
1. Proportion of population below $1 (1993 PPP) per day (World Bank)
2. Poverty gap ratio [incidence x depth of poverty] (World Bank)
3. Share of poorest quintile in national consumption (World Bank)

Target 2. Halve, between 1990 and 2015, the proportion of people who suffer from hunger

Indicators
4. Prevalence of underweight children under five years of age (UNICEF-WHO)
5. Proportion of population below minimum level of dietary energy consumption (FAO)

- **Goal 2: Achieve Universal Primary Education**

Target 3. Ensure that, by 2015, children everywhere, boys and girls alike, will be able to complete a full course of primary schooling

Indicators
6. Net enrolment ratio in primary education (UNESCO)
7. Proportion of pupils starting grade 1 who reach grade 5 (UNESCO)
8. Literacy rate of 15–24 years old (UNESCO)

- **Goal 3: Promote Gender Equality and Empower Women**

Target 4. Eliminate gender disparity in primary and secondary education, preferably by 2005, and in all levels of education no later than 2015.

Indicators
9. Ratio of girls to boys in primary, secondary and tertiary education (UNESCO)
10. Ratio of literate women to men, 15–24 years old (UNESCO)
11. Share of women in wage employment in the non-agricultural sector (ILO)
12. Proportion of seats held by women in National Parliament (IPU)

- **Goal 4: Reduce Child Mortality**

Target 5. Reduce by two-thirds, between 1990 and 2015, the under-five mortality rate

Indicators
13. Under-five mortality rate (UNICEF-WHO)
14. Infant mortality rate (UNICEF-WHO)
15. Proportion of 1-year-old children immunized against measles (UNICEF-WHO)

- **Goal 5: Improve Maternal Health**

Target 6. Reduce by three-quarters, between 1990 and 2015, the maternal mortality ratio

Indicators
16. Maternal mortality ratio (UNICEF-WHO)
17. Proportion of births attended by skilled health personnel (UNICEF-WHO)

- **Goal 6: Combat HIV/AIDS, Malaria and TB**

Target 7. Have halted by 2015 and begun to reverse the spread of HIV/AIDS

Indicators
18. HIV prevalence among pregnant women aged 15–24 years (UNAIDS-WHO-UNICEF)
19. Condom use rate of the contraceptive prevalence rate (UN Population Division)
19a. Condom use at last high-risk sex (UNICEF-WHO)
19b. Percentage of population aged 15–24 years with comprehensive correct knowledge of HIV/AIDS (UNICEF-WHO)
19c. Contraceptive prevalence rate (UN Population Division)
20. Ratio of school attendance of orphans to school attendance of non-orphans aged 10–14 years (UNICEF-UNAIDS-WHO)

Target 8. Have halted by 2015 and begun to reverse the incidence of malaria and other major diseases

Indicators
21. Prevalence and death rates associated with malaria (WHO)
22. Proportion of population in malaria-risk areas using effective malaria prevention and treatment measures (UNICEF-WHO)
23. Prevalence and death rates associated with tuberculosis (WHO)
24. Proportion of tuberculosis cases detected and cured under DOTS (internationally recommended TB control strategy) (WHO)

- ## Goal 7: Ensure Environmental Sustainability

Target 9. Integrate the principles of sustainable development into country policies and programmes and reverse the loss of environmental resources

Indicators

25. Proportion of land area covered by forest (FAO)
26. Ratio of area protected to maintain biological diversity to surface area (UNEP-WCMC)
27. Energy use (kg oil equivalent) per $1 GDP (PPP) (IEA, World Bank)
28. Carbon dioxide emissions per capita (UNFCCC, UNSD) and consumption of ozone-depleting CFCs (ODP tons) (UNEP-Ozone Secretariat)
29. Proportion of population using solid fuels (WHO)

Target 10. Halve, by 2015, the proportion of people without sustainable access to safe drinking water and basic sanitation

Indicators

30. Proportion of population with sustainable access to an improved water source, urban and rural (UNICEF-WHO)
31. Proportion of population with access to improved sanitation, urban and rural (UNICEF-WHO)

Target 11. Have achieved by 2020 a significant improvement in the lives of at least 100 million slum dwellers

Indicators

32. Proportion of households with access to secure tenure (UN-HABITAT)

- ## Goal 8: Develop Global Partnership for Development

Target 12. Develop further an open, rule-based, predictable, nondiscriminatory trading and financial system (includes a commitment to good governance, development, and poverty reduction, both nationally and internationally)

Target 13. Address the special needs of the Least Developed Countries (includes tariff- and quota-free access for Least Developed Countries exports, enhanced programme of debt relief for heavily indebted poor countries [HIPCs] and cancellation of official bilateral debt, and more generous official development assistance for countries committed to poverty reduction)

Target 14. Address the special needs of landlocked developing countries and small island developing states (through the Programme of Action for the Sustainable Development of Small Island Developing States and 22nd General Assembly provisions)

Target 15. Deal comprehensively with the debt problems of developing countries through national and international measures in order to make debt sustainable in the long term

Indicators
Official development assistance (ODA)

33. Net ODA, total and to LDCs, as percentage of OECD/Development assistance committee (DAC) donors gross national income (GNI)(OECD)
34. Proportion of total bilateral, sector-allocable ODA of OECD/DAC donors to basic social services (basic education, primary health care, nutrition, safe water and sanitation) (OECD)
35. Proportion of bilateral ODA of OECD/DAC donors that is untied (OECD)
36. ODA received in landlocked developing countries as a proportion of their GNIs (OECD)
37. ODA received in small island developing states as proportion of their GNIs (OECD)

India's MDG framework is based on UNDG's MDG 2003 framework, and it includes all the eight goals and 12 out of the 18 Targets (Targets 1 to 11 and 18) which are relevant for India and related 35 indicators. The MDG framework of the country was contextualized through a concordance with the existing official indicators of corresponding dimensions in the national statistical system. This process witnessed dropping some targets and indicators, which are not relevant for India or due to non-availability of sufficiently reliable data and modifying/including some indicators found better suited to the Indian context.

IMPORTANT MODIFICATIONS IN THE MDG FRAMEWORK

Some of the important modifications in the MDG framework of India vis-à-vis the UN MDG framework of 2003 are as follows:

- Targets 12 to 17 of Goal 8 (related to least developed, landlocked and small island countries) were dropped as they were not relevant for India.
- Target 2, indicator 5: Proportion of population below minimum level of dietary energy consumption was dropped due to non-availability of data.
- Target 7, indicator 20: Ratio of school attendance of orphans to school attendance of nonorphans aged 10–14 was dropped due to non-availability of data.
- Target 2, indicator 4: Prevalence of underweight children under 5 years of age has modified as 'prevalence of underweight children under 3 years of age' as per the comparative data availability in national context.
- Target 4, indicator 9: Ratio of girls to boys in primary, secondary and tertiary education was modified as 'Ratio of gross enrolment ratio (GER) of girls to GER of boys in primary, secondary and tertiary education—gender parity index (GPI) of gross enrolment ratio' as the specified indicator 'ratio of girls to boys in primary, secondary and tertiary education' shows only the gender parity in school population, whereas the GPI of GER is adequately reflecting the actual difference between girls and boys enrolment taking into account the population structure of the country.
- Target 7, indicator 19: Condom use rate of the contraceptive prevalence rate was modified as 'Condom use to overall contraceptive use among currently married women 15–49 years' by specifying the age group as per data availability and which covered the reproductive age group.
- In addition to the above, there are minor modifications in some other indicators.

Chapter 41

Rashtriya Bal Swasthya Karyakram

INTRODUCTION

Rashtriya Bal Swasthya Karyakram (RBSK) is an important initiative aiming at early identification and early intervention for children from birth to 18 years to cover 4 'D's viz. Defects at birth, Deficiencies, Diseases, Development delays including disability.

TARGET AGE GROUP

The services aim to cover children of 0–6 years of age in rural areas and urban slums in addition to children enrolled in classes I to XII in Government and Government-aided schools. It is expected that these services will reach to about 27 crores children in a phased manner. The broad category of age group and estimated beneficiary are shown below in the Table 1. The children have been grouped into three categories owing to the fact that different sets of tools would be used and also different set of conditions could be prioritized.

Table 1: Target group under child health screening and intervention service categories

Categories	Age Group	Estimated Coverage
Babies born at public health facilities and home	Birth to 6 weeks	2 crores
Preschool children in rural areas and urban slum	6 weeks to 6 years	8 crores
School children enrolled in class 1st to 12th in government and government-aided schools	6 years to 18 years	17 crores

Health Conditions to be Screened

Child health screening and early intervention services under RBSK envisage to cover 30 selected health conditions for screening, early detection and free management. States and UTs may also include diseases namely hypothyroidism, sickle cell anemia and beta thalassemia based on epidemiological situation and availability of testing and specialized support facilities within State and UTs.

Selected Health Conditions for Child Health Screening and Early Intervention Services

Defects at Birth

- Neural tube defect
- Down syndrome
- Cleft lip and palate
- Talipes club foot
- Developmental dysplasia of the hip
- Congenital cataract
- Congenital deafness
- Congenital heart disease
- Retinopathy of prematurity
- Deficiencies
- Anemia specially severe anemia
- Vitamin A deficiency
- Vitamin D deficiency (Rickets)
- Severe acute malnutrition
- Goiter

Diseases of Childhood

- Skin conditions (Scabies, fungal infection and eczema)
- Otitis media
- Rheumatic heart disease
- Reactive airway disease
- Dental conditions
- Convulsive disorders

Developmental Delays and Disabilities

- Vision impairment
- Hearing impairment
- Neuromotor impairment
- Motor delay
- Cognitive delay
- Language delay
- Behavior disorder
- Learning disorder
- Attention deficit hyperactivity disorder
- Congenital hypothyroidism, sickle cell anemia, beta thalassemia (Optional)

MECHANISMS FOR SCREENING AT COMMUNITY AND FACILITY LEVEL

Child screening under RBSK is at two levels, community level and facility level. While facility-based newborn screening at public health facilities like PHCs/CHCs/DH, will be by existing health manpower like Medical Officers, Staff Nurses and ANMs, the community level screening will be conducted by the mobile health teams at *Anganwadi* centers and Government and Government-aided schools.

Screening at *Anganwadi* center: All pre-school children below 6 years of age would be screened by mobile block health teams for deficiencies, diseases, developmental delays including disability at the *Anganwadi* center at least twice a year. Tool for screening for 0–6 years is supported by pictorial, job aids specifically for developmental delays. For developmental delays children would be screened using age specific tools specific and those suspected would be referred to DEIC for further management.

Screening at Schools-Government and Government-aided: School children aged 6–18 years would be screened by mobile health teams for deficiencies, diseases, developmental delays including disability, adolescent health at the local schools at least once a year. The tool used is questionnaire (preferably translated to local or regional language) and clinical examination.

Composition of mobile health team: The mobile health team will consist of four members—two Doctors (AYUSH) one male and one female, at least with a bachelor degree from an approved institution, one ANM/Staff nurse and one pharmacist with proficiency in computer for data management.

DISTRICT EARLY INTERVENTION CENTER (DEIC)

Following the initial step of screening of children from birth to 18 years of age group for selected health conditions including defects at birth, deficiencies, diseases and developmental delays including disabilities under Rashtriya Bal Swasthya Karyakram (RBSK) through trained and dedicated mobile health teams, the next vital step is confirmation of preliminary findings, referral support, management and follow-up. Under RBSK, these activities viz. confirmation, management, referral, tracking and follow-up, need to be planned according to the age group of the child. The early intervention centers are to be established at the district hospital level across the country as district early intervention centers (DEIC). The purpose of DEIC is to provide referral support to children detected with health conditions during health screening, primarily for children up to 6 years of age group. A team consisting of pediatrician, medical officer, staff nurses, paramedics will be engaged to provide services. There is also a provision for engaging a manager who would carry out mapping of tertiary care facilities in Government institutions for ensuring adequate referral support. The funds will be provided under NHM for management at the tertiary level at the rates fixed by State Governments in consultation with Ministry of Health and Family Welfare. Thus, the DEIC will be the hub of all activities, will act as a clearing house and also provide referral linkages.

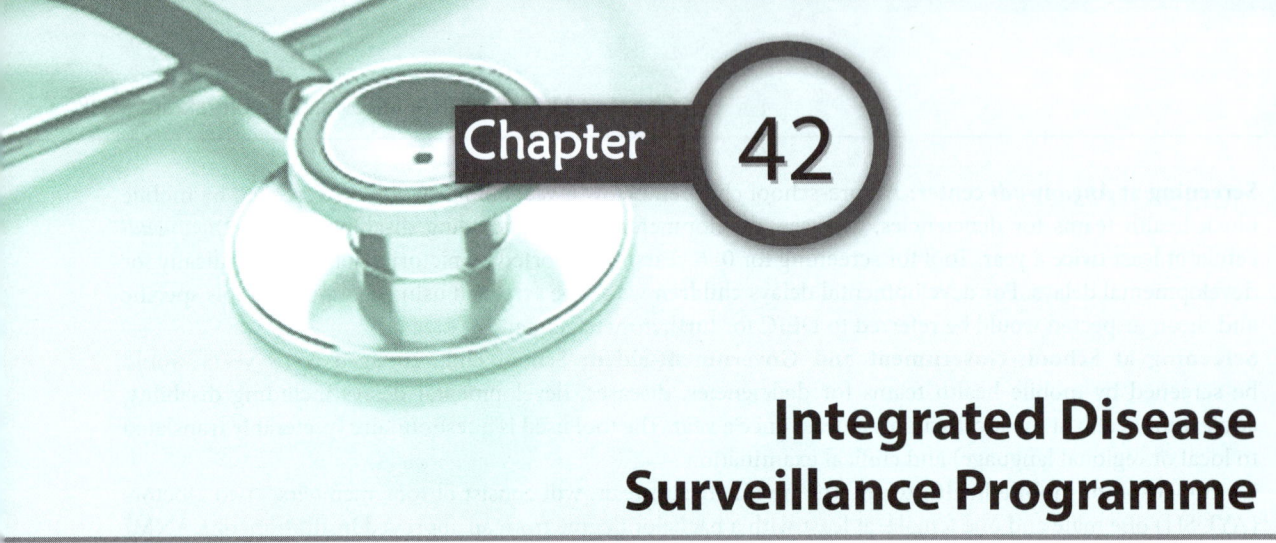

Chapter 42

Integrated Disease Surveillance Programme

INTRODUCTION

Integrated disease surveillance programme (IDSP) was launched with World Bank assistance in November 2004 to detect and respond to disease outbreaks quickly. The project was extended for 2 years in March 2010. From April 2010 to March 2012, World Bank funds were available for Central Surveillance Unit (CSU) at NCDC and 9 identified states (Uttarakhand, Rajasthan, Punjab, Maharashtra, Gujarat, Tamil Nadu, Karnataka, Andhra Pradesh and West Bengal) and the rest 26 States/UTs were funded by domestic budget. The programme will continue during 12th plan under NRHM with outlay of ₹640.40 crore from domestic budget only.

A central surveillance unit (CSU) at Delhi, State surveillance units (SSU) at all States/UT headquarters and district surveillance units (DSU) at all districts in the country have been established (Fig. 1).

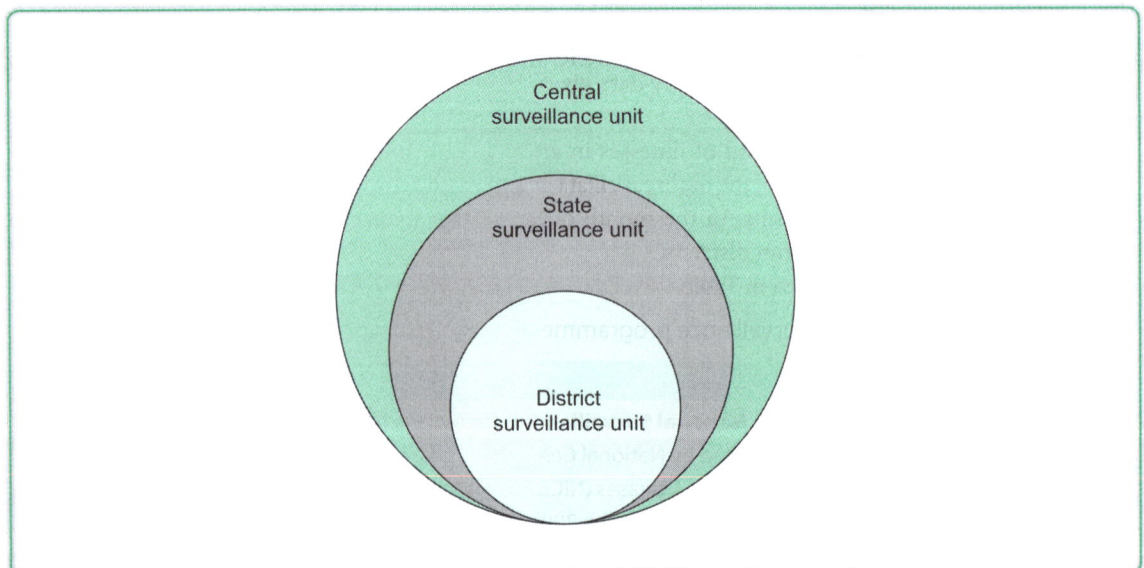

Figure 1: Organization structure of integrated disease surveillance programme

MISSION

To strengthen the disease surveillance in the country by establishing a decentralized state-based surveillance system for epidemic prone diseases to detect the early warning signals, so that timely and effective public health actions can be initiated in response to health challenges in the country at the District, State and National level.

OBJECTIVES

To strengthen/maintain decentralized laboratory-based IT enabled disease surveillance system for epidemic prone diseases to monitor disease trends and to detect and respond to outbreaks in early rising phase through trained rapid response team (RRTs).

PROGRAMME COMPONENTS

- Integration and decentralization of surveillance activities through establishment of surveillance units at Center, State and District level.
- Human resource development: Training of state surveillance officers, district surveillance officers, rapid response team and other medical and paramedical staff on principles of disease surveillance.
- Use of information communication technology for collection, collation, compilation, analysis and dissemination of data.
- Strengthening of public health laboratories.
- Intersectoral coordination for zoonotic diseases.

DATA MANAGEMENT

- Under IDSP, data is collected on epidemic prone diseases on weekly basis (Monday–Sunday). The information is collected on three specified reporting formats, namely "S" (suspected cases), "P" (presumptive cases) and "L" (laboratory confirmed cases) filled by health workers, clinicians and laboratory staff respectively. The weekly data gives information on the disease trends and seasonality of diseases.
- Whenever there is a rising trend of illnesses in any area, it is investigated by the rapid response teams (RRT) to diagnose and control the outbreak. Data analysis and actions are being undertaken by respective state/district surveillance units. In the month of June 2016, about 94% districts have reported weekly disease surveillance data from districts.

The milestones of IDSP are given in Table 1.

Table 1: Integrated disease surveillance programme (IDSP) milestones

Year	Events
1997–98	A pilot project titled **National Surveillance Programme for Communicable Diseases (NSPCD)** initiated and coordinated by National Center for Disease Control (NCDC) formerly National Institute of Communicable Diseases (NICD) and was implemented in 5 districts on a pilot basis. This was expanded to 101 districts by 2004
1998	In 1998, the **Government of India approached the World Bank** to initiate a disease surveillance project

Contd…

Year	Events
September, 2000	The **project preparation commenced** with a meeting at Hyderabad in September 2000, attended by representatives from Central Government, 4 State Governments, WHO, CDC, NIH, USAID, DFID and other national agencies like NCDC (formerly NICD) and ICMR
June, 2001	In June 2001, a **National level workshop** was conducted in New Delhi to reach the consensus
March, 2003	**Central surveillance unit (CSU) was established (at Nirman Bhawan)** in Ministry of Health and Family Welfare
March, 2004	**Expenditure finance committee** approved the proposal for IDSP on 23rd March 2004 with an outlay of ₹ 408.36 crore with 75% share coming from World Bank through soft credit under IDA
September, 2004	Approval from **Cabinet Committee on Economic Affairs (CCEA)** was got on 17th September 2004. The project development credit agreement (DCA) was signed by the GOI and the World Bank on September 23, 2004
November, 2004	World Bank funded project titled **Integrated Disease Surveillance Project (IDSP)** was launched
July, 2005	Development of comprehensive **guidelines for involvement of private sector and medical colleges**
2005	For the operational ease, the **administrative unit was relocated at NICD** under the leadership of director NICD as project director (PD). A Senior officer (ADG level) was designated as National project officer (NPO) to coordinate the project activities
September, 2005	VSAT installations initiated by IDSP through ISRO in phased manner
March, 2006	EDUSAT earth station with central hub established and inaugurated by Hon'ble Health Minister along with SSUs
April, 2006	Data reporting through e-mail started
June, 2006	IDSP was administratively and financially merged with NCDC
August, 2006	National informatics center (NIC) requested to provide feasible solution for ICT component after ISRO communicated that the allotted bandwidth of 8 Mhz is not sufficient for 800 sites planned initially
November, 2006	**Focus state Strategy** was applied to monitor the success of the project implementation in 14 identified states
January, 2007	The fifth component was added to IDSP's component, i.e. **Avian influenza**
February, 2007	Tri-partite MoU signed with NIC, NICSI and IDSP for ICT support. And architecture of IDSP portal for weekly reporting was initiated
September, 2007	**CDC review** of the IDSP, 6–17 September 2007
September, 2007	**Weekly reporting of disease alerts/outbreaks** through IDSP by States/UTs initiated
November, 2007	A **weekly compilation/summary of outbreak reports** was introduced, which became boon in the management of epidemics like Avian Influenza (H5N1), H1N1 Pandemic, Chikungunya, JE, Dengue, etc.
2007–08	Making of IDSP as part of **National Rural Health Mission (NRHM)** in 2007–08

Contd…

Year	Events
2007–08	IDSP initially aimed to support peripheral laboratories and microscopy centers also but discontinued as these are being strengthened by disease specific programmes, like NVBDCP and RNTCP. In 2007–08, it was decided that the programme would only support district public health laboratories (DPHL) and above (state, regional and national)
2007–08	**Infectious disease hospital network** and **urban surveillance in 4 metro cities** were included
February, 2008	**24 × 7, toll free call center (1075)** established to receive disease alerts from all over the country
March, 2008	IDSP/NCDC in consultation with WHO designed a **special 2 week FETP**
April/May, 2008	Data reporting started on Portal as a pilot in April 2008 and in May 2008 the portal was uploaded for all the sites. Data reporting formats (P and L) were revised
June, 2008	Sharing of **weekly summary of outbreaks** reported through IDSP with the stakeholders and other higher officials including Prime Minister's Office (PMO), started
July, 2008	**Media scanning and verification cell** (MSVC) established for detection of early warning signals/unusual health events through various media. The information is shared with the districts affected to investigate and take action
August 2008	Government approved the proposal of **contractual appointments of 766 positions** in January 2008 and the same was approved in 4th NRHM-MSG in August 2008 meeting. MoU signed with NHSRC for recruitment of the approved positions in August 2008. Interviews were held in November and December 2008
2008–09	Due to limited availability of microbiologists to operate the labs and availability of equipment it was decided in 2008–09 to initially support only **50 district public health laboratories**
January, 2009	**Revision of "P" and "L":** During 2008–09, it was decided that in P form, age and gender specific data for cases will not be collected; and also the data element on deaths was deleted as it was being captured in the new NRHM-HMIS formats. List of conditions under surveillance were also revised giving more focus for outbreak prone conditions. Decision was taken to limit the analysis of "S" form data at PHC and district only
March, 2009	Reporting surveillance data through portal started.
June, 2009	**Competency assessment tool** for monitoring the quality of outbreak investigations by IDSP was introduced
2009	Draft plan prepared and initial ground work done during 2009 to initiate **referral laboratory network** for diagnostic support during outbreaks by involving medical colleges and other apex public and private laboratories
2009	Inclusion of 19 regional director (RD) offices and 8 NCDC branches for IT connectivity under IDSP
November, 2009	Restructuring mission of the World Bank for restructuring and extension of project
March, 2010	Project restructured
April, 2010	**Restructured IDSP** project implemented. As per the re-structured project, the World Bank provided funds from 1st April 2010 for Central Surveillance Unit and 9 States (**Tamil Nadu, Karnataka, Gujarat, Punjab, West Bengal, Maharashtra, Uttarakhand, Andhra Pradesh and Rajasthan**). The domestic funds used for the remaining 26 States/UTs

Contd...

Year	Events
April, 2010	The referral laboratory network initiated in the World Bank funded 9 States
May, 2010	Ministry authorized all State Health Societies for **decentralized recruitment** of sanctioned positions at state/districts levels w.e.f. 1/6/2010
September–November, 2010	Exercise for assessment of consistency in data reporting done at CSU for Uttarakhand State as a pilot in September 2010. In November 2010, automated report was developed and uploading on portal to generate the consistency for different levels data reporting for monitoring
Jan, 2011	Since, January 2011, only portal data are being monitored and used for outcome indicators and for sending feedback report to SSU/DSU
February, 2011	The restructuring and extension of the IDSP for 2010–11 and 2011–12 was approved by **expenditure finance committee (EFC) on 28th February 2011**
May, 2011	Block level data entry module in portal developed and piloted in 2 blocks of Gujarat; Choryasi (Surat) and Babra (Amreli)
September, 2011	Data entry at block level started in Chhattisgarh
September, 2011	Recruited **additional contractual manpower in CSU of IDSP** for the speedy progress of the project
February–March, 2012	A **joint implementation review (JIR)** of the integrated disease surveillance project (IDSP) was conducted by the World Bank with technical support from the world health organization (WHO) during February 20–March 16, 2012
October 2012	Continuation of the IDS project is integrated disease surveillance programme (IDSP) as a central scheme during 12th plan period (2012–17) was **approved by empowered programme committee (EPC) of NRHM** on 04.10.2012
January, 2013	Continuation of integrated disease surveillance programme (IDSP) was **approved by mission steering group (MSG) of NRHM and HFM on 04.01.2013 with an outlay of ₹640 crore** for all States/UTs in 12th plan period under NRHM
August 2013	**Strategic workshop on disease surveillance:** A two-day workshop was held on 8th and 9th August, 2013, Delhi, with the objective to develop a road map for strengthening IDSP implementation in 12th plan period and identifying the role to be played by public health institutes/medical colleges in disease surveillance
2013	The strategic health operations center (SHOC) is established under IDSP to strengthen the outbreak detection and response capacities of the states and districts by utilizing state-of-the-art information technology
2014–2015	National review workshop held from 26th to 28th November 2014, at NCDC, Delhi and 14th -16th May 2015 and JMM in November–December 2015
2015	Block level data entry in phased manner in the country
2015	Offline data entry at IDSP portal in phased manner in the country

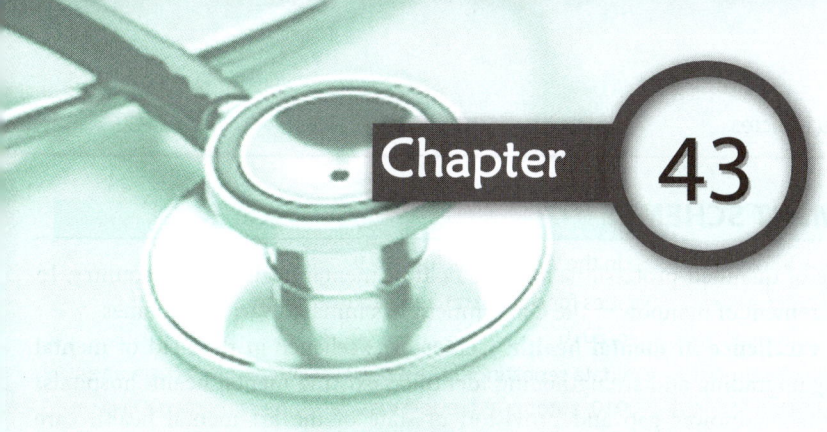

Chapter 43

National Mental Health Programme

INTRODUCTION

National Mental Health Programme (NMHP) was started in 1982 with the objectives to ensure availability and accessibility of minimum mental health care for all, to encourage mental health knowledge and skills and to promote community participation in mental health service development and to stimulate self-help in the community. Gradually the approach of mental health care services has shifted from hospital-based care (institutional) to community-based mental health care, as majority of mental disorders do not require hospitalization and can be managed at community level.

MENTAL HEALTH POLICY

A group of experts was constituted for the specific task of formulating a mental health policy (MHP) for the country in specific context of mental illness in India and Internationally accepted guidelines. On 10 October, 2014, this Ministry had launched for the first time the National Mental Health Policy with the vision of promoting mental health, preventing mental illnesses, enabling recovery and socioeconomic inclusion of persons affected by mental illness by providing accessible, affordable and quality health and social care to all persons through their life span. The goal is to reduce stress, disability, exclusion, morbidity and premature mortality associated with mental health problems.

DISTRICT MENTAL HEALTH PROGRAMME

District Mental Health Programme (DMHP) was initiated (1996) based on Bellary Model developed by NIMHANS, Bengaluru. In addition to early identification and treatment of mentally ill people, district mental health programme has now incorporated promotive and preventive activities for positive mental health which include:

- Life skills education in schools and counseling services
- College counseling trained services: Through teachers/councilors
- Work place stress management: Formal and informal sectors, including farmers, women, etc.
- Suicide prevention services: Counseling center at district level, sensitization workshops, IEC, helplines, etc. At present, DMHP has been extended to 241 districts in the country.

MANPOWER DEVELOPMENT SCHEMES

There has been an acute shortage of qualified professionals in the field of mental health in the country. In order to address the issue of requirement of manpower, the Government has initiated various schemes.

- **Establishment of center of excellence in mental health:** Center of excellence in the field of mental health is being established by upgrading and strengthening identified existing mental health hospitals/ institutes for addressing acute manpower gap and provision of state of the art mental health care facilities in the long run. Total budgetary support of up to ₹338 crore (up to ₹30 crore per center) to be provided for undertaking capital work, equipment, library, faculty induction and retention for the plan period. As of now 11 Mental Health Institutes have been funded for developing them as centers of excellence in mental health. It has been envisaged to establish 10 more centers of the excellence in mental health during the 12th Five-Year Plan with a total budgetary support of ₹360 crores (up to ₹36 crores per center).

- **Establishment/up-gradation of postgraduate training departments:** To provide an impetus to development of manpower in mental health, other training centers (Government Medical Colleges/ Government General Hospitals/State run Mental Health Institutes) were also to be supported for starting postgraduate (PG) courses or increasing the intake capacity for PG training in mental health. Till date 27 PG departments in mental health specialties viz. psychiatry, clinical psychology, psychiatric nursing and psychiatric social work have been provided support for their establishment/ strengthening. During the 12th Five-Year Plan, it has been envisaged to provide support for establishment/strengthening of 93 additional PG Departments in mental health specialties with a limit of ₹1.07 crore to ₹1.25 crore per PG department.

- **Research and training:** There is a gap in research in the field of mental health in the country. Funds will be provided to institutes and organizations for carrying basic, applied and operational research in mental health field. In order to address shortage of skilled mental health manpower, a short-term, skill-based training will be provided to the DMHP teams at identified institutes. Standard treatment guidelines, training modules, CME, distance learning courses in mental health, surveys etc. will also be supported.

- **Information, education and communication (IEC):** It has been observed that there is low awareness regarding mental illness and availability of treatment. There is also lot of stigma attached to mental illness leading to poor utilization of available mental health resources in the country. The awareness of mental health under provisions of Mental Health Act, 1987 is also very low among the public and implementing authorities. These issues are addressed through IEC activities at the district level by the district mental health programme. In addition to the district level activities, National Mental Health Programme Division conducts nationwide mass media campaign through audio-video and print media. An intensive national level mass media campaign on awareness generation regarding mental health problems and reduction of stigma attached to mental disorders was undertaken under NMHP.

- **Support for central and state mental health authorities:** As per Mental Health Act, 1987, there is provision for constitution of Central Mental Health Authority (CMHA) at central level and State Mental Health Authority (SMHA) at State level. These statutory bodies are entrusted with the task of development, regulation and coordination of mental health services in a State/UT and are also responsible for the implementation of Mental Health Act, 1987 in their respective States and Union Territories. States are required to have functional SMHAs to operationalize the mental health programme activities. Till date, funds have been provided to 32 State Mental Health Authorities in 32 States/UTs.

- **Monitoring and evaluation:** In order to strengthen the monitoring and improve implementation of existing NMHP schemes in states, support has been approved under the programme during 12th five-year plan period. A survey to ascertain the number of mentally ill patients and availability of mental health resources in the country has been commissioned through NIMHANS, Bengaluru.

Chapter 44

National Programme for Prevention and Control of Fluorosis

INTRODUCTION

Government of India started 100% centrally approved "National Programme for Prevention and Control of Fluorosis (NPPCF)" as a new health initiative during 11th Five-Year Plan in a phased manner. During the 11th Plan, 100 districts from 17 States were identified for programme implementation. During the 12th Five-Year Plan, it is proposed to add another 95 districts for prevention and control of fluorosis. Further, in the 12th Plan the programme has been brought under the NCD Flexi-pool of National Health Mission (NHM). The ratio of sharing of funds between Center and State accordingly would be 75 : 25 and in case of North Eastern States would be 90 : 10.

GOAL AND OBJECTIVES

The NPPCF aims to prevent and control fluorosis disease in the country.

Objectives of the national programme for prevention and control of fluorosis are as follows:

- To collect, assess and use the baseline survey data of fluorosis of Ministry of Drinking Water Supply for starting the project.
- Comprehensive management of fluorosis in the selected areas.
- Capacity building for prevention, diagnosis and management of fluorosis cases.

STRATEGIES

- **Capacity building** (Human resource) at different levels of health care delivery system for early detection, management and rehabilitation of fluorosis cases.
  - **Training:** Various types of training, advocacy and sensitization for various categories of health professionals/personnel at different levels of health care facilities such as health workers, ASHA, *Anganwadi* workers, policy makers, Panchayati Raj Institutions (PRI's), Village Health and Sanitation Committee (VHSC) and teachers will be undertaken at district level. There will be trainers training for state nodal officer, district nodal officers, district consultants at headquarter of any endemic state/ any recognized reference laboratory by National experts. Besides, laboratory monitoring/techniques

(estimation of fluoride in urine) training for laboratory technicians at any recognized national reference laboratory will be undertaken.

■ **Manpower support:** In order to implement the activities under the programme, manpower support at National level and district level, one national consultant and one data entry operator (DEO) at central level and one district consultant, one lab technician and three field investigators (for six months) on contractual basis in the district are provided. Surveillance of fluorosis in the community including school children survey will be conducted by the district contractual staff in association with district health officials as per surveillance guidelines for assessment and diagnosis of fluorosis cases including dental fluorosis in children in the age group of 6–11 years, skeletal and nonskeletal fluorosis at community level. After availability of baseline data, resurvey after three months of intervention activities.

● **Establishment of diagnostic facilities in the district/medical hospitals:** It is proposed to strengthen the laboratory diagnostic facilities in district/hospitals/medical college for early detection and confirmation of fluorosis cases.

● **Management of fluorosis cases including treatment, surgery, rehabilitation:**

■ **Early detection:** The identified cases shall be confirmed by
  ❖ Physical examination, i.e. dental changes, pain and stiffness in peripheral joints, skeletal deformities.
  ❖ Laboratory tests, i.e. urine, and drinking water analysis for fluoride level and where possible.
  ❖ Radiological examination, i.e. X-ray of forearm, X-ray of most affected part.

■ **Prompt intervention:** The prompt intervention is planned in the following manner:
  ❖ **Health education** is very important aspect of management. Creating awareness about fluorosis disease, drinking water (safe/unsafe), diet editing and diet counseling through interpersonal communication, group discussions, media, posters, wall paintings, etc. Fluorosis is mainly caused due to excess intake of fluoride through drinking water/food products/industrial pollutants over a long period. Fluorosis is not diagnosed as fluorosis even by several of the medical professionals. This is because there is not much awareness of the problem from the health point of view. There is need to create awareness and skills among the medical as well as paramedical health workers to detect the disease in the community.
  ❖ **Provision of safe drinking** water, water harvesting (rain water), other measures in collaboration with public health engineering department.
  ❖ **Referral** effective linkages would be developed from village level to district with the help of functionaries and personnel from grass-roots level (AWW, ASHA, PRIs, etc.) PHC/CHC level medical officers, health personnel, school teachers and district level officers.
  ❖ **Medical management:** Efforts are aimed to reduce the fluorosis induced disability and to improve quality of life of affected patients. Medical treatment is mainly supplementation of vitamins C and D, calcium, antioxidants and treatment of malnutrition. Treatment of deformity includes physiotherapy, corrective plasters, orthosis (appropriate appliances).

The programme commenced implementation in 100 endemic districts in 17 States/UTs in a phased manner during the 11th Five-Year Plan. During 2008–09, six districts were selected from each of the six zones of the country based on the information collected from Ministry of Drinking Water and Sanitation. The activities included baseline survey, diagnosis of fluorosis afflicted areas, capacity building by setting up/ strengthening laboratory for fluoride estimation, training of medical and laboratory manpower, early detection and rapid management and awareness generations through Informative Education Communications (IEC).

ACTIVITIES

Activities required to initiate the NPPCF:
- Procurement of ion meter and other items for fluoride testing.
- Training of laboratory technicians for five days in a reputed institution, where fluoride testing is a regular activity.
- Training of consultants on all aspects of fluorosis—two days

Programme Activities

- Community diagnosis of fluorosis village/block/cluster wise.
- Facility mapping for prevention, health promotion, diagnostic facilities, reconstructive surgery and medical rehabilitation point of view—village/block/district wise.
- Gap analysis in facilities and organization of physical and financial support for bridging the gaps, as per strategies listed above.
- Behavioral changes through appropriate IEC strategy.
- All members having fluorosis should be introduced to interventions and monitored to improve health. Three months later, health complaints and UFL to be reassessed.
- Referrals for severe cases and their follow-up.

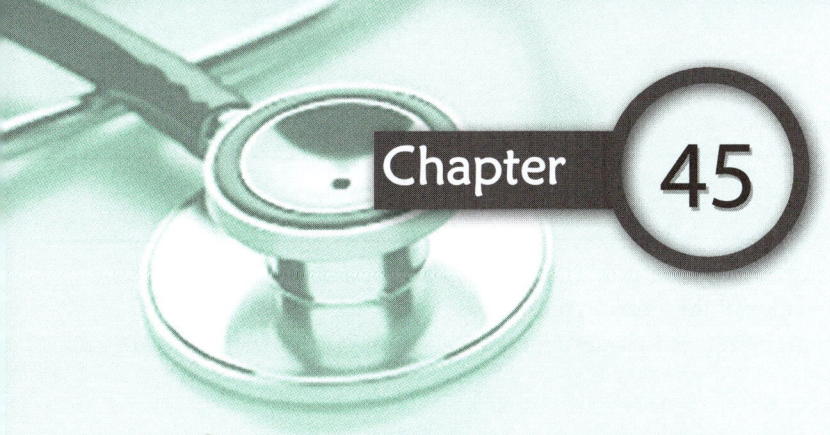

Chapter 45

National Tobacco Control Programme

INTRODUCTION

The National Tobacco Control Programme (NTCP) was launched by the Ministry of Health and Family Welfare (MoHFW), Government of India in 2007–08, during the 11th Five-Year Plan, with the following objectives:

- To bring about greater awareness about the harmful effects of tobacco use and about the tobacco control laws.
- To facilitate effective implementation of the tobacco control laws.

SCOPE

The interventions under the NTCP have been largely planned at the primordial and primary levels of prevention. The main thrust areas for the NTCP are as follows:

- Training of health and social workers, NGOs, school teachers, enforcement officers, etc.
- Information, education and communication (IEC) activities.
- School programmes.
- Monitoring tobacco control laws.
- Coordination with panchayati raj institutions for village level activities.
- Setting-up and strengthening of cessation facilities including provision of pharmacological treatment facilities at district level.

In order to improve the quality of implementation of the NTCP at the state and district levels, the National Tobacco Control Cell (NTCC) at the Ministry of Health and Family Welfare (MoHFW) has formulated the Operational Guidelines of the NTCP. These guidelines are to be used as a reference document by the various agencies working at the state and district levels to further the goal of tobacco control.

The Government of India enacted the national tobacco-control legislation namely the Cigarettes and Other Tobacco Products (Prohibition of Advertisement and Regulation of Trade and Commerce, Production, Supply and Distribution) Act in May, 2003.

India also ratified the WHO-Framework Convention on Tobacco Control (WHO-FCTC) in February 2004. Further, in order to facilitate the effective implementation of the tobacco control law, to bring about greater awareness about the harmful effects of tobacco as well as to fulfill the obligations under the WHO-FCTC, the Ministry of Health and Family Welfare, Government of India launched the National Tobacco Control Programme (NTCP) in 2007–08 in 42 districts of 21 States/Union Territories of the country.

OBJECTIVES

- To bring about greater awareness about the harmful effects of tobacco use and tobacco control laws.
- To facilitate effective implementation of the tobacco control laws.

The objective of this programme is to control tobacco consumption and minimize the deaths caused by it.

GOALS

The goals of NTCP are to eliminate exposure to environmental tobacco smoke; promote quitting among adults and youth; prevent initiation among youth; identify and eliminate disparities among population groups.

COMPONENTS

The four components of NTCP are:
- Population-based community interventions
- Counter-marketing
- Programme policy/regulation
- Surveillance and evaluation

ACTIVITIES

The various activities planned to control tobacco use are as follows:
- Training and capacity building
- IEC activity
- Monitoring tobacco control laws and reporting
- Survey and surveillance

Major Components and Activities at National Level

National level public awareness/mass media campaigns for awareness building and behavioral change: Mass media plays a key role in shaping tobacco-related knowledge, opinion, attitude and behavior, and is an extremely powerful tool for influencing both individuals and policy-makers. It is effective for disseminating information on the ill-effects of tobacco, discouraging the use of tobacco products, encouraging tobacco cessation and creating awareness about the provisions of COTPA and the need to comply with them. One of the key objectives of NTCP is to create public awareness about the harmful effects of tobacco usage, second hand smoke and various provisions under COTPA (2003). This can be only achieved through sustained public awareness/mass media campaigns targeting in particular the youth, women and vulnerable population through appropriate communication strategies, using a combination of the media and other grass-roots level interventions/approaches. Various TV/Radio spots and publicity materials (posters, stickers, handouts, factsheets) have been developed by Ministry of Health and Family Welfare (MoHFW) focusing on different themes and the same are being used to carry out sustained campaign at regular intervals. These TV/Radio spots have been translated in over 15 Regional languages for a wide variety of audience and can be downloaded from the Ministry's website at www.mohfw.nic.in.

Establishment of Tobacco Product Testing Laboratories

As a statutory obligation to COTPA, Ministry of Health and Family Welfare is in the process of setting up one apex laboratory and four regional tobacco testing laboratories. These laboratories will test the contents and emissions of all the tobacco products (both smoking and smokeless forms) as per the extant Rules.

Mainstreaming research and training on alternative crops and livelihoods with other nodal Ministries: Tobacco control is a multisectoral subject since there are a number of cross-cutting issues which do not lie within the domain of the Ministry of Health and Family Welfare. Issues like alternative crops (Ministry of Agriculture) and alternative livelihood for bidi rollers (Ministry of Labor/Ministry of Rural Development) need involvement of other Government Departments/Ministries. Hence, there is a need to bring on-board these stakeholder Departments/Ministries. The MoHFW has already collaborated with Central Tobacco Research Institute (CTRI) for a pilot project on alternative cropping system to tobacco growing. The MoHFW is also in discussion with Ministry of Rural Development to work out special projects for the bidi workers under the National Rural Livelihood Mission (NRLM). In addition, research on critical and cross cutting issues like alternative livelihoods for people engaged in the tobacco sector and alternative cropping system need to be taken up to build scientific evidence.

Monitoring and Evaluation Including Surveillance

As part of surveillance of tobacco use, Global Adult Tobacco Survey (GATS), India was undertaken in 2009–10 with technical support of WHO and the center for disease control (CDC), USA, to systematically monitor adult tobacco use and track key tobacco control indicators. The data from GATS is being used to map the extent of tobacco epidemic across states, to facilitate formulation of region/state specific strategies and provide clear direction for future interventions. The GATS-India provides us baseline data and can also be used as a tool to evaluate the implementation of NTCP, if repeated on a regular basis. There is a need to integrate the data on tobacco use and other key indicators in the ongoing health surveys like District Level Household and Facility Survey (DLHS), National Sample Survey Organization (NSSO), NCD Steps survey, etc. Further, in order to monitor the implementation of the NTCP at State/District level, NTCC has developed a reporting format in which data is collated at state/district cells and compiled by NTCC on a quarterly basis for regular monitoring of key parameters of the programme.

Integrating NTCP as a part of health care delivery mechanism under the National Rural Health Mission (NRHM) Framework and with other national health programmes: Tobacco has been identified as a risk factor for a number of communicable as well as noncommunicable diseases. Hence, it is suggested that the activities of NTCP at state/district level be synergized with NRHM and other national programmes by utilizing the existing manpower and infrastructure. For capacity building of States/Districts, awareness generation through mass media and monitoring/enforcement of anti-tobacco law, the states must explore the possibilities of integrating it as part of the NRHM activities and through the existing state health care delivery mechanism. Similarly, the manpower available under National Programme for Prevention and Control of Cancer, Diabetes, Cardiovascular Diseases and Stroke (NPCDCS), National Mental Health Programme (NMHP) and National Programme for Health care of Elderly (NPHCE) may be synergized for tobacco control measures as well. The tobacco cessation services may be included as part of the counseling services under NPCDCS, NMHP/Drug-de-addiction Programme(s), Integrated Counseling cum Testing Center (ICTC) under the National AIDS control programme.

NTCP AT STATE LEVEL

Every identified State/UT has a state tobacco control cell (STCC) in the state health department. The space for setting up the STCC is provided by the State Government. The STCC is responsible for overall planning, implementation and monitoring of different activities, and achievement of physical and financial targets planned under the programme in the state.

The STCC is headed by a State Nodal Officer, who is a Senior Officer from State Department of Health preferably on a full time basis, to look after all the NCD programmes like [NPCDCS, NTCP, NMHP, NPHCE]. Other team members of this cell include programme assistant and data entry operator appointed under NTCP. This cell may be placed as a subset of national rural health mission under the overall supervision of MD NRHM in the states.

Activities of STCC

Activities of State Tobacco Control Cell (STCC): The major activities of STCC are:

- **Training:** STCCs should train multiple stakeholders for tobacco control through state level advocacy workshops/sensitization programmes. Efforts should be made to involve all the state government departments for tobacco control. Specific/tailor made trainings should be organized for academicians, health/medical professionals, students, police, food and drug safety authorities, judiciary, media, etc. For this purpose, they should work very closely with NGO partners and involve them in advocacy workshops.
- **Integrating tobacco control with other health programmes/activities:** The tobacco control initiatives may be integrated with NCD programmes like NPCDCS, NMHP and NPHCE and also RNTCP being implemented in the states. The state team should also collaborate and cooperate with the team members of other health programmes under NRHM.
- **Incorporating tobacco control in the state level IEC campaign:** The IEC material developed by the NTCC can be locally adapted by the state team. The STCC is expected to guide and organize extensive IEC activities including health melas, bill boards, hand bills, posters, street plays, local cable network, etc. Efforts should also be made to integrate the IEC under NTCP with the State Health IEC under NRHM/NPCDCS/RNTCP or other similar health programmes to have better focus and to derive greater benefits.
- **Manpower for STCC:** There is provision of recruitment of two contractual staff at the state level to assist the State Nodal Officer in tobacco control initiatives. The two personnel are: Programme assistant and data entry operator. The terms of reference of the above personnel is at Annexure-IV. The state teams should be trained at the national level by the staff involved in NTCP through training workshops organized at regional level. They should also be given the opportunity to participate in trainings and meetings organized by MoHFW or by other agencies working on tobacco control.

Roles and Responsibilities

Roles and responsibilities of STCC: The following roles and responsibilities of STCC are indicative and not exhaustive:

- Implementation, supervision and monitoring of the various activities of the programme as per the quarterly report format.
- Recruitment of the staff at the state/district tobacco control cells, training of the staff and guidance to the district cells.
- Establishing tobacco cessation clinics in health care facilities and up-scaling tobacco cessation facilities through training of health care providers.

- Organizing state level training/sensitization programmes on tobacco control.
- Sharing and disseminating all the government orders and best practices to the districts.
- Enforcement of COTPA:
  - Display the Act and the rules on the official website of the state and regular communication to the officers of other departments who are authorized for enforcement of various provisions of the Act and the rules.
  - Open a separate head of account, printing of challan and receipt books and sending the same to districts.
  - Constitution of a state level monitoring committee for section–5 of COTPA and to take cognizance of the direct/indirect advertisement of tobacco products.
  - Conducting regular checks at public places, public conveyances, point of sale, etc. for compliance with COTPA.
- Adapting IEC materials developed by NTCC and disseminating it to districts.
- Advocacy and networking with NGOs, Nehru Yuva Kendras Sangathan, National Service Scheme, National Cadet Corps (NCC), Indian Medical Association, Indian Dental Association, Rotary International, SHGs, etc. for creating awareness against tobacco. Coordination with Departments of Agriculture, Social Welfare, Rural Development, Labor and other stakeholders for developing sustainable alternative crops and livelihood for tobacco growers/workers and bidi rollers.
- Coordination with the Finance/Taxation department for progressive increase of taxes on tobacco, tobacco products and inputs thereon.
- Coordination with department of education for reaching out to the youth and young children.
- Ensuring regular reporting to NTCC and assisting districts in timely submission of utilization certificate (UC) to ensure regular fund flow.
- Documentation of the best practices on tobacco control in the state and sharing thereof within the state and beyond.

NTCP AT DISTRICT LEVEL

Every identified district should have a District Tobacco Control Cell (DTCC) in the district hospital. The space for setting up the DTCC should be provided by the district authorities. The DTCC is responsible for overall planning, implementation, and monitoring of the different activities and achievement of physical and financial targets under the programme at the district level. The role of the DTCC is crucial as most of the activities under NTCP are to be implemented at district and sub district level. The DTCC is headed by District Nodal Officer preferably Chief Medical Officer/Civil Surgeon on a full time basis. For achieving synergy, it is desirable that the District Nodal Officer under NTCP is also given the responsibility to look after the NCD programmes like NPCDCS, NMHP and NPHCE. Other team members of this cell include a psychologist/counselor, social worker and data entry operator appointed on contract basis under NTCP. Every district should constitute an enforcement squad preferably under the Collector/District Magistrate (DM). The squad will be responsible for monitoring compliance with COTPA and taking action against any violations in the district.

District level coordination committee (DLCC): Each district should have a DLCC chaired by Collector or District Magistrate, and District Nodal Officer as the member secretary, who should convene the meetings of the committee.

Activities of DTCC

The major activities of DTCC are:

Training and Capacity Building of Relevant Stakeholders

- **Target trainees:** Training and capacity building is an important activity of DTCC. DTCC, under its initiative, should organize training programmes for multiple stakeholders in the district, which include doctors, nurses, community health workers, ASHAs, civil society organizations, NCC, NSSO, IMA, IDA, teachers, officials from enforcement departments, like police, food authorities, municipal officers, etc.
- **Training modules:** The key areas/topics to be covered for the training programmes should include: introduction of and key provisions under the National Tobacco Control Programme, Tobacco Control Act; prevalence of tobacco use; types and forms of tobacco; adverse health effects of tobacco use; socioeconomic consequences of tobacco use; benefits of quitting tobacco; role of civil society and other stakeholders in tobacco control at district level. The participants should be provided with existing training modules and other necessary resource material.
- **Resource persons for training:** The resource persons for the training sessions should be carefully selected according to their areas of interest. Effort should be made to identify local resource persons along with a few experts from the state as well as from the national levels.
- **Number and duration of trainings:** There should be three categories of trainings at the district level:
  - One district level advocacy and capacity building workshop for multiple stakeholders at district level. This should be a full day workshop and the number of participants should be 100. Efforts should be made to involve members from the district administration and the District Magistrate/ Collector may be invited as the chief guest in the workshop. Local politicians and policymakers may also be included in the guest list.
  - Ten training workshops for target groups should be organized throughout the year with 50 participants in each group. These trainings should be of half-a-day and the staff of DTCC should organize them in the workplaces/offices of the trainees/groups.
  - Integrating a session on tobacco control laws and related issues in existing training programmes or organized by NRHM or other departments like police, food and drugs administration, excise, department of women and child development, etc. The members of DTCC should make efforts to include a session on tobacco control in the agenda in the existing training programmes under different national programmes (both health and nonhealth).

School Awareness Programmes

School awareness programmes should be conducted to help the youth and the adolescents to acquire the knowledge, attitude and skills that are required to make informed choices and decisions and understand the consequences of tobacco use. It will empower students to contribute to the creation of tobacco-free environment in which they can learn and live. It is important to sensitize children at an early age and reinforce the same message at later stage. There can be two models in school programme:

- Integrate tobacco control activities in the schools already having/existing school health programme; and
- Initiate tobacco control programmes in 50 schools in a district.
  - Number of schools in a district: 50 schools in one district per year should be adopted and included in school awareness programme. Selection of the schools should be done carefully with a combination of government and private schools. The programme should target the students of middle school and onwards.

- Implementation of school programme: NGOs working on tobacco control issues or health programmes may be identified by DTCC and engaged for implementing the school programmes. The district nodal officer should regularly guide and monitor the activities of NGOs. He/she should also monitor the activities conducted in the schools covered under the programme. [(Guidelines for selection of NGOs under the National Tobacco Control Programme (NTCP) are at Annexure- VIII and four steps for implementation of school programme refer Annexure-IX.]
- Training module and guidelines for teachers: The following training module for teachers along with other training material has been developed:
  - ❖ A guide for teachers by Directorate General of Health Services and MoHFW.
  - ❖ Other IEC/Campaign materials developed by MoHFW.
- The annual budget for school programme per school should be ₹8000/- (Total ₹8000 × 50 = ₹4,00,000).

Setting up and Expansion of Tobacco Cessation Facilities

Tobacco contains nicotine, which is a highly addictive substance and leads to chronic nicotine dependency. To overcome this dependency, the tobacco users need help and counseling to gradually quit tobacco use. Thus, death and debilitating disease due to tobacco use can be reduced significantly through an increased emphasis on cessation programmes. Studies have indicated that by 2050, if the focus is only on prevention of initiation and not cessation of tobacco use, the result will be an additional 160 million deaths among smokers.

- Information, education and communication (IEC)/media campaign
  - The DTCC should use a mix of media methods to reach different target audience. The message on harmful effects of tobacco use should be communicated through health melas, billboards, hand bills, posters, street plays, local cable network, wall writings, traditional/folk media, etc. Specific IEC strategies should be developed by DTCC keeping in consideration the local needs. The support of NGOs and other partners may be enlisted to play an important role in organizing IEC activities.
  - The district teams can synergize their campaign with the national level media campaign. To make the campaigns cost-effective, the IEC material developed at national level will be sent to states/districts for adaptation/translation in local language.
  - The district team may develop a mobile exhibition kit with posters and standees. This will have a small tent/kiosk which can be set-up in any conspicuous location or in any exhibition. Some audio-visuals may also be shown which will have an immediate impact. This mobile exhibition kit can be easily carried from one place to another throughout the year and may be run in a cost effective manner.
  - Wall paintings/writings in local languages are also useful and a cost effective strategy of reaching out to the people to educate them about adverse effects of tobacco use and also to communicate about the tobacco control law. Wall writings/paintings on the provisions under COTPA and the signages may be made at all sub-centers, PHCs, CHCs, and school walls.
  - Directorate of field publicity (DFP) and song and drama division of DAVP should be approached for developing some popular communications which can be aired on radio or shown in the local channels of Doordarshan through audio-video spots.

Monitoring the Enforcement of Tobacco Control Law

- Every district should have enforcement squads/teams that will be responsible for regular enforcement drives/raids to monitor any violation of the provisions of COTPA. Regular raids should be conducted in public places like public transports, restaurants, Government buildings, health facilities, educational institutions, etc. The collected amount from the penalties should be deposited in a separate head of account. It is recommended that the funds so generated should be further utilized in tobacco control initiatives or awareness campaigns in the state/district.

- The DTCC should maintain a record of violations and prepare the violation report which can be submitted to the enforcement authorities. DTCC should coordinate at district level so that COTPA review is included in the monthly crime review meetings of the police authorities and the data is collected as per the format circulated.
- The MoHFW has developed guidelines for implementation of sections 4, 6 and 7 of COTPA. The said guidelines have been prepared to facilitate the states in implementing the various provisions of the Act. The guidelines also enlist key activities that the state needs to carry out towards implementation of sections 4, 6 and 7 of COTPA. The DTCC can train the enforcement officials as per the guidelines for law enforcers.
- People should be encouraged to report any violations (of COTPA provisions) to the national toll-free helpline No. 1800 110 456. The violations reported on this helpline will be disseminated to the States/ Districts (STCC/DTCC) for proper action and follow-up.

Manpower for District Tobacco Control Programme

In each DTCC, there is provision for recruiting contractual staff to assist the District Nodal Officer in the implementation of the programme. The three personnel are psychologist/counselor, social worker and data entry operator. The terms of reference of the above personnel are at Annexure-X. The district level staff should be trained in their respective states. In case there is a training programme organized by any of the neighboring states, a few district teams may collectively participate in the common training programmes.

Roles and Responsibilities

The following roles and responsibilities of DTCC are indicative and not exhaustive:
- Implementation, supervision and monitoring of the various activities of the programme as per the standard quarterly format.
- Recruitment of the staff at the district tobacco control cell and their training.
- Establish tobacco cessation services in health care facilities and up-scale them through training of health care providers.
- Organize outreach activities in collaboration with different departments and programmes.
- Organize district level trainings/sensitization programmes on tobacco control.
- Regular compilation of the data related to enforcement, preparation of reports and documenting the best practices and timely submission of quarterly reports to STCC.
- Enforcement of COTPA:
  - Display the Tobacco Control Act and the rules on the official district website and regular communication to the different departments of the government at district level about the provisions of the Act and the role of these departments.
  - Constitution of an enforcement squad preferably under the chairmanship of Collector/DM or his nominee for monitoring compliance with COTPA provisions and taking action on violations.
  - Constitution of District Level Monitoring committee for monitoring enforcement of section-5 of COTPA and for taking cognizance of all the direct/indirect advertisement of tobacco products.
  - Inclusion of COTPA in monthly crime review meetings.
- Advocacy by involving Nehru Yuva Kendras, NSS, NCC, SHGs, IMA, IDA, Rotary International, etc. for creating awareness at district/sub-district level.

- Develop awareness campaigns using the local media, cable channels, local festivals/traditional media/ wall writing and integrating the same with the existing mass media campaign under the district health budget for achieving the desired impact in awareness generation.
- Coordination with departments of agriculture, social welfare, rural development, labor and other stakeholders for developing sustainable alternative crops and livelihood for tobacco growers/workers and bidi rollers.
- Documentation of the best practices on tobacco control in the district and sharing them with STCC.

Supervision and Monitoring of Staff

The district nodal officer will supervise the district staff at the DTCC. The DTCC should be closely monitored and supervised by the STCC. The DTCC should prepare the quarterly report as per the prescribed format and submit it to the STCC.

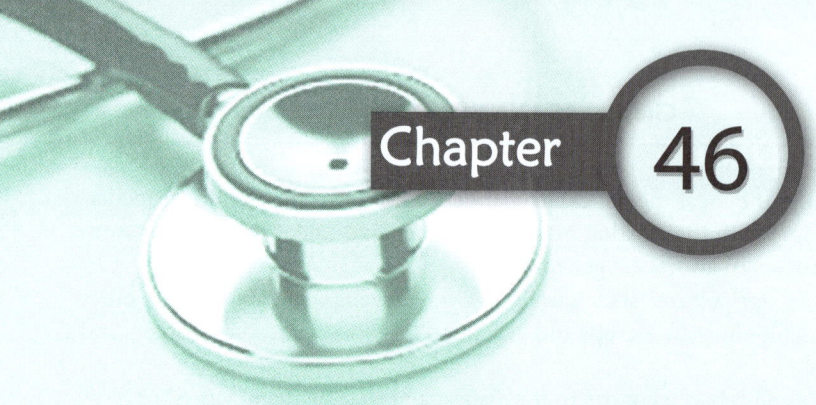

Chapter 46

National Programme on Prevention and Control of Viral Hepatitis

OBJECTIVES

- To establish laboratory network for laboratory-based surveillance of viral hepatitis in different geographical locations of India.
- To ascertain the prevalence of different types of viral hepatitis in different zones of the country.
- To provide laboratory support for outbreak investigation of hepatitis through established network of laboratories.
- To develop technical material for generating awareness among health care providers and in the community about water borne and blood borne hepatitis.

TARGETS

- Establishment of laboratory-based surveillance for viral hepatitis in the country for collection of data. Development of testing and surveillance guidelines and its dissemination.
- A total of 10 labs will be strengthened by the end of 12th Five-Year Plan.
- Training of manpower/health care providers in 10 regional labs including NCDC, i.e. the reference laboratory.
- A total of 10 working group meetings and 10 technical advisory group meetings will be conducted.
- Development of IEC for providers and community.
- Establishment of baseline data for hepatitis to see the impact.

ACTIVITIES

- Development of surveillance of viral hepatitis.
- Surveillance for prevalence of viral hepatitis in various geographical regions: Concept plan has been developed to carry out surveillance for prevention and control of viral hepatitis in various geographical regions and will initiate surveillance through 10 laboratory networks in a phase manner.

   A handbook on safe injection practices guidelines has been developed as a part of IEC for prevention and control of blood transmitted pathogens and has been circulated to different states.

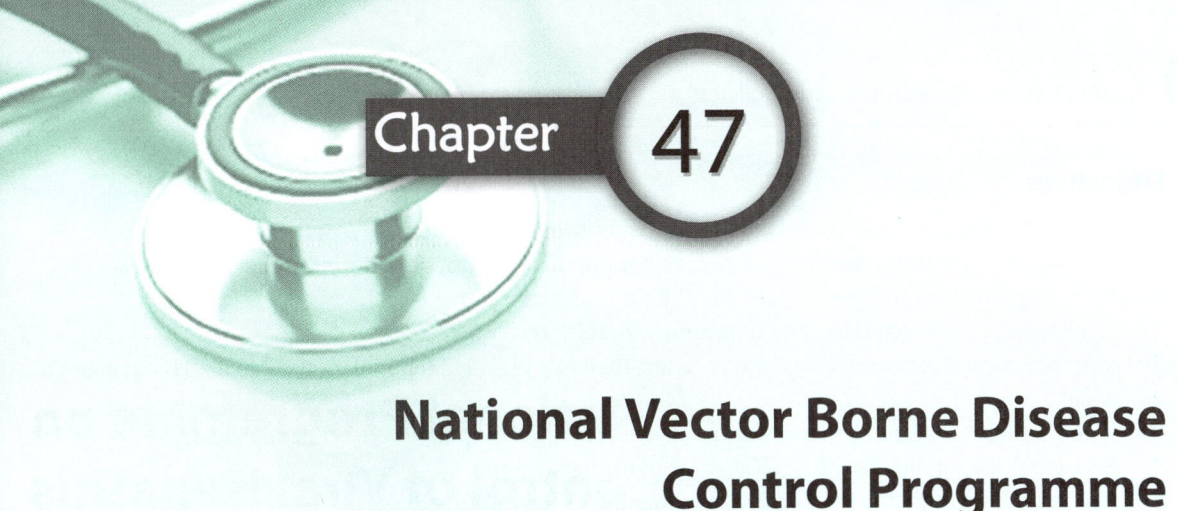

Chapter 47

National Vector Borne Disease Control Programme

INTRODUCTION

Launched in 2003–04 by merging National Anti-malaria Control Programme, National Filaria Control Programme and Kala-azar Control Programmes. Japanese B Encephalitis and Dengue/DHF have also been included in this Programme Directorate of NAMP. It is the nodal agency for prevention and control of major vector-borne diseases.

List of vector-borne diseases control programme legislations:
- National anti-malaria programme
- Kala-azar control programme
- National filaria control programme
- Japanese encephalitis control programme
- Dengue and dengue hemorrhagic fever

NATIONAL ANTIMALARIA PROGRAMME

Malaria is one of the serious public health problems in India. At the time of independence, malaria was contributing 75 million cases with 0.8 million deaths every year prior to the launching of National Malaria Control Programme in 1953. A countrywide comprehensive programme to control malaria was recommended in 1946 by the Bhore Committee report that was endorsed by the Planning Commission in 1951. The national programme against malaria has a long history since that time. In April 1953, Government of India launched a National Malaria Control Programme (NMCP).

Objective

To bring down malaria transmission to a level at which it would cease to be a major public health problem.

KALA-AZAR CONTROL PROGRAMME

Kala-azar or visceral leishmaniasis (VL) is a chronic disease caused by an intracellular protozoan (Leishmania species) and transmitted to man by bite of a female phlebotomus sandfly. Currently, it is a main problem in Bihar, Jharkhand, West Bengal and some parts of Uttar Pradesh. In view of the growing problem, planned control measures were initiated to control Kala-azar.

Objectives

The strategy for Kala-azar control broadly included three main activities:

1. Interruption of transmission by reducing vector population through indoor residual insecticides.
2. Early diagnosis and complete treatment of Kala-azar cases; and
3. Health education programme for community awareness.

To reduce the annual incidence of Kala-azar to less than one per 10,000 population at block PHC level by the end of 2015 by:

- Reducing Kala-azar in the vulnerable, poor and unreached populations in endemic areas;
- Reducing case-fatality rates from Kala-azar to negligible level;
- Reducing cases of PKDL to interrupt transmission of Kala-azar; and
- Preventing the emergence of Kala-azar and HIV/TB coinfections in endemic areas.

Kala-azar has been a serious medical and public health problem in India since historical times. Bengal is the oldest known Kala-azar endemic area of the world. After the initial success, Kala-azar resurged in 70s. Concerned with the increasing problem of Kala-azar in the country, the Government of India (GoI) launched a centrally sponsored Kala-azar control programme in the endemic states in 1990–91. The GoI provided drugs, insecticides and technical support and state governments provided costs involved in implementation. The programme was implemented through State/District Malaria Control Offices and the primary health care system. The programme brought a significant decline in Kala-azar morbidity, but could not sustain the pace of decline for long.

The National Health Policy-2002 set the goal of Kala-azar elimination in India by the year 2010 which was revised to 2015. Continuing focused activities with high political commitment, India signed a Tripartite Memorandum of Understanding (MoU) with Bangladesh and Nepal to achieve Kala-azar elimination from the South-East Asia Region (SEAR). Elimination is defined as reducing the annual incidence of Kala-azar to less than 1 case per 10,000 population at the sub-district (block PHCs) level in Bangladesh and India and at the district level in Nepal.

Presently all programmatic activities are being implemented through the National Vector Borne Disease Control Programme (NVBDCP) which is an umbrella programme for prevention and control of vector borne diseases and is subsumed under National Health Mission (NHM).

Goal

To improve the health status of vulnerable groups and at-risk population living in Kala-azar endemic areas by the elimination of Kala-azar so that it no longer remains a public health problem.

Target

To reduce the annual incidence of Kala-azar to less than one per 10,000 population at block PHC level.

The Elimination Strategy

The national strategy for elimination of Kala-azar is a multipronged approach which is in line with WHO Regional Strategic Framework for elimination of Kala-azar from the South-East Asia Region (2011–2015) and includes:

- Early diagnosis and complete case management
- Integrated vector management and vector surveillance
- Supervision, monitoring, surveillance and evaluation
  - Strengthening capacity of human resource in health

- ▪ Advocacy, communication and social mobilization for behavioral impact and intersectoral convergence
- ▪ Programme management.

Early Diagnosis and Complete Case Management

This is done for eliminating the human reservoir of infection through early case detection. Effective case management includes diagnosing a case early along with complete treatment and monitoring of adverse effects. This strategy will reduce case-fatality and will improve utilization of health services by people suspected to be suffering from the disease.

The starting point of early diagnosis is to follow uniform suspect case definition.

- A 'suspect' case: History of fever of >2 weeks and enlarged spleen and liver not responding to anti- malaria in a patient from an endemic area.
- All patients with above symptoms should be screened with rapid diagnostic test and if found positive should be treated with an effective drug.
- In cases with past history of Kala-azar or in those with high suspicion of Kala-azar but with negative RDT test result, confirmation of Kala-azar can be done by examination of bone marrow/spleen aspirate for Leishmania donovani (LD) bodies at appropriate level (district hospital) equipped with such skills and facilities.

Treatment

In 2010, the WHO Expert Committee on Leishmaniasis, and subsequently the Regional Technical Advisory Group (RTAG) of WHO South-East Asia Region (SEAR) recommended Liposomal Amphotericin B (LAMB) in a single dose of 10 mg/kg as the first choice treatment regimen for the Indian Subcontinent (ISC) within the current elimination strategy, given its high efficacy, safety, ease of use and assured compliance. The decision to use Liposomal Amphotericin B for Kala-azar was taken by the technical advisory committee based on the available evidences and approved by Ministry of Health and Family Welfare, Government of India. In selected districts, Amphotericin B emulsion has been approved. The combination regimen (Injection Paromomycin-Miltefosine for 10 days) is also recommended. Miltefosine 28 days regime and Amphotericin B as multiple doses may also be used.

Within the Indian National Programme, assuming availability of drugs, appropriate training of health personnel, infrastructure and indication, the following drugs will thus be used in order of preference at all levels:

- Single dose 10 mg/kg bw Liposomal Amphotericin B (LAMB)
- Combination regimens (e.g., Miltefosine and Paromomycin)
- Amphotericin B emulsion
- Miltefosine
- Amphotericin B deoxycholate in multiple doses
- Post-Kala-azar Dermal Leishmaniasis (PKDL) patients are to be treated with
  - ▪ Liposomal amphotericin B: 5 mg/kg/day by infusion two times per week for 3 weeks for a total dose of 30 mg/kg, or
  - ▪ Miltefosine: 100 mg orally per day for 12 weeks, or
  - ▪ Amphotericin B deoxycholate: 1 mg/kg over 4 months 60–80 doses, [as per WHO guidelines on diagnosis and management of PKDL, 2012].
- Case management of special conditions like relapse, HIV-VL co-infection and others will follow NVBDCP operational guidelines of Kala-azar.

It is to be noted that Miltefosine cannot be given to pregnant and lactating women, nor in young children. In women of child-bearing age, Miltefosine should not be prescribed unless contraception is guaranteed during treatment and for two months after the treatment is completed. In women suffering from PKDL treated with Miltefosine, this period is extended to 5 months following completion of treatment.

Integrated Vector Management (IVM) Including Indoor Residual Spraying (IRS)

Integrated vector management (IVM) is a rational decision-making process for the optimal use of resources for vector control. The main objective is to reduce longevity of the adult vectors, eliminate the breeding sites, decrease contact of vector with humans, and reduce the density of the vector. This approach improves the efficacy, cost-effectiveness, ecological soundness and sustainability of disease-vector control. The five key elements of IVM include capacity building and training, advocacy, collaboration, evidence-based decision-making and integrated approach. IRS is the main stay of vector control for breaking the human-vector-human cycle of transmission.

The current strategy is to do IRS twice a year in all houses (up to six feet height) and complete coverage of cattle sheds in villages, which had a Kala-azar case reported in the last three years including the current year supplemented with focused IRS in villages reporting KA cases. The spray is usually organized in two rounds, 1st round during February–March when sandflies are fairly active and 2nd round during May– June (months may vary from district-to-district based on entomological data) to limit sandfly population supplemented with focused IRS in the villages reporting KA cases.

Supervision, Monitoring, Surveillance and Evaluation

Supervision, monitoring and surveillance are essential components to ensure success of the programme. There is a need to strengthen surveillance for KA and PKDL including line listing of cases at village level to identify hot spot areas (villages reporting five or more KA cases in previous or current year) and update areas for micro planning for spray operations. As per WHO's Fifth Regional Technical Advisory Meeting of South-East Asia Region, 15–20% of KA patients seek treatment in the private sector. Information from private sector is essential to have better picture of burden of disease and sustain the gains achieved towards elimination. Since the emergence of VL-HIV co-infection and posing threat on the achievements, surveillance of VL-HIV cases is important apart from early and long term follow-up of KA and PKDL cases (six and 12 months respectively) as well as information on relapses. Independent evaluation or validation of elimination will pave the pathway towards further reducing KA burden in the community to the lowest level.

Strengthening Capacity of Human Resource in Health

Kala-azar elimination will require effective involvement of health personnel at all levels in the continuum of care, right from the early identification of a suspect case to diagnosis and management, including complications. This can be achieved by orientation of human resource in health appropriate for different levels. There are multiple actors engaged in KA control programme like ASHA at community level, ANM at sub-health center level, laboratory technicians and supervisory staff in the form of Kala-azar technical supervisors at primary health care center level, district VBD consultants, PHC and district medical and programme officers. In addition, other stakeholders like BMGF/CARE has also made provisions for human resource support at the district and block level (district programme manager and link workers at block PHC respectively). Roles and responsibilities at each level need to be defined and followed.

Advocacy, Communication and Social Mobilization for Behavioral Impact and Intersectoral Convergence

The population at risk for Kala-azar is among the poorest in the community and often poorly nourished. Access to care remains an issue in at-risk population and other under privileged sections of communities. Inadequate utilization of health services and lack of faith in public health systems by the affected population are major barriers in achieving elimination. This can be addressed by intensive awareness campaigns with the involvement of communities and community health volunteers. Awareness about the disease, its features, diagnostic and treatment options, prevention, existing schemes and incentives and other aspects of the disease are not widely known. Therefore, there is a need for advocacy, communication and social mobilization through all the existing methods (wall writing, hoardings, banner, pamphlets, radio jingles, etc.) as per the local context. Opportunities should be explored to spread the messages during weekly market or any other mass gathering (Chath puja, fairs, melas, etc.) Display of messages particularly during campaigns which are community-based and inter-personal communication are considered the best methods for spreading awareness.

Programme Management

Programme management is the most important operational component for success of Kala-azar elimination. It involves coordination between center and state level offices as well as effective coordination and harmonization of activities with different partners in the programme. Day-to-day management of the programme activities like cold chain maintenance, drug requests, procurement and transportation of drugs, diagnostics and commodities, planning and monitoring need to be strengthened at all levels of implementation.

NATIONAL FILARIA CONTROL PROGRAMME

Bancroftian filariasis, caused by Wuchereria bancrofti, which is transmitted to man by the bites of infected mosquitoes - Culex, Anopheles, Mansonia and Aedes. Lymphatic filaria is prevalent in 18 states and union territories. Bancroftian filariasis is widely distributed while Brugian filariasis caused by Brugia malayi is restricted to six States—UP, Bihar, Andhra Pradesh, Odisha, Tamil Nadu, Kerala, and Gujarat. After pilot project in Odisha from 1949 to 1954, the National Filaria Control Programme (NFCP) was launched in the country in 1955 with the objective of delimiting the problem, to undertake control measures in endemic areas and to train personnel to man the programme. The main control measures were mass DEC administration, antilarval measures in urban areas and indoor residual spray in rural areas. The activities were mainly confined to urban areas. However, the programme has been extended to rural areas since 1994.

Objectives

- Reduction of the problem in un-surveyed areas
- Control in urban areas through recurrent anti-larval and anti-parasitic measures.

JAPANESE ENCEPHALITIS CONTROL PROGRAMME

Japanese encephalitis (JE) is a zoonotic disease caused by an arbovirus, group B (Flavivirus) and transmitted by Culex mosquitoes. This disease has been reported in 26 States and UTs since 1978, only 15 States are reporting JE regularly. The case fatality in India is 35% which can be reduced by early detection, immediate referral to hospital and proper medical and nursing care. The total population at risk is estimated 160 million. The most disturbing feature of JE has been the regular occurrence of outbreak in different parts of the country.

Government of India has constituted a task force at national level which is in operation and reviews the JE situations and its control strategies from time to time. Though Directorate of National Anti-Malaria Programme is monitoring JE situation in the country.

Objectives

- Strengthening early diagnosis and prompt case management at PHCs, CHCs and hospitals through training of medical and nursing staff.
- IEC for community awareness to promote early case reporting, personal protection, isolation of amplifier host, etc.
- Vector control measures mainly fogging during outbreaks, space spraying in animal dwellings, and antilarval operation where feasible.
- Development of a safe and standard indigenous vaccine. Vaccination for high risk population particularly children below 15 years of age.

DENGUE AND DENGUE HEMORRHAGIC FEVER

One of the most important resurgent tropical infectious disease, is dengue. Dengue fever and dengue hemorrhagic fever (DHF) are acute fevers caused by four antigenically related but distinct dengue virus serotypes (DEN 1, 2, 3 and 4) are transmitted by the infected mosquitoes, Aedes aegypti. Dengue outbreaks have been reported from urban areas from all states. All the four serotypes of dengue virus (1, 2, 3 and 4) exist in India. The Vector Aedes aegypti breed in peridomestic fresh water collections and is found in both urban and rural areas.

Objectives

- Surveillance for disease and outbreaks
- Early diagnosis and prompt case management
- Vector control through community participation and social mobilization
- Capacity building.

Prevention and Control

Government of India has taken various steps for prevention and control of dengue and chikungunya in the country as follows:

- Developed a **long-term action plan** for prevention and control of dengue in the country and sent to the State(s) in January 2007 for implementation.
- **National guidelines for clinical management of dengue fever, dengue hemorrhagic fever, Dengue Shock syndrome** has been sent to the State(s) in April 2007 for circulation in all hospitals.
- Established **110 sentinel surveillance hospitals** with laboratory support for augmentation of diagnostic facility for dengue in endemic State(s) in 2007 which has been increased to 170 in 2009. All these are linked with **13 apex referral laboratories** with advanced diagnostic facilities for back up support.
- To maintain the uniformity and standard of diagnostics in these laboratories, IgM MAC ELISA test kits are provided through National Institute of Virology (NIV), Pune. Cost is borne by GoI.
- Diagnosis of dengue and chikungunya is provided to the community at free of cost.
- Since 2007, every year in the 1st quarter, Directorate of NVBDCP prepares the tentative allocation of test kits based on the previous epidemiological situation of dengue and chikungunya in the states and communicate to both NIV, Pune and States.

- Kits are supplied by NIV, Pune on receipt of requirement from the respective states.
- Buffer stocks are also maintained to meet any exigency.
- State wise allocation of **dengue** and **chikungunya** during 2010 was communicated to the states on 15th February 2010.
- Ensuring the diagnostic facility and availability of kits is the responsibility of the respective State Programme Officers, NVBDCP.

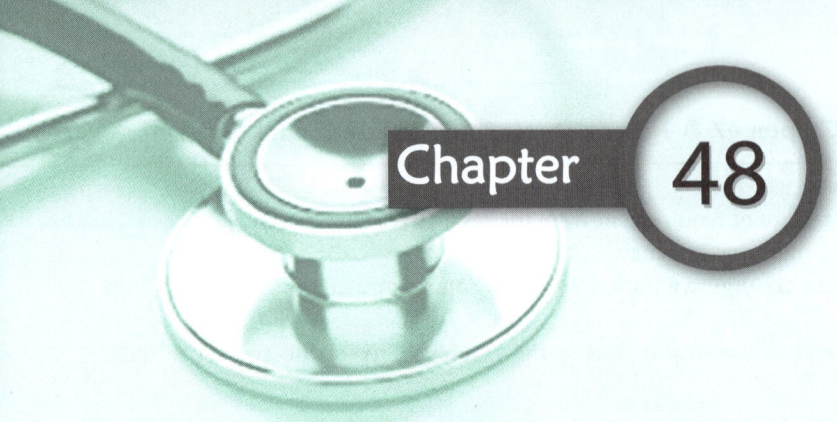

Chapter 48

Urban Vector Borne Disease Scheme

OBJECTIVES

- Prevention of malaria mortality and reduction of morbidity in identified urban areas.
- Effective management and control of other VBDs targets:
  - To improve vector surveillance and elimination of breeding at the source
  - To bring down cases of malaria and other VBDs in urban areas

STRATEGIES

- Detection and management of malaria cases and other VBDs
- Integrated vector management
- Capacity building and BCC
- Intersectional coordination

ACTIVITIES

- **Diagnosis and case management**
  - Diagnostic and treatment facilities will be strengthened by establishing malaria clinics @ 1 clinic per 20,000 population with special focus to urban slums.
  - Involvement of other sectors/private providers for diagnosis, treatment and reporting.
  - Sentinel sites will be equipped with necessary diagnostic kits for diagnosis of VBDs.
- **Integrated vector management by**
  - Larval control through source reduction, chemical larviciding and use of larvivorous fish and minor engineering.
  - Space spray during the outbreaks/epidemic.
  - LLINs in targeted vulnerable population of identified wards/burroughs under municipal corporations of mega cities.
- **Capacity building and BCC**
  - Training of personnels involved in antimalaria activities in urban areas including engineers and town planners.
  - Focused BCC.
  - Advocacy workshops for NGOs/CBOs/FBOs/stakeholders for their involvement in VBD control activities.
  - Social mobilization through intersectoral collaboration.
  - Intersectoral coordination.
  - Adoption of Model civic bye-laws for prevention and control of vector breeding.
  - Health impact assessment (HIA) of developmental projects.

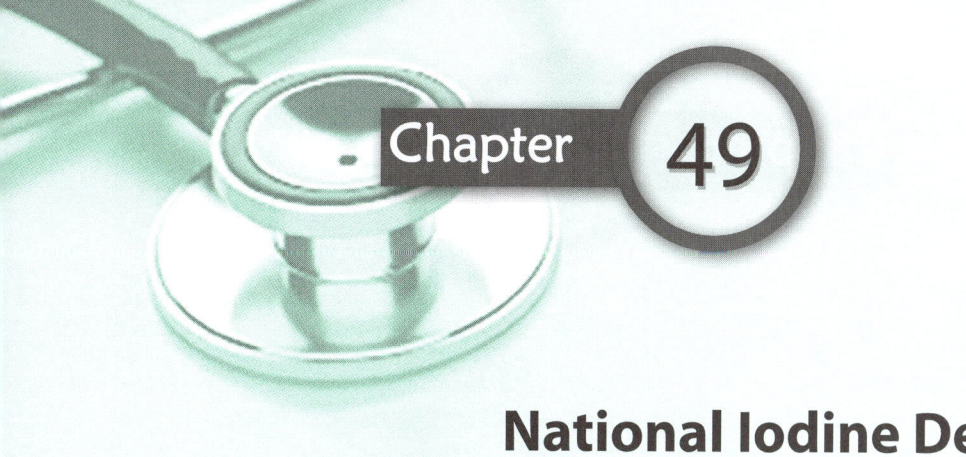

Chapter 49

National Iodine Deficiency Disorders Control Programme

INTRODUCTION

In 1962, the Government of India implemented the National Goiter Control Programme, now called the National Iodine Deficiency Disorders Control Programme (NIDDCP). In 1982, the government made a policy decision to iodate all edible salt in India by 1992. In 1992, the National Goiter Control Programme (NGCP) was renamed as National Iodine Deficiency Disorders Control Programme (NIDDCP).

GOALS

- Universal consumption of iodized salt.
- Universalization of access to iodized salt.

OBJECTIVES

The important objectives and components of NIDDCP are as follows:
- Surveys to assess the magnitude of the iodine-deficiency disorders.
- Supply of iodized salt in place of common salt.
- Resurvey after every 5 years to assess the extent of iodine-deficiency disorders and the impact of iodated salt.
- Laboratory monitoring of iodized salt and urinary iodine excretion.
- Health education and publicity.
- Mapping out IDD prevalent areas in the State.
- Creating awareness to use only iodized salt to prevent IDD.
- Re-survey on IDD.

During 1994–1995, India's private sector produced 34 lakh metric tons of iodized salt per year. The government expects iodized salt production to increase to 50 lakh metric tons in the near future. Iodized salt is transported on the railways under a priority category that is second only to defense. In 19 States and six Union Territories, the sale of noniodized salt has been completely banned. The remaining state governments have been urged to ban the sale of noniodized salt and to include iodized salt under the public distribution system. Each State Health Directorate has been advised to set up an IDD control cell. The biochemistry division of the National Institute of Communicable Diseases has a national reference laboratory for monitoring of IDD, and it also trains medical and paramedical personnel. District health officers in all endemic states have test kits to conduct on-the-spot qualitative testing to ensure quality control of iodized salt at the consumption level. NIDDCP provides IDD surveys, health education, and publicity campaigns. Its information, education, and campaign activities include video films, posters, and radio/TV spots.

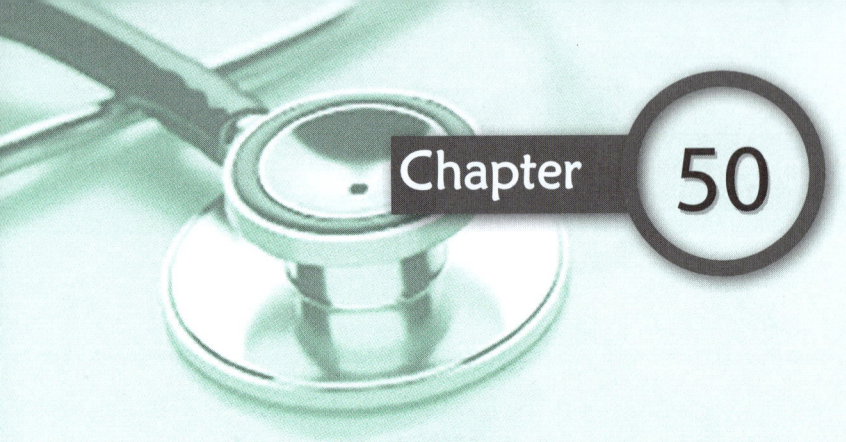

Chapter 50

Rashtriya Swasthya Bima Yojana

INTRODUCTION

Rashtriya Swasthya Bima Yojana (RSBY) was launched in early 2008 and was initially designed to target only the Below Poverty Line (BPL) households, but has been expanded to cover other defined categories of unorganized workers, covering:

- Building and other construction workers registered with the welfare boards
- Licensed railway porters
- Street vendors
- MGNREGA workers who have worked for more than 15 days during the preceding financial year
- Beedi workers
- Domestic workers
- Sanitation workers
- Mine workers
- Rickshaw pullers
- Rag pickers
- Auto/taxi driver.

The premium cost for enrolled beneficiaries under the scheme is shared by Government of India and the State Governments. The programme had the target to cover 70 million households by the end of the Twelfth Five-Year Plan (2012–17). Its main service delivery model remained as demand financing, freedom of choice among accredited government and private hospitals, and cashless service reimbursable to provide on a predetermined package rates on family floater basis, could become a strong pillar for the universal health care system laid down by Government of India.

Since 1st April, 2015, the Scheme Rashtriya Swasthya Bima Yojana (RSBY) has been transferred to Ministry of Health and Family Welfare on "as is where is" basis. Ministry of Health and Family Welfare is administering and implementing the scheme through a decentralized implementation structure at the state level.

OBJECTIVES

RSBY has two fold objectives:

1. To provide financial protection against catastrophic health costs by reducing out.
2. To improve access to quality health care for below poverty line households of pocket expenditure for hospitalization and other vulnerable groups in the unorganized sector.

The beneficiaries under RSBY are entitled to hospitalization coverage up to ₹30,000/- per annum on family floater basis, for most of the diseases that require hospitalization. The benefit will be available under the defined diseases in the package list. The government has framed indicative package rates for the hospitals for a large number of interventions. Pre-existing conditions are covered from day one and there is no age limit. The coverage extends to maximum five members of the family which includes the head of household, spouse and up to three dependents. Additionally, transport expenses of ₹100/- per hospitalization will also be paid to the beneficiary subject to a maximum of ₹1000/- per year per family. The beneficiaries need to pay only ₹30/- as registration fee for a year while Central and State Government pays the premium as per their sharing ratio to the insurer selected by the State Government on the basis of a competitive bidding. At every state, the State Government sets up a State Nodal Agency (SNA) that is responsible for implementing, monitoring, supervision and part-financing of the scheme by coordinating with insurance company, hospital, district authorities and other local stake holders.

FEATURES

The RSBY scheme is not the first attempt to provide health insurance to low income workers by the Government in India. The RSBY scheme, however, differs from these schemes in several important ways.

- **Empowering the beneficiary:** RSBY provides the participating BPL household with freedom of choice between public and private hospitals and makes it a potential client worth attracting on account of the significant revenues that hospitals stand to earn through the scheme.
- **Business model for all stakeholders:** The scheme has been designed as a business model for a social sector scheme with incentives built for each stakeholder. This business model design is conducive both in terms of expansion of the scheme as well as for its long run sustainability.
- **Insurers:** The insurer is paid premium for each household enrolled for RSBY. Therefore, the insurer has the motivation to enroll as many households as possible from the BPL list. This will result in better coverage of targeted beneficiaries.
- **Hospitals:** A hospital has the incentive to provide treatment to large number of beneficiaries as it is paid per beneficiary treated. Even public hospitals have the incentive to treat beneficiaries under RSBY as the money from the insurer will flow directly to the concerned public hospital which they can use for their own purposes. Insurers, in contrast, will monitor participating hospitals in order to prevent unnecessary procedures or fraud resulting in excessive claims.
- **Intermediaries:** The inclusion of intermediaries such as NGOs and MFIs which have a greater stake in assisting BPL households. The intermediaries will be paid for the services they render in reaching out to the beneficiaries.
- **Government:** By paying only a maximum sum up to ₹750/- per family per year, the Government is able to provide access to quality health care to the below poverty line population. It will also lead to a healthy competition between public and private providers which in turn will improve the functioning of the public health care providers.
- **Information technology (IT) intensive:** For the first time IT applications are being used for social sector scheme on such a large scale. Every beneficiary family is issued a biometric enabled smart card containing their fingerprints and photographs. All the hospitals empanelled under RSBY are IT enabled and connected to the server at the district level. This will ensure a smooth data flow regarding service utilization periodically.
- **Safe and foolproof:** The use of biometric enabled smart card and a key management system makes this scheme safe and foolproof. The key management system of RSBY ensures that the card reaches the

correct beneficiary and there remains accountability in terms of issuance of the smart card and its usage. The biometric enabled smart card ensures that only the real beneficiary can use the smart card.

- **Portability:** The key feature of RSBY is that a beneficiary who has been enrolled in a particular district will be able to use his/her smart card in any RSBY empanelled hospital across India. This makes the scheme truly unique and beneficial to the poor families that migrate from one place to another. Cards can also be split for migrant workers to carry a share of the coverage with them separately.
- **Cashless and paperless transactions:** A beneficiary of RSBY gets cashless benefit in any of the empanelled hospitals. He/she only needs to carry his/her smart card and provide verification through his/her finger print. For participating providers, it is a paperless scheme as they do not need to send all the papers related to treatment to the insurer. They send online claims to the insurer and get paid electronically.
- **Robust monitoring and evaluation:** RSBY is evolving a robust monitoring and evaluation system. An elaborate backend data management system is being put in place which can track any transaction across India and provide periodic analytical reports. The basic information gathered by government and reported publicly should allow for mid-course improvements in the scheme. It may also contribute to competition during subsequent tender processes with the insurers by disseminating the data and reports.

BENEFICIARIES

The beneficiary is any below poverty line (BPL) family, whose information is included in the district BPL list prepared by the State Government and the family falling into any of the above defined (point number 1) eleven categories are eligible. The eligible family needs to come to the enrolment station, and the identity of the household head needs to be confirmed by the authorized government official.

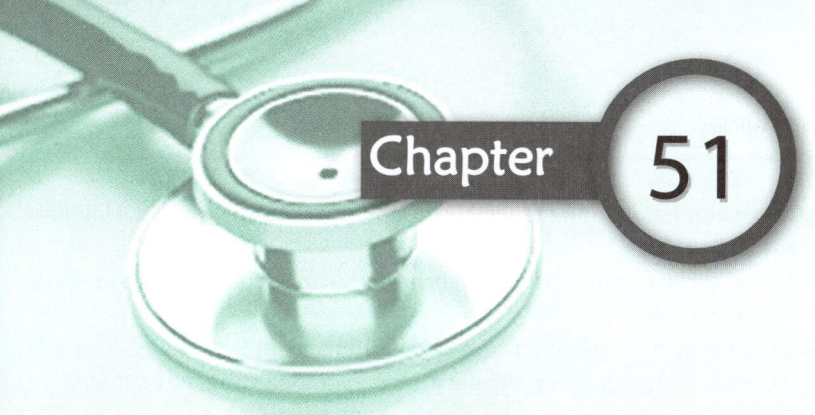

Chapter 51

National Programme for Burn Injuries

PILOT PROJECT DURING THE 11TH FIVE-YEAR PLAN: PPPBI

A pilot programme was initiated in the year 2010 by Ministry of Health and Family Welfare in the name of "Pilot Programme for Prevention of Burn Injuries" (PPPBI) with a total budget of ₹29 crores. The programme was initiated in the following three Medical Colleges and six Districts Hospitals:

- **Haryana:** Postgraduate Institute of Medical Sciences, Rohtak; General Hospital, Gurgaon; Civil Hospital, Panipat.
- **Himachal Pradesh:** Dr. Rajendra Prasad Medical College, Tanda at Kangra, District Hospital, Hamirpur; Zonal Hospital, Mandi.
- **Assam:** Guwahati Medical College; District Hospital, Nagaon; District Hospital, Dhubri.

The Goal of PPPBI was to ensure prevention of burn injuries, provide timely and adequate treatment in case burn injuries do occur, so as to reduce mortality, complications and ensuing disabilities and to provide effective rehabilitative interventions if disability has set in.

NATIONAL PROGRAMME DURING THE 12TH FIVE-YEAR PLAN

- The proposal for continuation of pilot project as full-fledged programme was approved by EFC on 17 May 2013 and subsequent to this approval, CCEA approved the programme on 6 February 2014.
- NPPPBI will now be an ongoing programme and will cover 67 State Government Medical Colleges and 19 District Hospitals during the 12th Five-Year Plan. The District Hospital component will be undertaken under National Health Mission (NHM)/National Rural Health Mission (NRHM).
- The programme will no more be a 100% centrally-sponsored scheme during the 12th plan. The programme will be part of the "Human resource in Health and Medical Education Scheme" and assistance to be provided to the states will be governed by the norms set under this parent scheme. One of the important criteria under the scheme is that the assistance proposed under the programme for various components will be shared between the Center and State Governments in the ratio of 75 : 25 (For North Eastern and hill States of Uttarakhand, Himachal Pradesh and Jammu and Kashmir, this ratio will be 90 : 10).

Objectives

The main objectives of the programme are:

- To reduce incidence, mortality, morbidity and disability due to burn injuries

- To improve awareness among the general masses and vulnerable groups especially the women, children, industrial and hazardous occupational workers.
- To establish adequate infrastructural facility and network for behavior change communication, burn management and rehabilitation interventions.
- To carry out research for assessing behavioral, social and other determinants of burn injuries in our country for effective need-based programme planning for burn injuries, monitoring and subsequent evaluation.

Guiding Principles of the NPPPBI

The National Programme for burn injuries shall be set up and function with the following guiding principles:
- To optimally and effectively utilize the existing health care and allied sectors, services and infrastructure.
- To elicit participation of Government, Nongovernment and private/corporate sector to avoid duplication of efforts and expenditures.
- To evolve three tier programme structure to have universal coverage and reach.
- The programme shall have balanced focus on preventive, curative and rehabilitative aspects of burn injuries.
- To establish a central burn registry.

Programme Structure of NPPPBI

To establish and manage the programme, a defined programme management will be structured under the following headings:
- Programme Division in Directorate General of Health Services.
  - A programme officer with public health.
  - Promotion and education qualifications.
  - Consultants in burns, rehabilitation and health promotion and education specialties.
  - Requisite support staff.
- A national burn case reporting mechanism.
  - Utilizing MIS in the country from sub-center > PHC > CHC > District Admn. > State > Center.
- A coordination committee.
  Experts from burns and plastic surgery, physical medicine and rehabilitation, health education and health promotion to guide, oversee, supervise and evaluate the NPPPBI programme activities.

Partners in the Programme

In the present set-up, there are many players working directly or indirectly for prevention of burns and other traumas, first aid and transportation facilities. Their services will be continued to be utilized for further improvements in the burn care. Various departments involved are:
- MoHFW through its Health services infrastructure, e.g., Departments of burns and plastic, causality services (Secondary and tertiary prevention/curative care)
- Fire Services, Ministry of Home Affairs
- Education Department (HRD)
- Women and Child Ministry (ICDS)
- Local Self Governments (PRI)
- Civil Defense and Home Guards (Ministry of Home Affairs)
- Police department
- Others.

Components of the Programme

The programme has following main components:

- Prevention programme (IEC)
- Treatment
- Rehabilitation
- Training
- Monitoring and evaluation
- Research

Preventive Programme

The key strategies of this programme would be:

- Development and implementation of an appropriate, need-based communication/behavioral change communication (BCC) strategy.
- Advocacy with the policy makers, administrators in health and allied sectors, corporate and industry sectors.
- Developing key messages for general public and special target groups such as health care providers at primary, secondary and tertiary levels for vulnerable groups, e.g. women and children, industrial workers and so on. It would be necessary to maintain consistency in the messages throughout.
- Media engagement strategy.
- A National commemorative day/week for prevention of burn injuries.
- Communication organizational structure at center, state, district, PHC levels.
- Capacity building programme for IEC/BCC manpower at all the three levels.
- Monitoring and evaluation of communication interventions for prevention.

Programme Activities

- **Audience research (Formative research):** To be undertaken by institution like ICMR/MCI to provide a base line data pertaining to the specific behavior to be changed for communication/BCC strategy.
- Advocacy with policy makers, administrators, MP/MLA/Local Self Government.
- Campaigns during Parliament/Assembly sessions. Printing informative brochures, etc.
- **Networking with active partners:** Bureaucrats, Stakeholders from Private and Corporate sectors and NGOs, Professional associations.
  - Integration with ongoing educational and training activities.
  - Fulfilling personnel requirement at different levels.
  - Capacity development of available manpower.
  - Health communication through media mix as per local needs.
  - Commemorative burn prevention week to be observed across the country.

Monitoring and Evaluation

Routine monitoring shall be done through existing monitoring system at National and State level or evaluation by an external agency.

BURN INJURY MANAGEMENT PROGRAMME

The main strategies for burn care would be to provide physical infrastructure and manpower for burn care at all three levels of health delivery system through inter agency coordination and public-private partnership.

This will be achieved through provision of material resources and capacity building programmes for easy accessibility, equity and universal coverage. Quality management and monitoring would be done to ensure maintenance of standards.

For quality burn injury management at all the three levels of health care delivery system, there would be certain additional requirements as following:

- **Primary level:** The existing space available will be utilized for various activities and the existing staff (such as ANMs, nurses, dressers, etc.) will be sensitized and trained on burn first aid.
- **District level:** A small 4–6 bedded burn unit will be set up in district hospitals. The existing operation theater and other facilities will be utilized but will be augmented by providing basic equipment such as vital parameter monitor, skin graft masher, Humby's knife, portable light, etc. and partly the consumables will also be provided. One advanced life support ambulance per district with manpower will be provided.
- **Tertiary level:** Capacity building will be done where there are no existing facilities or strengthening will be done if there are some existing facilities by providing additional infrastructure and manpower. A burn unit of 12 beds including an ICU of four beds will be created. The existing operation theater and other facilities will be utilized but will be augmented by providing basic equipment such as ventilators, vital parameter monitors, skin graft mesher, humby's knife, portable lights, dermatome etc.

TRAINING PROGRAMME FOR CAPACITY BUILDING OF BURN CARE MANPOWER

For smooth and efficient burn care management, capacity building of the relevant health care manpower would be undertaken as per plan detailed below:

- The Surgeons/Medical officers at the district level, two from each district shall be trained by the burns and plastic surgeons at the medical college/selected training centers.
- Training of the district level workers will be done at district hospitals by the trained surgeons and medical officers in burn care.
- Orientation training of the primary level workers will be done at district center by the surgeon/medical officers.
- On the job training of the medical college workers will be done at existing burn centers routinely.

BURN INJURY REHABILITATION PROGRAMME

The essential components of rehabilitation of burn injuries would encompass development of infrastructures—physical, manpower and materials with capacity and skill development initiatives. It will be equitable, accessible and with universal outreach. Inter-agency coordination and public private partnership will be used. Monitoring and quality control will be done. Services to be provided at three levels will be as follows:

- **Primary Level:** The main stress would be to integrate with the villagers through the *Aanganwadi* workers and other community level functionaries for awareness generation regarding scar management, therapeutic exercises with home exercise programme, splinting, electrotherapy modalities (Cold, Heat, etc.) and activities of daily living (modifications and equipment).

- **District level:** To set up fully equipped burns rehabilitation center in approximately 300 sq ft area with a basic team consisting of a surgeon, physiotherapist/occupational therapist and members like multi rehabilitation workers who can be a pivotal link between the three tiers of the system. The services of a psychologist and vocational counselor can be utilized on fixed days' basis. Equipment such as diathermy, ultrasound, electrical stimulators and traction equipment will be provided.
- **Tertiary level:** At this level, every possible facility and information related to complete burn rehabilitation should be available. This includes issues on pre- and post-operative assessments and planning and execution of treatments. Disability certificates, vocational guidance and placements, monetary assistance through various resources, functional prosthesis and compilation of various government and non-government organizations working in this sector. A special group of burn care professionals should be allotted with the work of patient outcome assessments.

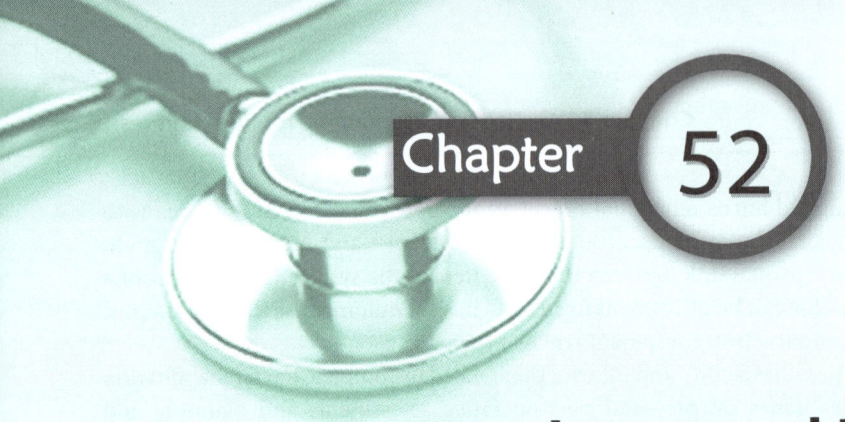

Chapter 52

Integrated Management of Neonatal and Childhood Illness

INTRODUCTION

Government of India recognizes the need to strengthen child health activities in the country. In order to do so and introduce IMCI in the country, a Core Group was constituted which included representatives from Indian Academy of Pediatrics (IAP), National Neonatology Forum of India (NNF), National Antimalaria Programme (NAMP), Department of Women and Child Development (DWCD), Child-in-Need Institute (CINI), WHO, UNICEF, eminent Pediatricians and Neonatologists, and the representatives from Ministry of Health and Family Welfare, Government of India. The Adaptation Group developed Indian version of IMCI guidelines and renamed it as Integrated Management of Neonatal and Childhood Illness (IMNCI). The major components of this strategy are:

- Strengthening the skills of the health care workers
- Strengthening the health care infrastructure
- Involvement of the community.

Although the major reason for developing the IMCI strategy stemmed from the needs of curative care, the strategy also addresses aspects of nutrition, immunization, and other important elements of disease prevention and health promotion. The objectives of the strategy are to reduce death and the frequency and severity of illness and disability, and to contribute to improved growth and development. This strategy has been adapted for India as Integrated Management of Neonatal and Childhood Illness (IMNCI). The IMNCI clinical guidelines target children less than 5-year-old—the age group that bears the highest burden of deaths due to common childhood diseases. The guidelines take an evidence-based, syndromic approach to case management that supports the rational, effective and affordable use of drugs and diagnostic tools. Evidence-based medicine stresses the importance of evaluation of evidence from clinical research and cautions against the use of intuition, unsystematic clinical experience, and untested pathophysiologic reasoning for medical decision-making. In situations where laboratory support and clinical resources are limited, the syndromic approach is a more realistic and cost-effective way to manage patients. Careful and systematic assessment of common symptoms and well-selected clinical signs provide sufficient information to guide rational and effective actions. An evidence-based syndromic approach can be used to determine the:

- Health problem(s) the child may have
- Severity of the child's condition
- Actions that can be taken to care for the child (e.g. refer the child immediately, manage with available resources, or manage at home). In addition, IMNCI promotes:
  - Adjustment of interventions to the capacity and functions of the health system; and
  - Active involvement of family members and the community in the health care process.

The major highlights of Indian adaptation are:
- Incorporation of neonatal care as it now constitutes two-thirds of infant mortality.
- Inclusion of 0–7 days.
- Incorporating national guidelines on malaria, anemia, vitamin A supplementation and immunization schedule.
- Training schedule reduced from 11 days to 8 days.
- Training begins with sick young infant up to two months.
- Proportion of training time devoted to sick young infant and sick child is almost equal. The Government has initiated implementation of the IMNCI strategy in four districts each in nine selected states of Odisha, Rajasthan, Madhya Pradesh, Haryana, Delhi, Gujarat, Uttaranchal, Tamil Nadu and Rajasthan.

COMPONENTS OF THE INTEGRATED APPROACH

The IMNCI strategy includes both preventive and curative interventions that aim to improve practices in health facilities, the health system and at home. At the core of the strategy is integrated case management of the most common childhood problems with a focus on the most common causes of death. The strategy includes three main components:
- Improvements in the case-management skills of health staff through the provision of locally-adapted guidelines on Integrated Management of Neonatal and Childhood illness and activities to promote their use.
- Improvements in the overall health system required for effective management of childhood illness.
- Improvements in family and community health care practices.

THE PRINCIPLES OF INTEGRATED CARE

The IMNCI guidelines are based on the following principles:
- All sick young infants age up to two months must be examined for signs of "possible serious bacterial infection" and all children two months to five years must be examined for "general danger signs" which indicate the need for immediate referral or admission to a hospital.
- All sick children must be routinely assessed for major symptoms (for young infants up to 2 months: diarrhea; and for children age two months up to five years: Cough or difficulty in breathing, diarrhea, fever and ear problem). They must also be routinely assessed for nutritional and immunization status, feeding problems, and other potential problems.
- Only a limited number of carefully selected clinical signs are used, based on evidence of their sensitivity and specificity to detect disease. These signs were selected considering the conditions and realities of first-level health facilities.
- A combination of individual signs leads to a child's classification(s) rather than a diagnosis. Classification(s) indicate the severity of condition(s). They call for specific actions based on whether the young infant or the child:
  - Should be urgently referred to another level of care.
  - Requires specific treatments (such as antibiotics or antimalarial treatment),
  - May be safely managed at home.
- **The classifications are color coded:** "Pink" suggests hospital referral or admission, "yellow" indicates initiation of treatment, and "green" calls for home treatment.

- The IMNCI guidelines address most, but not all, of the major reasons for which a sick child is brought to a clinic. A child returning with chronic problems or less common illnesses may require special care. The guidelines do not describe the care at birth and the management of trauma or other acute emergencies due to accidents or injuries.
- IMNCI management procedures use a limited number of essential drugs and encourage active participation of caretakers in the treatment of children.
- An essential component of the IMNCI guidelines is the counseling of caretakers about home care, including counseling about feeding, fluids and when to return to a health facility.

THE CASE MANAGEMENT PROCESS

The case management process is presented on a series of charts, which show the sequence of steps and provide information for performing them. The charts describe the following steps:

- Assess the young infant or child
- Classify the illness
- Identify treatment
- Treat the infant or child
- Counsel the mother
- Give follow-up care.

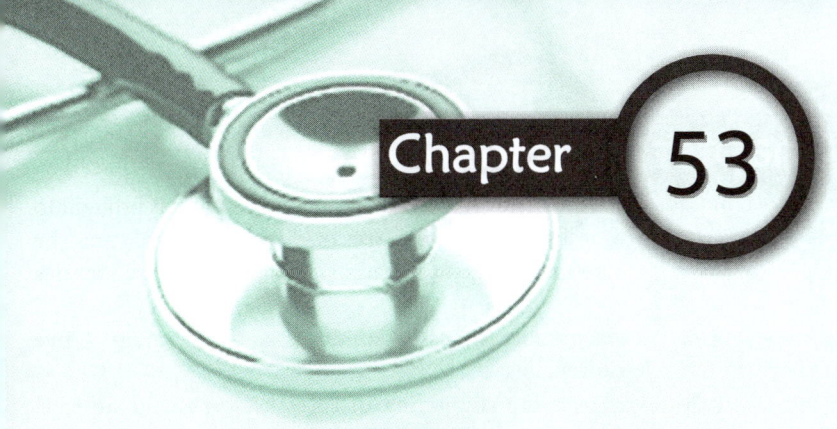

Chapter 53

National Rabies Control Programme

INTRODUCTION

Rabies is endemic throughout the country with the exception of Andaman and Nicobar and Lakshadweep Islands. Dog rabies is a major public health problem accounting for about 96% of the mortality and morbidity. Estimates suggest that annual human rabies death incidence to be around 20,000 and the annual incidence of animal bites to be 1.7% (17.5 million per year). Control of rabies involves two components viz. elimination of human deaths and control of canine rabies to break down the transmission.

Government of India, Ministry of Health and Family Welfare is implementing "National Rabies Control Programme" approved during 12th Five-Year Plan, with an objective to prevent the human deaths due to rabies and to prevent transmission of rabies through canine (dogs) rabies control. The programme has two components human component and animal component. A brief description of the two components of the programme is as under.

COMPONENTS OF THE PROGRAMME

Human Component

Human component is being implemented in all the States and UTs. National center for the diseases control is the nodal agency for the human component of the programme. The strategies for the human component are:

- Training of health professionals.
- Implementing use of intradermal route of inoculation of cell culture vaccines.
- Strengthening surveillance of human rabies.
- Information education and communication.
- Laboratory strengthening.

Animal Component

Animal component is being pilot tested in Haryana and Chennai. The Animal Welfare Board of India, Ministry of Environment and Forests is the Nodal agency for the animal component of the programme. The strategies for the animal component are:

- Population survey of dogs
- Mass vaccination of dogs
- Dog population management
- Strengthening surveillance.

Pulse Polio Programme

INTRODUCTION

With the global initiative of eradication of polio in World Health Assembly resolution in 1988, pulse polio immunization programme was launched in India in 1995. Children in the age group of 0–5 years are administered polio drops during national and sub-national immunization rounds (in high risk areas) every year. About 170 million children are immunized during each National Immunization Day (NID).

Additionally, multiple rounds (at least two) of Sub-National Immunization Day (SNID) have been conducted over the years in high risk states/areas. In these campaigns, children in the age group of 0–5 years are administered polio drops. Over 170 million children are immunized during each NID and 77 million in SNID. Surveillance for detection of polio virus transmission is being done through acute flaccid paralysis (AFP surveillance) with laboratory network since 1997. Oral polio drops are being provided to all children less than five years of age in routine immunization programme.

BACKGROUND

In 1985, the Universal Immunization Programme (UIP) was launched to cover all the districts of the country. UIP became a part of Child Survival and Safe Motherhood Programme (CSSM) in 1992 and Reproductive and Child Health Programme (RCH) in 1997. This programme led to a significant increase in coverage, up to 95%. The number of reported cases of polio also declined from 28,757 during 1987 to 3,265 in 1995.

In 1995, following the **Global Polio Eradication Initiative** of the World Health Organization (1988), India launched pulse polio immunization programme with universal immunization programme which aimed at 100% coverage.

OBJECTIVE

The pulse polio initiative (PPI) was started with an objective of achieving hundred percent coverage under oral polio vaccine. It aimed to immunize children through improved social mobilization, plan mop-up operations in areas where poliovirus has almost disappeared and maintain high level of morale among the public.

AIMS

The PPI aims at covering every individual in the country. It aspires to reach even children in remote communities through an improved social mobilization plan.

- Not a single child should miss the immunization, leaving no chance of polio occurrence.
- Cases of Acute Flaccid Paralysis (AFP) to be reported in time and stool specimens of them to be collected within 14 days. Outbreak Response Immunization (ORI) to be conducted as early as possible.
- Maintaining a high level of surveillance.
- Performance of good mop-up operations where polio has disappeared.

ACTIVITIES

- Setting up of booths in all parts of the country.
- Initializing walk-in cold rooms, freezer rooms, deep freezers, ice-lined refrigerators and cold boxes for a steady supply of vaccine to booths.
- Arranging employees, volunteers, and vaccines.
- Ensuring vaccine vial monitor on each vaccine vial.
- Immunizing children with Oral Poliovirus (OPV) on national immunization days.
- Identifying missing children from immunization process.
- Surveillance of efficacy.

PROGRESS

- South-East Asia Region of WHO including India has been certified polio free by "The Regional Certification Commission (RCC)" on 27th March 2014.
- India reported its last polio case from district Howrah, West Bengal on 13th January, 2011.
- WHO on 24th February 2012 removed India from the list of "endemic countries with active polio virus transmission."
- There are 24 lakh vaccinators and 1.5 lakh supervisors involved in the successful implementation of the Pulse Polio Programme (NID).

Steps Taken by the Government to Maintain Polio Free Status in India

- Maintaining community immunity through high quality National and Sub-National polio rounds each year.
- An extremely high level of vigilance through surveillance across the country for any importation or circulation of poliovirus and VDPV is being maintained. Environmental surveillance (sewage sampling) have been established to detect poliovirus transmission and as a surrogate indicator of the progress as well for any programmatic interventions strategically in Mumbai, Delhi, Patna, Kolkata, Punjab and Gujarat.
- All States and Union Territories in the country have developed a Rapid Response Team (RRT) to respond to any polio outbreak in the country. Emergency Preparedness and Response Plans (EPRP) have also been developed by all States indicating steps to be undertaken in case of detection of a polio case.
- To reduce risk of importation from neighboring countries, international border vaccination is being provided through Continuous Vaccination Teams (CVT) to all eligible children round the clock. These are provided through special booths set up at the international borders that India shares with

Pakistan, Bangladesh, Bhutan, Nepal and Myanmar. 7.8 million children have been vaccinated with OPV as on August 31, 2015.

- Government of India has issued guidelines effective since March 2014, for mandatory requirement of polio vaccination to all international travelers for travel to India and other affected countries namely Afghanistan, Nigeria, Pakistan, Ethiopia, Kenya, Somalia, Syria and Cameroon.
- A rolling emergency stock of OPV is being maintained to respond to detection/importation of Wild Poliovirus (WPV) or emergence of Circulating Vaccine Derived Poliovirus (cVDPV).
- National Technical Advisory Group on Immunization (NTAGI) has recommended injectable polio vaccine (IPV) introduction as an additional dose along with 3rd dose of DPT in the entire country in the last quarter of 2015 as a part of polio endgame strategy.

India to Introduce Injectable Inactivated Poliovirus Vaccine (IPV)

- In May 2012, the World Health Assembly endorsed the polio eradication and endgame strategic plan 2013–2018, calling on countries to strengthen routine immunization programmes and introduce at least one dose of injectable IPV in all countries using OPV.
- India joins 125 other countries to introduce IPV into routine immunization as part of polio eradication and endgame strategic plan in 2015. IPV would be given along with third dose of oral polio vaccine (OPV) at 14 weeks of age for children under one year of age.

Inactivated Poliovirus Vaccine

Injectable IPV will be introduced in the ongoing universal immunization programme (UIP) simultaneously with the existing OPV. IPV launch is a giant leap in India public health programme.

The main aim behind this ambitions programme is to strengthen the immune systems of children and to provide double protection against polio. IPV injection will be given to children below one year of age along with the third dose of the OPV in addition to the existing doses of OPV. Unit polio is abdicated globally, OPV is still the main preventive measure against polio. Thus, IPV is recommended in addition to OPV and does not replace OPV.

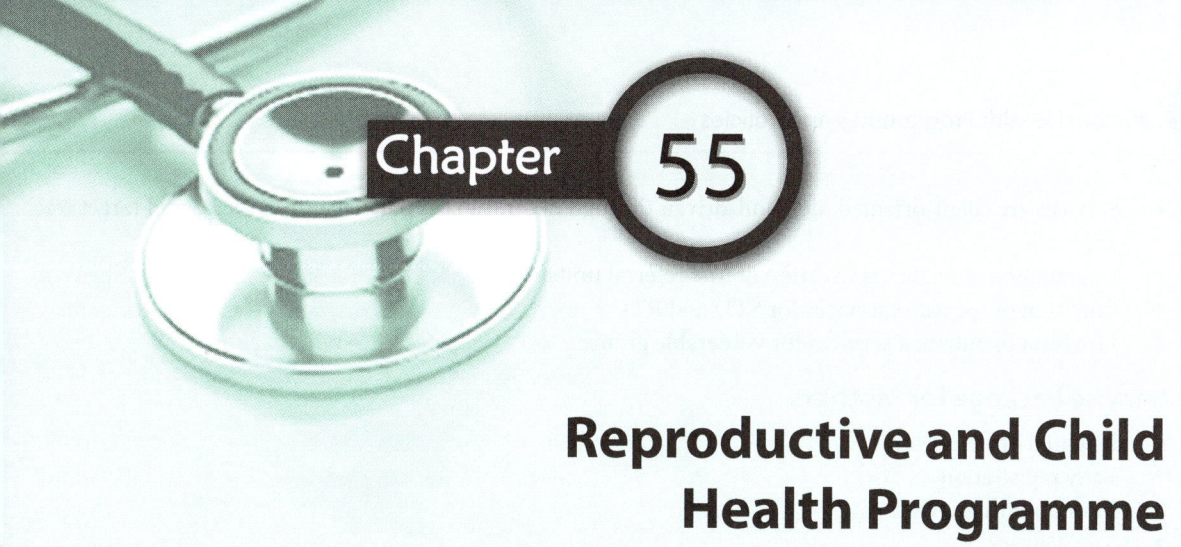

Chapter 55

Reproductive and Child Health Programme

INTRODUCTION

The Reproductive and Child Health (RCH) programme incorporated the earlier existing programmes, i.e. National family welfare programme and Child Survival and Survival and Safe Motherhood Programme (CSSM) and added two more components one relating to sexually transmitted disease and the other relating to reproductive tract infections. The programme was formally launched on 15 October 1997.

OBJECTIVES

- Promotion of MCH to ensure safe motherhood and child survival.
- Reduction of maternal and child morbidity and mortality.
- Attainment of population stabilization.

AIMS

- To bring down the birth rate below 21 per 1,000 population.
- To reduce the infant mortality rate below 60 per 1000 live births.
- To bring down the maternal mortality rate <400/10,000 lakhs.

ESSENTIAL COMPONENTS

- Prevention and management of unwanted pregnancy.
- Maternal care that includes antenatal, delivery and postpartum services.
- Child survival services for newborns and infants.
- Management of reproductive tract infections (TRIs) and sexually transmitted infections (STIs).
  - The Government has power to restrict any unit, and to take samples of effluents and to get them analyzed in Central or State laboratories. Whoever fails to comply with any provision of this Act is punishable with the imprisonment or with fine or with both. Second or third time breaking of the law is further punishable. Under the provision of this Act, Central Pollution Control Board was established to fulfil its object.

HIGHLIGHTS

- Integration of all programmes related fertility regulation, maternal and child health and reproductive health.

- Services are client-oriented, demand-driven through decentralized participatory process and target free approach.
- Upgradation of facilities: Creation of first referral units.
- Provision of specialist services for STD and RTI.
- Provision of outreach services for vulnerable groups.

Service Package for Mothers

- Essential obstetric care
- Early registration
- Minimum three ANC
- Safe delivery
- Three PNC
- Referral
- More relevant for Assam, Bihar, Rajasthan, Odisha, Uttar Pradesh, Madhya Pradesh
- Emergency obstetric care
- Strengthen FRUs
- Supply of kits and skilled manpower
- Traditional Birth Attendants (TBA) Dai training
- NGOs involved: More local specific
- 24-hour delivery services at PHCs/CHCs:
    - Promote institutional deliveries
    - Additional honorarium to staff
    - Safe deliveries
    - Deliveries by trained personnel in safe and hygienic surroundings are encouraged
    - Institutional deliveries are encouraged for women having complications.
    - In case of complication, referrals are made to first referral units for management of obstetric emergencies.
    - Three postnatal checkups are given to mothers after the delivery.

Spacing of at least three years between children are encouraged.

Service Package for Children

- Essential newborn care like keeping the baby warm, checking the baby's weight and giving the baby mother's first milk are encouraged.
- Babies that are premature or have low birth weight are provided special care.
- Babies with any complications are referred to the health center.
- Exclusive breastfeeding is encouraged for the first three months.
- Immunization is administered to every child meticulously to prevent death and disabilities.
- Vitamin A prophylaxis.
- ORT.
- Acute respiratory infection in children is treated by co-trimoxazole tablets.
- Treatment of anemia.

Service Package for Eligible Couple

- Promoting use of contraceptive methods among eligible couples is important to prevent unwanted pregnancies. Couples should be able to choose from various contraceptive methods including condoms, oral pills, IUDs, male and female sterilization.

- Safe services for medical termination of pregnancies should be encouraged for women desiring abortions.
- **Other new services:**
    - Treatment of RTI/STI is given.
    - Promotion activities for adolescent health.

STRATEGIES

- Bottom-up planning
- Decentralized participatory planning and implementation
- Strengthening infrastructure
- Integrated training package
- Improved management.

REPRODUCTIVE AND CHILD HEALTH PROGRAMME PHASE II

Reproductive and Child Health-II is a comprehensive programme under the National Rural Health Mission (NRHM) commenced with the main objective to bring about an improvement in mainly three critical health indicators, i.e. reducing total fertility rate, infant mortality rate and maternal mortality rate. The programme is consistent with the outcomes envisioned in the Millennium Development Goals, National Population Policy 2000, the National Health Policy 2002, the Tenth Plan Document, and Vision 2020 India. The target group of the programme is women in the reproductive age group and children up to 5 years of age.
Reproductive and Child Health Programme Phase II began on 1 April 2005.

Aims

To bring about outcomes as envisioned in the Millennium Development Goals, the National Population Policy 2000 (NPP 2000), the 10th Plan, the National Health Policy 2002 and Vision 2020 India.
- Minimizing the regional variations in the areas of RCH and population stabilization through an integrated, focused, participatory programme meeting the unmet needs of the target population, and provision of assured, equitable, responsive quality services.

Objectives of RCH Phase-II

- Reduction of maternal morbidity and mortality
- Reduction of infant morbidity and mortality
- Reduction of under-5 morbidity and mortality
- Promotion of adolescent health
- Control of reproductive tract infections and sexually transmitted infections.

Salient Features of RCH-II Programme

- Adoption of sector vide approach which effectively extends the programme reach beyond RCH to the entire family welfare sector.
- Building State ownership by involving States and UT's from the outset in development of the programme.
- Decentralization through development of District and State level need-based plans.
- Flexible programming with a view to moving away from prescriptive scheme-based micro planning and instead allowing States to develop need-based work plans with freedom to decide upon programme inputs.

- Capacity building at the District, State and the Central levels to ensure improved programme implementation. In particular, the emphasis being on strengthening financial management systems and monitoring and evaluation capabilities at different levels.
- Adoption of the logical frameworks as a programme management tour to support and outcome-driven approach.
- Performance-based funding to ensure adherence to programme objectives, reward good performance and support weak performers through enhance technical performance.
- Pool financing by the development partners to simplify and rationalize the process of assessing external assistance.
- Convergence, both intersectoral as well as intrasectoral to optimize utilization of resource as well as infrastructural facilities.

Components

- Essential obstetrical care
- Emergency obstetrical care
- Strengthening referral system
- Strengthening project management
- Strengthening infrastructure
- Capacity building
- Improving referral system
- Strengthening MIS
- Innovative schemes

Chapter 56

Reproductive, Maternal, Newborn, Child and Adolescent Health

INTRODUCTION

The Ministry of Health and Family Welfare is bringing out an integrated approach document for reproductive, maternal, newborn, child and adolescent health (RMNCH+A) in India. RMNCH+A approach essentially looks to address the major causes of mortality among women and children as well as the delays in accessing and utilizing health care and services. The RMNCH+A strategic approach document has been developed to provide an understanding of 'continuum of care' to ensure equal focus on various life stages.

The RMNCH+A document appropriately directs the States to focus their efforts on the most vulnerable population and disadvantaged groups in the country. The document also emphasizes on the need to reinforce efforts in the poor performing districts which have already been identified as the high focus districts. The document will serve as a hands-on guide for Mission Directors and State Programme Managers in the planning, implementation and monitoring of the new and existing RMNCH+A interventions.

The RMNCH+A approach document has been especially prepared for Health Secretaries, Mission Directors, Directors of Health Services and senior programme planners and implementers, with the purpose of providing an understanding of the comprehensive approach to improving child survival and safe motherhood, and operational guidance to implement this approach during the next phase of the NRHM (2012–2017). The document provides the programmers with direction, which when followed in earnest would lead to significant improvement in adolescent, woman and child health over the next five years. Individual states and districts would still need to translate the approach proposed here to specific actions within their own context in order to achieve state-specific targets. The document mainly refers to the measures taken so far to improve the health of women, mother and children; however, the national health programme is a dynamic and evolving programme, hence new measures will be included as more evidence emerges from pilot states and from intervention research and implementation experiences from across the country. Major changes and modifications in the flagship programmes of Ministry of Women and Child Development and other Ministries and sectors are also envisaged in the 12th Plan, and these are likely to have an impact on many indicators and social determinants of health and development that affect maternal and child survival. The RMNCH+A strategy aims to reduce child and maternal mortality through strengthening health care delivery system.

GOALS

The 12th Five-Year Plan has defined the national health outcomes and the three goals that are relevant to RMNCH+A strategic approach as follows:

Health outcome goals established in the 12th Five-Year Plan.
- Reduction of infant mortality rate (IMR) to 25 per 1,000 live births by 2017.
- Reduction in maternal mortality ratio (MMR) to 100 per 100,000 live births by 2017.
- Reduction in total fertility rate (TFR) to 2.1 by 2017.

COVERAGE TARGETS FOR KEY RMNCH+A INTERVENTIONS FOR 2017

- Increase facilities equipped for perinatal care (designated as 'delivery points') by 100%.
- Increase proportion of all births in government and accredited private institutions at annual rate of 5.6% from the baseline of 61% (SRS 2010).
- Increase proportion of pregnant women receiving antenatal care at annual rate of 6% from the baseline of 53% (CES 2009).
- Increase proportion of mothers and newborns receiving postnatal care at annual rate of 7.5% from the baseline of 45% (CES 2009).
- Increase proportion of deliveries conducted by skilled birth attendants at annual rate of 2% from the baseline of 76% (CES 2009).
  - Increase exclusive breastfeeding rates at annual rate of 9.6% from the baseline of 36% (CES 2009).
  - Reduce prevalence of under-five children who are underweight at annual rate of 5.5% from the baseline of 45% (NFHS 3).
  - Increase coverage of three doses of combined diphtheria-tetanus-pertussis (DTP3) (12–23 months) at annual rate of 3.5% from the baseline of 7% (CES 2009).
  - Increase ORS use in under-five children with diarrhea at annual rate of 7.2% from the baseline of 43% (CES 2009).

5 x 5 Matrix for RMNCH+A				
Let's make every mother and child healthy Transformational Leadership can do it				
Reproductive Health	**Maternal Health**	**Newborn Health**	**Child Health**	**Adolescent Health**
• Focus on spacing methods, particularly PPIUCD at high case load facilities • Interval IUCD at sub-centers on fixed days • Doorstep delivery of contraceptives by ASHA • Strengthening Safe abortion services • Maintaining sterilization services	• Use MCTS to ensure early registration of pregnancy and provide full ANC • Detect high risk pregnancies and line list and manage severely anemic mothers • Equip delivery points with trained HR & other infrastructure • Review maternal, infant and child deaths for corrective actions • Notify sub-centers with less institutional delivery load, distribute mesoprostol and incentivize ANMs for domiciliary deliveries	• Early initiation and exclusive breastfeeding • Home based newborn care through ASHA • Essential Newborn Care and resuscitation services at all delivery points • Equip special newborn care units with highly trained HR and other infrastructure • Empower ANM for community level use of Gentamycin	• Complementary feeding, IFA supplementation and focus on nutrition • Diarrhea management at community level using ORS and Zinc • Management of pneumonia • Full immunization coverage • Rashtriya Baal Swasthya Karyakram (RBSK): screening of children for 4D's (birth defects, development delays, deficiencies and disease) and its management	• Community-based services through peer educators • Delay in age of marriage • Strengthen ARSH clinics • Weekly IFA Supplementation (WIFS) under national Iron plus initiative • Promote menstrual hygiene
Health Systems			**Cross cutting**	
• Case load based deployment of HR at all levels • Ambulances, drugs, diagnostics, reproductive health commodities • Behavior change communication • Supportive supervision and use of scorecards based on HMIS • Public grievances redressal mechanism			• Equip nurses to provide specialized and quality care • Address social determinants of health through convergence • Introduce difficult area and performance based incentives • Focus on un-served and underserved villages, urban slums and blocks • Bring down out of pocket expenses	

(Source: nrhm.gov.in/nrhm-components)

- Reduce unmet need for family planning methods among eligible couples, married and unmarried, at annual rate of 8.8% from the baseline of 21% (DLHS 3).
- Increase met need for modern family planning methods among eligible couples at annual rate of 4.5% from the baseline of 47% (DLHS 3).
- Reduce anemia in adolescent girls and boys (15–19 years) at annual rate of 6% from the baseline of 56% and 30%, respectively (NFHS 3).
- Decrease the proportion of total fertility contributed by adolescents (15–19 years) at annual rate of 3.8% per year from the baseline of 16% (NFHS 3).
- Raise child sex ratio in the 0–6 years age group at annual rate of 0.6% per year from the baseline of 914 (Census 2011).

ADOLESCENCE

Adolescent health and nutrition status has an intergenerational effect. Therefore, adolescence is one of the important stages of life cycle in terms of health interventions. Although adolescence is considered to be a healthy phase, more than 33% of the disease burden and almost 60% of premature deaths among adults can be associated with behaviors or conditions that begin or occur during adolescence—for example, tobacco and alcohol use, poor eating habits, sexual abuse and risky sex (WHO 2002). Within the age group of 10–19 years, the profile of disease burden is significantly different for younger and older adolescents. While injuries and communicable diseases are prominent causes of disability and death in the 10–14 age group, outcomes of sexual behaviors and mental health become significant for the 15–19 years age group.

Taking cognizance of the diverse nature of adolescent health needs, a comprehensive adolescent health strategy has been developed. The priority under adolescent health include nutrition, sexual and reproductive health, mental health, addressing gender-based violence, non-communicable diseases and substance use. The strategy proposes a set of interventions (health promotion, prevention, diagnosis, treatment and referral) across levels of care. These interventions and approaches work toward building protective factors that can help adolescents and young people develop 'resilience' to resist negative behaviors and operate at four major levels: individual, family, school and community by providing a comprehensive package of information, commodities and services.

Priority Interventions

- Adolescent nutrition; iron and folic acid supplementation
- Facility-based adolescent reproductive and sexual health services (Adolescent health clinics)
- Information and counseling on adolescent sexual reproductive health and other health issues
- Menstrual hygiene
- Preventive health checkups.

PREGNANCY AND CHILDBIRTH

Pregnancy and childbirth are physiological events in the life of a woman. Though most pregnancies result in normal birth, it is estimated that about 15% may develop complications, which cannot be predicted. Majority of these complications can be averted by preventive care (such as antenatal checkups, birth preparedness), skilled care at birth, early detection of risk (like with use of partographs), appropriate and timely management of obstetric complications and postnatal care. The essential package of interventions needed for averting maternal mortality is well known. The challenge lies in ensuring that this package is delivered at a sufficient scale and with sufficient quality to have a significant impact.

Most of the services in this continuum are already in place; what is required is a stronger linkage between various levels, and tracking women and newborn to ensure the delivery of this package of services.

Priority Interventions

- Delivery of antenatal care package and tracking of high-risk pregnancies
- Skilled obstetric care
- Immediate essential newborn care and resuscitation
- Emergency obstetric and newborn care
- Postpartum care for mother and newborn
- Postpartum IUCD and sterilization
- Implementation of PC and PNDT Act

NEWBORN AND CHILD CARE

The interventions in this phase of life mainly focus on children under 5 years of age and address the most common causes of mortality in this period, with some interventions extending to children older than 5 years. The objectives for newborn and child health under the NRHM are:

- Immediate, routine newborn care and care of sick newborns
- Child nutrition including essential micronutrients supplementation
- Immunization against common childhood diseases and
- Management of common neonatal and childhood illnesses.

A new initiative of child health screening and early intervention services offering comprehensive care to children (0–5; 6–9; 10–18 years) is also being introduced. As newer health challenges emerge, it will be important to set up a surveillance programme to provide estimates and trends of the NCD burden such as childhood epilepsy, juvenile diabetes, childhood injuries, birth defects, sickle cell anemia and thalassemia for future programming and policy direction. The relative disease burden in states must be taken into account for identifying a rational mix of interventions that reflect the changing health needs of this population. The child death review and the other systems of monitoring should guide this planning and prioritization process as also the evidence base, depicting that the intervention is known to have an impact on child mortality.

Priority Interventions

- Home-based newborn care and prompt referral
- Facility-based care of the sick newborn
- Integrated management of common childhood illnesses (diarrhea, pneumonia and malaria)
- Child nutrition and essential micronutrients supplementation
- Immunization
- Early detection and management of defects at birth, deficiencies, diseases and disability in children (0–18 years).

REPRODUCTIVE YEARS

Reproductive health needs exist across the reproductive years and therefore access to these services is required in various life stages starting from the adolescence phase. Reproductive health services include the provision for contraceptives, access to comprehensive and safe abortion services, diagnosis and management of sexually transmitted infections, including HIV. These services will be delivered at home, through community outreach and at all levels of health facilities and include adolescents and adults in the reproductive age group.

Priority Interventions

- Community-based promotion and delivery of contraceptives
- Promotion of spacing methods (interval IUCD)
- Sterilization services (vasectomies and tubectomies)
- Comprehensive abortion care (includes MTP Act)
- Prevention and management of sexually transmitted and reproductive infections (STI/RTI).

INFRASTRUCTURE

The key steps proposed for strengthening health facilities for delivery of RMNCH+A interventions are as follows:

- Prepare and implement facility specific plans for ensuring quality and meeting service guarantees as specified under IPHS.
- Assess the need for new infrastructure, extension of existing infrastructure on the basis of patient load and location of facility.
- Equip health facilities to support forty-eight-hour stay of mother and newborn.
- Engage private facilities for family planning services, management of sick newborns and children, and pregnancy complications.
- Strengthen referral mechanisms between facilities at various levels and communities.
- Provision for adequate infrastructure for waste management.

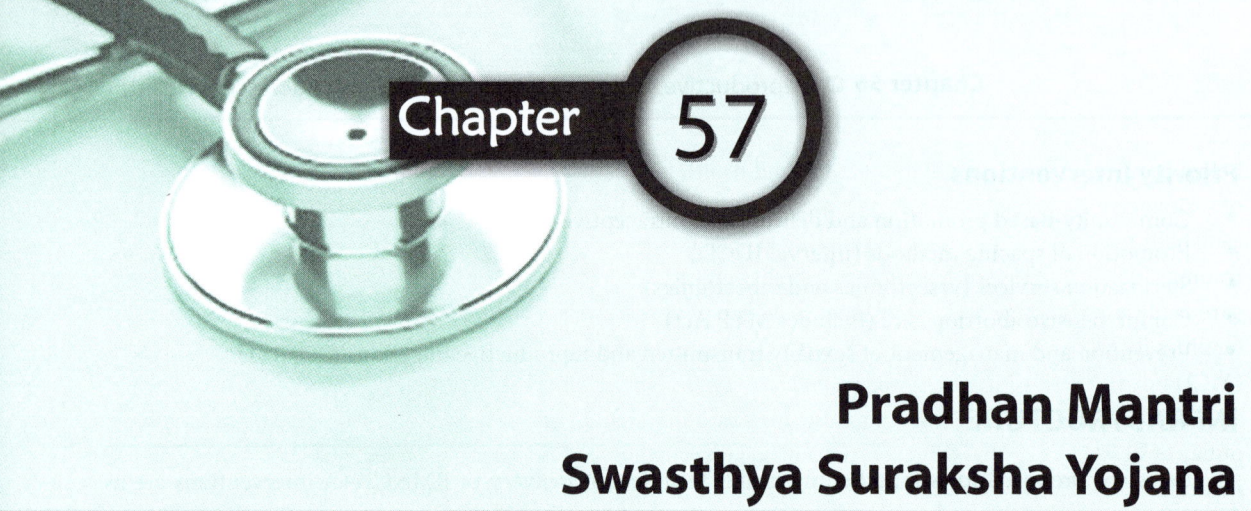

Chapter 57

Pradhan Mantri Swasthya Suraksha Yojana

INTRODUCTION

The Pradhan Mantri Swasthya Suraksha Yojana (PMSSY) was announced in 2003 with objectives of correcting regional imbalances in the availability of affordable/reliable tertiary health care services and also to augment facilities for quality medical education in the country.

PMSSY has two components:

- **Setting up new AIIMS:**
    - Six AIIMS are already functional.
    - AIIMS Raebareli is under construction.
    - Eleven more AIIMS are announced. Out of which, 5 AIIMS are approved by cabinet.
- **Upgradation of government medical colleges:**
    - Phase l : 13 GMCs
    - Phase ll: 06 GMCs
    - Phase lll : 39 GMCs
    - Phase lV : 13 GMCs

OBJECTIVES

The PMSSY aims at correcting the imbalances in the availability of affordable health care facilities in the different parts of the country in general, and augmenting facilities for quality medical education in the under-served states in particular. The scheme was approved in March 2006.

IMPLEMENTATION

First Phase

The first phase in the PMSSY has two components—setting up of six institutions in the line of AIIMS; and upgradation of 13 existing government medical college institutions.

It has been decided to set up 6 AIIMS-like institutions, one each in the States of Bihar (Patna), Chhattisgarh (Raipur), Madhya Pradesh (Bhopal), Odisha (Bhubaneswar), Rajasthan (Jodhpur) and Uttaranchal (Rishikesh) at an estimated cost of ₹840 crores per institution. These states have been identified on the basis of various socio-economic indicators like human development index, literacy rate, population below poverty line and per capital income and health indicators like population to bed ratio, prevalence rate of serious communicable diseases, infant mortality rate, etc. Each institution will have a 960-bedded hospital (500 beds for the medical college hospital; 300 beds for Specialty/Super Specialty; 100 beds for ICU/Accident trauma; 30 beds for physical medicine and rehabilitation and 30 beds for AYUSH) intended to provide health care facilities in 42 Specialty/Super-Specialty disciplines. Medical Colleges will have 100 UG intake besides facilities for imparting PG/doctoral courses in various disciplines, largely based on Medical Council of India (MCI) norms and also nursing college conforming to Nursing Council norms.

In addition to this, 13 existing medical institutions spread over 10 States will also be upgraded, with an outlay of ₹120 crores (₹100 crores from Central Government and ₹20 crores from State Government) for each institution. These institutions are:

- Government Medical College, Jammu, Jammu and Kashmir
- Government Medical College, Srinagar, Jammu and Kashmir
- Kolkata Medical College, Kolkata, West Bengal
- Sanjay Gandhi Post Graduate Institute of Medical Sciences, Lucknow, Uttar Pradesh
- Institute of Medical Sciences, BHU, Varanasi, Uttar Pradesh
- Nizam's Institute of Medical Sciences, Hyderabad, Telangana
- Sri Venkateshwara Institute of Medical Sciences, Tirupati, Andhra Pradesh
- Government Medical College, Salem, Tamil Nadu
- B.J. Medical College, Ahmedabad, Gujarat
- Bangalore Medical College, Bengaluru, Karnataka
- Government Medical College, Thiruvananthapuram, Kerala
- Rajendra Institute of Medical Sciences (RIMS), Ranchi
- Grants Medical College and Sir J.J. Group of Hospitals, Mumbai, Maharashtra

Second Phase

In the second phase of PMSSY, the Government has approved the setting up of two more AIIMS-like institutions, one each in the States of West Bengal and Uttar Pradesh and upgradation of six medical college institutions namely:

- Government Medical College, Amritsar, Punjab
- Government Medical College, Tanda, Himachal Pradesh
- Government Medical College, Madurai, Tamil Nadu
- Government Medical College, Nagpur, Maharashtra
- Jawaharlal Nehru Medical College of Aligarh Muslim University, Aligarh, Uttar Pradesh
- Pt. B.D. Sharma Postgraduate Institute of Medical Sciences, Rohtak, Haryana

The estimated cost for each AIIMS-like institution is ₹823 crore. For upgradation of medical college institutions, Central Government will contribute ₹125 crore each.

Third Phase

In the third phase of PMSSY, it is proposed to upgrade the following existing medical college institutions namely:

- Government Medical College, Jhansi, Uttar Pradesh
- Government Medical College, Rewa, Madhya Pradesh
- Government Medical College, Gorakhpur, Uttar Pradesh

- Government Medical College, Darbhanga, Bihar
- Government Medical College, Kozhikode, Kerala
- Vijaynagar Institute of Medical Sciences, Bellary, Karnataka
- Government Medical College, Muzaffarpur, Bihar

The project cost for upgradation of each medical college institution has been estimated at ₹150 crores per institution, out of which Central Government will contribute ₹125 crores and the remaining ₹25 crore will be borne by the respective State Governments.

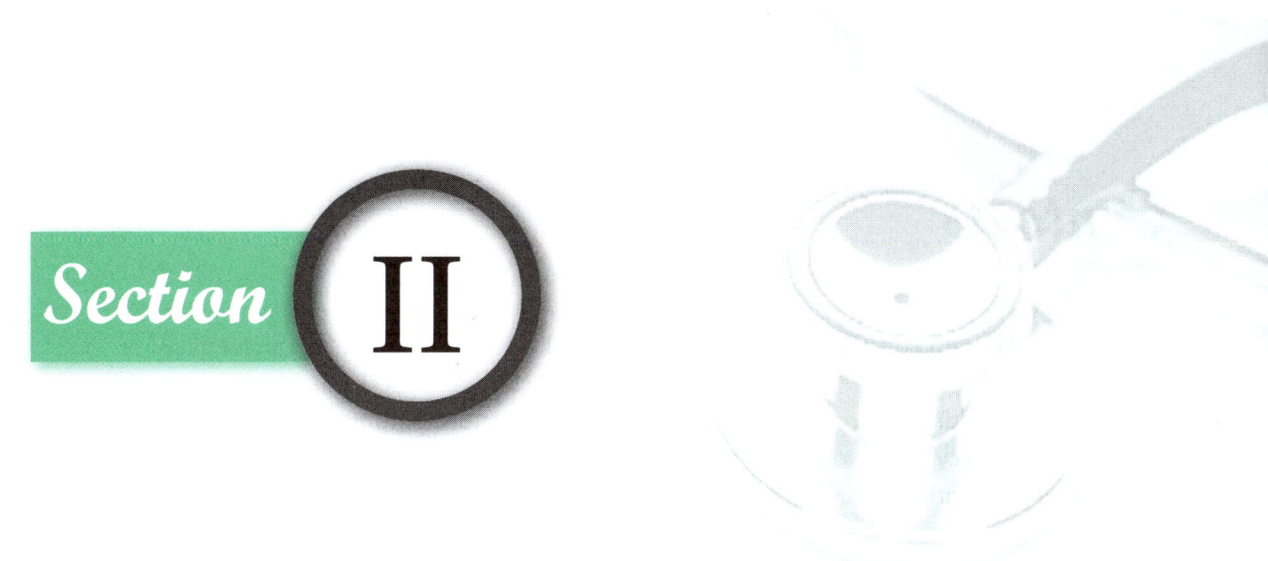

Section II

HEALTH RELATED POLICIES IN INDIA

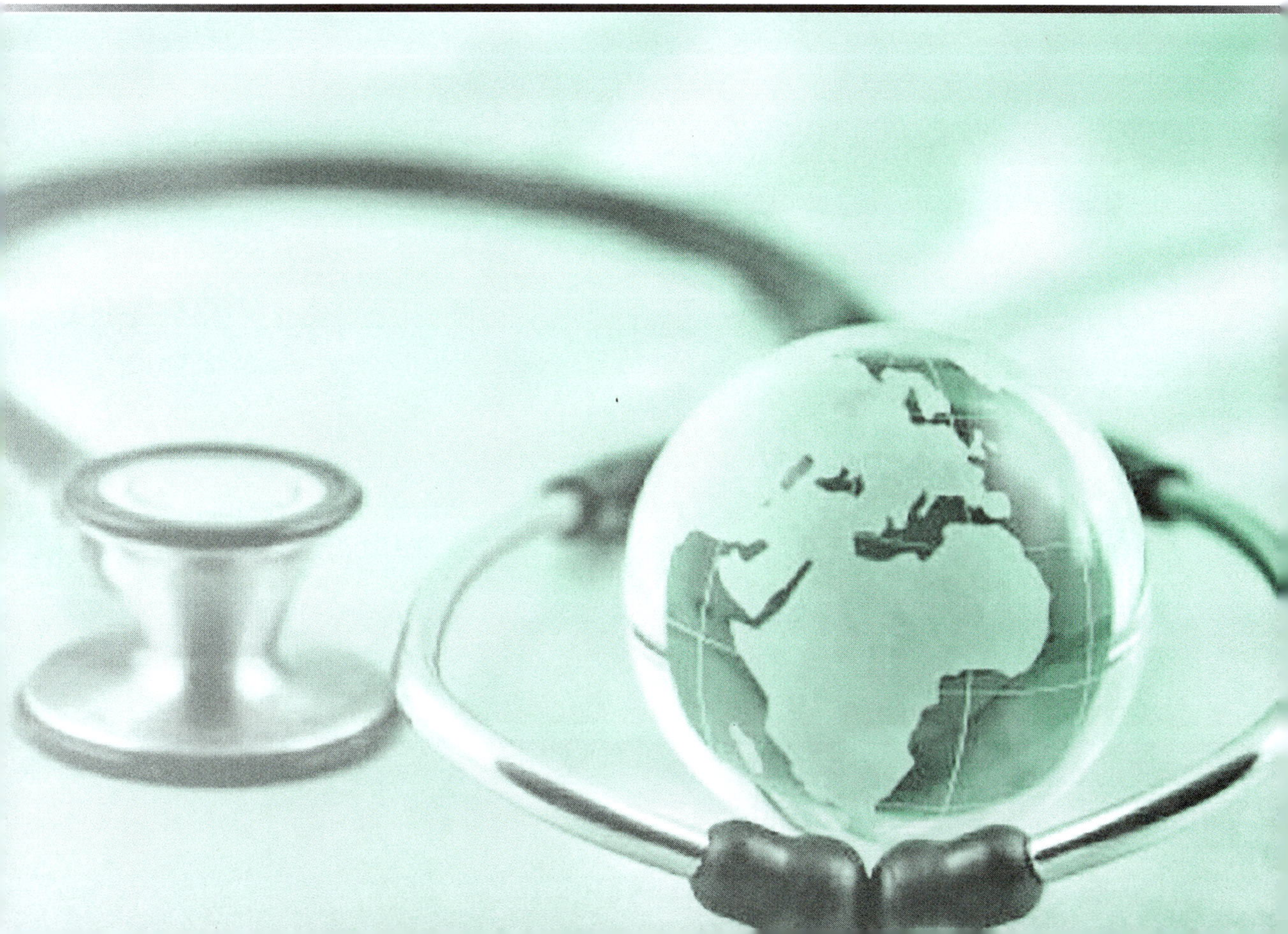

Contents

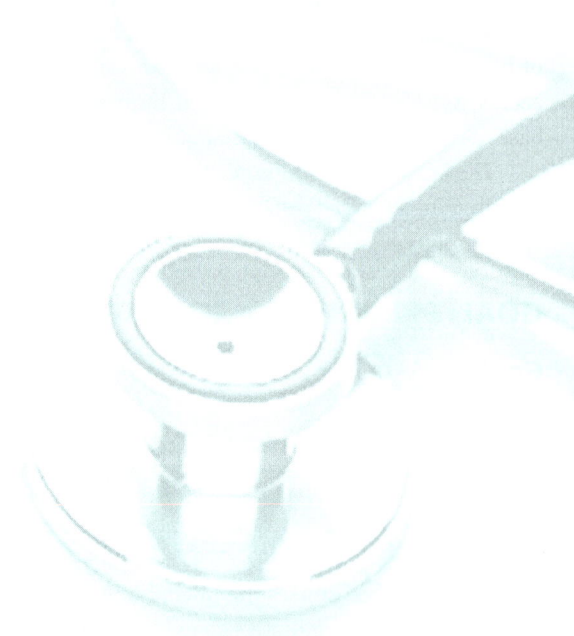

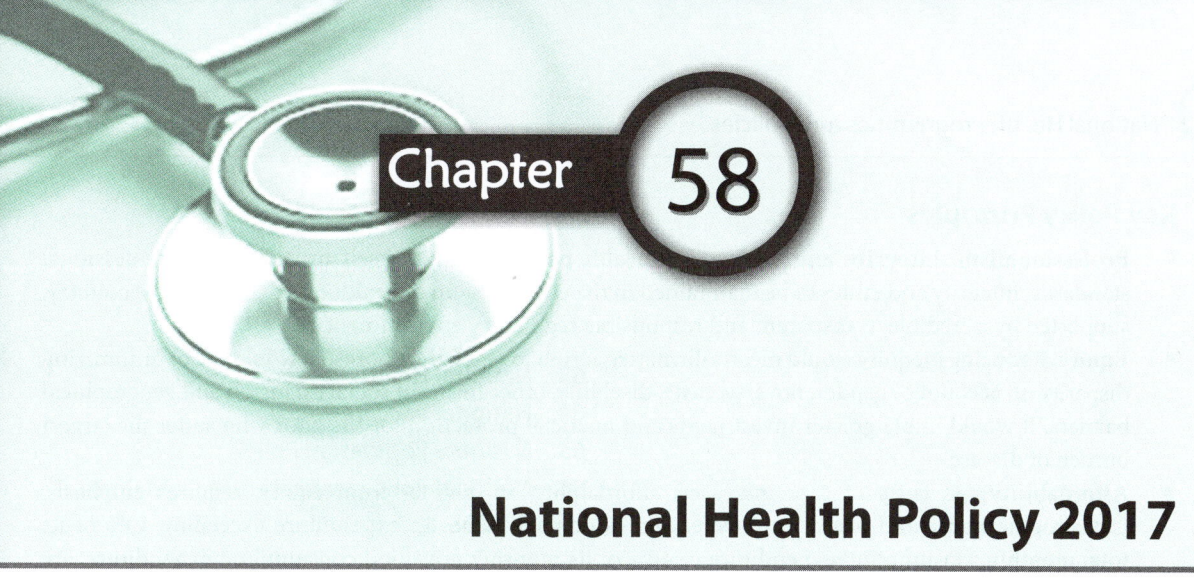

Chapter 58

National Health Policy 2017

INTRODUCTION

The National Health Policy (NHP) of 1983 and the National Health Policy of 2002 have served well in guiding the approach for the health sector in the Five-Year Plans. Fourteen years after the last health policy, the context has changed in four major ways. First, the health priorities are changing. Although maternal and child mortality have rapidly declined, there is growing burden on account of non-communicable diseases and some infectious diseases. The second important change is the emergence of a robust health care industry estimated to be growing at double digit. The third change is the growing incidence of catastrophic expenditure due to health care costs, which are presently estimated to be one of the major contributors to poverty. Fourth, a rising economic growth enables enhanced fiscal capacity. Therefore, a new health policy responsive to these contextual changes is required.

The primary aim of the National Health Policy 2017, is to inform, clarify, strengthen and prioritize the role of the Government in shaping health systems in all its dimensions—investments in health, organization of healthcare services, prevention of diseases and promotion of good health through cross sectoral actions, access to technologies, developing human resources, encouraging medical pluralism, building knowledge base, developing better financial protection strategies, strengthening regulation and health assurance.

The NHP 2017 builds on the progress made since the last NHP 2002. The developments have been captured in the document "Backdrop to National Health Policy 2017—Situation Analyses", Ministry of Health and Family Welfare, Government of India.

GOAL, PRINCIPLES AND OBJECTIVES

Goal

The policy envisages as its goal the attainment of the highest possible level of health and well-being for all at all ages, through a preventive and promotive health care orientation in all developmental policies, and universal access to good quality health care services without anyone having to face financial hardship as a consequence. This would be achieved through increasing access, improving quality and lowering the cost of healthcare delivery.

The policy recognizes the pivotal importance of Sustainable Development Goals (SDGs). An indicative list of time bound quantitative goals aligned to ongoing national efforts as well as the global strategic directions is given in detail at the end of this section.

Key Policy Principles

- **Professionalism, integrity and ethics:** The health policy commits itself to the highest professional standards, integrity and ethics to be maintained in the entire system of health care delivery in the country, supported by a credible, transparent and responsible regulatory environment.
- **Equity:** Reducing inequity would mean affirmative action to reach the poorest. It would mean minimizing disparity on account of gender, poverty, caste, disability, other forms of social exclusion and geographical barriers. It would imply greater investments and financial protection for the poor who suffer the largest burden of disease.
- **Affordability:** As costs of care increases, affordability, as distinct from equity, requires emphasis. Catastrophic household health care expenditures defined as health expenditure exceeding 10% of its total monthly consumption expenditure or 40% of its monthly non-food consumption expenditure, are unacceptable.
- **Universality:** Prevention of exclusions on social, economic or on grounds of current health status. In this backdrop, systems and services are envisaged to be designed to cater to the entire population—including special groups.
- **Patient centered and quality of care**: Gender sensitive, effective, safe, and convenient healthcare services to be provided with dignity and confidentiality. There is need to evolve and disseminate standards and guidelines for all levels of facilities and a system to ensure that the quality of healthcare is not compromised.
- **Accountability:** Financial and performance accountability, transparency in decision making, and elimination of corruption in health care systems, both in public and private.
- **Inclusive partnerships**: A multistakeholder approach with partnership and participation of all non-health ministries and communities. This approach would include partnerships with academic institutions, not for profit agencies, and health care industry as well.
- **Pluralism:** Patients who so choose and when appropriate, would have access to AYUSH care providers based on documented and validated local, home and community-based practices. These systems, inter alia, would also have Government support in research and supervision to develop and enrich their contribution to meeting the national health goals and objectives through integrative practices.
- **Decentralization:** Decentralization of decision making to a level as is consistent with practical considerations and institutional capacity. Community participation in health planning processes, to be promoted side by side.
- **Dynamism and adaptiveness:** Constantly improving dynamic organization of health care based on new knowledge and evidence with learning from the communities and from national and international knowledge partners is designed.

Objectives

Improve health status through concerted policy action in all sectors and expand preventive, promotive, curative, palliative and rehabilitative services provided through the public health sector with focus on quality.

Progressively Achieve Universal Health Coverage

- Assuring availability of free, comprehensive primary health care services, for all aspects of reproductive, maternal, child and adolescent health and for the most prevalent communicable, non-communicable and occupational diseases in the population. The Policy also envisages optimum use of existing manpower and infrastructure as available in the health sector and advocates collaboration with non-government sector on pro bono basis for delivery of health care services linked to a health card to enable every family to have access to a doctor of their choice from amongst those volunteering their services.

- Ensuring improved access and affordability, of quality secondary and tertiary care services through a combination of public hospitals and well-measured strategic purchasing of services in health care deficit areas, from private care providers, especially the not-for profit providers.
- Achieving a significant reduction in out of pocket expenditure due to health care costs and achieving reduction in proportion of households experiencing catastrophic health expenditures and consequent impoverishment.

Reinforcing Trust in Public Health Care System

Strengthening the trust of the common man in public health care system by making it predictable, efficient and patient-centric, affordable and effective, with a comprehensive package of services and products that meet immediate health care needs of most people.

Align the Growth of Private Health Care Sector with Public Health Goals

Influence the operation and growth of the private health care sector and medical technologies to ensure alignment with public health goals. Enable private sector contribution to making health care systems more effective, efficient, rational, safe, affordable and ethical. Strategic purchasing by the Government to fill critical gaps in public health facilities would create a demand for private health care sector, in alignment with the public health goals.

Specific Quantitative Goals and Objectives

The indicative, quantitative goals and objectives are outlined under three broad components, viz.
- Health status and programme impact
- Health systems performance
- Health system strengthening.

These goals and objectives are aligned to achieve sustainable development in health sector in keeping with the policy thrust.

Health Status and Programme Impact

Life expectancy and healthy life
- Increase life expectancy at birth from 67.5 to 70 by 2025.
- Establish regular tracking of Disability Adjusted Life Years (DALY) Index as a measure of burden of disease and its trends by major categories by 2022.
- Reduction of TFR to 2.1 at national and sub-national level by 2025.

Mortality by age and/or cause
- Reduce Under-Five Mortality to 23 by 2025 and MMR from current levels to 100 by 2020.
- Reduce infant mortality rate to 28 by 2019.
- Reduce neonatal mortality to 16 and still birth rate to "single digit" by 2025.

Reduction of disease prevalence/incidence
- Achieve global target of 2020 which is also termed as target of 90:90:90, for HIV/AIDS, i.e.,—90% of all people living with HIV know their HIV status,—90% of all people diagnosed with HIV infection receive sustained antiretroviral therapy and 90% of all people receiving antiretroviral therapy will have viral suppression.
- Achieve and maintain elimination status of Leprosy by 2018, Kala-azar by 2017 and lymphatic filariasis in endemic pockets by 2017.
- To achieve and maintain a cure rate of >85% in new sputum positive patients for TB and reduce incidence of new cases, to reach elimination status by 2025.

- To reduce the prevalence of blindness to 0.25/1000 by 2025 and disease burden by one-third from current levels.
- To reduce premature mortality from cardiovascular diseases, cancer, diabetes or chronic respiratory diseases by 25% by 2025.

Health Systems Performance

Coverage of health services
- Increase utilization of public health facilities by 50% from current levels by 2025.
- Antenatal care coverage to be sustained above 90% and skilled attendance at birth above 90% by 2025.
- More than 90% of the newborn are fully immunized by one year of age by 2025.
- Meet need of family planning above 90% at national and subnational level by 2025.
- 80% of known hypertensive and diabetic individuals at household level maintain, 'controlled disease status' by 2025.

Cross-sectoral goals related to health
- Relative reduction in prevalence of current tobacco use by 15% by 2020 and 30% by 2025.
- Reduction of 40% in prevalence of stunting of under-five children by 2025.
- Access to safe water and sanitation to all by 2020 (Swachh Bharat Mission).
- Reduction of occupational injury by half from current levels of 334 per lakh agricultural workers by 2020.
- National/State level tracking of selected health behavior.

Health Systems Strengthening

Health finance
- Increase health expenditure by Government as a percentage of GDP from the existing 1.15–2.5% by 2025.
- Increase State sector health spending to > 8% of their budget by 2020.
- Decrease in proportion of households facing catastrophic health expenditure from the current levels by 25%, by 2025.

Health Infrastructure and Human Resource
- Ensure availability of paramedics and doctors as per Indian Public Health Standard (IPHS) norm in high priority districts by 2020.
- Increase community health volunteers to population ratio as per IPHS norm, in high priority districts by 2025.
- Establish primary and secondary care facility as per norms in high priority districts (population as well as time to reach norms) by 2025.

Health Management Information
- Ensure district-level electronic database of information on health system components by 2020.
- Strengthen the health surveillance system and establish registries for diseases of public health importance by 2020.
- Establish federated integrated health information architecture, Health Information Exchanges and National Health Information Network by 2025.

POLICY THRUST

Ensuring Adequate Investment

The policy proposes a potentially achievable target of raising public health expenditure to 2.5% of the GDP in a time-bound manner. It envisages that the resource allocation to States will be linked with State development indicators, absorptive capacity and financial indicators. The States would be incentivized for incremental State resources for public health expenditure. General taxation will remain the predominant means for financing care. The Government could consider imposing taxes on specific commodities—such as the taxes on tobacco, alcohol and foods having negative impact on health, taxes on extractive industries and pollution cess. Funds available under Corporate Social Responsibility would also be leveraged for well-focused programmes aiming to address health goals.

Preventive and Promotive Health

The policy articulates to institutionalize intersectoral coordination at national and subnational levels to optimize health outcomes, through constitution of bodies that have representation from relevant non-health ministries. This is in line with the emergent international "Health in All" approach as complement to Health for All. The policy prerequisite is for an empowered public health cadre to address social determinants of health effectively, by enforcing regulatory provisions.

The policy identifies coordinated action on seven priority areas for improving the environment for health:
* The *Swachh Bharat Abhiyan*
* Balanced, healthy diets and regular exercises.
* Addressing tobacco, alcohol and substance abuse
* *Yatri Suraksha*—preventing deaths due to rail and road traffic accidents
* *Nirbhaya Nari*—action against gender violence
* Reduced stress and improved safety in the work place
* Reducing indoor and outdoor air pollution

The policy also articulates the need for the development of strategies and institutional mechanisms in each of these seven areas, to create Swasth Nagrik Abhiyan—a social movement for health. It recommends setting indicators, their targets as also mechanisms for achievement in each of these areas.

The policy recognizes and builds upon preventive and promotive care as an under-recognized reality that has a two-way continuity with curative care, provided by health agencies at same or at higher levels. The policy recommends an expansion of scope of interventions to include early detection and response to early childhood development delays and disability, adolescent and sexual health education, behavior change with respect to tobacco and alcohol use, screening, counseling for primary prevention and secondary prevention from common chronic illness—both communicable and non-communicable diseases. Additionally, the policy focus is on extending coverage as also quality of the existing package of services. Policy recognizes the need to frame and adhere to health screening guidelines across age groups. Zoonotic diseases like rabies need to be addressed through concerted and coordinated action, at the national front and through strengthening of the National Rabies Control Programme.

The policy lays greater emphasis on investment and action in school health—by incorporating health education as part of the curriculum, promoting hygiene and safe health practices within the school environment and by acting as a site of primary health care. Promotion of healthy living and prevention strategies from AYUSH systems and Yoga at the work-place, in the schools and in the community would also be an important form of health promotion that has a special appeal and acceptability in the Indian context.

Recognizing the risks arising from physical, chemical, and other workplace hazards, the policy advocates for providing greater focus on occupational health. Work-sites and institutions would be encouraged and monitored to ensure safe health practices and accident prevention, besides providing preventive and promotive healthcare services.

ASHA will also be supported by other frontline workers like health workers (male/female) to undertake primary prevention for non-communicable diseases. They would also provide community or home-based palliative care and mental health services through health promotion activities. These workers would get support from local self-government and the Village Health Sanitation and Nutrition Committee (VHSNC).

In order to build community support and offer good healthcare to the vulnerable sections of the society like the marginalized, the socially excluded, the poor, the old and the disabled, the policy recommends strengthening the VHSNCs and their equivalent in the urban areas.

"Health Impact Assessment" of existing and emerging policies, of key non-health departments which directly or indirectly impact health would be taken up.

Organization of Public Health Care Delivery

The policy proposes seven key policy shifts in organizing health care services:
- In primary care—from selective care to assured comprehensive care with linkages to referral hospitals.
- In secondary and tertiary care—from an input oriented to an output-based strategic purchasing.
- In public hospitals—from user fees and cost recovery to assured free drugs, diagnostic and emergency services to all.
- In infrastructure and human resource development—from normative approach to targeted approach to reach underserviced areas.
- In urban health—from token interventions to on-scale assured interventions, to organize Primary Health Care delivery and referral support for urban poor. Collaboration with other sectors to address wider determinants of urban health is advocated.
- In National Health Programmes—integration with health systems for programme effectiveness and in turn contributing to strengthening of health systems for efficiency.
- In AYUSH services—from stand-alone to a three-dimensional mainstreaming.

Free primary care provision by the public sector, supplemented by strategic purchase of secondary care hospitalization and tertiary care services from both public and from non-government sector to fill critical gaps would be the main strategy of assuring healthcare services. The policy envisages strategic purchase of secondary and tertiary care services as a short-term measure. Strategic purchasing refers to the Government acting as a single payer. The order of preference for strategic purchase would be public sector hospitals followed by not for profit private sector and then commercial private sector in underserved areas, based on the availability of services of acceptable and defined quality criteria. In the long run, the policy envisages to have fully-equipped and functional public sector hospitals in these areas to meet secondary and tertiary health care needs of population, especially the poorest and marginalized. Public facilities would remain the focal point in the healthcare delivery system and services in the public health facilities would be expanded from current levels. The policy recognizes the special health needs of tribal and socially vulnerable population groups and recommends situation specific measures in provisioning and delivery of services. The policy advocates enhanced outreach of public healthcare through Mobile Medical Units (MMUs), etc. Tribal population in the country is over 100 million (Census 2011), and hence deserves special attention keeping in mind their geographical and infrastructural challenges. Keeping in view the high cost involved in provisioning and managing orphan diseases, the policy encourages active engagement with non-government sector for addressing the situation. In order to provide access and financial protection at secondary and tertiary care levels, the policy proposes free drugs, free diagnostics and free emergency care services in all public hospitals. To address the growing challenges of urban health, the policy advocates scaling up National Urban Health Mission (NUHM) to cover the entire urban population within the next five-years with sustained financing.

For effectively handling medical disasters and health security, the policy recommends that the public healthcare system retains a certain capacity in terms of health infrastructure, human resources, and technology which can be mobilized in times of crisis.

In order to leverage the pluralistic health care legacy, the policy recommends mainstreaming the different health systems. This would involve increasing the validation, evidence and research of the different health care systems as a part of the common pool of knowledge. It would also involve providing access and informed choice to the patients, providing an enabling environment for practice of different systems of medicine, an enabling regulatory framework and encouraging cross referrals across these systems.

Primary Care Services and Continuity of Care

This policy denotes important change from very selective to comprehensive primary health care package which includes geriatric health care, palliative care and rehabilitative care services. The facilities which start providing the larger package of comprehensive primary health care will be called "Health and Wellness Centers." Primary care must be assured. To make this a reality, every family would have a health card that links them to primary care facility and be eligible for a defined package of services anywhere in the country. The policy recommends that health centers be established on geographical norms apart from population norms. To provide comprehensive care, the policy recommends a matching human resources development strategy, effective logistics support system and referral backup. This would also necessitate upgradation of the existing subcenters and reorienting PHCs to provide comprehensive set of preventive, promotive, curative and rehabilitative services. It would entail providing access to assured AYUSH healthcare services, as well as support documentation and validation of local home and community-based practices. The policy also advocates for research and validation of tribal medicines. Leveraging the potential of digital health for two-way systemic linkages between the various levels of care viz., primary, secondary and tertiary, would ensure continuity of care. The policy advocates that the public health system would put in place a gatekeeping mechanism at primary level in a phased manner, accompanied by an effective feedback and follow-up mechanism.

Secondary Care Services

The policy aspires to provide at the district level most of the secondary care which is currently provided at a medical college hospital. Basic secondary care services, such as cesarean section and neonatal care would be made available at least at subdivisional level in a cluster of few blocks.

To achieve this, policy therefore aims:

- To have at least two beds per thousand population distributed in such a way that it is accessible within golden hour rule. This implies an efficient emergency transport system. The policy also aims that ten categories of what are currently specialist skills be available within the district. Additionally, four or at least five of these specialist skill categories be available at subdistrict levels. This may be achieved by strengthening the district hospital and a well-chosen, well-located set of subdistrict hospitals.
- Resource allocation that is responsive to quantity, diversity and quality of caseloads provided.
- Purchasing care after due diligence from non-government hospitals as a short-term strategy till public systems are strengthened.

Policy proposes a responsive and strong regulatory framework to guide purchasing of care from non-government sector so that challenges of quality of care, cost escalations and impediments to equity are addressed effectively.

In order to develop the secondary care sector, comprehensive facility development and obligations with regard to human resources, especially specialist's needs, are to be prioritized. To this end, the policy recommends a scheme to develop human resources and specialist skills.

Access to blood and blood safety has been a major concern in district healthcare services. This policy affirms in expanding the network of blood banks across the country to ensure improved access to safe blood.

Reorienting Public Hospitals

Public hospitals have to be viewed as part of tax financed single payer health care system, where the care is prepaid and cost-efficient. This outlook implies that quality of care would be imperative and the public hospitals and facilities would undergo periodic measurements and certification of level of quality. The policy endorses that the public hospitals would provide universal access to a progressively wide array of free drugs and diagnostics with suitable leeway to the States to suit their context. The policy seeks to eliminate the risks of inappropriate treatment by maintaining adequate standards of diagnosis and treatment. Policy recognizes the need for an information system with comprehensive data on availability and utilization of services not only in public hospitals but also in non-government sector hospitals. State public health systems should be able to provide all emergency health services other than the services covered under National Health Programmes.

Closing Infrastructure and Human Resources/Skill Gaps

The policy duly acknowledges the roadmap of the 12th Five-Year Plan for managing human resources for health. The policy initiatives aim for measurable improvements in quality of care. Districts and blocks which have wider gaps for development of infrastructure and deployment of additional human resources would receive focus. Financing for additional infrastructure or human resources would be based on needs of outpatient and inpatient attendance and utilization of key services in a measurable manner.

Urban Health Care

National Health Policy prioritizes addressing the primary health care needs of the urban population with special focus on poor populations living in listed and unlisted slums, other vulnerable populations such as homeless, rag-pickers, street children, rickshaw pullers, construction workers, sex workers and temporary migrants. Policy would also prioritize the utilization of AYUSH personnel in urban health care. Given the large presence of private sector in urban areas, policy recommends exploring the possibilities of developing sustainable models of partnership with for profit and not for profit sector for urban health care delivery. An important focus area of the urban health policy will be achieving convergence among the wider determinants of health—air pollution, better solid waste management, water quality, occupational safety, road safety, housing, vector control, and reduction of violence and urban stress. These dimensions are also important components of smart cities. Healthcare needs of the people living in the peri-urban areas would also be addressed under the NUHM. Further, non-communicable diseases (NCDs) like hypertension, diabetes which are predominant in the urban areas would be addressed under NUHM, through planned early detection. Better secondary prevention would also be an integral part of the urban health strategy. Improved health seeking behavior, influenced through capacity building of the community-based organizations and establishment of an appropriate referral mechanism, would also be important components of this strategy.

NATIONAL HEALTH PROGRAMMES

RMNCH+A Services

Maternal and child survival is a mirror that reflects the entire spectrum of social development. This policy aspires to elicit developmental action of all sectors to support maternal and child survival. The policy strongly recommends strengthening of general health systems to prevent and manage maternal complications, to ensure continuity of care and emergency services for maternal health. In order to comprehensively address factors affecting maternal and child survival, the policy seeks to address the social determinants through developmental action in all sectors.

Child and Adolescent Health

The policy endorses the national consensus on accelerated achievement of neonatal mortality targets and "single digit" stillbirth rates through improved home-based and facility-based management of sick newborns. District hospitals must ensure screening and treatment of growth related problems, birth defects, genetic diseases and provide palliative care for children. The policy affirms commitment to pre-emptive care (aimed at pre-empting the occurrence of diseases) to achieve optimum levels of child and adolescent health. The policy envisages school health programmes as a major focus area as also health and hygiene being made a part of the school curriculum. The policy gives special emphasis to the health challenges of adolescents and long-term potential of investing in their health care. The scope of reproductive and sexual health should be expanded to address issues like inadequate calorie intake, nutrition status and psychological problems inter alia linked to misuse of technology, etc.

Interventions to Address Malnutrition and Micronutrient Deficiencies

Malnutrition, especially micronutrient deficiencies, restricts survival, growth and development of children. It contributes to morbidity and mortality in vulnerable population, resulting in substantial diminution in productive capacity in adulthood and consequent reduction in the nation's economic growth and well-being. Recognizing this, the policy declares that micronutrient deficiencies would be addressed through a well-planned strategy on micronutrient interventions. Focus would be on reducing micronutrient malnourishment and augmenting initiatives like micronutrient supplementation, food fortification, screening for anemia and public awareness. A systematic approach to address heterogeneity in micronutrient adequacy across regions in the country with focus on the more vulnerable sections of the population is needed. Hence, screening for multiple micronutrient deficiencies is advocated. During the critical period of pregnancy, lactation, early childhood, adolescence and old age, the consequences of deficiencies are particularly severe and many are irreversible. While dietary diversification remains the most desirable way forward, supplementation and fortification require to be considered as short and medium-term solutions to fill nutrient gaps. The present efforts of iron folic acid (IFA) supplementation, calcium supplementation during pregnancy, iodized salt, zinc and oral rehydration salts/solution (ORS), vitamin A supplementation, need to be intensified and increased. Sustained efforts are to be made to ensure outreach to every beneficiary, which in turn necessitates that intensive monitoring mechanisms are put in place. The policy advocates developing strong evidence base, of the burden of collective micronutrient deficiencies, which should be correlated with disease burden and in particular for understanding the etiology of anemia. Policy recommends exploring fortified food and micronutrient sprinkles for addressing deficiencies through Anganwadi centers and schools. Recognizing the complementary role of various nutrition-sensitive interventions from different platforms, the policy calls for synergy of inputs from departments like Women and Child Development, Education, WASH, Agriculture and Food and Civil Supplies. Policy envisages that the MoHFW would take on the role of convener to monitor and ensure effective integration of both nutrition-sensitive and nutrition-specific interventions for coordinated optimal results.

Universal Immunization

Priority would be to further improve immunization coverage with quality and safety, improve vaccine security as per National Vaccine Policy 2011 and introduction of newer vaccines based on epidemiological considerations. The focus will be to build upon the success of Mission Indradhanush and strengthen it.

Communicable Diseases

The policy recognizes the interrelationship between communicable disease control programmes and public health system strengthening. For Integrated Disease Surveillance Programme, the policy advocates the need for districts to respond to the communicable disease priorities of their locality. This could be through network of well-equipped laboratories backed by tertiary care centers and enhanced public health capacity to collect, analyze and respond to the disease outbreaks.

Control of Tuberculosis

The policy acknowledges HIV and TB coinfection and increased incidence of drug resistant tuberculosis as key challenges in control of tuberculosis. The policy calls for more active case detection, with a greater involvement of private sector supplemented by preventive and promotive action in the workplace and in living conditions. Access to free drugs would need to be complemented by affirmative action to ensure that the treatment is carried out, dropouts reduced and transmission of resistant strains are contained.

Control of HIV/AIDS

While the current emphasis on prevention continues, the policy recommends focused interventions on the high-risk communities (MSM, Transgender, FSW, etc.) and prioritized geographies. There is a need to support care and treatment for people living with HIV/AIDS through inclusion of 1st, 2nd and 3rd line antiretroviral (ARV), Hep-C and other costly drugs into the essential medical list.

Leprosy Elimination

To carry out leprosy elimination, the proportion of grade-2 cases amongst new cases will become the measure of community awareness and health systems capacity, keeping in mind the global goal of reduction of grade 2 disability to less than 1 per million by 2020. Accordingly, the policy envisages proactive measures targeted toward elimination of leprosy from India by 2018.

Vector Borne Disease Control

The policy recognizes the challenge of drug resistance in Malaria, which should be dealt with by changing treatment regimens with logistics support as appropriate. New National Programme for prevention and control of Japanese Encephalitis (JE)/Acute Encephalitis Syndrome (AES) should be accelerated with strong component of intersectoral collaboration.

The policy recognizes the interrelationship between communicable disease control programmes and public health system strengthening. Every one of these programmes requires a robust public health system as its core delivery strategy. At the same time, these programmes also lead to strengthening of healthcare systems.

Non-communicable Diseases

The policy recognizes the need to halt and reverse the growing incidence of chronic diseases. The policy recommends to set-up a National Institute of Chronic Diseases including Trauma, to generate evidence for adopting cost-effective approaches and to showcase best practices. This policy will support an integrated approach where screening for the most prevalent NCDs with secondary prevention would make a significant impact on reduction of morbidity and preventable mortality. This would be incorporated into the comprehensive primary health care network with linkages to specialist consultations and follow-up at the primary level. Emphasis on medication and access for select chronic illness on a 'round the year' basis would be ensured. Screening for oral, breast and cervical cancer and for chronic obstructive pulmonary disease (COPD) will be focused in addition to hypertension and diabetes. The policy focus is also on research. It emphasizes developing protocol for mainstreaming AYUSH as an integrated medical care. This has a huge potential for effective prevention and therapy that is safe and cost-effective. Further the policy commits itself to support programmes for prevention of blindness, deafness, oral health, endemic diseases like fluorosis and sickle cell anemia/thalassemia, etc. The National Health Policy commits itself to culturally appropriate community-centered solutions to meet the health needs of the aging community in addition to compliance with constitutional obligations as per the Maintenance and Welfare of Parents and Senior Citizens Act, 2007. The policy recognizes the growing need for palliative and rehabilitative care for all geriatric illnesses and advocates the continuity of care across all levels. The policy recognizes the critical need of meeting the growing demand of tissue and organ transplant in the country and encourages widespread public awareness to promote voluntary donations.

Mental Health

- This policy will take into consideration the provisions of the National Mental Health Policy 2014 with simultaneous action on the following fronts:
  - Increase creation of specialists through public financing and develop special rules to give preference to those willing to work in public systems.
  - Create network of community members to provide psychosocial support to strengthen mental health services at primary level facilities.
  - Leverage digital technology in a context where access to qualified psychiatrists is difficult.

Population Stabilization

The National Health Policy recognizes that improved access, education and empowerment would be the basis of successful population stabilization. The policy imperative is to move away from camp-based services with all its attendant problems of quality, safety and dignity of women, to a situation where these services are available on any day of the week or at least on a fixed day. Other policy imperatives are to increase the proportion of male sterilization from <5% currently, to at least 30% and if possible much higher.

WOMEN'S HEALTH AND GENDER MAINSTREAMING

There will be enhanced provisions for reproductive morbidities and health needs of women beyond the reproductive age group (40+). This would be in addition to package of services covered in the previous paragraphs.

GENDER-BASED VIOLENCE (GBV)

Women's access to healthcare needs to be strengthened by making public hospitals more women-friendly and ensuring that the staff have orientation to gender—sensitivity issues. This policy notes with concern the serious and wide ranging consequences of GBV and recommends that the health care to the survivors/victims need to be provided free and with dignity in the public and private sector.

SUPPORTIVE SUPERVISION

For supportive supervision in more vulnerable districts with inadequate capacity, the policy will support innovative measures such as use of digital tools and HR strategies like using nurse trainers to support field workers.

EMERGENCY CARE AND DISASTER PREPAREDNESS

Better response to disasters, both natural and man-made, requires a dispersed and effective capacity for emergency management. It requires an army of community members trained as first responder for accidents and disasters. It also requires regular strengthening of their capacities in close collaboration with the local self-government and community-based organizations. The policy supports development of earthquake and cyclone resistant health infrastructure in vulnerable geographies. It also supports development of mass casualty management protocols for CHC and higher facilities and emergency response protocols at all levels. To respond to disasters and emergencies, the public healthcare system needs to be adequately skilled and equipped at defined levels, so as to respond effectively during emergencies. The policy envisages creation of a unified emergency response system, linked to a dedicated universal access number, with network of emergency care that has an assured provision of life support ambulances, trauma management centers—

- One per 30 lakh population in urban areas.
- One for every 10 lakh population in rural areas.

MAINSTREAMING THE POTENTIAL OF AYUSH

For persons who so choose, this policy ensures access to AYUSH remedies through colocation in public facilities. Yoga would be introduced much more widely in school and work places as part of promotion of good health as adopted in National AYUSH Mission (NAM). The policy recognizes the need to standardize and validate Ayurvedic medicines and establish a robust and effective quality control mechanism for AUSH drugs. Policy recognizes the need to nurture AYUSH system of medicine, through development of infrastructural facilities of teaching institutions, improving quality control of drugs, capacity building of institutions and professionals. In addition, it recognizes the need for building research and public health skills for preventive and promotive healthcare. Linking AYUSH systems with ASHAs and VHSNCs would be an important plank of this policy. The National Health Policy would continue mainstreaming of AYUSH with general health system but with the addition of a mandatory bridge course that gives competencies to mid-level care provider with respect to allopathic remedies. The policy further supports the integration of AYUSH systems at the level of knowledge systems, by validating processes of health care promotion and cure. The policy recognizes the need for integrated courses for Indian System of Medicine, Modern Science and Ayurgenomics. It puts focus on sensitizing practitioners of each system to the strengths of the others.

Further the development of sustainable livelihood systems through involving local communities and establishing forward and backward market linkages in processing of medicinal plants will also be supported by this policy. The policy seeks to strengthen steps for farming of herbal plants. Developing mechanisms for certification of 'prior knowledge' of traditional community health care providers and engaging them in the conservation and generation of the raw materials required, as well as creating opportunities for enhancing their skills are part of this policy.

TERTIARY CARE SERVICES

The policy affirms that the tertiary care services are best organized along lines of regional, zonal and apex referral centers. It recommends that the Government should set up new Medical Colleges, Nursing Institutions and AIIMS in the country following this broad principle. Regional disparities in distribution of these institutions must be addressed. The policy supports periodic review and standardization of fee structure and quality of clinical training in the private sector medical colleges. The policy enunciates the core principle of societal obligation on the part of private institutions to be followed.

This would include:

- Operationalization of mechanisms for referral from public health system to charitable hospitals.
- Ensuring that deserving patients can be admitted on designated free/subsidized beds.

The policy proposes to consider forms of resource generation, where corporate hospitals and medical tourism earnings are through a high degree of associated hospitality arrangements and on account of certain procedures and services, as a form of resource mobilization towards the health sector. The policy recommends establishing National Healthcare Standards Organization and to develop evidence-based standard guidelines of care applicable both to public and private sector. The policy shows the way forward in developing partnership with non-government sector through empaneling the socially motivated and committed tertiary care centers into the Government efforts to close the specialist gap.

To expand public provisioning of tertiary services, the Government would additionally purchase select tertiary care services from empaneled non-government sector hospitals to assist the poor. Coverage in terms of population and services will expand gradually. The policy recognizes development of evidence-based standard guidelines of care, applicable both to public and private sector as essential.

HUMAN RESOURCES FOR HEALTH

There is a need to align decisions regarding judicious growth of professional and technical educational institutions in the health sector, better financing of professional and technical education, defining professional boundaries and skill sets, reshaping the pedagogy of professional and technical education, revisiting entry policies into educational institutions, ensuring quality of education and regulating the system to generate the right mix of skills at the right place. This policy recommends that medical and paramedical education be integrated with the service delivery system, so that the students learn in the real environment and not just in the confines of the medical school. The key principle around the policy on human resources for health is that, workforce performance of the system would be best when we have the most appropriate person, in terms of both skills and motivation, for the right job in the right place, working within the right professional and incentive environment.

Medical Education

The policy recommends strengthening existing medical colleges and converting district hospitals to new medical colleges to increase number of doctors and specialists, in States with large human resource deficit. The policy recognizes the need to increase the number of postgraduate seats. The policy supports expanding the number of AIIMS like centers for continuous flow of faculty for medical colleges, biomedical and clinical research. National Knowledge Network shall be used for Tele-education, Tele-CME, Teleconsultations and access to digital library. A common entrance exam is advocated on the pattern of NEET for UG entrance at All India level; a common national-level Licentiate/exit exam for all medical and nursing graduates; a regular renewal at periodic intervals with continuing medical education (CME) credits accrued, are important recommendations. This policy recommends that the current pattern of Multiple Choice Question (MCQ) based entrance test for postgraduates' medical courses—that drive students away from practical learning—should be reviewed. The policy recognizes the need to revise the undergraduate and postgraduate medical curriculum keeping in view the changing needs, technology and the newer emerging disease trends. Keeping in view the rapid expansion of medical colleges in public and private sector, there is an urgent need to review existing institutional mechanisms to regulate and ensure quality of training and education being imparted. The policy recommends that the discussion on recreating a regulatory structure for health professional education be revisited to address the emerging needs and challenges.

Attracting and Retaining Doctors in Remote Areas

Policy proposes financial and nonfinancial incentives, creating medical colleges in rural areas; preference to students from underserviced areas, realigning pedagogy and curriculum to suit rural health needs, mandatory rural postings, etc. Measures of compulsion—through mandatory rotational postings dovetailed with clear and transparent career progression guidelines are valuable strategies. A constant effort, therefore, needs to be made to increase the capacity of the public health systems to absorb and retain the manpower. The total sanctioned posts of doctors in the public sector should increase to ensure availability of doctors corresponding to the accepted norms. Exact package of policy measures would vary from State to State and would change over time.

Specialist Attraction and Retention

Proposed policy measures include—recognition of educational options linked with National Board of Examination and College of Physicians and Surgeons, creation of specialist cadre with suitable pay scale, upgradation of short-term training to medical officers to provide basic specialist services at the block and district level, performance linked payments and popularize Doctor of Medicine (MD) course in Family Medicine or General Practice. The policy recommends that the National Board of Examinations should expand the postgraduate training up to the district level. The policy recommends creation of a large number of distance and continuing education options for general practitioners in both the private and the public sectors, which would upgrade their skills to manage the large majority of cases at local level, thus avoiding unnecessary referrals.

Mid-level Service Providers

For expansion of primary care from selective care to comprehensive care, complementary human resource strategy is the development of a cadre of mid-level care providers. This can be done through appropriate courses like a BSc in community health and/or through competency-based bridge courses and short courses. These bridge courses could admit graduates from different clinical and paramedical backgrounds like AYUSH doctors, BSc Nurses, Pharmacists, GNMs, etc. and equip them with skills to provide services at the subcenter and other peripheral levels. Locale-based selection, a special curriculum of training close to the place where they live and work, conditional licensing, enabling legal framework and a positive practice environment will ensure that this new cadre is preferentially available where they are needed most, i.e., in the underserved areas.

Nursing Education

The policy recognizes the need to improve regulation and quality management of nursing education. Other measures suggested are—establishing cadres like Nurse Practitioners and Public Health Nurses to increase their availability in most needed areas. Developing specialized nursing training courses and curriculum (critical care, cardiothoracic vascular care, neurological care, trauma care, palliative care and care of terminally ill), establishing nursing school in every large district or cluster of districts of about 20–30 lakh population and establishing Centers of Excellence for Nursing and Allied Health Sciences in each State. States which have adequate nursing institutions have flexibility to explore a gradual shift to three year nurses even at the subcenter level to support the implementation of the comprehensive primary health care agenda.

Accredited Social Health Activist (ASHA)

This policy supports certification programme for ASHAs for their preferential selection into ANM, nursing and paramedical courses. While most ASHAs will remain mainly voluntary and remunerated for time spent, those who obtain qualifications for career opportunities could be given more regular terms of engagement. Policy also supports enabling engagements with NGOs to serve as support and training institutions for ASHAs and to serve as learning laboratories on future roles of community health workers. The policy recommends revival and strengthening of multipurpose male health worker cadre, in order to effectively manage the emerging infectious and non-communicable diseases at community level. Adding a second Community Health Worker would be based on geographic considerations, disease burdens, and time required for multiple tasks to be performed by ASHA/Community Health Worker.

Paramedical Skills

Training courses and curriculum for super specialty paramedical care (perfusionists, physiotherapists, occupational therapists, radiological technicians, audiologists, MRI technicians, etc.) would be developed. The policy recognizes the role played by physiotherapists, occupational and allied health professionals keeping in view the demographic and disease transition the country is faced with and also recognizes the need to address their shortfall. Planned expansion of allied technical skills—radiographers, laboratory technicians, physiotherapists, pharmacists, audiologists, optometrists, occupational therapists with local employment opportunities, is a key policy direction. The policy would allow for multiskilling with different skill sets so that when posted in more peripheral hospitals there is more efficient use of human resources.

Public Health Management Cadre

The policy proposes creation of Public Health Management Cadre in all States based on public health or related disciplines, as entry criteria. The policy also advocates an appropriate career structure and recruitment policy to attract young and talented multidisciplinary professionals. Medical and health professionals would form a major part of this, but professionals coming in from diverse backgrounds such as sociology, economics, anthropology, nursing, hospital management, communications, etc., who have since undergone public health management training would also be considered. States could decide to locate these public health managers, with medical and nonmedical qualifications, into same or different cadre streams belonging to Directorates of health. Further, the policy recognizes the need to continuously nurture certain specialized skills like entomology, housekeeping, biomedical waste management, biomedical engineering, communication skills, management of call centers and even ambulance services.

Human Resource Governance and Leadership Development

The policy recognizes that human resource management is critical to health system strengthening and healthcare delivery and therefore the policy supports measures aimed at continuing medical and nursing education and on the job support to providers, especially those working in professional isolation in rural areas using digital tools and other appropriate training resources. Policy recommends development of leadership skills, strengthening human resource governance in public health system, through establishment of robust recruitment, selection, promotion and transfer postings policies.

FINANCING OF HEALTH CARE

The policy advocates allocating major proportion (up to two-thirds or more) of resources to primary care followed by secondary and tertiary care. Inclusion of cost-benefit and cost-effectiveness studies consistently in programme design and evaluation would be prioritized. This would contribute significantly to increasing efficiency of public expenditure. A robust National Health Accounts System would be operationalized to improve public sector efficiency in resource allocation/payments. The policy calls for major reforms in financing for public facilities—where operational costs would be in the form of reimbursements for care provision and on a per capita basis for primary care. Items like infrastructure development and maintenance, nonincentive cost of the human resources, i.e., salaries and much of administrative costs, would however continue to flow on a fixed cost basis. Considerations of equity would be factored in—with higher unit costs for more difficult and vulnerable areas or more supply side investment in infrastructure. Total allocations would be made on the basis of differential financial ability, developmental needs and high priority districts to ensure horizontal equity through targeting specific population subgroups, geographical areas, health care services and gender related issues. A higher unit cost or some form of financial incentive payable to facilities providing a measured and certified quality of care is recommended.

Purchasing of Healthcare Services

The existing Government financed health insurance schemes shall be aligned to cover selected benefit package of secondary and tertiary care services purchased from public, not for profit and private sector in the same order of preference, subject to availability of quality services on time as per defined norms. The policy recommends creating a robust independent mechanism to ensure adherence to standard treatment protocols by public and non-government hospitals. In this context the policy recognizes the need of mandatory disclosure of treatment and success rates across facilities in a transparent manner. It recommends compliance to right of patients to access information about their condition and treatment. For need-based purchasing of secondary and tertiary care from non-government sector, multistakeholder institutional mechanisms would be created at Center and State levels—in the forms of trusts or registered societies with institutional autonomy. These agencies would also be charged with ensuring that purchasing is strategic—giving preference to care from public facilities where they are in a position to do so—and developing a market base through encouraging the creation of capacity in services in areas where they are needed more. Private 'not for profit' and 'for profit' hospitals would be empanelled with preference for the former, for comparable quality and standards of care. The payments will be made by the trust/society on a reimbursement basis for services provided.

COLLABORATION WITH NON-GOVERNMENT SECTOR/ENGAGEMENT WITH PRIVATE SECTOR

The policy suggests exploring collaboration for primary care services with 'not for profit' organizations having a track record of public services where critical gaps exist, as a short-term measure. Collaboration can also be done for certain services where team of specialized human resources and domain specific organizational experience is required. Private providers, especially those working in rural and remote areas or with underserved communities, could be offered encouragement through provision of appropriate skills to meet public health goals, opportunities for skill upgradation to serve the community better, participation in disease notification and surveillance efforts, sharing and supporting certain high value services. The policy supports voluntary service in rural and underserved areas on pro bono basis by recognized healthcare professionals under a 'giving back to society' initiative. The policy advocates a positive and proactive engagement with the private sector for critical gap filling toward achieving National goals. One form is through engagement in public goods, where the private sector contributes to preventive or promotive services without profit—as part of CSR work or on contractual terms with the Government. The other is in areas where the private sector is encouraged to invest—which implies an adequate return on investment, i.e., on commercial terms which may entail contracting, strategic purchasing, etc. The policy advocates for contracting of private sector in the following activities:

- **Capacity building:** Outsourcing of training of teachers to strengthen school health programmes by adopting neighborhood schools for quarterly training modules.
- **Skill development programmes:** Recognizing that there are huge gaps in technicians, nursing and para-nursing, paramedical staff and medical skills in select areas, the policy advocates coordination between National Council for Skill Development, MoHFW and State Government(s) for engaging private hospitals/private general medical practitioners in skill development.
- **Corporate social responsibility (CSR):** CSR is an important area which should be leveraged for filling health infrastructure gaps in public health facilities across the country. The private sector could use the CSR platform to play an active role in the awareness generation through campaigns on occupational health, blood disorders, adolescent health, safe health practices and accident prevention, micronutrient adequacy, antimicrobial resistance, screening of children and antenatal mothers, psychological problems

linked to misuse of technology, etc. The policy recommends engagement of private sector through adoption of neighborhood schools/colonies/slums/tribal areas/backward areas for healthcare awareness and services.

- **Mental healthcare programmes:** Training community members to provide psychological support to strengthen mental health services in the country. Collaboration with Government would be an important plank to develop a sustainable network for community/locality toward mental health.
- **Disaster management:** Is another area where collaboration with private sector would enable better outcomes especially in the areas of medical relief and post-trauma counseling/treatment. A pool of human resources from private sector could be generated to act as responders during disasters. The private sector could also pool their infrastructure for quick deployment during disasters and emergencies and help in creation of a unified emergency response system. Additionally, sharing information on infrastructure and services deployable for disaster management would enable development of a comprehensive information system with data on availability and utilization of services, for optimum use during golden hour and other emergencies.
- **Strategic purchasing as stewardship:** Directing areas for investment for the commercial health sector.
  - The health policy recognizes that there are many critical gaps in public health services which would be filled by 'strategic purchasing'. Such strategic purchasing would play a stewardship role in directing private investment toward those areas and those services for which currently there are no providers or few providers. The policy advocates building synergy with 'not for profit' organizations and private sector subject to availability of timely quality services as per predefined norms in the collaborating organization for critical gap filling.
  - The main mechanisms of strategic purchasing are insurance and through trusts. Schemes like Aarogyasri and Rashtriya Swasthya Bima Yojana (RSBY) have been able to increase private participation significantly. Payment is by reimbursement on a fee for service basis and many private providers have been able to benefit greatly by these schemes. The aim would be to improve health outcomes and reduce out of pocket payments while minimizing moral hazards and—so that these schemes can be scaled up and made more effective. The policy provides for preferential treatment to collaborating private hospitals/institutes for CGHS empanelment and in proposed strategic purchase by Government subject to other requirements being met.
  - For achieving the objective of having fully functional primary healthcare facilities—especially in urban areas to reach underserviced populations and on a fee basis for middle class populations, Government would collaborate with the private sector for operationalizing such health and wellness centers to provide a larger package of comprehensive primary health care across the country. Partnerships that address specific gaps in public services: These would inter alia include diagnostics services, ambulance services, safe blood services, rehabilitative services, palliative services, mental healthcare, telemedicine services, managing of rare and orphan diseases.
  - The policy advocates building synergy with 'not for profit' organizations and private sector subject to availability of timely quality services as per predefined norms in the collaborating organization for critical gaps.

Enhancing Accessibility in Private Sector

The policy recommends a better public private healthcare interface and recognizes the need for engagement in operationalization of mechanisms for referrals from public health system. Charitable hospitals and 'not for profit' hospitals may volunteer for accepting referrals from public health facilities. The private sector could also provide increased designated free/subsidized beds in their hospitals for the downtrodden, poor and others toward societal cause.

- **Role in immunization:** The policy recognizes the role of the private sector in immunization programmes and advocates their continued collaboration in rendering immunization service as per protocol.
- **Disease surveillance:** Toward strengthening disease surveillance, the private sector laboratories could be engaged for data pooling and sharing. All clinical establishments would be encouraged to notify diseases and provide information of public health importance.
- **Tissue and organ transplantations:** Tissue and organ transplantations and voluntary donations are areas where private sector provides services—but it needs public interventions and support for getting organ donations. Recognizing the need for awareness, the private sector and public sector could play a vital role in awareness generation.
- **Make in India:** Towards furthering 'Make in India', the private domestic manufacturing firms/industry could be engaged to provide customized indigenous medical devices to the health sector and in creation of forward and backward linkages for medical device production. The policy also seeks assured purchase by Government health facilities from domestic manufacturers, subject to quality standards being met.
- **Health information system:** The objective of an integrated health information system necessitates private sector participation in developing and linking systems into a common network/grid which can be accessed by both public and private healthcare providers. Collaboration with private sector consistent with Meta Data and Data Standards and Electronic Health Records would lead to developing a seamless health information system. The private sector could help in creation of registries of patients and in documenting diseases and health events.
- **Incentivizing private sector:** To encourage participation of private sector, the policy advocates incentivizing the private sector through inter alia (i) reimbursement/fees (ii) preferential treatment to collaborating private hospitals/institutes for CGHS empanelment and in proposed strategic purchase by Government, subject to other requirements being met (iii) Nonfinancial incentives like recognition/ acknowledgement/felicitation and skill upgradation to the private sector hospitals/practitioners for providing public health services and for partnering with the Government of India/State Governments in health care delivery and (iv) through preferential purchase by Government health facilities from domestic manufacturers, subject to quality standards being met.
- **Private sector engagement goes beyond contracting and purchasing:** Private providers, especially those working in rural and remote areas, or with underserviced communities, require access to opportunities for skill upgradation to meet public health goals, to serve the community better, for participation in disease notification and surveillance efforts, and for sharing and support through provision of certain high value services—like laboratory support for identification of drug resistant tuberculosis or other infections, supply of some restricted medicines needed for special situations, building flexibilities into standards needed for service provision in difficult contexts and even social recognition of their work. This would greatly encourage such providers to do better. Hitherto all public training and skill provision has been only to public providers. The policy recognizes the need for training and skilling of many small private providers and recommends the same.

REGULATORY FRAMEWORK

The regulatory role of the Ministry of Health and Family Welfare—which includes regulation of clinical establishments, professional and technical education, food safety, medical technologies, medical products, clinical trials, research and implementation of other health related laws—needs urgent and concrete steps toward reform. This will entail moving toward a more effective, rational, transparent and consistent regime.

Professional Education Regulation

The policy calls for a major reform in this area. It advocates strengthening of six professional councils (Medical, Ayurveda, Unani and Siddha, Homeopathy, Nursing, Dental and Pharmacy) through expanding membership of these councils between three key stakeholders—doctors, patients and society in balanced numbers. The policy supports setting up of National Allied Professional Council to regulate and streamline all allied health professionals and ensure quality standards.

Regulation of Clinical Establishments

A few States have adopted the Clinical Establishments Act 2010. Advocacy with the other States would be made for adoption of the Act. Grading of clinical establishments and active promotion and adoption of standard treatment guidelines would be one starting point. Protection of patient rights in clinical establishments (such as rights to information, access to medical records and reports, informed consent, second opinion, confidentiality and privacy) as key process standards, would be an important step. Policy recommends the setting up of a separate, empowered medical tribunal for speedy resolution to address disputes/complaints regarding standards of care, prices of services, negligence and unfair practices. Standard Regulatory framework for laboratories and imaging centers, specialized emerging services such as assisted reproductive techniques, surrogacy, stem cell banking, organ and tissue transplantation and nanomedicine will be created as appropriate.

Food Safety

The policy recommends putting in place and strengthening necessary network of offices, laboratories, e-governance structures and human resources needed for the enforcement of Food Safety and Standards (FSS) Act, 2006.

Drug Regulation

Prices and availability of drugs are regulated by the Department of Pharmaceuticals. However, with regard to other areas of drugs and pharmaceuticals, this policy encourages the streamlining of the system of procurement of drugs; a strong and transparent drug purchase policy for bulk procurement of drugs; and facilitating spread of low cost pharmacy chain such as Jan Aushadhi stores linked with ensuring prescription of generic medicines. It further recommends education of public with regard to branded and nonbranded generic drugs. The setting up of common infrastructure for development of the pharmaceutical industry will also be promoted. The policy advocates strengthening and rationalizing the drug regulatory system, promotion of research and development in the pharmaceutical sector and building synergy and evolving a convergent approach with related sectors.

Medical Devices Regulation

The policy recommends strengthening regulation of medical devices and establishing a regulatory body for medical devices to unleash innovation and the entrepreneurial spirit for manufacture of medical device in India. The policy supports harmonization of domestic regulatory standards with international standards. Building capacities in line with international practices in our regulatory personnel and institutions, would have the highest priority. Post-market surveillance program for drugs, blood products and medical devices shall be strengthened to ensure high degree of reliability and to prevent adverse outcomes due to low quality and/or refurbished devices/health products.

Clinical Trial Regulation

Clinical trials are essential for new product discovery and development. With the objective of ensuring the rights, safety and well-being of clinical trial participants, while facilitating such trials as are essential, specific clause(s) be included in the Drugs and Cosmetics Act for its regulation. Transparent and objective procedures shall be specified, and functioning of ethics and review committees will be strengthened. The Global Good Clinical Practice Guidelines, which specifies standards, roles and responsibilities of sponsors, investigators and participants would be adhered to. Irrational drug combination will continue to be monitored and controlled and appropriate regulatory framework for standardization of ASU & H drugs will be ensured. Clear and transparent guidelines, with independent monitoring mechanisms, are the ways forward to foster a progressive and innovative research environment, while safeguarding the rights and health of the trial participants.

Pricing—Drugs, Medical Devices and Equipment

The regulatory environment around pricing requires a balance between the patients' concern for affordability and industry's concern for adequate returns on investment for growth and sustainability. Timely revision of National List of Essential Medicines (NLEM) along with appropriate price control mechanisms for generic drugs shall remain a key strategy for decreasing costs of care for all those patients seeking care in the private sector. An approach on the same lines but suiting specific requirements of the sectors would be considered for price control with regard to a list of essential diagnostics and equipment.

VACCINE SAFETY

Vaccine safety and security would require effective regulation, research and development for manufacturing new vaccines in accordance with National Vaccine Policy 2011. The policy advocates commissioning more research and development for manufacturing new vaccines, including against locally prevalent diseases. It recommends building more public sector manufacturing units to generate healthy competition; uninterrupted supply of quality vaccines, developing innovative financing and creating assured supply mechanisms with built in flexibility. Units such as the integrated vaccine complex at Chengalpattu would be set up and vaccine antisera manufacturing units in the public sector upgraded with increase in their installed capacity.

MEDICAL TECHNOLOGIES

India is known as the pharmacy of the developing world. However, its role in new drug discovery and drug innovations including biopharmaceuticals and biosimilar for its own health priorities is limited. This needs to be addressed in the context of progress toward universal health care. Making available good quality, free essential and generic drugs and diagnostics, at public health care facilities is the most effective way for achieving the goal. The free drugs and diagnostics basket would include all that is needed for comprehensive primary care, including care for chronic illnesses, in the assured set of services. At the tertiary care level too, at least for inpatients and outpatients in geriatric and chronic care segments, most drugs and diagnostics should be free or subsidized with fair price selling mechanisms for most and some copayments for the 'well-to-do'.

PUBLIC PROCUREMENT

Quality of public procurement and logistics is a major challenge to ensuring access to free drugs and diagnostics through public facilities. An essential prerequisite that is needed to address the challenge of providing free drugs through public sector, is a well-developed public procurement system.

AVAILABILITY OF DRUGS AND MEDICAL DEVICES

The policy accords special focus on production of Active Pharmaceutical Ingredient (API) which is the backbone of the generic formulations industry. Recognizing that over 70% of the medical devices and equipment are imported in India, the policy advocates the need to incentivize local manufacturing to provide customized indigenous products for Indian population in the long run. The goal with respect to medical devices shall be to encourage domestic production in consonance with the 'Make in India' national agenda. Medical technology and medical devices have a multiplier effect in the costing of healthcare delivery. The policy recognizes the need to regulate the use of medical devices so as to ensure safety and quality compliance as per the standard norms.

ALIGNING OTHER POLICIES FOR MEDICAL DEVICES AND EQUIPMENT WITH PUBLIC HEALTH GOALS

For medical devices and equipment, the policy recommends and prioritizes establishing sufficient labeling and packaging requirements on part of industry, adequate medical devices, testing facility and effective port—clearance mechanisms for medical products.

IMPROVING PUBLIC SECTOR CAPACITY FOR MANUFACTURING ESSENTIAL DRUGS AND VACCINES

Public sector capacity in manufacture of certain essential drugs and vaccines is also essential in the long-term for the health security of the country and to address some needs which are not attractive commercial propositions. These public institutions need more investment, appropriate HR policies and governance initiatives to enable them to become comparable with their benchmarks in the developed world.

ANTIMICROBIAL RESISTANCE

The problem of antimicrobial resistance calls for a rapid standardization of guidelines, regarding antibiotic use, limiting the use of antibiotics as Over-the-Counter medication, banning or restricting the use of antibiotics as growth promoters in animal livestock. Pharmacovigilance including prescription audit inclusive of antibiotic usage, in the hospital and community, is a must in order to enforce change in existing practices.

HEALTH TECHNOLOGY ASSESSMENT

Health Technology assessment is required to ensure that technology choice is participatory and is guided by considerations of scientific evidence, safety, consideration on cost-effectiveness and social values. The National Health Policy commits to the development of institutional framework and capacity for Health Technology Assessment and adoption.

DIGITAL HEALTH TECHNOLOGY ECOSYSTEM

Recognizing the integral role of technology (eHealth, mHealth, Cloud, Internet of things, wearable, etc.) in the healthcare delivery, a National Digital Health Authority (NDHA) will be set up to regulate, develop and deploy digital health across the continuum of care. The policy advocates extensive deployment of digital tools for improving the efficiency and outcome of the healthcare system. The policy aims at an integrated health information system which serves the needs of all stakeholders and improves efficiency, transparency, and citizen experience. Delivery of better health outcomes in terms of access, quality, affordability, lowering of disease burden and efficient monitoring of health entitlements to citizens, is the goal. Establishing federated national health information architecture, to roll-out and link systems across public and private health providers at State and national levels consistent with Metadata and Data Standards (MDDS) and Electronic Health Record (EHR), will be supported by this policy. The policy suggests exploring the use of 'Aadhaar' (Unique ID) for identification. Creation of registries (i.e., patients, provider, service, diseases, document and event) for enhanced public health/big data analytics, creation of health information exchange platform and national health information network, use of National Optical Fiber Network, use of smartphones/tablets for capturing real time data, are key strategies of the National Health Information Architecture.

Application of Digital Health

The policy advocates scaling of various initiatives in the area of teleconsultation which will entail linking tertiary care institutions (medical colleges) to District and Sub- district hospitals which provide secondary care facilities, for the purpose of specialist consultations. The policy will promote utilization of National Knowledge Network for Tele-education, Tele-CME, Teleconsultations and access to digital library.

Leveraging Digital Tools for AYUSH

Digital tools would be used for generation and sharing of information about AYUSH services and AYUSH practitioners, for traditional community level healthcare providers and for household level preventive, promotive and curative practices.

HEALTH SURVEYS

The scope of health, demographic and epidemiological surveys would be extended to capture information regarding costs of care, financial protection and evidence-based policy planning and reforms. The policy recommends rapid programme appraisals and periodic disease specific surveys to monitor the impact of public health and disease interventions using digital tools for epidemiological surveys.

HEALTH RESEARCH

The National Health Policy recognizes the key role that health research plays in the development of a Nation's health. In knowledge-based sector like health, where advances happen daily, it is important to increase investment in health research.

Strengthening Knowledge for Health

The policy envisages strengthening the publicly funded health research institutes under the Department of Health Research, the apex public health institutions under the Department of Health and Family Welfare, as well as those in the Government and private medical colleges. The policy supports strengthening health research in India in the following fronts—health systems and services research, medical product innovation (including point of care diagnostics and related technologies and internet of things) and fundamental research in all areas relevant to health—such as Physiology, Biochemistry, Pharmacology, Microbiology, Pathology, Molecular Sciences and Cell Sciences. Policy aims to promote innovation, discovery and translational research on drugs in ASU & H and allocate adequate funds toward it. Research on social determinants of health along with neglected health issues such as disability and transgender health will be promoted. For drug and devices discovery and innovation, both from Allopathy and traditional medicines systems would be supported. Creation of a Common Sector Innovation Council for the Health Ministry that brings together various regulatory bodies for drug research, the Department of Pharmaceuticals, the Department of Biotechnology, the Department of Industrial Policy and Promotion, the Department of Science and Technology, etc. would be desirable. Innovative strategies of public financing and careful leveraging of public procurement can help generate the sort of innovations that are required for Indian public health priorities. Drug research on critical diseases such as TB, HIV/AIDS, and Malaria may be incentivized, to address them on priority. For making full use of all research capacity in the nation, grant-in-aid mechanisms which provide extramural funding to research efforts is envisaged to be scaled up.

Drug Innovation and Discovery

Government policy would be to both stimulate innovation and new drug discovery as required, to meet health needs as well as ensure that new drugs discovered and brought into the market are affordable to those who need them most. Similar policies are required for discovering more affordable, more frugal and appropriate point of care diagnostics as also robust medical equipment for use in our rural and remote areas. Public procurement policies and public investment in priority research areas with greater coordination and convergence between drug research institutions, drug manufacturers and premier medical institutions must also be aligned to drug discovery.

Development of Information Databases

There is also a need to develop information data-bases on a wide variety of areas that researchers can share. This includes ensuring that all unit data of major publicly funded surveys related to health, are available in public domain in a research-friendly format.

Research Collaboration

The policy on international health and health diplomacy should leverage India's strength in cost-effective innovations in the areas of pharmaceuticals, medical devices, health care delivery and information technology. Additionally, leveraging international cooperation, especially involving nations of the Global South, to build domestic institutional capacity in green-field innovation and for knowledge and skill generation could be explored.

GOVERNANCE

Role of Center and State

One of the most important strengths and at the same time challenges of governance in health is the distribution of responsibility and accountability between the Center and the States. The policy recommends equity sensitive resource allocation, strengthening institutional mechanisms for consultative decision-making and coordinated implementation, as the way forward. Besides, better management of fiduciary risks, provision of capacity building, technical assistance to States to develop State-specific strategic plans, through the active involvement of local self-government and through community-based monitoring of health outputs is also recommended. The policy suggests State Directorates to be strengthened by HR policies, central to which is the issue that those from a public health management cadre must hold senior positions in public health.

Role of Panchayati Raj Institutions

Panchayati Raj Institutions would be strengthened to play an enhanced role at different levels for health governance, including the social determinants of health. There is need to make Community-Based Monitoring and Planning (CBMP) mandatory, so as to place people at the center of the health system and development process for effective monitoring of quality of services and for better accountability in management and delivery of health care services.

Improving Accountability

The policy would be to increase both horizontal and vertical accountability of the health system by providing a greater role and participation of local bodies and encouraging community monitoring, programme evaluations along with ensuring grievance redressal systems.

LEGAL FRAMEWORK FOR HEALTH CARE AND HEALTH PATHWAY

One of the fundamental policy questions being raised in recent years is whether to pass a health rights bill making health a fundamental right—in the way that was done for education. The policy question is whether we have reached the level of economic and health systems development so as to make this a justiciable right—implying that its denial is an offense. Questions that need to be addressed are manifold, namely, (a) whether when health care is a State subject, is it desirable or useful to make a Central law, (b) whether such a law should mainly focus on the enforcement of public health standards on water, sanitation, food safety, air pollution, etc., or whether it should focus on health rights—access to health care and quality of health care—i.e., whether focus should be on what the State enforces on citizens or on what the citizen demands of the State? Right to healthcare covers a wide canvas, encompassing issues of preventive, curative, rehabilitative and palliative healthcare across rural and urban areas, infrastructure availability, health human resource availability, as also issues extending beyond health sector into the domain of poverty, equity, literacy, sanitation, nutrition, drinking water availability, etc. Excellent health care system needs to be in place to ensure effective implementation of the health rights at the grassroots level. Right to health cannot be perceived unless the basic health infrastructure like doctor-patient ratio, patient-bed ratio, nurses-patient ratio, etc. are near or above threshold levels and uniformly spread-out across the geographical frontiers of the country. Further, the procedural guidelines, common regulatory platform for public and private sector, standard treatment protocols, etc. need to be put in place. Accordingly, the management, administrative and overall governance structure in the health system needs to be overhauled. Additionally, the responsibilities and liabilities of the providers, insurers, clients, regulators and Government in administering the right to health need to be clearly spelt out. The policy while supporting the need for moving in the direction of a rights-based approach to healthcare is conscious of the fact that threshold levels of finances and infrastructure is a precondition for an enabling environment, to ensure that the poorest of the poor stand to gain the maximum and are not embroiled in legalities. The policy therefore advocates a progressively incremental assurance-based approach, with assured funding to create an enabling environment for realizing health care as a right in the future.

IMPLEMENTATION OF FRAMEWORK AND WAY FORWARD

A policy is only as good as its implementation. The National Health Policy envisages that an implementation framework be put in place to deliver on these policy commitments. Such an implementation framework would provide a roadmap with clear deliverables and milestones to achieve the goals of the policy.

Chapter 59

National Blood Policy

INTRODUCTION

The policy aims to ensure easily accessible and adequate supply of safe and quality blood and blood components collected/procured from a voluntary, non-remunerated regular blood donor in well-equipped premises, which is free from transfusion transmitted infections, and is stored and transported under optimum conditions. Transfusion under supervision of trained personnel for all who need it irrespective of their economic or social status through comprehensive, efficient and a total quality management approach will be ensured under the policy.

OBJECTIVES

To achieve the above aim, the following objectives are drawn:
- To reiterate firmly the government commitment to provide safe and adequate quantity of blood, blood components and blood products.
- To make available adequate resources to develop and reorganize the blood transfusion services in the entire country.
- To make latest technology available for operating the blood transfusion services and ensure its functioning in an updated manner.
- To launch extensive awareness programmes for donor information, education, motivation, recruitment and retention in order to ensure adequate availability of safe blood.
- To encourage appropriate clinical use of blood and blood products.
- To strengthen the manpower through human resource development.
- To encourage research and development in the field of transfusion medicine and related technology.
- To take adequate regulatory and legislative steps for monitoring and evaluation of blood transfusion services and to take steps to eliminate profiteering in blood banks.

STRATEGIES

To reiterate firmly the government commitment to provide safe and adequate quantity of blood, blood components and blood products.
- A national blood transfusion programme shall be developed to ensure establishment of non-profit integrated national and state blood transfusion services in the country.

- Trading in blood, i.e., sale and purchase of blood shall be prohibited.
- Transfusion services shall be promoted for making available the safe blood to the people.
- Due to the special requirement of armed forces in remote border areas, necessary amendments shall be made in the Drugs and Cosmetics Act/Rules to provide special licenses to small garrison units. These units shall also be responsible for the civilian blood needs of the region.

To make available adequate resources to develop and reorganize the blood transfusion services in the entire country.

- National and State/UT Blood Transfusion Councils (NBTC/SBTC) shall be supported/strengthened financially by pooling resources from various existing programmes and if possible by raising funds from international/bilateral agencies.
- Efforts shall be directed to make the blood transfusion service viable through nonprofit recovery system.

To make latest technology available for operating the blood transfusion services and ensure its functioning in an updated manner.

- Minimum standards for testing, processing and storage shall be set and ensured.
- A quality system scheme shall be introduced in all blood centers.
- Regular proficiency testing of personnel shall be introduced in all the blood centers.
- An external quality assessment scheme (EQAS) through the referral laboratories approved by the National Blood Transfusion Council shall be introduced to assist participating centers in achieving higher standards and uniformity.
- Efforts shall be made towards indigenization of kits, equipment and consumables used in blood banks.
- Use of automation shall be encouraged to manage higher workload with increased efficiency.
- A mechanism for transfer of technology shall be developed to ensure the availability of state-of-the-art technology from outside of India.
- Each blood center shall develop its own standard operating procedures on various aspects of blood banking.
- All blood centers shall adhere to bio-safety guidelines as provided in the Ministry of Health and Family Welfare manual 'Hospital acquired Infections: Guidelines for Control' and disposal of biohazardous waste as per the provisions of the existing Biomedical Wastes (Management and Handling) Rules- 1996 under the Environmental Protection Act, 1986.

To launch extensive awareness programmes for donor information, education, motivation, recruitment and retention in order to ensure adequate availability of safe blood.

- Efforts shall be directed towards recruitment and retention of voluntary, non-remunerated blood donors through education and awareness programmes.
- Enrolment of safe donors shall be ensured.
- State/UT blood transfusion councils shall recognize the services of regular voluntary, non-remunerated blood donors and donor organizers appropriately.
- National/State/UT Blood Transfusion Councils shall develop and launch an IEC campaign using all channels of communication including mass-media for promotion of voluntary blood donation and generation of awareness regarding dangers of blood from paid donors and procurement of blood from unauthorized blood banks/laboratories.
- National/State/UT blood transfusion councils shall involve other departments/sectors for promoting voluntary blood donations.

To encourage appropriate clinical use of blood and blood products.

- Blood shall be used only when necessary. Blood and blood products shall be transfused only to treat conditions leading to significant morbidity and mortality that cannot be prevented or treated effectively by other means.
- National guidelines on 'clinical use of blood' shall be made available and updated as required from time to time.
- Effective and efficient clinical use of blood shall be promoted in accordance with guidelines.
- Education and training in effective clinical use of blood shall be organized.
- Blood and its components shall be prescribed only by a registered medical practitioner as per the provisions of Medical Council Act–1956.
- Availability of blood components shall be ensured through the network of regional centers, satellite centers and other blood centers by creating adequate number of blood component separation units.
- Appropriate steps shall be taken to increase the availability of plasma fractions as per the need of the country through expanding the capacity of existing center and establishing new centers in the country.
- Adequate facilities for transporting blood and blood products including proper cold-chain maintenance shall be made available to ensure appropriate management of blood supply.
- Guidelines for management of blood supply during natural and manmade disasters shall be made available.

To strengthen the manpower through human resource development.

- Transfusion Medicine shall be treated as a specialty.
- In all the existing courses for nurses, technicians and pharmacists, transfusion medicine shall be incorporated as one of the subjects.
- In-service training programmes shall be organized for all categories of personnel working in blood centers as well as drug inspectors and other officers from regulatory agencies.
- Appropriate modules for training of donor organizers/donor recruitment officers shall be developed to facilitate regular and uniform training programmes to be conducted in all States.
- Short orientation training cum advocacy programmes on donor motivation and recruitment shall be organized for community.
- Community Based Organizations (CBOs) and NGOs who wish to participate in Voluntary Blood Donor Recruitment Programme.
- Inter-country and intra-country exchange for training and experience of personnel associated with blood centers shall be encouraged to improve quality of Blood Transfusion Service.
- States/UTs shall create a separate cadre and opportunities for promotions for suitably trained medical and para medical personnel working in blood transfusion services.

To encourage research and development in the field of transfusion medicine and related technology

- A corpus of funds shall be made available to NBTC/SBTCs to facilitate research in transfusion medicine and technology related to blood banking.
- A technical resource core group at national level shall be created to coordinate research and development in the country. This group shall be responsible for recommending implementation of new technologies and procedures in coordination with DC(I).
- Multi-centric research initiatives on issues related to blood transfusion shall be encouraged.

- To take appropriate decisions and/or introduction of policy initiatives on the basis of factual information, operational research on various aspects such as various aspects of transfusion transmissible diseases, knowledge, attitude and practices (KAP) among donors, clinical use of blood, need assessment, etc. shall be promoted.
- Computer-based information and management systems shall be developed which can be used by all the centers regularly to facilitate networking.

To take adequate regulatory and legislative steps for monitoring and evaluation of blood transfusion services and to take steps to eliminate profiteering in blood banks.

- For grant/renewal of blood bank licenses including plan of a blood bank, a committee, comprising members from State/UT Blood Transfusion Councils including transfusion medicine expert, central and State/UT FDAs shall be constituted which will scrutinize all applications as per the guidelines provided by Drugs Controller General (India).
- Fresh licenses to stand-alone blood banks in private sector shall not be granted. Renewal of such blood banks shall be subjected to thorough scrutiny and shall not be renewed in case of noncompliance of any condition of license.
- A separate blood bank cell shall be created under a senior officer not below the rank of DDC(I) in the office of the DC(I) at the headquarter.
- As a deterrent to paid blood donors who operate in the disguise of replacement donors, institutions who prescribe blood for transfusion shall be made responsible for procurement of blood for their patients through their affiliation with licensed blood centers.
- States/UTs shall enact rules for registration of nursing homes wherein provisions for affiliation with a licensed blood bank for procurement of blood for their patients shall be incorporated.

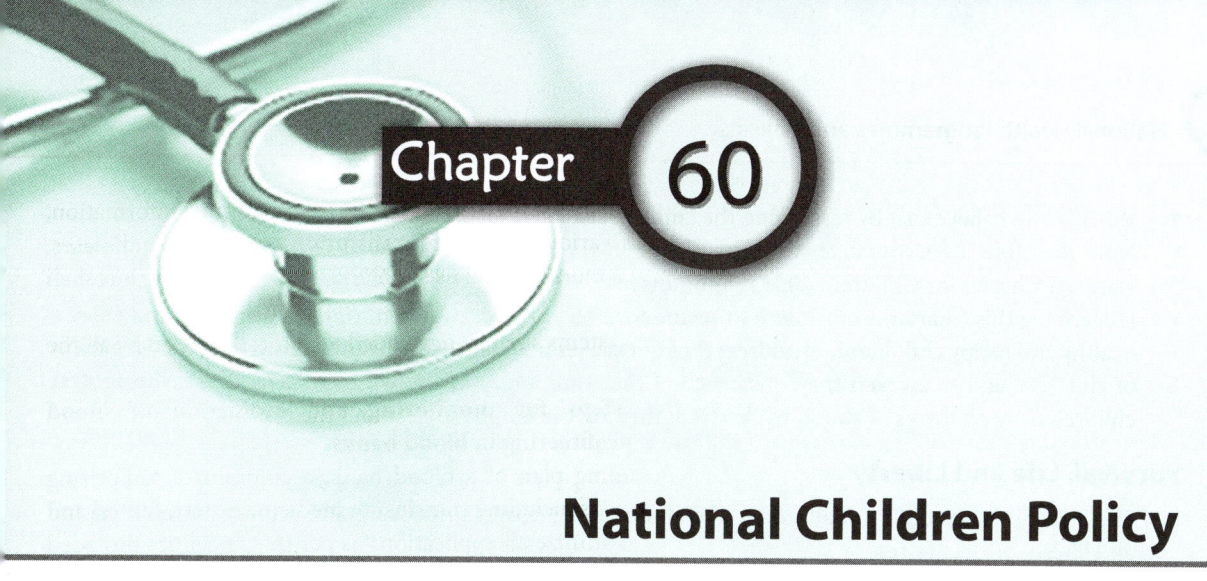

Chapter 60

National Children Policy

INTRODUCTION

The Government of India have had for consideration the question of adopting a National Charter for Children to reiterate its commitment to the cause of the children in order to see that no child remains hungry, illiterate or sick. After the consideration, it has been decided to adopt the National Charter for Children enunciated below.

NATIONAL CHARTER FOR CHILDREN, 2003

Whereas the Constitution of India enshrines both in Part III and IV the cause and the best interest of children, in so far that:

- The State can make special provisions for children [Art 15 (3)] and shall provide free and compulsory education to all children of the age of six to fourteen years, (Art 21A).
- No child below the age of 14 years shall be employed to work in a factory, mine or any other hazardous employment, (Art. 24).
- The tender age of children is not abused and that citizens are not forced by economic necessity to enter avocations unsuited to their age or strength (Art. 39 e), and that children are given opportunities and facilities to develop in a healthy manner and in conditions of freedom and dignity and that youth are protected against exploitation and against moral and material abandonment, (Art. 39 f).
- The State shall endeavor to provide early childhood care and education for all children until they complete the age of six years, (Art. 45).
- Whereas it is a fundamental duty of a parent or guardian to provide opportunities for education to his child or ward between the age of six and fourteen years (Art. 51A).
- Whereas through the National Policy for Children, 1974, we are committed to providing for adequate services to children, both before and after birth and throughout the period of growth, to ensure their full physical, mental and social development.
- Whereas we affirm that the best interest of children must be protected through combined action of the State, civil society, communities and families in their obligations in fulfilling children's basic needs.
- Whereas we also affirm that while state, society, community and family have obligations towards children, these must be viewed in the context of intrinsic and attendant duties of children and inculcating in children a sound sense of values directed towards preserving and strengthening the family, society and the Nation.

- Whereas we believe that by respecting the child, society is respecting itself.
- Now, therefore, in accordance with our pledge in the National Agenda of Governance, the following National Charter for Children, 2003 is announced.
- Underlying this Charter is our intent to secure for every child its inherent right to be a child and enjoy a healthy and happy childhood, to address the root causes that negate the healthy growth and development of children, and to awaken the conscience of the community in the wider societal context to protect children from all forms of abuse, while strengthening the family, society and the Nation.

Survival, Life and Liberty

- The State and community shall undertake all possible measures to ensure and protect the survival, life and liberty of all children.
- In particular, the State and community will undertake all appropriate measures to address the problems of infanticide and feticide, especially of female child and all other emerging manifestations that deprive the girl child of her right to survive with dignity.

Promoting High Standards of Health and Nutrition

- The State shall take measures to ensure that all children enjoy the highest attainable standards of health, and provide for preventive and curative facilities at all levels especially immunization and prevention of micronutrient deficiencies for all children.
- The State shall take measures to cover, under primary health facilities and specialized care and treatment, all children of families below the poverty line.
- The State shall take measures to provide adequate pre-natal and postnatal care for mothers along with immunization against preventable diseases.
- The State shall undertake measures to provide for a national plan that will ensure that the mental health of all children is protected.
- The State shall take steps to ensure protection of children from all practices that are likely to harm the child's physical and mental health.
- The State shall take steps to provide all children from families below the poverty line with adequate supplementary nutrition and undertake adequate measures for ensuring access to safe drinking water and environmental sanitation and hygiene.

Assuring Basic Minimum Needs and Security

- The State recognizes that the basic minimum needs of every child must be met, that foster full development of the child's faculties.
- In order to ensure this, the State shall in partnership with the community provide social security to children, especially to abandoned children and street children.
- State and community shall try and remove the fundamental causes which result in abandoned children and children living on streets, and provide infrastructural and material support by way of shelter, education, nutrition and recreation.

Play and Leisure

- The State and community shall recognize that all children require adequate play and leisure for their healthy development and must ensure means to provide for recreational facilities and services for children of all ages and social groups.

Early Childhood Care for Survival, Growth and Development

- The State shall in partnership with the community provide early childhood care for all children and encourage programmes which will stimulate and develop their physical and cognitive capacities.
- The State shall in partnership with the community aim at providing a child care center in every village where infants and children of working mothers can be adequately cared for.
- The State shall make special efforts to provide these facilities to children from SCs/STs and marginalized sections of society.

Free and Compulsory Primary Education

- The State recognizes that all children shall have access to free and compulsory education. Education at the elementary level shall be provided free of cost and special incentives should be provided to ensure that children from disadvantaged social groups are enrolled, retained and participate in schooling.
- At the secondary level, the State shall provide access to education for all and provide supportive facilities from the disadvantaged groups.
- The State shall in partnership with the community ensure that all the educational institutions function efficiently and are able to reach universal enrolment, universal retention, universal participation and universal achievement.
- The State and community recognize that a child be educated in its mother tongue.
- The State shall ensure that education is child-oriented and meaningful. It shall also take appropriate measures to ensure that education is sensitive to the healthy development of the girl child and to children of varied cultural backgrounds.
- The State shall ensure that school discipline and matters related thereto do not result in physical, mental, psychological harm or trauma to the child.
- The State shall formulate special programmes to spot, identify, encourage and assist the gifted children for their development in the field of their excellence.

Protection from Economic Exploitation and All Forms of Abuse

- The State shall provide protection to children from economic exploitation and from performing tasks that are hazardous to their well-being.
- The State shall ensure that there is appropriate regulation of conditions of work in occupations and processes where children perform work of a nonhazardous nature and that their rights are protected.
- The State shall move towards a total ban of all forms of child labor.
- All children have a right to be protected against neglect, maltreatment, injury, trafficking, sexual and physical abuse of all kinds, corporal punishment, torture, exploitation, violence and degrading treatment.
- The State shall take legal action against those committing such violations against children even if they are legal guardians of such children.
- The State shall in partnership with the community set up mechanisms for identification, reporting, referral, investigation and follow-up of such acts, while respecting the dignity and privacy of the child.
- The State shall in partnership with the community take up steps to draw up plans for the identification, care, protection, counseling and rehabilitation of child victims and ensure that they are able to recover, physically, socially and psychologically, and re-integrate into society.
- The State shall take strict measures to ensure that children are not used in the conduct of any illegal activity, namely, trafficking of narcotic drugs and psychotropic substances, begging, prostitution, pornography

or violence. The State in partnership with the community shall ensure that such children are rescued and immediately placed under appropriate care and protection.

- The State and community shall ensure protection of children in distress for their welfare and all round development.
- The State and community shall ensure protection of children during the occurrence of natural calamities in their best interest.

Protection of the Girl Child

- The State and community shall ensure that crimes and atrocities committed against the girl child, including child marriage, discriminatory practices, forcing girls into prostitution and trafficking are speedily eradicated.
- The State shall in partnership with the community undertake measures, including social, educational and legal, to ensure that there is greater respect for the girl child in the family and society.
- The State shall take serious measures to ensure that the practice of child marriage is speedily abolished.

Empowering Adolescents

- The State and community shall take all steps to provide the necessary education and skills to adolescent children so as to equip them to become economically productive citizens. Special programmes will be undertaken to improve the health and nutritional status of the adolescent girl.

Equality, freedom of expression, freedom to seek and receive information, freedom of association and peaceful assembly.

- The State and community shall ensure that all children are treated equally without discrimination on grounds of the child's or the child's parents' or legal guardian's race, color, caste, sex, language, religion, political or other opinion, national, ethnic or social origin, disability, birth, political status, or any other consideration.
- All children shall be given every opportunity for all round development of their personality, including expression of creativity.
- Every child shall have the freedom to seek and receive information and ideas. The State and community shall provide opportunities for the child to access information that will contribute to the child's development.
- The State and community shall undertake special measures to ensure that the linguistic needs of children are taken care of and encourage the production and dissemination of child-friendly information and material in various forms.
- The State and community shall be responsible for formulating guidelines for the mass media in order to ensure that children are protected from material injuries to their well-being.
- All children shall enjoy freedom of association and peaceful assembly, subject to reasonable restrictions and in conformity with social and family values.

Strengthening family

- Every child has a right to a family. In case of separation of children from their families, the State shall ensure that priority is given to re-unifying the child with its parents. In cases where the State perceives adverse impact of such a reunification, the State shall make alternate arrangements immediately, keeping in mind the best interests and the views of the child.
- All children have a right to maintain contact with their families, even when they are within the custody of the State for various reasons.

- The State shall undertake measures to ensure that children without families are either placed for adoption, preferably intra-country adoption, or foster care or any other family substitute services.
- The State shall ensure that appropriate rules with respect to the implementation of such services are drafted in a manner that are in the best interest of the child and that regulatory bodies are set up to ensure the strict enforcement of these rules.
- All children shall have the right to meet their parents and other family members who may be in custody.

Responsibilities of Both Parents

The State recognizes the common responsibilities of both parents in rearing their children.

Protection of Children with Disabilities

- The State and community recognize that all children with disabilities must be helped to lead a life with dignity and respect. All measures would be undertaken to ensure that children with disabilities are encouraged to be integrated into the mainstream society and actively participate in all walks of life.
- State and community shall also provide for their education, training, health care, rehabilitation, recreation in a manner that will contribute to their overall growth and development.
- State and community shall launch preventive programmes against disabilities and early detection of disabilities so as to ensure that the families with disabled children receive adequate support and assistance in bringing up their children.
- The State shall encourage research and development in the field of prevention, treatment and rehabilitation of various forms of disabilities.

Care, protection, and welfare of children of marginalized and disadvantaged communities.

- The State and community shall provide care, protect and ensure the welfare of children from marginalized and disadvantaged communities, support them in preserving their identity, and encourage them to adopt practices that promote their best interest. The State recognizes that children from disadvantaged communities and weaker/vulnerable sections of the society are in need of special interventions and support in all matters pertaining to education, health, recreation and supportive services. It shall make adequate provisions for providing such groups with special attention in all its policies and programmes.

Ensuring Child-Friendly Procedures

- All matters and procedures relating to children, viz. judicial, administrative, educational or social, should be child-friendly. All procedures laid down under the juvenile justice system for children in conflict with law and for children in need of special care and protection shall also be child-friendly.

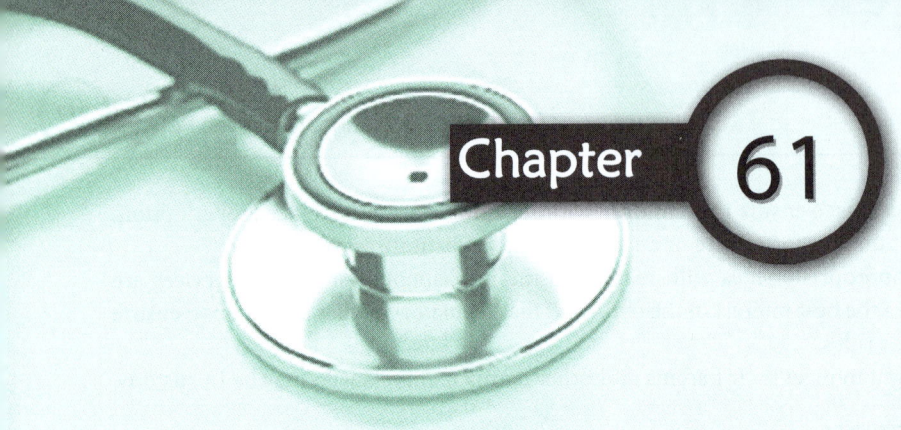

Chapter 61

National Policy on Senior Citizens 2011

INTRODUCTION

The National Policy on older persons was announced by the Government of India in the year 1999. It was a step in the right direction in pursuance of the UN General Assembly Resolution 47/5 to observe 1999 as International Year of older persons and in keeping with the assurances to older persons contained in the Constitution. The well-being of senior citizens is mandated in the Constitution of India under Article 41—The State shall, within the limits of its economic capacity and development, make effective provision for securing the right to public assistance in cases of old age. The Right to Equality is guaranteed by the Constitution as a fundamental right. Social security is the concurrent responsibility of the Central and State Governments.

Subsequent international efforts made an impact on the implementation of the National Policy on older persons. The Madrid Plan of Action and the United Nations principles for senior citizens adopted by the UN General Assembly in 2002, the proclamation on aging and the global targets on aging for the year 2001 adopted by the General Assembly in 1992, the Shanghai Plan of Action 2002 and the Macau Outcome document 2007 adopted by UNESCAP form the basis for the global policy guidelines to encourage governments to design and implement their own policies from time to time. The Government of India is a signatory to all these documents demonstrating its commitment to address the concerns of the elderly.

The policy and plans were put in place by Central and State Governments for the welfare of older persons. The State Governments issued their policies and programmes for the welfare of older persons. While some States and Union Territories implemented their policies with vigor, most states—particularly the big ones—were behind perhaps due to financial and operational deficiencies.

Pensions, travel concessions, income tax relief, medical benefit, extra interest on savings, security of older persons through an integrated scheme of the Ministry of Social Justice and Empowerment as well as financial support was provided for homes, day care centers, medical vans, helplines, etc. are extended currently.

The Ministry of Social Justice and Empowerment coordinates programmes to be undertaken by other Ministries in their relevant areas of support to older persons.

The Ministry of Social Justice and Empowerment piloted landmark legislation the Maintenance and Welfare of Parents and Senior Citizens Act 2007 which is being promulgated by the States and Union Territories in stages.

This policy looks at the increasing longevity of people and lack of care giving.

OBJECTIVES

The foundation of the new policy, known as the—National Policy for Senior Citizens 2011 is based on several factors. These include the demographic explosion among the elderly, the changing economy and social milieu, advancement in medical research, science and technology and high levels of destitution among the elderly rural poor (51 million elderly live below the poverty line). A higher proportion of elderly women than men experience loneliness and are dependent on children. Social deprivations and exclusion, privatization of health services and changing pattern of morbidity affect the elderly. All those of 60 years and above are senior citizens. This policy addresses issues concerning senior citizens living in urban and rural areas, special needs of the oldest old and older women.

In principle, the policy values an age integrated society. It will endeavor to strengthen integration between generations, facilitate interaction between the old and the young as well as strengthen bonds between different age groups. It believes in the development of a formal and informal social support system, so that the capacity of the family to take care of senior citizens is strengthened and they continue to live in the family. The policy seeks to reach out in particular to the bulk of senior citizens living in rural areas who are dependent on family bonds and intergenerational understanding and support.

THE FOCUS OF THE NEW POLICY

- Mainstream senior citizens, especially older women, and bring their concerns into the national development debate with priority to implement mechanisms already set by governments and supported by civil society and senior citizen associations. Support promotion and establishment of senior citizen associations, especially amongst women.
- Promote the concept of aging in place or aging in own home, housing, income security and home care services, old age pension and access to health care insurance schemes and other programmes and services to facilitate and sustain dignity in old age. The thrust of the policy would be preventive rather than cure.
- The policy will consider institutional care as the last resort. It recognizes that care of senior citizens has to remain vested in the family which would partner the community, government and the private sector.
- Being a signatory to the Madrid Plan of Action and barrier free framework it will work towards an inclusive, barrier-free and age-friendly society.
- Recognize that senior citizens are a valuable resource for the country and create an environment that provides them with equal opportunities, protects their rights and enables their full participation in society. Towards achievement of this directive, the policy visualizes that the states will extend their support for senior citizens living below the poverty line in urban and rural areas and ensure their social security, health care, shelter and welfare. It will protect them from abuse and exploitation so that the quality of their lives improves.
- Long-term savings instruments and credit activities will be promoted to reach both rural and urban areas. It will be necessary for the contributors to feel assured that the payments at the end of the stipulated period are attractive enough to take care of the likely erosion in purchasing power.
- Employment in income generating activities after superannuation will be encouraged.
- Support and assist organizations that provide counseling, career guidance and training services.
- States will be advised to implement the Maintenance and Welfare of Parents and Senior Citizens Act, 2007 and set up tribunals so that elderly parents unable to maintain themselves are not abandoned and neglected.

- States will set up homes with assisted living facilities for abandoned senior citizens in every district of the country and there will be adequate budgetary support.

AREAS OF INTERVENTION

The concerned ministries at central and state level as mentioned in the "Implementation Section" would implement the policy and take necessary steps for senior citizens as under:

Income Security in Old Age

A major intervention required in old age relates to financial insecurity as more than of the elderly live below the poverty line. It would increase with age uniformly across the country.

Indira Gandhi National Old Age Pension Scheme

- Old age pension scheme would cover all senior citizens living below the poverty line.
- Rate of monthly pension would be raised to ₹1000 per month per person and revised at intervals to prevent its deflation due to higher cost of purchasing.
- The oldest old would be covered under Indira Gandhi National Old Age Pension Scheme (IGNOAPS). They would be provided additional pension in case of disability, loss of adult children and concomitant responsibility for grandchildren and women. This would be reviewed every 5 years.

Public Distribution System

The public distribution system would reach out to cover all senior citizens living below the poverty line.

Income Tax

Taxation policies would reflect sensitivity to the financial problems of senior citizens which accelerate due to very high costs of medical and nursing care, transportation and support services needed at homes.

Microfinance

Loans at reasonable rates of interest would be offered to senior citizens to start small businesses. Microfinance for senior citizens would be supported through suitable guidelines issued by the Reserve Bank of India.

Health Care

With advancing age, senior citizens have to cope with health and associated problems some of which may be chronic, of a multiple nature, require constant attention and carry the risk of disability and consequent loss of autonomy. Some health problems, especially when accompanied by impaired functional capacity require long-term management of illness and nursing care.

- Health care needs of senior citizens will be given high priority. The goal would be good, affordable health service, heavily subsidized for the poor and a graded system of user charges for others. It would have a judicious mix of public health services, health insurance, health services provided by not-for-profit organizations including trusts and charities, and private medical care. While the first of these will need to be promoted by the State, the third category given some assistance, concessions and relief and the fourth encouraged and subjected to some degree of regulation, preferably by an association of providers of private care.
- The basic structure of public health care would be through primary health care. It would be strengthened and oriented to meet the health needs of senior citizens. Preventive, curative, restorative and rehabilitative

services will be expanded and strengthened and geriatric care facilities provided at secondary and tertiary levels. This will imply much larger public sector outlays, proper distribution of services in rural and urban areas, and much better health administration and delivery systems. Geriatric services for all age groups above 60—preventive, curative, rehabilitative health care will be provided. The policy will strive to create a tiered national level geriatric health care with focus on outpatient day care, palliative care, rehabilitation care and respite care.

- Twice in a year, the PHC nurse or the ASHA will conduct a special screening of the 80+ population of villages and urban areas and public/private partnerships will be worked out for geriatric and palliative health care in rural areas recognizing the increase of non-communicable diseases (NCD) in the country.
- Efforts would be made to strengthen the family system so that it continues to play the role of primary caregiver in old age. This would be done by sensitizing younger generations and by providing tax incentives for those taking care of the older members.
- Development of health insurance will be given priority to cater to the needs of different income segments of the population with provision for varying contributions and benefits. Packages catering to the lower income groups will be entitled to state subsidy. Concessions and relief will be given to health insurance to enlarge the coverage base and make it affordable. Universal application of health insurance—Rashtriya Swasthya Bima Yojana (RSBY) will be promoted in all districts and senior citizens will be compulsorily included in the coverage. Specific policies will be worked out for health care insurance of senior citizens.
- From an early age, citizens will be encouraged to contribute to a government created health care fund that will help in meeting the increased expenses on health care after retirement. It will also pay for the health insurance premium in higher socioeconomic segments.
- Special programmes will be developed to increase awareness on mental health and for early detection and care of those with Dementia and Alzheimer's disease.
- Restoration of vision and eyesight of senior citizens will be an integral part of the National Programme for Control of Blindness (NPCB).
- Use of science and technology such as web-based services and devices for the well-being and safety of senior citizens will be encouraged and expanded to under-serviced areas.
- National and regional institutes of aging will be set up to promote geriatric health care. Adequate budgetary support will be provided to these institutes and a cadre of geriatric health care specialists is created including professionally trained caregivers to provide care to the elderly at affordable prices.
- The current National Programme for Health Care of the Elderly (NPHCE) being implemented would be expanded immediately and, in partnership with civil society organizations, scaled up to all districts of the country.
- Public-private partnership models will be developed wherever possible to implement health care of the elderly.
- Services of mobile health clinics would be made available through PHCs or a subsidy would be granted to NGOs who offer such services.
- Health insurance cover would be provided to all senior citizens through public funded schemes, especially those over 80 years who do not pay income tax.
- Hospices and palliative care of the terminally ill would be provided in all district hospitals and the Indian protocol on palliative care will be disseminated to all doctors and medical professionals.
- Recognize gender-based attitudes towards health and develop programmes for regular health checkups especially for older women who tend to neglect their problems.

Safety and Security

- Provision would be made for stringent punishment for abuse of the elderly.
- Abuse of the elderly and crimes against senior citizens especially widows and those living alone and disabled would be tackled by community awareness and policing.
- Police would be directed to keep a friendly vigil and monitor programmes which will include a comprehensive plan for security of senior citizens whether living alone or as couples. They would also promote mechanisms for interaction of the elderly with neighborhood associations and enrolment in special programmes in urban and rural areas.
- Protective services would be established and linked to helplines, legal aid and other measures.

Housing

Shelter is a basic human need. The stock of housing for different income segments will be increased. Ten per cent of housing schemes for urban and rural lower income segments will be earmarked for senior citizens. This will include the Indira Awas Yojana and other schemes of the government.

- Age-friendly, barrier-free access will be created in buses and bus stations, railways and railway stations, airports and bus transportation within the airports, banks, hospitals, parks, places of worship, cinema halls, shopping malls and other public places that senior citizens and the disabled frequent.
- Develop housing complexes for single older men and women, and for those with need for specialized care in cities, towns and rural areas.
- Promote age-friendly facilities and standards of universal design by Bureau of Indian Standards.
- Since a multi-purpose center is a necessity for social interaction of senior citizens, housing colonies would reserve sites for establishing such centers. Segregation of senior citizens in housing colonies would be discouraged and their integration into the community supported.
- Senior citizens will be given loans for purchase of houses as well as for major repairs, with easy repayment schedules.

Productive Aging

- The policy will promote measures to create avenues for continuity in employment and/or post-retirement opportunities.
- Directorate of Employment would be created to enable seniors find re-employment.
- The age of retirement would be reviewed by the ministry due to increasing longevity.

Welfare

- A welfare fund for senior citizens will be set up by the government and revenue generated through a social security cess. The revenue generated from this would be allocated to the states in proportion to their share of senior citizens. States may also create similar funds.
- Non-institutional services by voluntary organizations will be promoted and assisted to strengthen the capacity of senior citizens and their families to deal with problems of the aging.
- All senior citizens, especially widows, single women and the "oldest old" would be eligible for all schemes of government. They would be provided universal identity under the Aadhaar scheme on priority.
- Larger budgetary allocations would be earmarked to pay attention to the special needs of rural and urban senior citizens living below the poverty line.

Multigenerational Bonding

- The policy would focus on promoting bonding of generations and multigenerational support by incorporating relevant educational material in school curriculum and promoting value education. School Value Education modules and textbooks promoting family values of caring for parents would be promoted by NCERT and State Educational Bodies.

Media

- Media has an important role to play in highlighting the changing situation of senior citizens and in identifying emerging issues and areas of action.
- Involve mass media as well as informal and traditional communication channels on aging issues.
- Provide equal access to food, shelter, medical care and other services to senior citizens during and after natural disasters and emergencies.
- Enhance financial grants and other relief measures to assist senior citizens to re-establish and reconstruct their communities and rebuild their social fabric following emergencies.

IMPLEMENTATION MECHANISM

There will be efforts to provide an identity for senior citizens across the country and the Aadhaar Unique Identity Number will be offered to them so that implementation of assistance schemes of Government of India and concessions can be offered to them. As part of the policy implementation, the Government will strive for:

- **Establishment of Department of Senior Citizens under the Ministry of Social Justice and Empowerment:** The Ministry of Social Justice and Empowerment will establish a—Department of Senior Citizens which will be the nodal agency for implementing programmes and services for senior citizens and the NPSC 2011. An inter-ministerial committee will pursue matters relating to implementation of the national policy and monitor its progress. Coordination will be by the nodal ministry. Each ministry will prepare action plans to implement aspects that concern them and submit regular reviews.
- **Establishment of Directorates of Senior Citizens in States and Union Territories:** States and Union Territories will set up separate Directorates of Senior Citizens for implementing programmes and services for senior citizens and the NPSC 2011.
- **National/State Commission for Senior citizens:** A National Commission for senior citizens at the center and similar commissions at the state level will be constituted. The Commissions would be set up under an Act of the Parliament with powers of civil courts to deal with cases pertaining to violations of rights of senior citizens.
- **Establishment of National Council for Senior Citizens:** A National Council for senior citizens, headed by the Minister for Social Justice and Empowerment will be constituted by the Ministry. With tenure of five-years, the Council will monitor the implementation of the policy and advise the government on concerns of senior citizens. A similar body would be established in every state with the concerned minister heading the State Council for senior citizens.
  - The Council would include representatives of relevant Central Ministries, the Planning Commission and 10 States by rotation.
  - Representatives of senior citizen associations from every State and Union Territory.
  - Representatives of NGOs, academia, media and experts on aging.
  - The Council would meet once in six months.

Responsibility for Implementation

The Ministries of Home Affairs, Health and Family Welfare, Rural Development, Urban Development, Youth Affairs and Sports, Railways, Science and Technology, Statistics and Programme Implementation, Labor, Panchayati Raj and Departments of Elementary Education and Literacy, Secondary and Higher Education, Road Transport and Highways, Public Enterprises, Revenue, Women and Child Development, Information Technology and Personnel and Training will setup necessary mechanism for implementation of the policy. A five-year perspective plan and annual plans setting targets and financial allocations will be prepared by each Ministry/Department. The annual report of these Ministries/Departments will indicate progress achieved during the year. This will enable monitoring by the designated authority.

Role of Block Development Offices, Panchayati Raj Institutions and Tribal Councils/ Gram Sabhas

Block development offices (BDO) would appoint nodal officers to serve as a one-point contact for senior citizens to ease access to pensions and handle documentation and physical presence requirements, especially by the elderly women. Panchayati Raj Institutions would be directed to implement the NPSC 2011 and address local issues and needs of the aging population. In rural/tribal areas, the tribal council or gram sabha or the relevant Panchayati Raj Institution would be responsible for implementation of the policy. The provisions of the 13th Finance Commission for special funding to them would be made applicable.

Chapter 62

National Nutrition Policy

INTRODUCTION

National nutrition policy (NNP) has been adopted by the Government in 1993. The NNP identified key action in various areas having impact on nutrition such as agriculture, food production, food supply, education, information, health care, social justice, tribal welfare, urban development, rural development, labor, women and child development, people with special needs and monitoring and surveillance.

The core strategy is to tackle the problem of nutrition through direct nutrition interventions for vulnerable groups as well as through various development policy instruments which will improve access and create conditions for improved nutrition.

The direct short-term nutrition interventions suggested by NNP include:

- Nutrition interventions for especially vulnerable group such as children below six years, adolescent girls and pregnant and lactating women, expanding the safety nets, facilitating behavior change among mothers, reaching the adolescent girls and ensuring better coverage of expectant women.
- Fortification of essential food items with appropriate nutrients.
- Popularization of low cost nutritious foods prepared from indigenous and locally available raw materials.
- Control of micronutrient deficiencies among vulnerable groups.

The indirect long-term nutrition interventions leading to institutional and structural changes include:

- Food security for improved availability of food grains.
- Improvement of dietary patterns through production and demonstration.
- Policies for effective income transfers so as to improve the entitlement package of the rural and urban poor—improving the purchasing power and strengthening public distribution system.
- Land reforms measures for reducing vulnerabilities of landless and landed poor.
- Strengthen health and family welfare programme.
- Imparting basic health and nutrition knowledge.
- Prevention of food adulteration.
- Improvement in nutrition surveillance.
- Monitoring of nutrition programmes.
- Research into various aspects of nutrition.
- Equal remuneration for women.
- Communication through established media.
- Minimum wage administration to ensure its strict enforcement and timely revision and linking it with price rise through a suitable nutrition formula—a special legislation for providing agricultural women laborers the minimum support, and at least 60 days leave by the employer in the last trimester of her pregnancy.

- Community participation for generating awareness on NNP—active participation of community members in management of nutrition programmes and related interventions through beneficiaries, committees, participation of women in food production and processing, promoting kitchen gardens, food preservation, preparation of weaning food, and generating demand of nutrition services.
- Education and literacy.
- Improvement in status of women.

Further to this, a National Plan of Action on Nutrition (NPAN) 1995 was laid down focusing on reducing under nutrition which entails a multisectoral approach for accelerated action on determinants of malnutrition.

POLICY DETAILS

Nutrition intervention net through ICDS so as to cover all vulnerable children in the age group 0–6 years. Presently, India's child population for 0–6 years is around 18% of the total population and, out of this 30.76 million comprise the children from the households living below the poverty line in rural areas. Presently, ICDS covers around 15.3 million children (most of them in the rural areas). It should be our conscious policy to cover the remaining 15.46 million children who are nutritionally at risk, by extending ICDS to all the remaining 2388 blocks (5153 minus 2765 blocks existing) of the country by the year 2000.

With the objective of reducing the incidence of severe and moderate malnutrition by half by the year 2000 a concerted effort needs to be made to trigger appropriate behavioral changes among the mothers. Improving growth monitoring between the age group 0–3 years in particular with closer involvement of the mothers is a key intervention. Presently growth monitoring has become a one-way process and the mothers are mere passive observers of the entire process. This needs to be changed because after all nutrition management of the children will have to be done by the mothers at home. Getting involved in the growth monitoring of her child will give her a feeling of control. In the decentralized processes of salt marketing in the country, there is the need to identify a vehicle which can be better controlled. Research in iron fortification of rice and other cereals should be intensified. The distribution of iodized salt should cover all the population in endemic areas of the country to reduce the iodine deficiency to below endemic levels.

- **Popularization of low cost nutritious food:** Efforts to produce and popularize the cost of nutritious foods from indigenous and locally available raw material shall be intensified. It is necessary to involve women particularly in this activity.
- **Control of micronutrient deficiencies among vulnerable groups:** Deficiencies of vitamins, iron, folic acid and iodine among children, pregnant women and nursing mothers shall be controlled through intensified programmes.
- Iron supplementation to adolescent girls shall be introduced. The programme shall be expanded to cover all eligible members of the community.
- The prophylaxis programme, at present, do not cover all children. For example, the vitamins and micronutrient programme covers only 30 out of about 80 million. It is necessary to intensify all these efforts and work on a specific time frame. Nutritional blindness should be completely eradicated by the year 2000 AD.
- The National Nutritional Anemia Prophylaxis Programme should be extended and strengthened to reduce anemia in expectant women to 25% by 2000 AD.

INDIRECT POLICY INSTRUMENTS

- **Long-term institutional and structural changes:**
  - **Food security:** In order to ensure aggregate food security, a per capita availability of 215 kg/person/year of food grains needs to be attained. This requires production of 250 million tons of food grains

per year by 2000 AD and buffer stocks of 30–35 million tons in order to guard against exigencies such as flood and droughts. However, taking into account the present trends and the possibility of improved availability of non-cereal food items, there should be a target of at least attaining 230 million tons food grains production by 2000 AD.

- **Improvement of dietary pattern through production and demonstration:** Improving the dietary pattern by promoting the production and increasing the per capita availability of nutritionally rich foods. The production of pulses, oilseeds and other food crops will be increased with a view to attain self-sufficiency and building surplus and buffer stocks.

  - ❖ The production of protective food crops such as vegetables, fruits, milk, meat, fish and poultry shall be augmented. Preference shall be given to growing foods, such as millets, legumes, vegetables and fruits (carrots, green leafy vegetables, guava, papaya and amla) for this purpose. The latest and improved techniques shall be increasingly applied, high-yielding varieties of food crops developed and extensively cultivated, and adequate extension services made available to farmers.

  - ❖ Wastage of food in transit and storage reduced to the minimum available food conserved and effectively utilized and adequate buffer stocks built up. Certain imbalances and anomalies in our agricultural policy need to be redressed immediately. Our agricultural policy has been hitherto concerned with production exclusively and not nutrition which is the ultimate end. While the green revolution has largely remained a cereal revolution, with bias towards wheat, coarse grains and pulses, which constitute the poor man's staple and protein requirements, have not received adequate attention.

  - ❖ The prices of pulses, which were below cereal prices before the green revolution are now almost double the price of cereals. Our food policy should be consistent with our national nutritional needs.

Policies for effective income transfers so as to improve the entitlement package of the rural and urban poor.

- **Improving the purchasing power:** Poverty alleviation programmes, like the Integrated Rural Development Programme (IRDP) and employment generation schemes like Jawahar Rozgar Yojana, Nehru Rozgar Yojana and DWCRA are to be re-oriented and restructured to make a forceful dent on the purchasing, power of the lowest economic segments of the population. In all poverty alleviation programmes, nutritional objectives shall be incorporated explicitly and the nutritional benefits of income genuine shall be taken for granted, existing programmes shall be scrutinized for their nutrition component. It is necessary to improve the purchasing power of the landless and the rural and urban poor by implementing employment generation programmes so that additional employment of at least 100 days is created for each rural landless family and employment opportunities are created in urban areas for slum dwellers and the urban poor.

- **Public distribution system:** Ensuring an equitable food distribution, through the expansion of the public distribution system. The Public distribution system shall ensure availability of essential food articles such as coarse grains, pulses and jaggery, beside rice, wheat, sugar and oil; conveniently and at reasonable prices to the public. Particularly to those living below the poverty line not only in urban areas but throughout the country. For this purpose, encouragement shall be given to the consumer cooperatives and fair price shops shall be opened in adequate number in all areas. Effective price and quality control shall be exercised over the cooked foods in restaurants and other eating places. The Public Distribution system should be strengthened especially during the monsoon months for giving special rations at specially subsidized rates for at least four months (July–October) to the seasonally high risk population. The beneficiaries of this programme should include landless laborers and their families and the migrant laborers and their families.

- **Land reforms:** Implementing land reform measures so that the vulnerability of the landless and the landed poor could be reduced. This will include both tenures' reforms as well as implementation of ceiling laws.
- **Health and family welfare:** The health and family welfare programmes are an inseparable part of the strategy. Through "Health for All by 2000 AD" programme increased health and immunization facilities shall be provided to all. Improved pre-natal and post-natal care to ensure safe motherhood shall be made accessible to all women. The population in the reproductive age group shall be empowered through education to be responsible for their own family size. Through intensive family welfare and motivational measures, small family norm and adequate spacing shall be encouraged so that the food available to the family is sufficient for proper nutrition of the members.
- **Basic health and nutrition knowledge:** Basic health and nutrition knowledge with special focus on wholesome infant feeding practices, shall be imparted to the people extensively and effectively. Nutrition and health education concepts shall be effectively integrated into the school curricula, as well as into 211 nutrition programmes. Nutrition and health education are very important in the context of the problems of overnutrition also.
- **Prevention of food adulteration:** Prevention of food adulteration must be strengthened by gearing up the enforcement machinery.
- **Nutrition surveillance:** Nutritional status is another weak area requiring immediate attention. The NNMB/NIN of ICMR needs to be strengthened so that periodical monitoring of the nutritional status of adolescent girls, and pregnant and lactating mothers below the poverty line takes place through representative samples and results are transmitted to all agencies concerned. The NNMB should not only try and assess the impact of ongoing nutrition and development programmes but also serve as an early warning system for initiating prompt action. Since the department of women and child development is the nodal department for national nutrition policy, it is necessary for the NNMB to be accountable to this department in so far as nutrition surveillance is concerned.
- **Monitoring of nutrition programmes:** Monitoring of nutrition programmes (viz ICDS), and of nutrition education and demonstration by the Food and Nutrition Board, through all its 67 centers and field units, should be continued. The transfer of Food and Nutrition Board to the department of women and child development has already been approved by the Prime Minister. This will ensure an integrated set up to deal with the problem of nutrition with adequate technical and field-level set up.
- **Research:** Research into various aspects of nutrition, both on the consumption side as well as the supply side, is another essential aspect of the strategy. Research must accurately identify those who are suffering from various degrees of malnutrition. Research should enable selection of new varieties of food with high nutrition value which can be within the purchasing power of the poor.
- **Equal remuneration:** Special efforts should be made to improve the effectiveness of programmes related to women. The wages of women shall be at par with that of men in order to improve women's economic status. This requires a stricter enforcement of the equal remuneration with special emphasis that will have to be given for expanding employment opportunities for women.
- **Communication:** Communication through established media is one of the most important strategies to be adopted for the effective implementation of the nutrition policy. The department of women and child development will have a well-established, permanent communications division with adequate staff and fund support.
  - While using the communication tools, both mass communication as well as group or inter-personal communication should be used. Not only the electronic media but also folk and print media should be used extensively. The existing facilities in the song and drama division and the Directorate of

Advertising and Visual Publicity (DAVP) in the Ministry of Information and Broadcasting could help in a big way to improve nutrition and health education.

- To give a new direction to communication and media, efforts will be made for promoting sound feeding practices, which are culturally acceptable and based on local food habits. Alongside the information gap, existing social attitudes and prejudices, inherent in our milieu, which discriminate against girls and women and affect their health and nutrition, need to be countered through educational programmes. Further, the media policy shall focus on ways and means to combat malnutrition among girl children, adolescent girls and women in the reproductive age group.
- Educational programmes will be made meaningful and interesting to meet the growing needs of the population. The role of information is crucial for nutrition. Such information is not only important with regard to improved health and nutrition practices but can also have a vital influence on the market, particularly during natural calamities, war, etc.
- The role of information during such exigencies is to ensure that the market remain stable without any panic being created. This also needs to be carefully monitored.

- **Minimum wage administration:** Closely related to the market, is the need to ensure an effective minimum wage administration to ensure its strict enforcement and timely revision and linking it with price rise through a suitable nutrition formula. A special legislation should be introduced for providing agricultural women laborers the minimum support, and at least 60 days leave by the employer in the last trimester of her pregnancy. Excessive loss of energy during the working sessions has serious nutritional implications. The legislation should take care of this problem also.

- **Community participation:** The active involvement of the community is essential not only in terms of being aware of the services available to the community but also for deriving the maximum benefit from such services by giving timely feedback necessary at all levels. After all, communication must form an essential part of all services and people themselves are the best communicators. Community participation will include:
  - Generating awareness among the community regarding the National Nutrition Policy and its major concerns.
  - Involving the community through their Panchayats or where Panchayat do not exist, through beneficiary committees in the management of nutrition programmes and interventions related to nutrition such as employment generation land reforms, health, education, etc.
  - Actual participation particularly of women in food production and processing activities,
  - Promoting schemes relating to kitchen gardens, food preservation preparation of weaning foods and other food processing units both at the home level as well as the commodity levels.
  - Generation of effective demand at the level of the community for all services relating to nutrition.

- **Education literacy:** It has been shown that education and literacy particularly that of women, are the key determinants for better nutritional status. For instance, Kerala State which has the highest literacy level, also has the best nutrition status despite the fact that calorie intake in Kerala is not the highest among all States in the country.
  - **Improvement of the status of women:** The most effective way to implement nutrition with mainstream activities in agriculture, health, education and rural development is to focus on improving the status of women, particularly the economic status. After all, women are the ultimate providers of nutrition to both through acquisition of food as well as preparation of food for consumption.
    - ❖ There is evidence that women's employment does beneficial household nutrition both through increase in household income as well as through an increase in women's status, autonomy and decision-making power. Moreover, female education also has a strong inverse relationship with IMR.

- ❖ Educated women have greater roles in household decision making, particularly those relating to nutrition and feeding practices. Therefore, emphasis on women's employment and education particularly nutrition and health education should provide the bedrock of the nation's nutritional intervention.
- ❖ If a self-sustaining development model is to be pursued in which the community is able to manage its nutrition and health needs on its own, socioeconomic security of women is sine qua non. This underscores the importance of improving the employment status of women.
- ❖ The groundswell of voluntary action created through the National Literacy Mission should be harnessed and channelized into the areas of child survival and nutrition.

- **Administration and monitoring implementation of national nutrition policy:**
  - ■ The measures enumerated above have to be administered by several ministries/departments of the Government of India and various governmental and non-governmental organizations. There should be a close collaboration between the Food Policy, the Agricultural Policy, the Health Policy, the Education Policy, the Rural Development Programme and the Nutrition Policy as each complements the other.
    - ❖ The NNP should immediately be translated into forceful, viable and realistic sectoral action programmes. Special working groups shall be constituted in the Departments of Agriculture, Rural Development, Health, Education, Food and Women and Child Development to analyze the nutritional relevance of Sectoral proposals and to incorporate nutritional considerations in the light of the Nutrition Policy wherever necessary.
    - ❖ Each concerned Central Ministry shall implement the measures for which it has direct or nodal responsibility.
  - ■ An Inter-Ministerial Coordination Committee will function in the Ministry of Human Resource Development under the Chairmanship of Secretary, Department of Women and Child Development, to oversee and review the implementation of nutrition intervention measures.
    - ❖ Sectoral Ministries Departments concerned, like Health and Family Welfare, Education and Agriculture, Food and Civil supplies, etc. will be represented in the Inter-Ministerial Coordination Committee. The Committee will meet once or twice a year.
    - ❖ The Coordination Committee would be constituted with the sectoral representatives or administrators essential for decision making on policy matters to analyze and discuss and resolve the technical use and nutrition aspects of all plans and strategies during the implementation stage, technical experts from concerned areas would be associate members.
  - ■ A National Nutrition Council will be constituted in the Planning Commission, with Prime Minister as President. Members will include concerned Union Ministers, a few State Ministers by rotation, and experts, and representatives of non-governmental organizations.
    - ❖ The Council will be the national forum for policy coordination, review and direction at the national level. The Council will meet once a year.
    - ❖ The National Nutrition Council will be the highest body for overseeing the implementation of the National Nutrition Policy through the various sectoral plans of action and will issue policy guidelines based on latest nutritional surveillance feedback.
- **Monitoring of nutrition situation:** Nutritional surveillance of the country's population especially children and mothers, shall be the responsibility of the National Institute of Nutrition/NNMB who in turn may involve the National Institute of Health and Family Welfare, Central Health Education Bureau, Home Science, Medical Colleges and NGOs.
  - ■ There shall be a mechanism to utilize the services of Food/Nutrition science and medical graduates trained every year, to manage, the national nutrition programmes. NIN/NNMB should be accountable to the Department of Women and Child Development insofar as nutrition surveillance is concerned.

- The paucity of reliable and comparable data from all parts of the country is a definite obstacle toward a realistic and disaggregated problem definition.
- This calls for a nation-wide monitoring system. To achieve this, it is necessary to restructure and strengthen the existing National Nutrition Monitoring Bureau (NNMB) and to develop a mechanism for generating nation-wide disaggregated data within a short period for use by the center and the states for taking corrective action wherever necessary. This would ensure a regular monitoring and surveillance system and develop a reliable data base in the country not only to assess the impact of ongoing nutrition and development programmes but also to serve as an early warning system for initiating prompt action.

- **Role of state governments:** In a federal polity like ours, the cutting edge of governmental interventions commences from the state level. Therefore, the successful actualization of nutrition policy is largely dependent on the effective role of the state governments.
    - The formal structure at the state level should be similar to that envisaged under the Government of India. There should be an apex State level nutrition council to be chaired by the Chief Minister and to comprise concerned Minister of the State Government, representatives of leading NGOs working in the state, experts and representatives of related professional bodies.
    - There should be an inter-departmental coordinating Committee to function under the Chief Secretary which will coordinate, oversee and monitor the implementation of the national nutrition policy.
    - The committee would also focus on the State level targets for the various nutrition-related indicators based targets set under the NNP. The Secretary of the Department dealing with women and children should be the convener of this committee.
    - Special working groups will be set in the departments of agriculture, rural development, health, education, food and women and child development and this group will be responsible for vetting the various sectoral schemes from the point of view of nutrition before they are finalized.

- Given the problem of mounting delivery cost of various nutrition interventions, it is necessary to mobilize resources from within the community in order to ensure sustainability of these interventions. This is a major area of concern and the State Governments, local bodies (including Municipal and Panchayat bodies); NGOs, cooperatives and professional organizations and pressure groups must take this up as a challenge.
    - In a pluralistic society like ours, a concerted effort by all of them is the only way to build community support and ultimately community participation in these schemes. Successful examples of the community contributing the nutrition component of ICDS scheme exists in certain States. It is possible to replicate these examples.
    - Many State Governments have started a major mid-day meal programme funded out of the state resources. The other State Government and Union Territory Administration may also consider such an introduction in their primary and secondary schools.
    - The private schools and schools which are capable of mobilizing their own resources may be encouraged to introduce such schemes out of their own resources.
    - The State Governments may consider constituting similar bodies, i.e. State Coordination Committees and State Nutrition Councils, as well as such bodies at the district levels. In a massive country like India, with autonomous states, each with its characteristic problems, priorities, approaches and resources, the state level nutrition policies would be better able to deal with the problems.
    - After the NNP of India is operational with specific objectives, plans, operation, strategies, targets and time frame, development of state-level policies shall be encouraged.

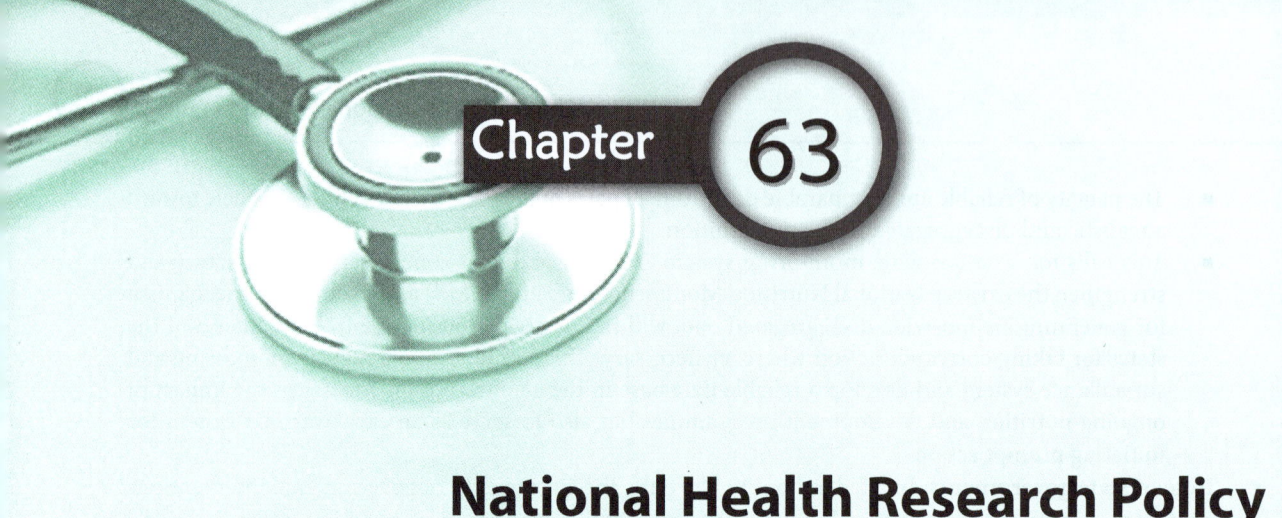

Chapter 63

National Health Research Policy

INTRODUCTION

The establishment of a Department of Health Research (DHR) in the Ministry of Health is recognition by the Government of India (GoI) about the key role that health research should play in the nation's development. The weakness of the publicly funded health structures and the research infrastructure is a key limiting factor in realizing the full benefits of this commitment to research. The fact that almost 300 medical colleges in the country are not contributing their best to health research is highlighted by the fact that in 2007, 96% of the research publications in India emanated from 9 medical colleges. Much of this published research is not on priority health concerns and the translational of key research findings into policy which could improve the health of the people is very limited and needs to be enhanced.

Epidemiological know-how, surveillance technology and diagnostic services which are essential for determining health priorities are very poorly developed. There is also a compelling need to build multidisciplinary research blending physical, medical and social sciences. Besides, there is also an equal urgency to establish regulations, strict ethical norms and transparency, standardize methodology and international standards of research. Such capacity is necessary for undertaking operational research as also large-scale evaluation of diagnostics and trials of drugs, devices of both modern and traditional systems of medicine. It is in this context that the DHR has formulated a draft National Health Research Policy.

VISION

To maximize the returns on investments in health research through creation of a health research system to prioritize, coordinate, facilitate conduct of effective and ethical health research and its translation into products, policies and programmes aimed at improving health especially of the vulnerable populations.

OBJECTIVES

The broad objectives of the national health research policy are:
- Identify priorities for effective and ethical health research to enable the achievement of the objectives of NHP 2002, NRHM, Bharat Nirman and National Food Security Act as well as global commitments such as MDG and IHR, ensuring that the results of health research are translated into action.
- Foster inter-sectoral coordination in health research including all departments within the government, private sector and the academia to promote innovation and ensure effective translation

to encourage/accelerate indigenous production of diagnostics, vaccines, therapeutics, medical devices, etc.
- Focus on the marginalized, the vulnerable and the disadvantaged sections of society.
- Strengthen national networks between research institutes, academia and service institutes, and encourage public private partnership (PPP).
- Put in place strategies and mechanisms for assessing the cost effectiveness and cost benefits of interventions for health.
- Develop and manage human resources and infrastructure for health research and ensure that international collaborative research contributes to national health.

PRESCRIPTION OF THE NATIONAL HEALTH RESEARCH POLICY

- Create a National Health Research System
- Establish a National Health Research Management Forum
- Operationalize a 10-point action programme.

National Health Research System (NHRS)

In order to achieve intersectoral coordination and to make national priorities for health research, a new architecture of national health research system is envisaged. Health research system is a concept that integrates and coordinates the objectives, structures, stakeholders, processes, cultures and outcomes of health research towards development of equity in health and in national health system. It is a system for planning, coordinating, monitoring and managing health research resources and activities, and for promoting research for effective and equitable national health development. Health Research in the country would be developed into a NHRS wherein all research agencies, cutting across Ministries and sectors identify priority areas of research and coordinate with each other to avoid duplication, fragmentation, redundancy and gaps in knowledge, in order to enable the results of research to transform health as a major driving force for development.

Goals

- To generate and communicate knowledge that helps to form the national health plan and guides its implementation, and thus contribute, directly or indirectly, to equitable health development in the country.
- To adapt and apply knowledge generated elsewhere to national health development; and
- To contribute to the global knowledge base on issues relevant to the country.

Functions

The national health research system would be responsible for:
- **Developing national health research plan:** The DHR is responsible for the National Health Research Plan for a National Plan aligned with the Five-Year Plans of GoI and its implementation and monitoring.
- **Set priorities:** A priority research agenda will be developed in tune with the national programmes, and relevant to national and local needs.
- **Engage with private sector:** The private sector, pharmaceutical industry, biotechnology and biomedical technology oriented industries, private educational institutions, hospitals and nursing homes, research foundations and institutions, private practitioners, NGO's and CBO's working on a not-for-profit basis etc. are now major stakeholders in health care research and delivery. The national health research system would recognize their important role in health research and shall foster their participation in the system as partners. These engagements have to be concurrent and intense rather than linear and loose.

- **Strengthen international linkages:** In the current global scenario, International collaborative efforts are recognized as one of the factors in successful research because of the complementarity of technology transfer, capacity building and access to diseased populations. There are a large number of potential partners and in the choice of partners the priorities of the NHRP and national interest shall be paramount. Linkages with International developmental partners and WHO and other UN agencies shall be further developed and strengthened to ensure that India plays a legitimate role as an emerging economy.
- **Ensure ethical research:** The Bill on Research on Human Subjects and establishment of the National Biomedical Research Authority therein along with the guidelines developed by other agencies shall regulate all research. The health research system shall review these guidelines from time to time, and harmonize them with International guidelines. Facilitation of training in ethical research shall be the responsibility of the DHR. A major achievement has been the establishment of a National Clinical Trial Registry and all clinical trials are mandated to be registered by the DCGI.
- **Ensure targeted financing:** The National Health Research System shall be responsible for ensuring equity in resource mobilization and allocation of public funds. It shall endeavor to ensure that the allocation/expenditure on health research is at least 2% of the allocation/expenditure on health. International funds will also be mobilized in keeping with the priorities. The NHRS would track the resources available and spent on research in the country and monitor its impact on health. Though a minimum of 2% of health expenditure has been achieved, this may be too small a figure considering that the allocation for health itself is meagre in relation to the population and health concerns of the country.
- **Monitor and evaluate impact of health research:** To ensure that resources are used efficiently and in line with agreed priorities there is a need for continuous monitoring and evaluation. The health research system will develop explicit policies and procedures for reviewing proposals, and for monitoring and evaluating the output and impact of those that are funded. Indicators will be developed to monitor the development and effectiveness of the health research system. Indicators would also be defined for assessing health status, health system effectiveness, efficiency and affordability, in order to capture the contribution of research in reducing inequities. Direct indicators of national development, would serve as indirect indicators of the efficacy of health system research as a vehicle of development. Set mechanisms to ensure that best practices are encouraged, and practices are evidence-based.
- **Partnership with state health system:** Encourage health research within states. Help set state level health research system by strengthening partnership between central and state systems.
- **Assess health research system:** The health research system would need to be assessed periodically to provide evidence that it is functioning optimally. The NHRS shall be managed by a National Health Research Management Forum (NHRMF).

The National Health Research Management Forum (NHRMF)

The National Health Research Policy envisages a system wherein all present and prospective players have their own space. However, an overarching National Health Research Management Forum is proposed, having representation of all key stakeholders, the DHR as its secretariat, and the following functions/ terms of reference:

- To advise on and evolve national health research policies and priorities and to evolve mechanisms and action plans for their implementation.
- To develop a five year projection of the plans for health research and to prepare an annual National health research plan.
- To do a mid-plan appraisal for course correction, as needed.

- To promote the development of health research activities in the country.
- To review biomedical and health research management, and suggest strategies to overcome problems in implementation of policies.
- To suggest mechanisms to nurture a scientific environment to attract talent and to develop human resources for biomedical and health research.
- To facilitate utilization and dissemination of research results and advocacy for health research.

Structure

The NHRMF will be chaired by the Minister of Health and Family Welfare and co-chaired by Minister of Science and Technology. The Minister(s) of State for Health would be the Vice-chairperson(s). The Secretariat shall be in the DHR and its secretary shall be the Member-Secretary. All secretaries of various departments in S and T would be the members, DGHS and 8–10 eminent scientists/ public health experts (numbers flexible) as well as selected representatives from State Governments would be the other members. These experts would also be the Chairmen of the various working groups which would be constituted to address the following areas:

- Development and evaluation of interventions for promotion, restoration, maintenance and protection of health.
- Human resource management and infrastructure development.
- Knowledge management.
- Encouragement to translational research and originality in basic science research, and innovations.
- Optimizing intra- and intersectoral networks, coordination and collaboration especially with private sector and industry.
- Track current resource flow and future requirements to address priority areas of health research.
- Establishment of priorities for health research.
- Implementation of health research policy, planning, monitoring and evaluation.

Responsibilities

Stewardship

- This would encompass a range of activities for the national health system intended to ensure quality leadership, productivity, strategic direction and coherent action.
- Sub-functions would include strategic vision, policy formulation, priority setting, performance and impact assessment promotion and advocacy, and the setting of norms, standards and frameworks for the sound practice of research.
- Provide best practices for research management.

Financing

- The essential functions of the system as regards, finances would be to address issues related to resource generation, targeted allocation and judicious utilization.
- On the basis of recommendations of the National Health Research Management Forum, funds would be allocated in ways that are consistent with national priorities.
- External partners would be apprised of these priorities, while a national capability to monitor where and how research funds are being spent, and the quantities involved, would be created and put in place. Ensure that funds are spent where the burden of disease is.

- Efforts would be made to invest at least 2% of national health expenditure in research and research capacity strengthening.

Knowledge Generation

The research system would generate knowledge relevant to the Indian health situation, appraise the measures available for dealing with health problems, and suggest the actions likely to produce the greatest improvement in health.

Utilization and Management of Knowledge

- The research system fully endorses the principle that the research process does not end with knowledge generation, but includes the translation of results into policy or action, or absorption into the existing knowledge/technology base. For this to happen, links will be strengthened between researchers, policy makers, health and development workers, nongovernmental organizations, communities, and media.
- Vertical and horizontal connectedness will be improved upon. More specifically, for better utilization and management of knowledge, an information culture would be fostered, supported by enhanced use of information technologies currently and likely to be available.
- A synergy with knowledge management policy would be made.

Capacity Development

- A long-term approach to the development and maintenance of research capacity will be adopted. Efforts will be focused on both the quantity and quality of skills available/needed, including research techniques, research priority setting, research management, use of research (demand, side), policy and systems analysis, communications, development of partnerships including medical colleges and rural health research centers.
- A situation analysis done periodically would ensure a phased and realistic plan for constructive and sustained capacity development. Thus, both the 'Supply' and 'Demand' sides of the research system needs will be addressed. Encourage policy research.

Operationalization of 10-point Action Programme

The 10-point action programme:

- Harmonize optimally national policies in a variety of areas (education, social sciences, population, agriculture, nutrition, science, etc.) to facilitate intersectoral collaboration and partnership, so that maximum developmental returns can occur from health research.
- Ensure true inter-sectorality of health research and harness the resources in areas such as social sciences, economics and traditional systems of medicine.
- Facilitate priority setting to guide the direction of health research and prepare Five-Year Plan and strategy documents.
- Encourage the development of fundamental and basic research in areas relevant to health to ensure that a national critical mass of scientists who can contribute the benefits of modern technology to health research is created.
- Foster translational research to ensure that the products of basic research can be appropriately utilized in health systems and services.
- Establish linkages between health research and national health programmes to identify key operational issues and facilitate the operationalization of evidence-based programmes and to obtain feedback for the optimization of health research.

- Build and integrate capacity for research in national health programmes, research institutions and in the private sector (profit and non-profit organizations) both in rural and urban research settings utilizing as far as possible areas of excellence already available in the country.
- Ensure that the global knowledge base is available for national programmes, and that research is channeled in relevant directions without unnecessary duplication by the optimal use of information, communication and networking technology.
- Manage global resources and transnational collaborations optimally to ensure that collaborative health research primarily facilitates the development of national health systems and services.
- Generate the evidence-based health systems and services, to be significant promoters of equity and contribute to national development so that health research becomes a poverty reduction tool.

Achievement

- The policy is under the consideration of the government for approval.
- Action has been initiated for setting up of necessary infrastructure for implementation.

Chapter 64

National Vaccine Policy

INTRODUCTION

In this backdrop, as a part of the broader national health policy, a national vaccine policy is needed, based on the principles of public health and comprehensive primary health care. This is to enable rational and evidence-based decisions for the development, entry, production, stable supply, pricing, promotion and use of appropriate vaccines on scientific grounds. Additionally, this is also needed to protect the national vaccine programmes and national health security, as well as to leverage indigenous capabilities to cater the domestic and overseas markets.

OBJECTIVES

- To contribute in the prevention of mortality and morbidity due to communicable diseases that affect large populations, especially children through the development/production and use of safe, effective and affordable vaccines, chosen rationally.
- To ensure consistent delivery and administration of vaccines to everyone in need.
- To achieve national self-reliance in vaccine R and D, as well as to maximize the national benefits of international sharing of indigenous biological diversity of pathogens, hosts and knowledge, to the Indian end-users of vaccines on terms that are fair and just.
- To achieve pre-eminence in the capabilities of the indigenous public sector for self-reliance and foster a leading role for them in all the aspects of vaccine development, production and immunization for national health security and biosecurity.
- To develop and use the interdisciplinary knowledge base needed for science-based policy and evidence-based medicine in the field of vaccines.
- To promote ethical conduct in the development, trials, adoption and administration of vaccines, especially aimed at children and pregnant women.
- To develop a system for monitoring and compensating adverse events following vaccination where required.
- To enable India to play a leading role in the supply of affordable vaccines to the emerging world, considering the declining interest of the multinational sector to make cost-effective vaccines for the emerging world.
- To synergize all other relevant policies for effective implementation of the national vaccine policy to fulfill the above objectives.

GUIDING PRINCIPLES, CONTEXT AND APPROACH

- A vaccine is just one among the many inputs needed for effective public health management of communicable diseases. Other measures like food security, safe drinking water, sanitation, primary education, gender sensitivity, and health education are known to be the most important factors in the control of communicable diseases. Even all the known vaccines put together cannot prevent all deaths due to the communicable diseases. However, amongst medicines, rationally selected vaccines are the most cost-effective in reducing morbidity and mortality and have an important role to play as a public health measure in the control of some communicable diseases.

- Most of the indigenous capabilities and strengths in this area were pioneered or sustained by the public sector. Strengthening the role of the public sector in the area of vaccines is crucial to ensure self-reliance and to protect national health security from the uncertainties of the local and global market forces, as well as from bio-terrorism and biological warfare.

- Vaccination should be need-based and all vaccines are deemed non-universal, unless specified otherwise based on scientific evidence. While therapeutic vaccines and antisera are administered only to patients diagnosed with a treatable condition (e.g., Tetanus, diphtheria, anti-snake and anti-rabies), preventive vaccines are generally administered to largely 'normal' populations and therefore need stronger medical and economic rationale. Even the so-called 'Universal' vaccines are universal only for the children and pregnant women. Most adult vaccines are not required for all the adults, and are often used for 'selective' immunization of high-risk groups.

- The mere availability of a safe and efficacious or even affordable vaccine cannot be good enough justification for its widespread use. Vaccines are not consumer goods and should not be given or taken, unless their necessity is proven based on the scientific principles of public health. As vaccines are given to a healthy population, their safety and efficacy should be thoroughly assessed based on various scientific parameters, before any vaccine is introduced into the national programme.

- Vaccines outside the UIP should not be unethically promoted through direct or surrogate advertising, advocacy by individuals, groups or aid agencies, on their own or funded directly or indirectly by the vaccine industry.

- The choice of which vaccine to give (or not to give), target population, and mode of administration (dosage, schedule, interval between doses, intramuscular or intradermal, etc.), are important policy decisions that must be guided by a strong scientific rationale, with rigorous inputs from multicentric field epidemiology, irrespective of whether it has been proven in populations abroad. Cost-benefit as well as risk-benefit assessment should be carried out in India taking into account local serotypes and variations in indigenous host-pathogen-environment interactions. These studies can be best done by one or more public sector institutions and the results be made available openly on the website of the concerned agency for wider peer review and public debate. The dosage and schedule should also be decided after wider scientific debate in the country.

- Vaccine choice, source of procurement and the quality standards of the products as well as of the production system should be based on sound principles to achieve maximum benefit to maximum number of people and are independent decisions of the national government guided by this national policy (not imposed by industry and international organizations). At the same time, it should be the endeavor of this policy to develop all the requisite indigenous capabilities in line with the evolving global standards, without compromising the national health security or self-reliance.

- Technological advances in vaccines, especially for mass immunization, have to be measured in terms of their improvements in efficacy, long-term protection, safety, and cost-competitiveness stability during storage and transport, and method of administration. Technological superiority of vaccine should not be assumed solely in terms of purity, sophisticated methods of production, combinations or other incremental innovations aimed at extension of intellectual property and commercial monopoly.

- Combination vaccines are convenient but useful and acceptable only when universal and nonuniversal vaccines are not combined, whether for public or private use. In any case, the safety and efficacy of every combination vaccine has to be freshly established in the target population and cannot be extrapolated from the safety and efficacy of its individual components. Cocktail combination vaccines and genetically engineered multivalent vaccines must be differentiated clearly. In case of cocktail combinations, the price of the combination may not exceed the sum of its individual components.

- Clinical trials and bio-safety regulations in vaccines targeting children and pregnant women pose special ethical concerns, due to the inability of fetuses and infants to decide for themselves, even if the parents are assumed to take decisions in the best interest of their children. Such issues can become more critical when foreign entities conduct clinical trials on Indian children. Phase lag is necessary in such situations. In addition, unless absolutely necessary, vaccine trials in children should begin with grown up children and then move downwards. Suitable amendments may be introduced in the proposed National Biotechnology Authority Act to address these and other public health concerns.

- The Government shall evolve a suitable legislation enabling adverse vaccine reaction monitoring and compensation for injuries to any person(s) arising out of vaccinations in India, including for those in the trial phase. This should apply to all vaccines, whether provided by the Government, public sector or by the private manufacturers/practitioners. The legislation would be designed to fix responsibility and deliver compensation adequately and promptly in the event of injuries/adverse events due to vaccines and vaccination.

- Pricing of all vaccines should be brought under the Drug Price Control Order (DPCO) and subjected to regulation in accordance with the objectives of this policy. Pricing of vaccines should be done on a transparent basis and agreed principles of reasonable returns on investment, rates of royalty and costing of R and D efforts. There should be no overhead taxes imposed on vaccines such as excise duty, value added tax (VAT), customs duty, etc. The difference between maximum retail price (MRP) and the price at which vaccines are supplied to wholesalers, retailers, hospitals or even to doctors will also be minimized to deter monetary incentives for unethical vaccine promotions.

- International sharing of indigenous biological diversity of pathogens, hosts and knowledge should be governed by the legal principles of prior informed consent and benefits sharing agreements set in the National Biodiversity Act. The material transfer agreement should have a clause preventing the recipient from seeking or claiming intellectual property rights over any inventions derived from Indian biodiversity or indigenous knowledge. It should also have copyleft style clauses for open sharing of the research results to develop vaccines and other technologies to combat diseases. Prior informed consent to any overseas individual or entity should be subject to the condition that Indian scientists, technologists and public sector manufacturing entities will have automatic royalty-free rights to use all the further improvement in that knowledge and any technology, product or process that comes out of the shared biological resource or knowledge, or to license it further to indigenous private firms if deemed necessary. This maximizes the national benefits of international sharing to the Indian end users of vaccines.

- Publicly funded R and D on vaccine technologies should be made available widely on a nonexclusive basis to promote manufacture of quality vaccines at competitive prices. Research papers emerging out of publicly funded R and D should also be made available freely through an open access policy. In all publicly funded vaccine research and development programmes, affordable access to vaccine technologies and the crucial role of the public sector manufacture for national programmes should be given priority over all IPR issues and other technology transfer considerations. Further, knowledge commons approach to R and D and other measures that enhance access to vaccine technologies identified under the National Vaccine Policy should be promoted.

- The above principles and public health concerns of the nation will have an overriding priority over any multilateral, bilateral or regional trade agreements.

POLICY MEASURES

- The success of vaccination or any other public health programme depends heavily on the disease surveillance and monitoring system in the country. Ideally, such a system should contain frequently collected information on the incidence and prevalence of diseases in the population, local variations in the pathogens including serotypes, resistance to drugs/antibiotics if any, host response to vaccination, efficacy and duration of protection, etc. These data form the basis for all decisions regarding whether to adopt vaccination as a strategy and if so, whether universal or selective and for how long. In order to augment the present mechanisms available for disease surveillance and monitoring as well as vaccination, the Panchayati Raj institutions should be strengthened, and training imparted to the Health Management Information System (HMIS), Integrated Disease Surveillance Project (IDSP), Accredited Social Health Activist (ASHA), Auxiliary Nurse Midwife (ANM) and health workers.

- To ensure selection of appropriate vaccines on scientific grounds, for the Universal Immunization programme, well-defined criteria of cost-efficacy and logistical feasibility, appropriateness should be formed based on the science of public health. A committee should do this selection after a broad-based debate amongst the concerned public health experts. No new vaccine should be introduced into the UIP unless adequate and sustained resources/efforts have been devoted to achieve universal coverage of the existing vaccines. The lure of external aid/loan cannot be a sufficient ground for introduction of new vaccines under UIP.

- In order to ensure stable and affordable supply of vaccines to the national immunization programme and also to address national health security and biosecurity concerns, all essential vaccines covered under UIP (TT, DT, DTP, BCG, Polio, and Measles) must continue to be produced by the public sector. Further, the presence of at least two functional PSUs per vaccine (as a backup for each other) must be ensured as a protection against market uncertainties.

- For patented vaccines and other interventions needed for public health, the government should take all necessary law and policy measures including government use and compulsory license provisions to ensure timely availability of vaccines at an affordable cost. For off-patented vaccines, suitable law and policy measures should be taken to promote competition by providing incentives to generic manufacturers.

- All the vaccine PSUs must be urgently revived and modernized to fill the demand-supply gaps in all essential vaccines and anti-sera, including the UIP vaccines. The Government purchase orders for safe and effective vaccines available from PSUs must not be diverted to the private sector under any pretext. For example, the recent introduction of a pentavalent vaccine (that combines DTP with Hepatitis B and Influenza Type B) into the UIP14 effectively diverts all the DTP purchase order from PSUs to private entities, as the PSUs do not manufacture them so far. Besides, the merits of universal vaccination against Hepatitis B and Influenza Type B are highly debatable.

- Various vaccine PSUs are currently under different managerial regimes—State and Central Governments, and even within the Central Government, under Ministry of Health and Family Welfare (MoHFW), Department of Biotechnology (DBT) and National Dairy Development Board (NDDB). In order to enhance functional coordination between them to meet the national vaccine needs, their governing bodies should be expanded to include public health experts, epidemiologists, microbiologists, immunologists, vaccine policy experts, pharmacologists, economists, sociologists and other interdisciplinary experts and non-governmental organizations (NGOs).

- The current National Technical Advisory Group on Immunization (NTAGI) should be restructured into a Central National Vaccine Regulatory Authority (NVRA) that allows wider representation to indigenous scientists, policy experts and indigenous public sector and civil society. Apart from invited membership, provision should also be made for voluntary participation of representatives from any non-commercial organization. This authority would be empowered to take all major decisions such as monitoring disease burden, vaccine development, adoption, production, procurement, distribution, immunization and follow-up.
- Indigenous vaccine R and D and production capacities must be strengthened to ensure a stable and affordable supply of all essential vaccines, especially the UIP vaccines. For this purpose, the core strengths of the vaccine PSUs must be preserved and nurtured with higher functional autonomy (at least at par with the Navratnas), incentives to attract interdisciplinary talent for R and D and production.
- Enhanced public funding and programme support for R and D into communicable diseases, especially neglected diseases and vaccine-preventable diseases.
- Further strengthening the integrated disease surveillance programme, critical appraisal of literature should be undertaken while considering new vaccine adoption in UI or SI decisions. Limited data on the actual prevalence of a disease may overestimate the actual disease burden. Large multicenter and community-based studies should confirm the real burden of any particular disease in the country.
- Improved logistics and supply chain system, including maintenance of cold-chain during periods of heavy load shedding, especially in rural areas. Emphasis on the outreach of vaccination programmes to remote areas and the marginalized populations, tribals, etc. Promotion of awareness and trust building in communities through various measures to ensure full vaccination coverage.
- Regulation of advertisements and other promotional marketing activities to prevent unethical means and kickbacks to doctors. Literature should not be cited selectively to base decisions. The role of the industry as the educators of the professionals, policy makers and people must be discouraged. Direct-to-consumer promotional advertisements on upcoming vaccines (e.g., rotavirus, HPV, Chickenpox, etc.) with incomplete and biased information must be banned.
- Government procurement of vaccines under UIP must be based on price and opportunity parity, and no PSU should be excluded from government vaccine procurement, as long as the product quality and affordable price are ensured. Similarly, no PSUs should be excluded from producing any vaccine, as long as it stakes a credible claim to manufacture it in compliance with all the regulatory and quality norms at competitive prices. The Government may make advance market commitments with vaccine PSUs subject to quality parameters, but not with any other private or foreign entity to the detriment of the vaccine PSU. No private firm should be paid higher prices than their PSU counterparts supplying to UIP. The whole process should be made transparent.
- Any private sector unit that wishes to produce new (non-UIP) or combination vaccines must produce some UIP vaccines (individually and not as combinations) to fill any shortfalls in PSU production and Government procurement.
- A critical review of the current UIP vaccines and new vaccines may be undertaken by the NVRA. Any new vaccine introduction in UIP must be qualified before its introduction for universal or selective immunization, based on epidemiological evidence, suitability and efficacy to the local pathogens and human populations, risk-benefit and cost-benefit analyses.

- Similarly, a critical review of the combination of UIP and non-UIP vaccines must be carried out in view of the stated policy objectives. Combining any UIP vaccine with any non-UIP vaccine needs rigorous scrutiny and public debate. Other combinations must be proven to be equivalent to or more effective and safer than single vaccines before adoption. In any case, cocktail combinations and multivalent vaccines must be clearly differentiated.

- The Government of India is solely responsible for the compliance of its PSUs for Good Manufacturing Practice (GMP) and all other regulatory norms, as well as to prevent stoppage of production on such counts. Therefore, the Government of India must provide all the necessary administrative and financial support for PSU compliance with GMP and all other regulations. The governing bodies and other technical committees of PSUs must be expanded to enable expert monitoring/advice from vaccine policy and public health experts, apart from scientists/technologists of relevance. Representatives from private vaccine manufacturers and industry-funded medical associations/academies must be specifically prohibited to prevent conflicts of interest.

- In order to make the essential vaccines more affordable to the indigenous end-consumers, measures such as tax concessions/exemptions may be considered.

- Rejuvenation of the existing institutions of research, education and training of public health workers. The NVRI will identify such aspects relevant to India and coordinate with existing agencies like Indian Council of Medical Research (ICMR), DBT, Council of Scientific and Industrial Research (CSIR) etc.

- Promotion of health systems research to formulate optimized health systems that can deliver vaccines efficiently and effectively.

- Strengthening of basic infrastructure and manpower in Primary Healthcare Centers (PHC) and ancillary programmes such as ICDS and the ASHA network, with emphasis on name-based tracking of individual children and women, ensuring planned fixed-day immunization sessions, reporting based on correct denominators and frequent decentralized monitoring of coverage independent of service reports are keystones of successful coverage. In addition, the regular audit of vaccine utilization is essential. Currently, all these are not subject to regular and independent scrutiny, and can be brought under the ambit of NVRA. A prevailing concern has been the tendency of immunization programmes to operate independently of other primary health care programmes. Maintaining this balance will be critical to the success of both, the UIP and the other PHC programmes.

- Increase in budgetary allocations for investment in proven cost-effective programmes.

- Private vaccine markets and also their use in private clinics should be regulated through a mechanism to be brought under NVRA supervision.

- A thorough and transparent review of all Public Private Partnerships (PPP) in vaccine development, production and delivery is needed, including the upcoming vaccine park at Chengalpattu. All measures should be taken to ensure that PPPs do not amount to public spending and private profiteering. The public private partnerships for developing and manufacturing new vaccines may be beneficial only when the state of art for making vaccines remains with public sector, while private sector is made to meet vaccines that are needed.

Chapter 65

National Population Policy

INTRODUCTION

The National Population Policy (NPP) finally came into force in 2000.

The policy states that the "immediate objective of the NPP 2000 is to address the unmet needs for contraception, health care infrastructure, and health personnel, and to provide integrated service delivery for basic reproductive and child health care. The medium-term objective is to bring the total fertility rate (TFR) to replacement levels by the year 2010, through vigorous implementation of intersectoral operational strategies. The long-term objective of the policy is to achieve a stable population by 2045, at a level consistent with the requirements of sustainable economic growth, social development, and environmental protection."

GOALS FOR 2010

The NPP listed the following goals for 2010:

- Address the unmet needs for basic reproductive and child health services, supplies, and infrastructure.
- Make school education up to age 14 free and compulsory, and reduce dropouts at the primary and secondary school levels to below 20% for both boys and girls.
- Reduce the infant mortality rate to below 30 per 1,000 live births.
- Reduce the maternal mortality ratio to below 100 per 100,000 live births.
- Achieve universal immunization of children against all vaccine preventable diseases.
- Promote delayed marriage for girls, not earlier than age 18 and preferably after 20 years of age.
- Achieve 80% institutional deliveries and 100% deliveries by trained persons.
- Achieve universal access to information/counseling, and services for fertility regulation and contraception with a wide basket of choices.
- Achieve 100% registration of births, deaths, marriages, and pregnancy.
- Contain the spread of the acquired immunodeficiency syndrome (AIDS) and promote greater integration between the management of reproductive tract infections (RTIs) and sexually transmitted infections (STIs) and the national AIDS control organization.
- Prevent and control communicable diseases.
- Integrate Indian Systems of Medicine (ISM) in the provision of reproductive and child health services, and in reaching out to households.

- Promote vigorously the small family norm to achieve replacement levels of TFR. Bring about convergence in implementation of related social-sector programmes so that family welfare becomes a people-centered programme.

The NPP 2000 anticipates that proper implementation of this policy will help limit the population to 1,107 million (110 crores) in 2010, instead of 1,162 million (116 crores) as projected by the technical group on population projections. It is hoped that the TFR will reach the replacement level of 2.1 by 2010.

The long-term objective of achieving a stable population by 2045, at a level consistent with the requirements of sustainable economic growth, social development, and environment protection will also require considerable effort and efficient implementation of the NPP.

As the existing NPP-2000 is uniformly applicable to all irrespective of religions and communities, etc., therefore, no proposal is under consideration of the government to formulate new uniform population policy. The steps taken by the government under various measures/programme are as follows:

STEPS/MEASURES TO CONTROL THE POPULATION GROWTH OF INDIA BY THE GOVERNMENT OF INDIA

On-Going Interventions

- More emphasis on spacing methods like IUCD.
- Availability of fixed day static services at all facilities.
- A rational human resource development plan is in place for provision of IUCD, minilap and NSV to empower the facilities (DH, CHC, PHC, SHC) with at least one provider each for each of the services and sub-centers with ANMs trained in IUD insertion.
- Quality care in family planning services by establishing quality assurance committees at state and district levels.
- Improving contraceptives supply management up to peripheral facilities.
- Demand generation activities in the form of display of posters, billboards and other audio and video materials in the various facilities.
- National Family Planning Indemnity Scheme (NFPIS) under which clients are insured in the eventualities of deaths, complications and failures following sterilization and the providers/ accredited institutions are indemnified against litigations in those eventualities.
- Compensation scheme for sterilization acceptors—under the scheme, MoHFW provides compensation for loss of wages to the beneficiary and also to the service provider (and team) for conducting sterilizations.
- Increasing male participation and promotion of non-scalpel vasectomy
- Emphasis on minilap tubectomy services because of its logistical simplicity and requirement of only MBBS doctors and not postgraduate gynecologists/surgeons.
- Accreditation of more private/NGO facilities to increase the provider base for family planning services under PPP.
- Strong political will and advocacy at the highest level, especially, in states with high fertility rates.

New Interventions under Family Planning Programme

- **Scheme for home delivery of contraceptives by ASHAs at doorstep of beneficiaries:** The government has launched a scheme to utilize the services of ASHA to deliver contraceptives at the doorstep of beneficiaries.

- **Scheme for ASHAs to ensure spacing in births:** The scheme is operational from 16th May, 2012, under this scheme, services of ASHAs to be utilized for counseling newly married couples to ensure delay of 2 years in birth after marriage and couples with 1 child to have spacing of 3 years after the birth of 1st child. ASHAs are to be paid the following incentives under the scheme:
  - ₹500/- to ASHA for ensuring spacing of 2 years after marriage.
  - ₹500/- to ASHA for ensuring spacing of 3 years after the birth of 1st child.
  - ₹1000/- in case the couple opts for a permanent limiting method up to 2 children only. The scheme is being implemented in 18 States of the country (8 EAG, 8 NE, Gujarat and Haryana).
- Boost to spacing methods by introduction of new method Post-Partum Intra Uterine Contraceptives Device (PPIUCD).
- Introduction of the new device Cu IUCD 375, which is effective for 5 years.
- Emphasis on Post-Partum Family Planning (PPFP) services with introduction of PPIUCD and promotion of minilap as the main mode of providing sterilization in the form of post-partum sterilization to capitalize on the huge cases coming in for institutional delivery under JSY.
  - Assured delivery of family planning services for both IUCD and sterilization.
- Compensation for sterilization acceptors has been enhanced for 11 High Focus States with high TFR.
- Compensation scheme for PPIUCD under which the service provider as well as the ASHAs who escorts the clients to the health facility for facilitating the IUCD insertion are compensated.
- Scheme for provision of pregnancy testing kits at the sub-centers as well as in the drug kit of the ASHAs for use in the communities to facilitate the early detection and decision making for the outcome of pregnancy.
- RMNCH Counselors (Reproductive Maternal Newborn and Child Health) availability at the high case facilities to ensure counseling of the clients visiting the facilities.
- **Celebration of World Population Day 11th July and fortnight:** The event is observed over a month long period, split into fortnight of mobilization/sensitization followed by a fortnight of assured family planning service delivery and has been made a mandatory activity from 2012–13 and starts from 27th June each year.
- **FP 2020—Family Planning Division** is working on the national and state wise action plans so as to achieve FP 2020 goals. The key commitments of FP 2020 are as under:
  - Increasing financial commitment on family planning whereby India commits an allocation of 2 billion USD from 2012–2020.
  - Ensuring access to family planning services to 48 million (4.8 crore) additional women by 2020 (40% of the total FP 2020 goal).
  - Sustaining the coverage of 100 million (10 crore) women currently using contraceptives.

Reducing the unmet need by an improved access to voluntary family planning services, supplies and information. In addition to above, Jansankhya Sthirata Kosh/National Population Stabilization Fund has adopted the following strategies as population control measures:

- **Prerna strategy:** JSK has launched this strategy for helping to push up the age of marriage of girls and delay in first child and spacing in between the birth of two children in the interest of health of young mothers and infants. The couple who adopt this strategy is awarded suitably. This helps to change the mindsets of the community.
- **Santushti strategy:** Under this strategy, Jansankhya sthirata kosh invites private sector gynecologists and vasectomy surgeons to conduct sterilization operations in public private partnership mode. The private hospitals/nursing homes who achieved target to 10 or more are suitably awarded as per strategy.

- **National helpline:** JSK is also running a call center for providing free advice on reproductive health, family planning, maternal health and child health, etc. Toll free no. is 1800116555.
- **Advocacy and IEC activities:** JSK as a part of its awareness and advocacy efforts on population stabilization, has established networks and partnerships with other ministries, development partners, private sectors, corporate and professional bodies for spreading its activities through electronic media, print media, workshop, walkathon, and other multi-level activities, etc. at the national, state, district and block levels.

NEW STRUCTURES

The NPP 2000 is to be largely implemented and managed at panchayat and nagar palika levels, in coordination with the concerned State/Union Territory administrations. Accordingly, the specific situation in each state/UT must be kept in mind. This will require comprehensive and multisectoral coordination of planning and implementation between health and family welfare on one hand, along with schemes for education, nutrition, women and child development, safe drinking water, sanitation, rural roads, communications, transportation, housing, forestry development, environmental protection, and urban development. Accordingly, the following structures are recommended:

National Commission on Population

A National Commission on Population, presided over by the Prime Minister, will have the Chief Ministers of all States and UTs, and the Central Minister in charge of the Department of Family Welfare and other concerned Central Ministries and Departments, for example, Department of Woman and Child Development, Department of Education, Department of Social Justice and Empowerment in the Ministry of HRD, Ministry of Rural Development, Ministry of Environment and Forest, and others as necessary, and reputed demographers, public health professionals, and NGOs as members. This Commission will oversee and review implementation of policy. The Commission Secretariat will be provided by the Department of Family Welfare.

State/UT Commissions on Population

Each State and UT may consider having a State/UT Commission on Population, presided over by the Chief Minister, on the analogy of the National Commission, to likewise oversee and review implementation of the NPP 2000 in the State/UT.

Coordination Cell in the Planning Commission

The Planning Commission will have a coordination cell for intersectoral coordination between Ministries for enhancing performance, particularly in States/UTs needing special attention on account of adverse demographic and human development indicators.

Technology Mission in the Department of Family Welfare

To enhance performance, particularly in states with currently below average socio-demographic indices that need focused attention, a Technology Mission in the Department of Family Welfare will be established to provide technology support in respect of design and monitoring of projects and programmes for reproductive and child health, as well as for IEC campaigns.

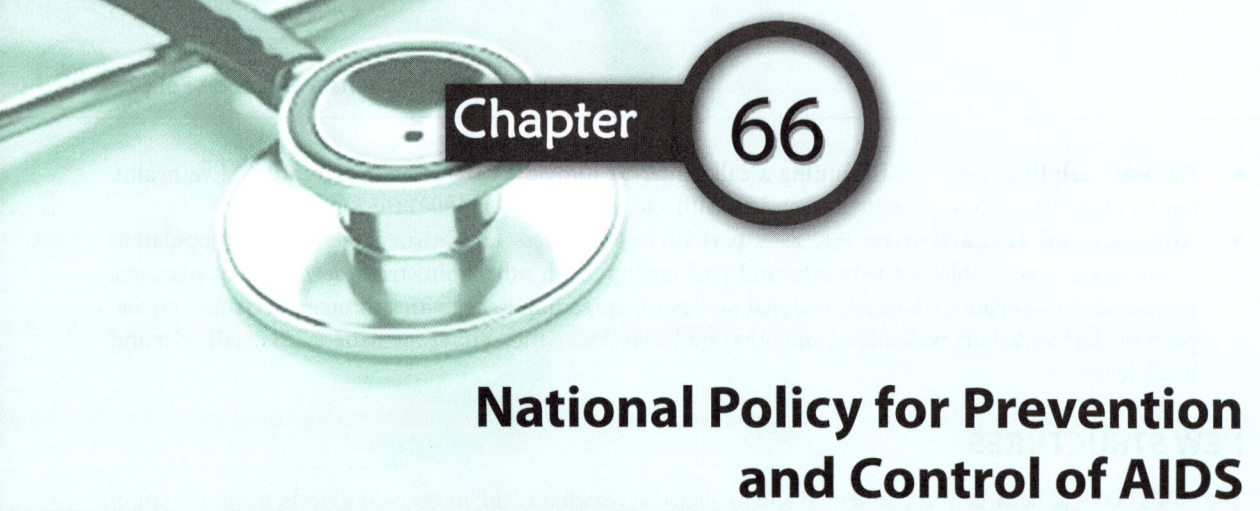

Chapter 66

National Policy for Prevention and Control of AIDS

INTRODUCTION

The inexorable spread of the disease from the initial epicenters to the rest of the country underscores the immediate need to have a paradigm shift in the response against HIV/AIDS at all levels making it imperative to formulate a comprehensive national policy on HIV/AIDS in order to cope effectively with the changed nature of the HIV/AIDS problem. The entire programme of prevention and control of HIV/AIDS needs to adopt a more holistic approach looking at AIDS as a developmental problem and not as a mere public health issue.

OBJECTIVES

The general objective of the policy is to prevent the epidemic from spreading further and to reduce the impact of the epidemic not only upon the infected persons but upon the health and socio-economic status of the general population at all levels. The policy envisages effective containment of the infection levels of HIV/AIDS in the general population in order to achieve zero-level of new infections by 2007.

The specific objectives of the policy are:
- To reiterate strongly the Government's firm commitment to prevent the spread of HIV infection and reduce personal and social impact.
- To generate a feeling of ownership among all the participants both at the Government and non-Government levels, like the Central Ministries and agencies of the Government of India, State Governments, city corporations, industrial undertakings in public and private sectors, panchayat institutions and local bodies to make it a truly national effort.
- To create an enabling socio-economic environment for prevention of HIV/AIDS, to provide care and support to people living with HIV/AIDS and to ensure protection/promotion of their human rights including right to access health care system, right to education, employment and privacy. To mobilize support of a large number of NGOs/Community-Based Organizations (CBOs) for an enlarged community initiative for prevention and alleviation of the HIV/AIDS problem.
- To decentralize HIV/AIDS control programme to the field level with adequate financial and administrative delegation of responsibilities.
- To strengthen programme management capabilities at the State Governments, municipal corporations, panchayat institutions and leading NGOs participating in the programme.

- To bring in horizontal integration at the implementation level with other national programmes like reproductive and child health, TB control, integrated child development scheme and with the primary health care system.
- To prevent women, children and other socially weak groups from becoming vulnerable to HIV infection by improving health education, legal status and economic prospects.
- To provide adequate and equitable provision of health care to the HIV-infected people and to draw attention to the compelling public health rationale for overcoming stigmatization, discrimination and seclusion in society.
- To constantly interact with international and bilateral agencies for support and cooperation in the field of research in vaccines, drugs, emerging systems of health care and other financial and managerial inputs.
- To ensure availability of adequate and safe blood and blood products for the general population through promotion of voluntary blood donation in the country.
- To promote better understanding of HIV infection among people, especially students, youth and other sexually active sections to generate greater awareness about the nature of its transmission and to adopt safe behavioral practices for prevention.

STRATEGY

The national AIDS control policy principally aims at the following strategy for prevention and control of the disease:

- Prevention of further spread of the disease by
  - Making the people aware of its implications and provide them with the necessary tools for protecting themselves.
  - Controlling STDs among vulnerable sections together with promotion of condom use as a preventive measure.
  - Ensuring availability of safe blood and blood products.
  - Reinforcing the traditional Indian moral values among youth and other impressionable groups of population.
- To create an enabling socio-economic environment so that all sections of population can protect themselves from the infection and families and communities can provide care and support to people living with HIV/AIDS.
- Improving services for the care of people living with AIDS in times of sickness both in hospitals and at homes through community health care.

POLICY INITIATIVES

One of the biggest lessons learnt globally as well as in the country is that national responses should not wait for HIV/AIDS cases to soar. Policies should not wait at a time when crucial prevention and care information and services are needed. HIV is particularly fueled by situations of injustice and poverty and its impact is felt beyond health sectors. Another important lesson learnt is that a multisectoral response must be designed in the context of the overall development strategy to ensure its sustainability and effectiveness. A substantial component of AIDS prevention and care relies on strong public health infrastructure in order to mount a more effective health sector response to AIDS. It includes early diagnosis and treatment of sexually transmitted infections using the syndromic approach, blood transfusion safety, epidemiological surveillance and research and a continuum of HIV/AIDS care linking health institutions, community and home. It can only be achieved if the programme is decentralized and owned up completely by States/UTs for implementation. NGO's and private sector have an equally critical role to play in an effective response. The challenge is to identify appropriate, locally relevant interventions and experienced community-based organizations to work with poor and marginalized populations who are particularly vulnerable to HIV infections. HIV/AIDS control programme, however, well planned and designed at the central level remains ineffective unless they reach out where people live, work, study and access health and other welfare services including information services.

For this purpose, the policy recognizes the following issues as critical for bringing in a paradigm shift in the response to HIV/AIDS at all levels both within and outside Government.

- Programme management
- Advocacy and social mobilization
- Participation of NGOs/CBOs
- Control of sexually transmitted diseases
- Use of condoms as a HIV/AIDS prevention measure
- HIV testing
- Counseling
- Care and support for people living with HIV/AIDS (PLWHAs)
- Surveillance
- HIV and injecting drug use
- Safety of blood and blood products
- Research and development
- Indigenous systems of medicine (ISM)
- Bilateral and international cooperation.

Government of India is fully committed to prevent the spread of HIV/AIDS at the initial stage itself before it emerges into a catastrophic epidemic. Government of India looks at HIV/AIDS prevention and control as a developmental issue with deep socio-economic implications. It touches all sections of the population, both infected and affected, irrespective of their regional, economic or social status. By following a concerted policy and an action plan that emerges out of it, Government hopes to control the epidemic and slow down its spread in the general population within the shortest possible time. All participating agencies in the Governmental and non-Governmental sectors, international and bilateral agencies, would need to adopt policies and programmes in conformity with this national policy in their effort to prevent and control HIV/AIDS in India.

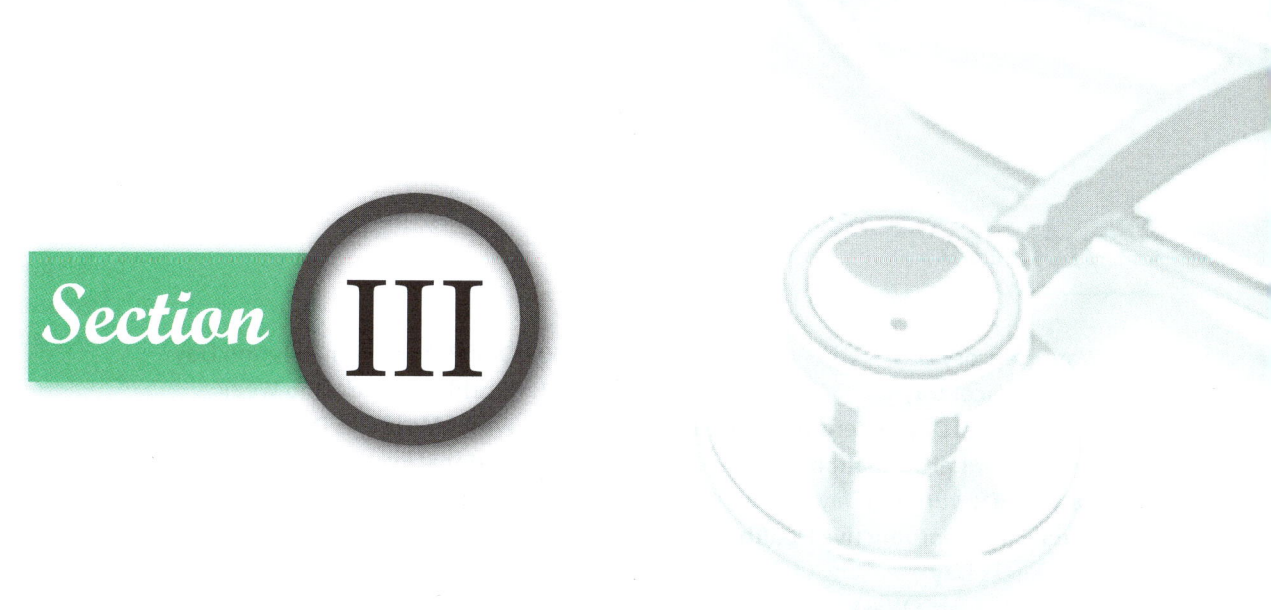

Section III

NATIONAL HEALTH DAYS

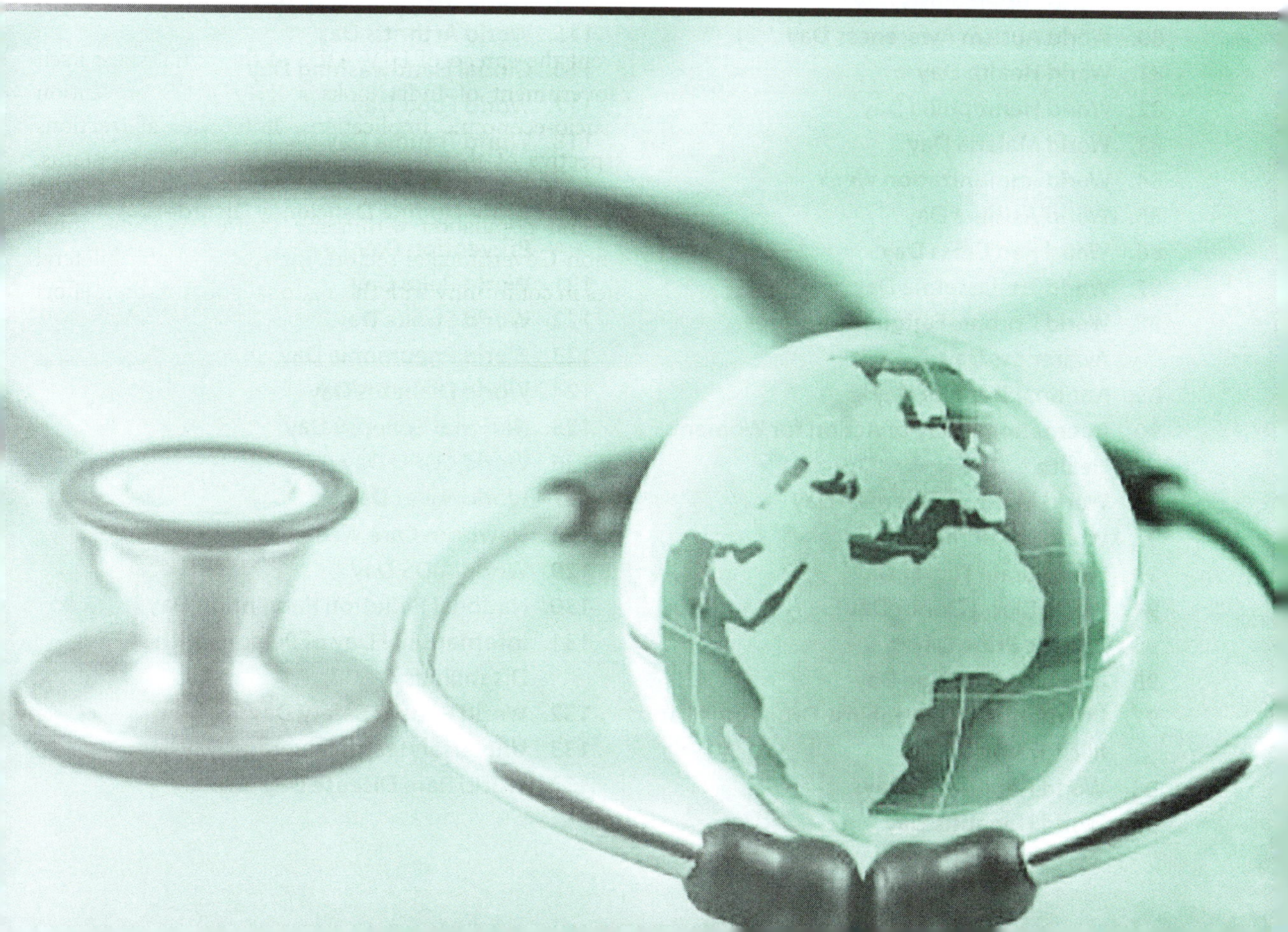

Contents

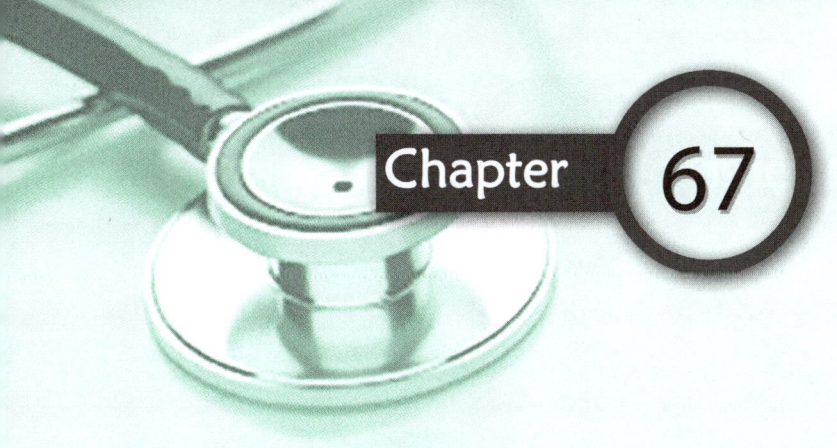

Chapter 67

World Leprosy Day

INTRODUCTION

World Leprosy Eradication Day is observed every year on last Sunday of January.

The aim of the day is to create awareness about leprosy, to help people living with the disease and to educate other people who take care of people suffering from this disease.

OBJECTIVES OF CELEBRATING ANTILEPROSY DAY

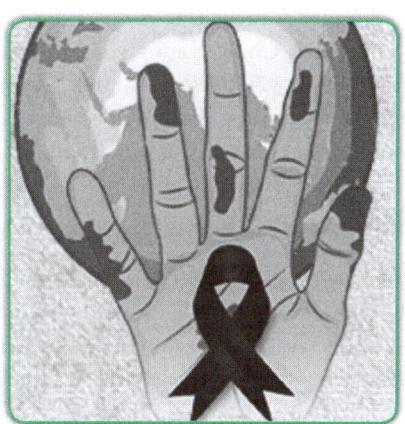

- To raise the leprosy awareness among people.
- To offer help to those affected by the disease through the regular and free of cost treatment they need.
- To make the diseased person psychologically strong and help them to cope up with physical impairments of skin sores and nerve damage.
- To ascertain that all affected persons are getting the necessary treatment, rehabilitation and care or not.
- To estimate the marked decrease or increase in the rate of spreading disease.

This is the day when people around the world stand in support of those suffering from the disease and raise funds for helping out people living with leprosy. Leprosy is a chronic infectious disease caused by *Mycobacterium leprae* which results in severe disfiguring skin sores and nerve damage in the arms and legs.

It is also known as Hansen's disease (named after Dr Armauer Hansen, who discovered the bacteria).

The disease has been around since ancient times, often surrounded by terrifying, negative stigmas and tales of leprosy patients being treated as outcasts.

Chapter 68

World Cancer Day

INTRODUCTION

World Cancer Day is observed every year on 4th February. World Cancer Day was established by the **Paris Charter** adopted at the **World Summit against Cancer for the New Millennium in Paris on 4th February 2000**. This Charter aimed at the promotion of the research for curing as well as preventing the disease, upgrading the provided services to the patients, the sensitization of the common opinion and the mobilization of the global community against cancer.

AIM

The aim to observe World Cancer Day is to reduce misconceptions about cancer and to help people in getting the right information about it. It also offers a chance to make an impact on the patients' lives.

This day aims to raise awareness regarding cancer and focuses upon the need of early detection and treatment of cancer. It also focuses upon removing social stigma against cancer and spread the message that one can fight cancer. Taking this in consideration, a three-year campaign with the theme **"We can, I can"** has been undertaken for reach and impact. This theme focuses that all people **have the power to take various actions** to reduce the impact that cancer has on individuals, families and communities. World Cancer Day 2016–2018 aimed to empower people **as individuals or as a community to do their part to reduce the global burden of cancer. The theme was "We can. I can."**

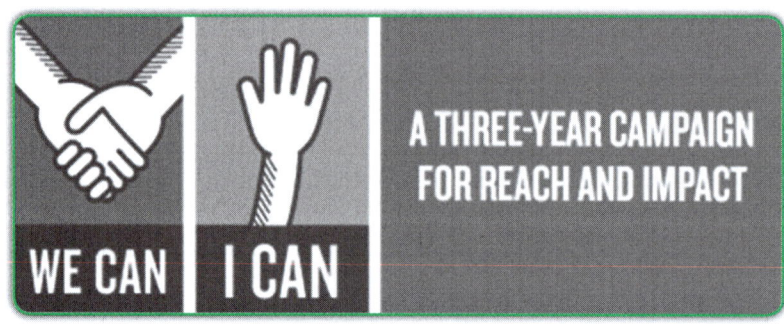

WE CAN | I CAN — A THREE-YEAR CAMPAIGN FOR REACH AND IMPACT

KEY MESSAGES

	Inspire action, take action		Make healthy lifestyle choices
	Prevent cancer		Understand that early detection saves lives
	Challenge perceptions		Ask for support
	Create healthy environments		Support others
	Improve access to cancer care		Take control of my cancer journey
	Build a quality cancer workforce		Love, and be loved

Contd…

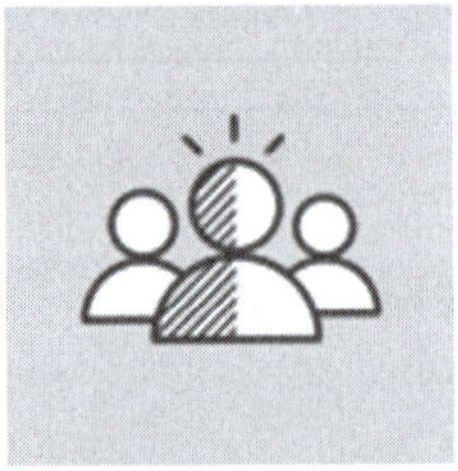	Mobilize our networks to drive progress	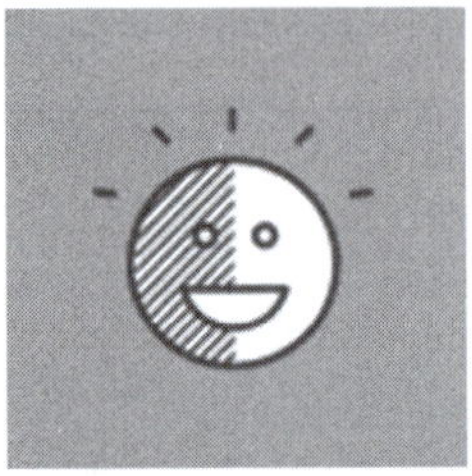	Be myself
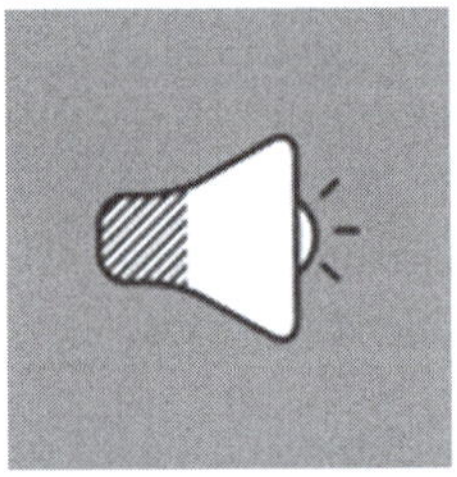	Shape policy change	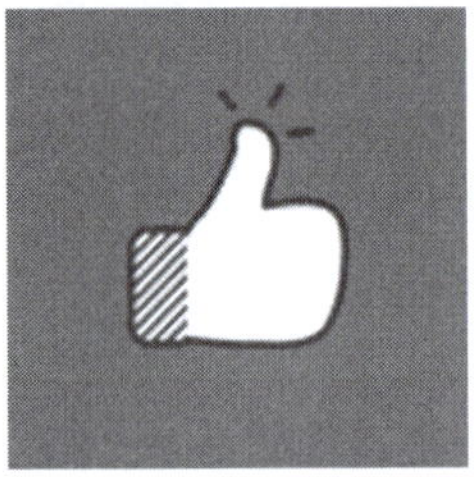	Return to work
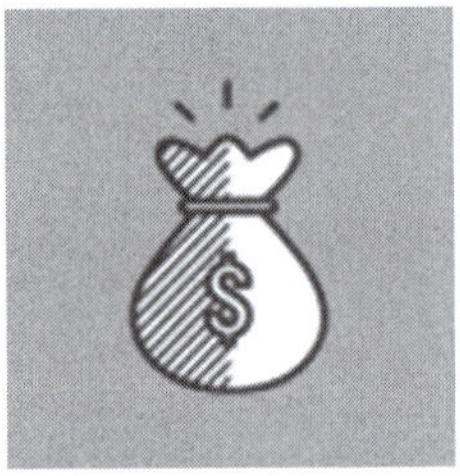	Make the case for investing in cancer control	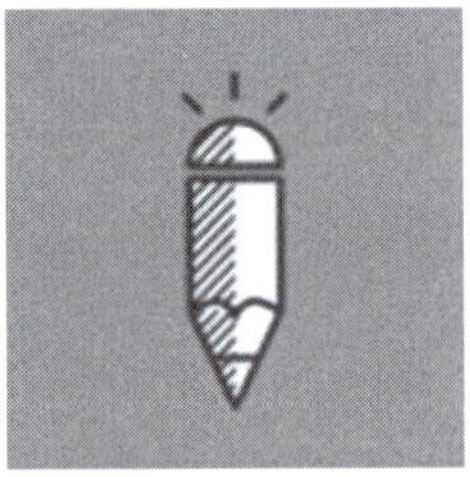	Share my story
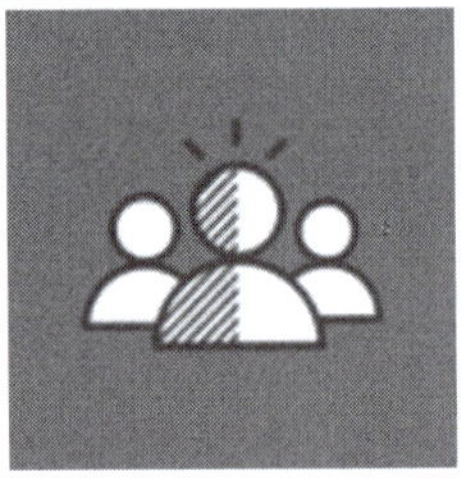	Work together for increased impact	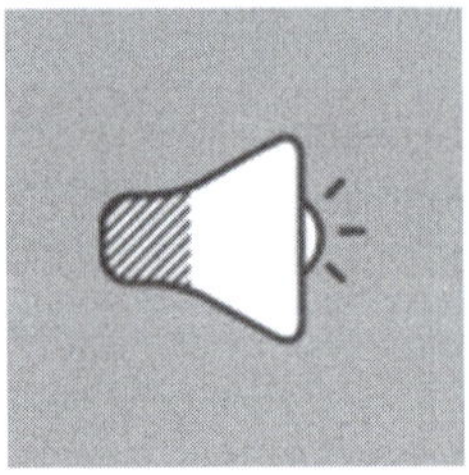	Speak out

World Cancer Day 2021 theme—I am and I will

- The theme for World Cancer Day 2021 is 'I Am and I Will.' It is a multi-year campaign that began in 2019 and this year will mark the last year. The theme represents an empowering call-to-action urging personal commitment, it also represents the power of action taken now to have a positive impact on the future. The theme clearly focuses on "together all our actions matter."

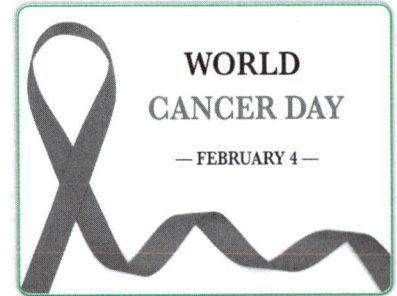

WORLD CANCER DAY
— FEBRUARY 4 —

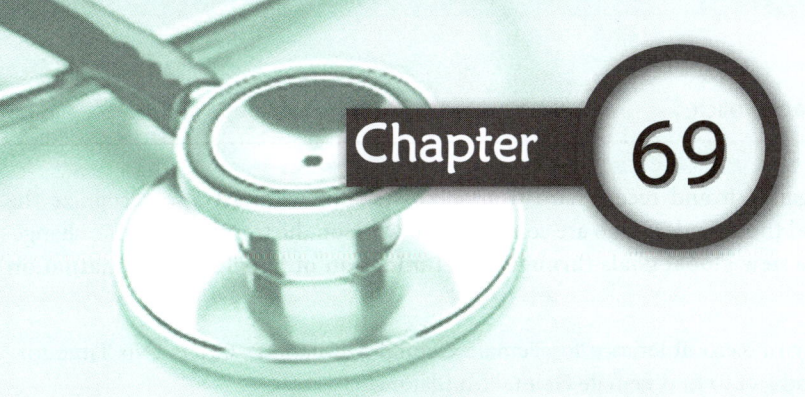

Chapter 69

International Day of Zero Tolerance for Female Genital Mutilation

INTRODUCTION

International day of zero tolerance for female genital mutilation is observed on **6th February** every year to create awareness on genital mutilation to girls and women and to promote its eradication.

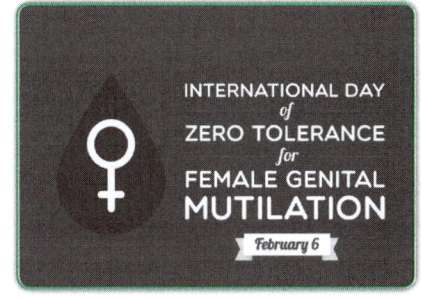

Female genital mutilation, also known as genital circumcision or genital cutting, includes partial and complete removal or injury to female reproductive organs for non-medical reasons, mainly in the name of cultural tradition. It is done using a razor blade or knife, causing serious health issues including severe bleeding, infections, infertility, complications in childbirth and newborn deaths.

According to World Health Organization, over 140 million girls and women have undergone some form of female genital mutilation and 3 million girls are at risk every year. This practice is primarily concentrated in 29 countries in Africa and the Middle East countries. It is carried out mainly between infancy (after birth) and puberty for cultural, religious and social reasons within families and communities. This brutal practice is recognized globally as violation of human rights of girls and women. It projects the deep-rooted gender inequality and violence against women and girls.

If the practice continues, around 86 million additional girls globally will be subjected to this torture by 2030. Thus, there was an urgent need to abandon this inhumane practice, for which United Nations International Children's Emergency Fund (UNICEF) and the United Nations Population Fund (UNFPA) have made efforts to run a global programme for the complete elimination of female genital mutilation.

ORIGIN OF INTERNATIONAL DAY OF ZERO TOLERANCE FOR FEMALE GENITAL MUTILATION

Zero Tolerance Day originated on 6th February, 2003, when the first lady of Nigeria, Mrs Stella Obasanjo, officially declared "Zero Tolerance to FGM" in Africa during a conference organized by the Inter-African Committee on Traditional Practices Affecting the Health of Women and Children. Since then, this day has been observed around the world. As we commemorate February 6, we should acknowledge the bravery of those who first spoke out against it and recent hard-won successes. But we must also recognize the still-overwhelming challenges and those leaders who are continuing to work on the frontline to make change. **Theme 2016 was "Achieving the new global goals through the elimination of female genital mutilation by 2030."**

The theme of International Day of Zero Tolerance for Female Genital Mutilation 2021 is "No Time for Global Inaction, Unite, Fund, and Act to End Female Genital Mutilation."

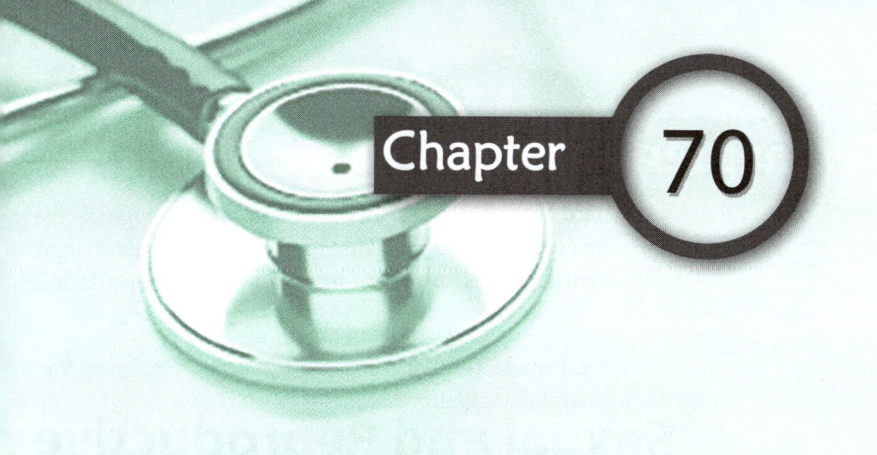

Chapter 70

National Deworming Day

INTRODUCTION

National Deworming Day is observed on 10th of February in India. The day was launched in the year 2015, by Ministry of Health and Family Welfare (MoHFW), Government of India.

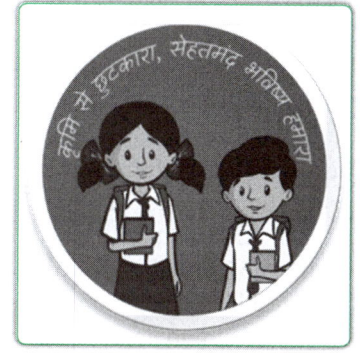

The aim of this day is to deworm all children between the ages of 1 and 19 years and to provide them good health and quality of life. The deworming drug is distributed free of cost at schools and *Anganwadi* centers.

National Deworming Day is a ground-breaking initiative focused on reducing the threat of parasitic worm infections, a widespread health issue affecting over 241 million children in India alone.

According to World Health Organization (WHO), in India, about 241 million children between 1 and 14 years of age are living at risk of parasitic intestinal worms also known as soil-transmitted helminths (STH).

A soil-transmitted helminth (Intestinal parasitic worm) infection is a sub-group within the group of helminth infections. It is caused specifically by those helminths (worms) which are transmitted through soil contaminated with fecal matter and therefore called soil-transmitted helminth infections.

OBJECTIVE OF NATIONAL DEWORMING DAY

The objective of National Deworming Day is to deworm all preschool and school-age children (enrolled and non-enrolled) between the ages of 1 and 19 years through the platform of schools and Anganwadi centers in order to improve their overall health, nutritional status, access to education and quality of life.

KEY STAKEHOLDERS

- The Ministry of Health and Family Welfare, Government of India is the nodal agency for providing all States/UTs with guidelines related to National Deworming Day (NDD) implementation at all levels.
- The programme is being implemented through the combined efforts of department of school education and literacy under Ministry of Human Resource and Development, Ministry of Women and Child Development and Ministry of Drinking Water and Sanitation.
- Ministry of Panchayati Raj, Ministry of Tribal Affairs, Ministry of Rural Development, Ministry of Urban Development, and Urban Local Bodies (ULBs) also provide support to deworming programme.

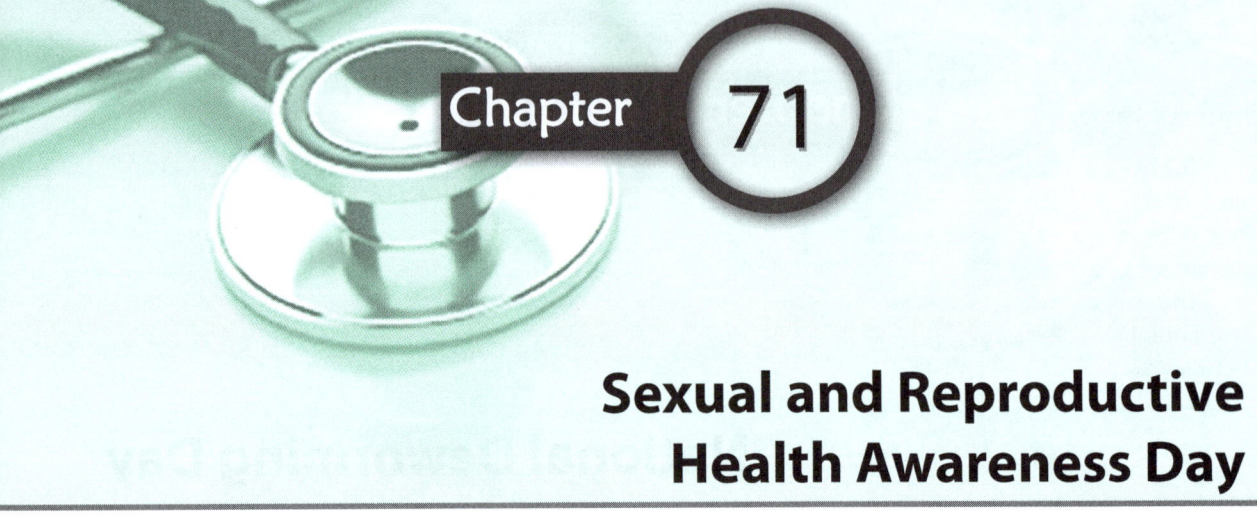

Chapter 71

Sexual and Reproductive Health Awareness Day

INTRODUCTION

This year in 2021, Sexual and Reproductive Health Awareness Week is focused on Youth!

Sexual and Reproductive Health Awareness Day is held annually on 12th February.

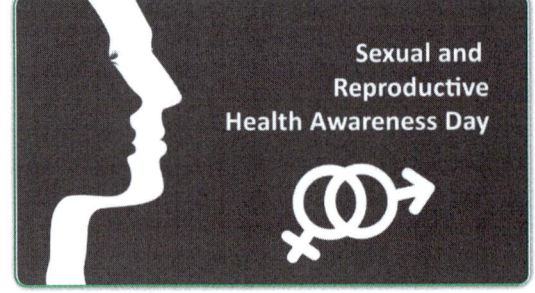

This day is an opportunity to raise awareness about sexual and reproductive health issues and to educate to reduce the spread of sexually-transmitted infections. Sexually-transmitted infections continue to be one of the major public health concerns.

Health awareness events create publicity for health issues and aim to improve the condition and help save lives, sometimes these events encourage preventative action against conditions becoming more serious.

Sexual health is a broad area that encompasses many inter-related challenges and problems.

KEY ISSUES AND CONCERNS

Key issues and concerns are human rights related to sexual health, sexual pleasure, eroticism and sexual satisfaction, diseases (HIV/AIDS, STIs, RTIs), violence, female genital mutilation, sexual dysfunction and mental health related to sexual health.

The National Population Stabilization Fund (Jansankhya Sthirata Kosh) has started a helpline to provide confidential counseling services and immediate answers to queries on sexual and reproductive health problems.

1800-11-6555 (Jansankhya Sthirata Kosh). This helpline operates daily from 9 am to 11 pm.

A team of health executives and doctors answer questions about sexual health concerns, sexually-transmitted infections, contraception, pregnancy, infertility, abortions, menopause and puberty and can explain the functioning of the reproductive systems of males and females.

The helpline will also work toward removing popular misconceptions about sex, important in a country such as India where the subject is still socially taboo.

When experimented within schools, confidential information services have been shown to be in high demand.

They can help in providing objective advice from a respected source rather than peers, the Internet and word of mouth, increase public knowledge of rights and trust in public facilities, and can reduce the bridge between users and services.

Chapter 72

World Glaucoma Week

INTRODUCTION

World Glaucoma week was celebrated from **March 6–12 in 2016**. The theme of the year 2016 was **"Beat Invisible Glaucoma."**

The main objective of this day is to eliminate glaucoma blindness by motivating people to have regular eye checks, including optic nerve examination.

Glaucoma is a term used to describe a group of diseases of the eye characterized by progressive and irreversible damage to the optic nerve (nerve of the eye responsible for vision) and which, if untreated, can lead to blindness. One of the important factors is increase in pressure of the eye, but people with normal eye pressure can also develop glaucoma. According to WHO, there are several types of glaucoma, however, the two most common are, Primary Open Angle Glaucoma (POAG), having a slow and insidious onset, and Angle Closure Glaucoma (ACG), which is less common and tends to be more acute.

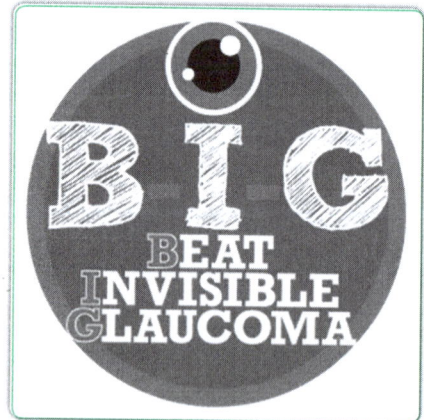

Glaucoma is the second most common cause of blindness worldwide. WHO has estimated that 4.5 million people are blind due to glaucoma. In India, glaucoma is the leading cause of irreversible blindness with at least 12 million people affected and nearly 1.2 million people blind from the disease. More than 90% of the cases of glaucoma remain undiagnosed in the community. Glaucoma is uncommon among persons under the age of 40, but the prevalence increases with age.

World Glaucoma Week is a global initiative of the World Glaucoma Association (WGA) in order to raise awareness on glaucoma.

THEME OF 2021

The 2021 theme reflects the hope that with regular testing, people continue to see the world around full of beauty, charm, and adventure. The world is bright, save your sight!

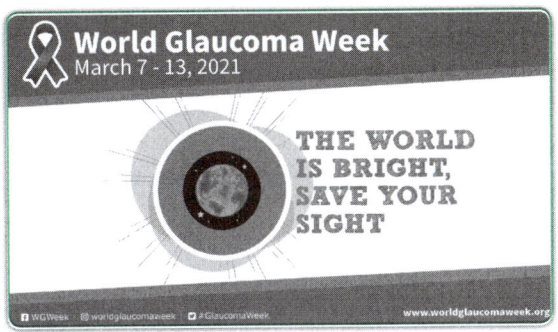

Chapter 73

International Women's Day

INTRODUCTION

International Women's Day (IWD) is celebrated worldwide every year on 8th March. In year 2016, the theme of the day is **"Planet 50-50 by 2030: Step It Up for Gender Equality."**

The United Nations observance on IWD will reflect on how to accelerate the 2030 agenda for sustainable development.

It will equally focus on new commitments under UN Women's 'Step It Up' initiative as well as existing commitments on gender equality, women empowerment and women human rights.

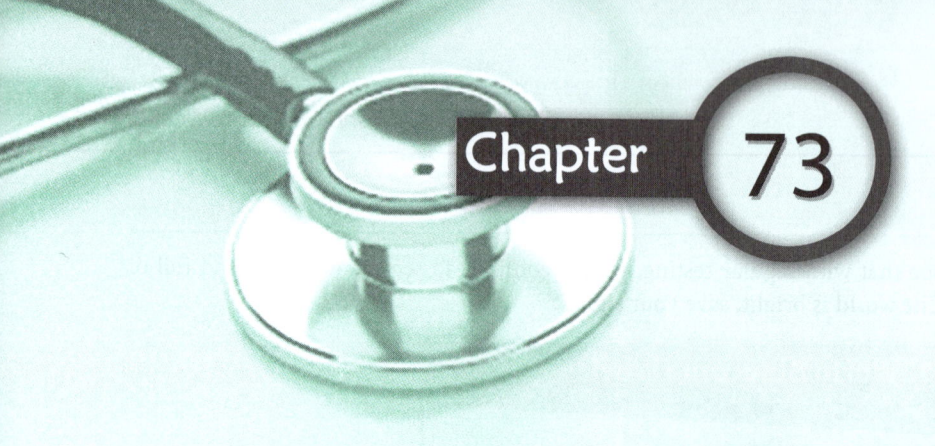

On this day, we should make a pledge for parity.

It is a day when women are recognized for their achievements without regard to divisions such as nation, ethnic, linguistic, cultural, economic or political.

The day also recognizes the role of women in peace efforts and development.

It urges the countries to put an end to the discrimination and support women's full and equal participation.

"UN Women announces the theme for International Women's Day, 8 March 2021 (IWD 2021) as, "Women in leadership: Achieving an equal future in a COVID-19 world."

HISTORY

- **1908:** Great unrest and critical debate was occurring amongst women. Women's oppression and inequality was spurring women to become more vocal and active in campaigning for change. Then in 1908, 15,000 women marched through New York City demanding shorter hours, better pay and voting rights.
- **1909:** In accordance with a declaration by the Socialist Party of America, the first National Women's Day (NWD) was observed across the United States on 28 February. Women continued to celebrate NWD on the last Sunday of February until 1913.
- **1910:** In 1910, a second International Conference of Working Women was held in Copenhagen. A woman named Clara Zetkin (Leader of the 'Women's Office' for the Social Democratic Party in Germany) tabled the idea of an International Women's Day. She proposed that every year in every country there should be a celebration on the same day—a Women's Day—to press for their demands. The conference of

over 100 women from 17 countries, representing unions, socialist parties, working women's clubs—and including the first three women elected to the Finnish parliament—greeted Zetkin's suggestion with unanimous approval and thus International Women's Day was the result.

- **1911:** Following the decision agreed at Copenhagen in 1911, IWD was honored the first time in Austria, Denmark, Germany and Switzerland on 19 March. More than one million women and men attended IWD rallies campaigning for women's rights to work, vote, be trained, to hold public office and end discrimination. However, less than a week later on 25 March, the tragic 'Triangle Fire' in New York City took the lives of more than 140 working women, most of them Italian and Jewish immigrants. This disastrous event drew significant attention to working conditions and labor legislation in the United States that became a focus of subsequent International Women's Day events. 1911 also saw women's **Bread and Roses**' campaign.

- **1913–1914:** On the eve of World War I, campaigning for peace, Russian women observed their first International Women's Day on the last Sunday in February 1913. In 1913, following discussions, International Women's Day was transferred to 8 March and this day has remained the global date for International Women's Day ever since. In 1914, further women across Europe held rallies to campaign against the war and to express women's solidarity. For example, in London in the United Kingdom there was a march from Bow to Trafalgar Square in support of women's suffrage on 8 March 1914. Sylvia Pankhurst was arrested in front of Charing Cross station on her way to speak in Trafalgar Square.

- **1917:** On the last Sunday of February, Russian women began a strike for "bread and peace" in response to the death of over 2 million Russian soldiers in World War 1. Opposed by political leaders, the women continued to strike until four days, later the Czar was forced to abdicate and the provisional Government granted women the right to vote. The date the women's strike commenced was Sunday 23 February on the Julian calendar then in use in Russia. This day on the Gregorian calendar in use elsewhere was 8 March.

- **1975:** International Women's Day was celebrated for the first time by the United Nations in 1975. Then in December 1977, the General Assembly adopted a resolution proclaiming a United Nations Day for Women's Rights and International Peace to be observed on any day of the year by Member States, in accordance with their historical and national traditions.

- **1996:** The UN commenced the adoption of an annual theme in 1996, which was "Celebrating the past, Planning for the Future". This theme was followed in 1997 with "Women at the Peace table", and in 1998 with "Women and Human Rights", and in 1999 with "World Free of Violence against Women", and so on each year until the current. More recent themes have included, for example, "Empower Rural Women, End Poverty and Hunger" and "A Promise is a Promise—Time for Action to End Violence against Women."

- **2000:** By the new millennium, IWD activity around the world had stalled in many countries. The world had moved on and feminism was not a popular topic. International Women's Day needed re-ignition. There was urgent work to do—battles had not been won and gender parity had still not been achieved.

- **2001:** The global internationalwomensday.com digital hub for everything IWD was launched to re-energize the day as an important platform to celebrate the successful achievements of women and to continue calls for accelerating gender parity. Each year, the IWD website sees vast traffic and is used by hundreds of thousands of people and organizations all over the world to learn about and share IWD activity. The IWD website is made possible each year through support from corporations committed to driving gender parity. The website's charity of choice for many years has been the World Association of Girl Guides and Girl Scouts (WAGGGS) whereby IWD fund raising is channeled. The IWD website adopts an annual theme that is globally relevant for groups and organizations. This theme, one of many around the world, provides a framework and direction for annual IWD activity and takes into account the wider agenda of both celebration as well as a broad call to action for gender parity. Recent themes have included "Make it happen", "The Gender Agenda: Gaining Momentum" and "Connecting Girls,

Inspiring Futures." Themes for the global IWD website are collaboratively and consultatively identified each year and widely adopted.

- **2011:** 2011 saw the 100-year centenary of IWD with the first IWD event held exactly 100 years ago in 1911 in Austria, Denmark, Germany and Switzerland. In the United States, President Barack Obama proclaimed March 2011 to be "Women's History Month", calling Americans to mark IWD by reflecting on "the extraordinary accomplishments of women" in shaping the country's history. The then Secretary of State, Hillary Clinton launched the "100 Women Initiative: Empowering Women and Girls through International Exchanges." In the United Kingdom, celebrity activist Annie Lennox lead a superb march across one of London's iconic bridges raising awareness in support for global charity Women for Women International. Further charities such as Oxfam have run extensive activity supporting IWD and many celebrities and business leaders also actively support the day.

- **2016 and beyond:** The world has witnessed a significant change and attitudinal shift in both women's and society's thoughts about women's equality and emancipation. Many from a younger generation may feel that 'all the battles have been won for women' while many feminists from the 1970s know only too well the longevity and ingrained complexity of patriarchy. With more women in the boardroom, greater equality in legislative rights, and an increased critical mass of women's visibility as impressive role models in every aspect of life, one could think that women have gained true equality. The unfortunate fact is that women are still not paid equally to that of their male counterparts, women still are not present in equal numbers in business or politics, and globally women's education, health and the violence against them is worse than that of men. However, great improvements have been made. We do have female astronauts and prime ministers, school girls are welcomed into university, women can work and have a family, women have real choices. And so each year the world inspires women and celebrates their achievements. IWD is an official holiday in many countries including Afghanistan, Armenia, Azerbaijan, Belarus, Burkina Faso, Cambodia, China (for women only), Cuba, Georgia, Guinea-Bissau, Eritrea, Kazakhstan, Kyrgyzstan, Laos, Madagascar (for women only), Moldova, Mongolia, Montenegro, Nepal (for women only), Russia, Tajikistan, Turkmenistan, Uganda, Ukraine, Uzbekistan, Vietnam and Zambia. The tradition sees men honoring their mothers, wives, girlfriends, colleagues, etc. with flowers and small gifts. In some countries IWD has the equivalent status of Mother's Day where children give small presents to their mothers and grandmothers.

A global web of rich and diverse local activity connects women from all around the world ranging from political rallies, business conferences, government activities and networking events through to local women's craft markets, theatric performances, fashion parades and more. Many global corporations actively support IWD by running their own events and campaigns. For example, on 8 March, search engine and media giant Google often changes its Google Doodle on its global search pages to honor IWD. Year on year, IWD is certainly increasing in status.

THEMES

International Women's Day is celebrated annually using a particular theme.

Themes of International Women's Day	
International Women's Day is celebrated annually using a particular theme	
1975	"United Nations recognizes International Women's Day"
1996	"Celebrating the Past, Planning for the Future"
1997	"Women and the Peace Table"

Contd…

Themes of International Women's Day	
1998	"Women and Human Rights"
1999	"World Free of Violence against Women"
2000	"Women Uniting for Peace"
2001	"Women and Peace: Women Managing Conflicts"
2002	"Afghan Women Today: Realities and Opportunities"
2003	"Gender Equality and the Millennium Development Goals"
2004	"Women and HIV/AIDS"
2005	"Gender Equality Beyond 2005; Building a More Secure Future"
2006	"Women in Decision-making"
2007	"Ending Impunity for Violence against Women and Girls"
2008	"Investing in Women and Girls"
2009	"Women and Men United to End Violence against Women and Girls"
2010	"Equal Rights, Equal Opportunities: Progress for All"
2011	"Equal Access to Education, Training, and Science and Technology: Pathway to Decent Work for Women"
2012	"Empower Rural Women, End Poverty and Hunger"
2013–2014	"A Promise is a Promise: Time for action to end Violence against Women"
2015	"Empowering Women—Empowering Humanity: Picture It!" (by UN), "Re-thinking Women's Empowerment and Gender Equality in 2015 and beyond" (by UNESCO) and "Breaking Through" (by Manchester City Council)
2016	"Make it Happen"
2017	"Women in the Changing World of Work: Planet 50-50 by 2030"
2018	"Time is Now: Rural and urban activists transforming women's lives"
2019	"Think equal, build smart, innovate for change"
2020	"I am Generation Equality: Realizing Women's Rights"
2021	"Choose to Challenge"

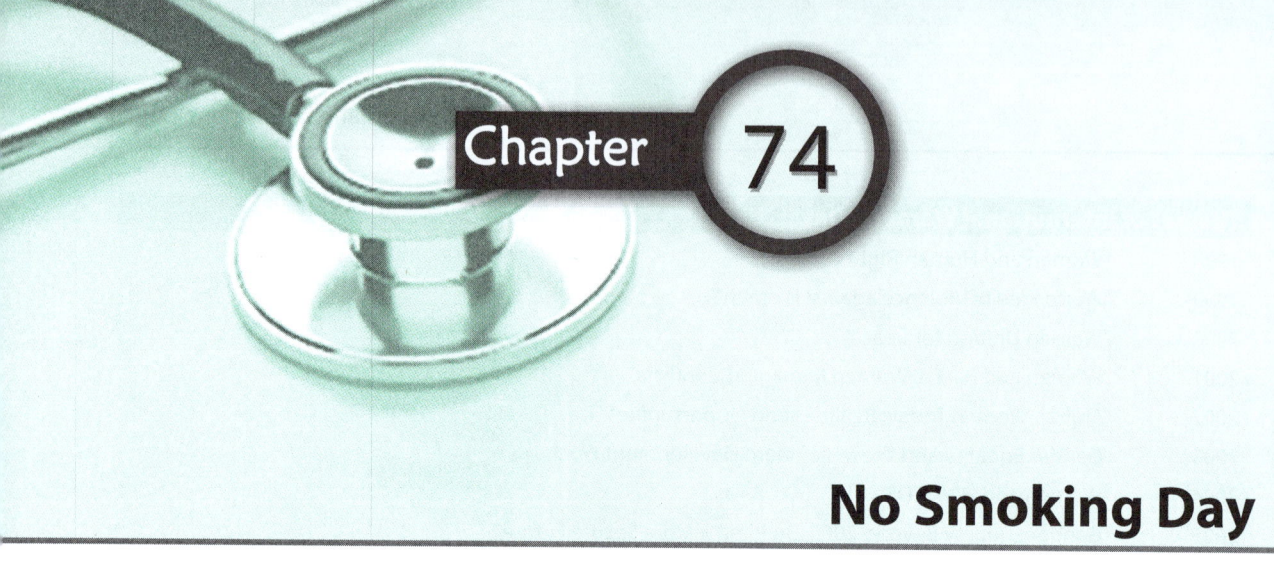

Chapter 74

No Smoking Day

INTRODUCTION

No Smoking Day is observed every year on the second Wednesday of March, to encourage people over the world to quit smoking. In year 2016, No Smoking Day was on 9th March, but you can quit smoking on any day of the year.

World No Tobacco Day was first introduced by the World Health Organization to be celebrated as the most recognized event all over the world in order to make people easily get aware of all the problems and health complications occurred by the tobacco chewing or smoking to prevent all the health hazards to make the whole world free of tobacco and a world full of healthy people.

The main purpose of this day is to spread awareness about the harmful effects of tobacco consumption through cigarette and other modes. Important message is to help smokers to get rid from the bad habit of smoking.

The main objective of celebrating the World No Tobacco Day all over the world is to promote and encourage the common public to reduce or stop the use of tobacco or consumption of its products as it may lead to the some lethal diseases (cancer, heart problem) or even death.

Smoking or chewing tobacco is one of the worst habits one can adopt. The health risks are known to all but still thousands of youth, between 12–17 years of age, start smoking each day. Some start it out of curiosity and others might just want to look like grown-ups.

Effect of smoking starts with coughing and throat irritation accompanied with bad breath and bad smelling clothes. It also leads to a patchy skin and discoloration of teeth.

Over the time, more serious conditions may develop, including health problems like heart disease, bronchitis, pneumonia, stroke, and many types of cancer, out of which, oral cancer being quite common.

STEPS TAKEN BY THE WHO ON WORLD NO TOBACCO DAY

World Health Organization (WHO) has taken many steps in reducing or banning the use of tobacco or its products by establishing an event called World No Tobacco Day and various other health awareness campaigns on world level. Some of the special steps taken by the WHO towards no tobacco use are mentioned below:

- WHO had passed a resolution called WHA40.38 in 1987 to celebrate an event called "World no-smoking day" on 7th of April in 1988 on its 40th anniversary aiming to request and aware tobacco users all over the world to reduce or quit the use of tobacco.
- WHO had passed another resolution called WHA 42.19 in 1988 to celebrate an event called World No Tobacco Day yearly on every 31st of May. It also supports the celebration by organizing various events and tobacco-related themes.

- WHO had established another event called Tobacco Free Initiative (TFI) in 1998 aiming to focus on international resources as well as draw people's attention towards the global health issues of tobacco use. It helps in creating the public health policies globally, encouraging people across societies, etc. for effective tobacco control.
- WHO FCTC is another public health treaty adopted globally in 2003 as an agreement of implementing policies for tobacco cessation.
- WHO had declared ban on tobacco advertisement, sponsorship and promotion on the eve of World No Tobacco Day celebration in 2008 by creating the theme "Tobacco-free youth."

WORLD NO TOBACCO DAY THEMES

For effectively celebrating the World No Tobacco Day all over the world, WHO selects a special theme every year as central component in order to distribute a global message to the people for more awareness. Other publicity materials for the theme like brochures, posters, fliers, press releases, websites, etc. are also provided by the WHO to the members organizing the celebration of World No Tobacco Day. Year wise themes from 1987 to the 2014 are listed below:

Themes of World No Tobacco Day	
1992	"Tobacco free workplaces: Safer and healthier"
1993	"Health services: Our windows to a tobacco free world"
1994	"Media and tobacco: Get the message across"
1995	"Tobacco costs more than you think"
1997	"United for a tobacco free world"
1996	"Sport and art without tobacco: Play it tobacco free"
1998	"Growing up without tobacco"
1999	"Leave the pack behind"
2000	"Tobacco kills, don't be duped"
2001	"Second-hand smoke kills"
2002	"Tobacco free sports"
2003	"Tobacco free film, tobacco free fashion"
2004	"Tobacco and poverty, a vicious circle"
2005	"Health professionals against tobacco"
2006	"Tobacco: deadly in any form or disguise"
2007	"Smoke free inside"
2008	"Tobacco-free youth"
2009	"Tobacco health warnings"
2010	"Gender and tobacco with an emphasis on marketing to women"
2011	"The WHO Framework Convention on Tobacco Control"
2012	"Tobacco industry interference"
2013	"Ban tobacco advertising, promotion and sponsorship"
2014	"Raise taxes on tobacco"
2015	"Stop illicit trade of tobacco products"
2016	Get ready for plain packaging
2017	Tobacco - a threat to development
2018	Tobacco and heart disease
2019	Tobacco and Lung Health
2020	Protecting youth from industry manipulation and preventing them from tobacco and nicotine use
2021	Commit to quit

Chapter 75

World Kidney Day

INTRODUCTION

World Kidney Day (WKD) is observed every year on the second Thursday in March. The day will be observed on 10th March. This day is a mutual initiative of International Society of Nephrology (ISN) and the International Federation of Kidney Foundations (IFKF). The aim of the day is to raise awareness about the role played by kidneys in maintaining overall health and to reduce the frequency and impact of kidney disease and its associated health problems worldwide.

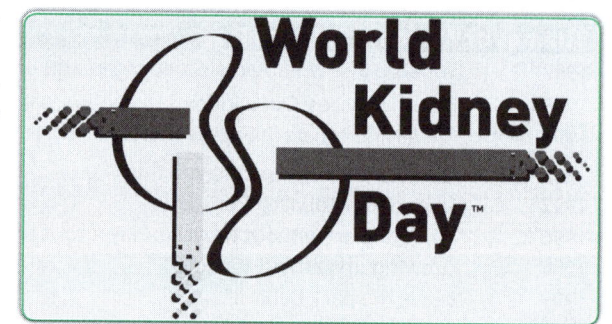

OBJECTIVES

- Raising awareness about kidney diseases.
- Highlighting that diabetes and high blood pressure are key risk factors for the Chronic Kidney Diseases (CKD).
- Encouraging systematic screening of all patients with diabetes and hypertension for CKD.
- Encouraging preventive behaviors.
- Briefing all medical professionals on their key role in detecting and reducing the risk of CKD, particularly in high risk populations.
- Stressing the important role of local and national health authorities in controlling the CKD. Health authorities worldwide have to deal with high costs of treatment in light of the increased number of kidney patients.
- Encouraging the act of organ donation as a life-saving initiative.
- Highlight the kidney problems related to the common health disorders like diabetes, high blood pressure which may lead to the CKD.
- Encourage the common public through the systematic screening of all patients having problems like diabetes or hypertension.
- Motivate and promote the common public for the better prevention by describing them all aspects of the prevention measures in order to get prevented from such kidney problems.

- Instruct the medical professionals about all aspects of the kidneys as well as teaching them to play their key role in the detection and prevention of kidney problems among the people of high risk populations.
- Get together of all the medical professionals from the local and national health authorities in order to control the spread of CKD.
- Deal with the high risk problems as well as implement the new strategies by motivating all the governments' authorities.
- Encourage people about kidney donation and transplantation as the best option of life saving for getting free from the kidney failure or other CKD.
- Encourage people for the early detection and prevention methods of the kidney problems to reduce the future complications and deaths and disability from the chronic renal and cardiovascular failure.

In year 2016, the theme of the event is Kidney Disease and Children: Act Early to Prevent it. It is very essential to prevent kidney damage in children. It is important to take early initiative to treat children with inborn and acquired disorders of the kidney.

Kidney disease in children can be acute or chronic. Acute kidney disease develops suddenly, either it may be short-lived and may improve completely after treatment or it may linger on and become chronic and serious. Chronic kidney disease cannot be treated easily and gets worse eventually.

THEMES

The celebration of World Kidney Day event was started in 2006. The every year campaign highlights a particular theme:

Themes of World Kidney Day	
2006	"Are your kidneys OK?"
2007	"CKD: Common, harmful and treatable"
2008	"Your amazing kidneys!"
2009	"Protect your kidneys: Keep your pressure down"
2010	"Protect your kidneys: Control diabetes"
2011	"Protect your kidneys: Save your heart"
2012	"Donate—Kidneys for Life—Receive"
2013	"Kidneys for Life—Stop Kidney Attack!"
2014	"Chronic Kidney Disease (CKD) and aging"
2015	"Kidney Health for All"
2016	"Kidney Disease and Children: Act Early to Prevent It"
2017	"Kidney Disease and Obesity"
2018	"Kidneys & Women's Health: Include, Value, Empower"
2019	"Kidney Health for Everyone Everywhere"
2020	"Kidney Health for Everyone Everywhere"
2021	"Living Well with Kidney Disease"

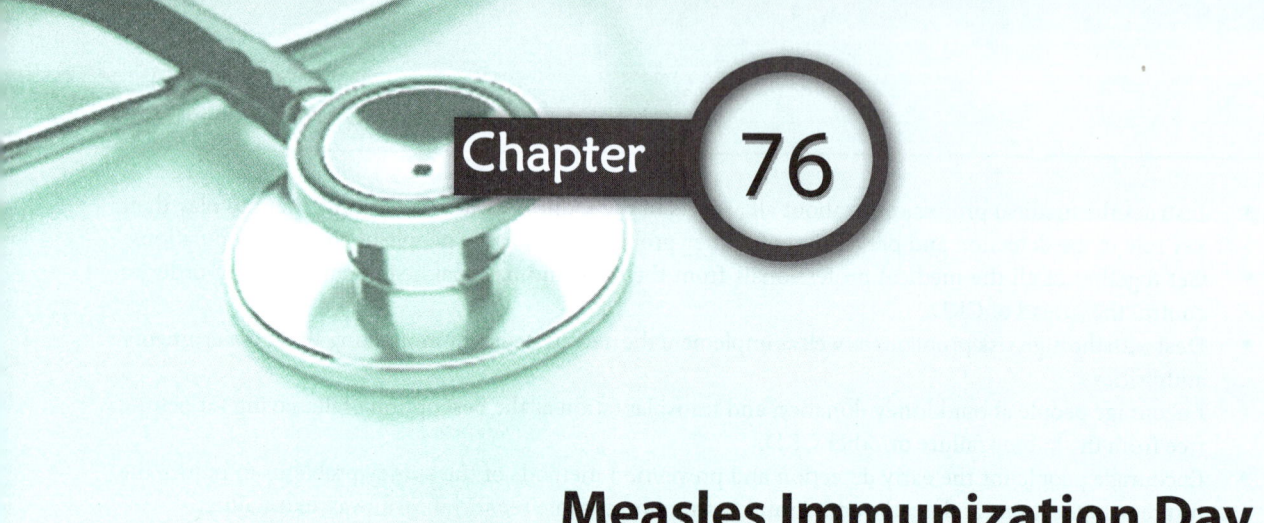

Chapter 76

Measles Immunization Day

INTRODUCTION

Measles (Khasra) is a highly contagious viral disease that affects mostly children. It is one of the leading causes of death and disability among young children. Measles Immunization Day is celebrated on 16th March every year to make people aware about this deadly disease and how they can deal with the same. There is no specific treatment for measles but there is a vaccine to protect from the disease, which is both safe as well as cost-effective. Young children, who do not receive measles immunization, are at highest risk of measles and its complications, including death.

In 2014, about 85% of the world's children received one dose of measles vaccine by their first birthday through routine health services. Measles vaccination resulted in a 79% drop in deaths that means it saved an estimated 17.1 million lives between 2000 and 2014 worldwide.

This day is celebrated to create awareness amongst people about different vaccines and how it is effective in fighting against different diseases. Diseases like measles, polio, hepatitis, diphtheria, tuberculosis, etc. are some diseases which usually attack children and parents are unaware of these types of diseases. So to create awareness amongst people about these disease, various programmes are organized.

The first symptom of measles is usually a high fever, which begins about 10–12 days after exposure to an infected person, along with, cold, redness of the eyes and rash. Measles spreads by coughing and sneezing, close personal contact or direct contact with infected nasal or throat secretions.

World Health Organization (WHO) recommends immunization for all children with two doses of measles vaccine, either alone, or in a measles-rubella (MR) or measles-mumps-rubella (MMR) combination. In India, measles vaccination is given under Universal Immunization Programme at 9–12 months of age and 2nd dose at 16–24 months of age.

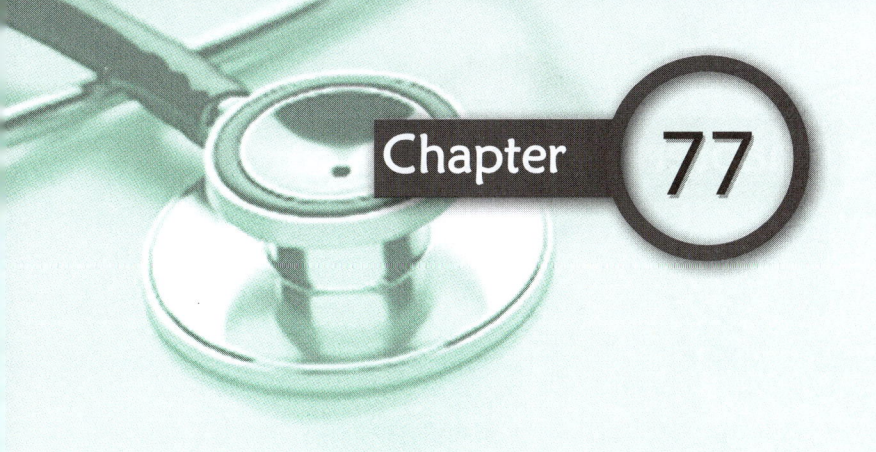

Chapter 77

World Oral Health Day

INTRODUCTION

World Oral Health Day is observed every year on 20th March. It focuses on highlighting the benefits of good oral health, spreads awareness about oral diseases and promotes maintenance of oral hygiene. This year the theme will be: It all starts here, "Healthy mouth, Healthy body." As we all know that our body's engine requires fuel of calories which we get from food and we eat food through mouth. If our mouth is not fit, no matter how much healthy we eat. It will not remain useful for us.

Oral health is as important as general health. It helps you maintain a healthy mouth, teeth and gums. It also helps to improve your appearance. Poor oral health does not only lead to oral diseases, but also major health problems like heart disease, diabetes mellitus, stroke, respiratory problems and premature births in pregnant women.

World Oral Health Day offers the global dental profession a platform to take action in a world wide effort to reduce tooth decay and organize programming and events under a single, unifying and simple message.

The theme of campaign from 2021–2023 is "Be proud of your mouth."

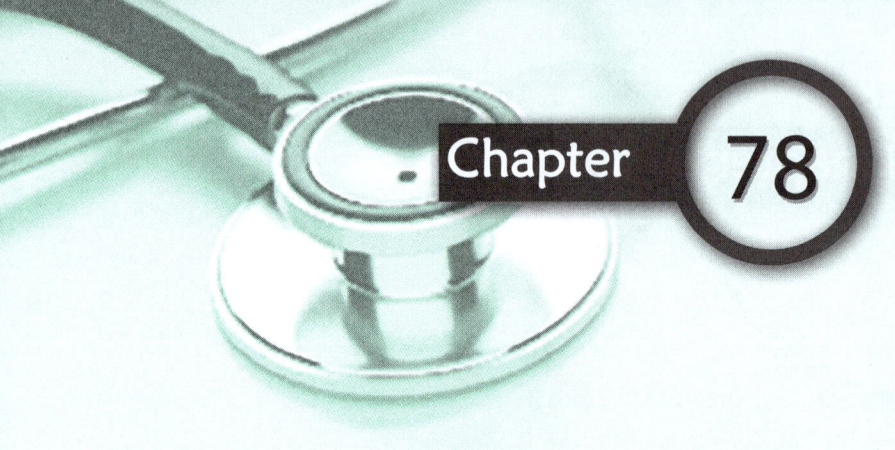

Chapter 78

World Down Syndrome Day

INTRODUCTION

March 21 is observed as World Down Syndrome Day. The aim of this day is to spread awareness about the syndrome.

For World Down Syndrome Day 2020, Down Syndrome International focused on the theme "We Decide": all people with Down syndrome should have full participation in decision making about matters relating to, or affecting, their lives.

The theme of 2021 is "Lots Of Socks".

Down syndrome, also called Trisomy 21, is a genetic disorder caused by the presence of extra chromosome 21. Down syndrome affects the child development, mentally as well as physically. According to World Health Organization (WHO), it is estimated that 1 out of every 1,000 or 1,100 children born are likely to suffer from Down syndrome.

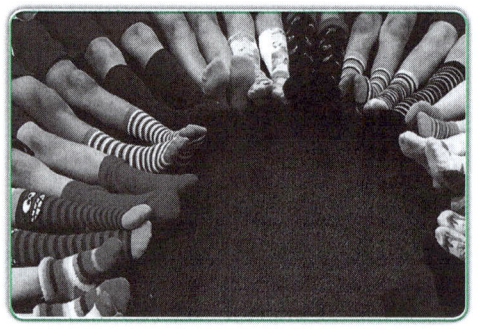

In the past, people with Down syndrome could not live a long life. Times have changed now. Pregnant women can go for screening tests to detect Down syndrome and be prepared for it. Although there is no cure for it, yet with the advancement in medical science, children with Down syndrome can receive appropriate medical care. As a result, such children can lead long lives with adequate medical attention and family support.

Children with Down syndrome need special attention, love and care. Parents can be the best people to understand and support their child.

FART, the French Association for Research on Trisomy 21, was created in 1990 for supporting research and information on medical and scientific advances in the field of Down syndrome (trisomy 21). In 2005, FART decided to select the date of March 21 (21/3 in French and 3/21 in English) as a symbolic date for the Day of Trisomy 21. The first meeting was organized by FART on March 21, 2005, in Paris, on the theme "From patient to research, better understand to better help."

When in June of the same year, Dr Juan Pereira organized an international meeting in Palma of Majorca on behalf of European Down Syndrome Association (EDSA), FART proposed them to choose the date of March 21 as a symbolic date for an International Day on trisomy 21 (DS). March 21 was then adopted as the symbolic date by both the EDSA and Down Syndrome International (DSI) boards.

On March 21, 2006, FART organized its second meeting in Paris on the theme, "How to approach the patient to cure mental deficiency." At the same time, professor Stylianos E. Antonarakis, from University of

Geneva Medical School, who knew FART, EDSA and DSI decisions, suggested to ART21, an association of parents from Swiss Alemanric regions concerned by DS, to organize a manifestation on March 21 in Geneva.

It was thus on March 21, 2006, that the first two manifestations took place in the world. Since then, FART organizes each year at this date a meeting.

On December 20, 2007, WHO recognized March 21 as the World Down Syndrome Day. The General Assembly of the United Nations recognized the same date on December 19, 2011(A/RES/66/149).

The General Assembly decided to "designate 21 March as World Down Syndrome Day, to be observed every year beginning in 2012" and "invites all Member States, relevant organizations of the United Nations system and other international organizations, as well as civil society, including non-governmental organizations and the private sector, to observe World Down Syndrome Day in an appropriate manner, in order to raise public awareness of Down syndrome." Thus, each year, on this symbolic date of March 21, persons concerned with DS organize demonstrations, scientific, social and/or medical meetings, exchange their knowledge as well as their requests at the National, European and International levels.

Chapter 79

World Tuberculosis Day

INTRODUCTION

The World Tuberculosis (TB) Day is observed every year on 24th March. It aims to increase the awareness of tuberculosis across the world. It also emphasizes upon finding solutions to eliminate the disease. The significance of the day is to change the gear and speed up global efforts to end TB altogether.

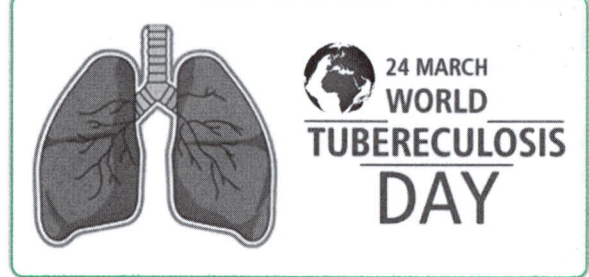

For World TB Day, 24th March 2016, WHO called on governments, communities, civil society, and the private sector to "Unite to End TB". The theme for World TB day 2020 was "It's time to End TB!" The theme of World TB Day 2021—"The Clock is Ticking"—conveys the sense that the world is running out of time to act on the commitments to end TB made by global leaders.

Four sub-themes under the "Unite to End TB" theme that WHO programmed:

1. Together we will tackle TB by stamping out poverty.
2. Together we will better test, treat, and cure.
3. Together we will stop stigma and discrimination.
4. Together we will drive research and innovation.

This annual event is marked on 24th March of every year to commemorate Dr Robert Koch's discovery, in 1882, for tubercle bacillus causing tuberculosis (TB), which was the first step towards diagnosing the disease and its treatment. Current efforts are focused on the diagnosis and treatment of this disease, as global studies indicate the following:

- One-third of the world's population is infected with TB.
- In 2014, 9.6 million people around the world became sick with TB disease. There were 1.5 million TB-related deaths worldwide.
- TB is a leading killer of people who are HIV infected.

Targeted Group:
- Patients with active tuberculosis.
- Patients suffering from latent tuberculosis (TB) infection.
- Persons in contact with tuberculosis patients for a long period of time.
- Workers in the health care sector, who are in direct contact with tuberculosis patients.
- The elderly.
- People suffering from diseases of the weak immune system, such as HIV/AIDS patients.
- People with low income, who live in unhealthy environments.

OBJECTIVES

- To detect the cases affected with tuberculosis early and treat them.
- To apply all preventive actions to tuberculosis patients.
- To render comprehensive care for patients.
- To provide effective vaccines to protect against tuberculosis.
- To free the community of tuberculosis.

HISTORY

On the 100th anniversary of tuberculosis presentation of the Dr Robert Koch, "the International Union Against Tuberculosis and Lung Disease (IUATLD)" had planned to establish 24th of March to be celebrated as an annual official event, the World TB Day. This was established by the effort of both the IUATLD and the WHO under the theme "Defeat TB: Now and forever". However, it was not announced as an official event to be celebrated annually by the WHO's World Health Assembly and the UN.

The first World TB Day celebration meeting was held by the WHO and the Royal Netherlands Tuberculosis. It was declared to be celebrated annually in Foundation in the year 1995 in Den Haag, Netherlands. Next year in 1996, various organizations like WHO, the IUATLD and KNCV had organized variety of events and activities to conduct the World TB Day celebration.

Directly Observed Treatment, Short-course (DOTS) was declared as the biggest step taken against tuberculosis by the WHO in the news conference of Berlin in 1997. According to the global situation of this epidemic disease, a really working health breakthrough was very necessary to make possible the control of TB across the world. Almost 200 organizations were joined to perform the awareness activities on the World TB Day of 1998 where top 22 most affected countries with TB were announced by the WHO in the news conference of London.

A new network "Stop TB Partnership" has been launched by various organizations to fight against TB by highlighting the scope of prevention and cure of this disease to the common public. International Committee of the Red Cross (ICRC) is helping people to fight against TB in prisons because of the overcrowding and poor nutrition.

World TB Day celebration provides a big opportunity to all the people to get aware about the causes and precautions of TB. It mobilizes the political and social authorities for further progress towards the disease prevention for the effective reduction in the TB cases and death rate in the coming years. Since 1990, the mortality rate of TB has decreased by 40% all over the world. Invention of various new TB tools has occurred for rapid diagnostic tests of TB. All this have become possible only because of this awareness campaign.

THEMES

Themes of the World TB Day	
1997	"Use DOTS more widely"
1998	"DOTS success stories"
1999	"Stop TB, use DOTS"
2000	"Forging new partnerships to Stop TB"
2001	"DOTS: TB cure for all"
2002	"Stop TB, fight poverty"
2003	"DOTS cured me—it will cure you too!"
2004	"Every breath counts—Stop TB now!"
2005	"Frontline TB care providers: Heroes in the fight against TB"
2006	"Actions for life—Towards a world free of TB"
2007	"TB anywhere is TB everywhere"
2008–2009	"I am stopping TB"
2010	"On the move against TB: Innovate towards action"
2011	"On the move against TB: Transforming the fight towards elimination"
2012–2013	"Stop TB in my lifetime Call for a world free of TB"
2014	"Reach the three million: A TB test, treatment and cure for all"
2015	"Reach, Treat, Cure Everyone"
2016	"Find TB. Treat TB. Working together to eliminate TB"
2017–2018	"Unite to end TB"
2019	"It's time"
2020	"It's time to End TB!"
2021	"The Clock is Ticking"

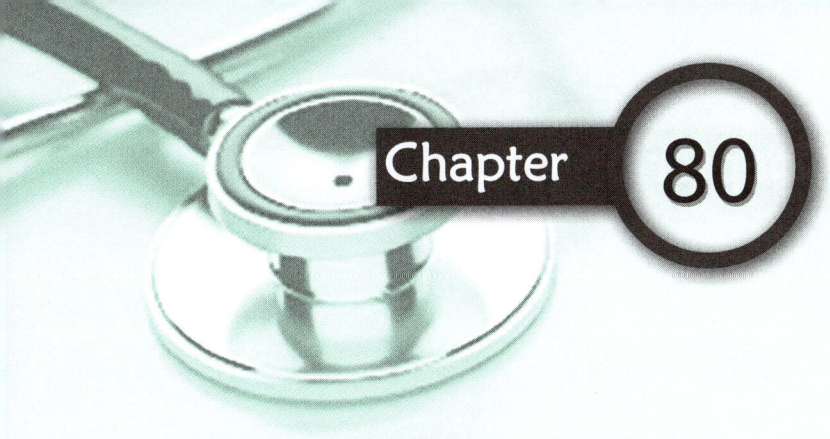

Chapter 80

World Autism Awareness Day

INTRODUCTION

- World Autism Awareness Day is observed every year on 2nd April to raise awareness about autism. In 2016, the theme was "Autism and the 2030 Agenda: Inclusion and Neurodiversity." The theme of 2020 was "The Transition to Adulthood". Theme of 2021 is "Light It Up Blue".
- As per United Nations (UN), it is estimated that more than 80% of the adults suffering with autism are unemployed. Autism is a developmental disability that manifests itself at or before the age of three years and lasts throughout a person's life. It affects the functions of brain. Autistic children may find it difficult to communicate with others or understand the world around them. They have unpredictable behavior, get easily irritated and may face difficulty in learning at school. But the good news is that autistic individuals pay great attention to minute details and may be better in some activities than many others.
- The exact cause of autism is not yet known, but scientists believe that it may be associated with genetic or environmental factors. There is no cure for the disease. However, it can be managed with the help of medications and special educators. Autistic individuals may need behavioral, speech, occupational or educational therapies depending upon their specific needs. Their symptoms may improve with time, if special care is provided to them.

EVENTS

Many events are organized on World Autism Awareness Day, they include:
- Panel discussions with autism experts, politicians and non-governmental organization (NGO) representatives.
- Informational events for parents of children with autism.
- Conferences and workshops for professionals working with people with autism.
- Artistic workshops for people with autism.
- Television and radio shows, as well as newspaper features, about people with autism and their lives.
- The launch of educational materials for parents and teachers.
- Exhibitions of art work by artists with autism.
- The display of posters and banners to increase public awareness of autism.
  Special clinics are also organized for families dealing with autism to obtain consultations with pediatricians, educational psychologists and social workers.

Chapter 81

World Health Day

INTRODUCTION

World Health Day is observed every year on 7th April on the foundation day of World Health Organization (WHO). Every year a different theme is selected keeping in mind the global public health concern.

It is an annual event being celebrated for years to raise the common public awareness towards the health issues and concerns. A particular theme is chosen to run the celebration and take care of the health for whole year. Global Polio Eradication was also one of the special themes of the year 1995 of World Health Day. Since then, most of the countries have become free of this fatal disease whereas in other parts of the world its awareness level has increased.

World Health Day targets all the health issues on global basis for which several programmes are organized yearly by the WHO and other related health organizations at various places like schools, colleges and other crowded places. It is celebrated to remember the establishment of the World Health Organization as well as draw the attention of people towards the major health issues in the world. WHO is a vast health organization working under UN for addressing the health issues on a global basis. Since its establishment, it has addressed serious health issues including chickenpox, polio, smallpox, TB, leprosy, etc. from various developing countries. It has played a significant role aiming to make the world a healthy place to live in. It has all the statistics about global health reports.

World Health Day celebration focuses on increasing the life expectancy by adding good health to the lives of people and promoting healthier living habits. Youths of the new era are also targeted by this event to prevent and make them healthy to make the world healthy and free from AIDS and HIV.

Disease spreading vectors like mosquitoes (malaria, dengue fever, filaria, chikungunya, yellow fever, etc.), ticks, bugs, sandflies, snails, etc. are also spotlighted by the WHO to make the world free from a wide range of diseases caused by parasites and pathogens. It provides better prevention and cure from the vector-borne diseases spread by vectors to travelers from one country to other. WHO supports various health authorities on global basis to make their own efforts for the prevention of public health problems to enhance better life without any diseases.

OBJECTIVES

- To increase the public awareness of various causes and prevention of high blood pressure.
- To provide detailed knowledge of getting prevented from various diseases and their complications.
- To encourage the most vulnerable group of people to frequently check their blood pressure and follow medications from the professionals.
- To promote self-care among people.

- To motivate the worldwide health authorities to make their own efforts in creating the healthy environments in their country.
- To protect families living in the vulnerable areas.
- To teach travelers and send them messages about how to get protected from the vector-borne diseases while travelling.

THEMES

Themes of World Health Day	
1950	"Know your Health Services"
1951	"Health for your Child and World's Children"
1952	"Healthy surroundings make Healthy people"
1953	"Health is Wealth"
1954	"The Nurse: Pioneer of Health"
1955	"Clean water means better Health"
1956	"Destroy disease carrying Insects"
1957	"Food for All"
1958	"Ten years of Health progress"
1959	"Mental Illness and Mental Health in the World of today"
1960	"Malaria Eradication—A world challenge"
1961	"Accidents and their prevention"
1962	"Preserve Sight—Prevent Blindness"
1963	"Hunger: Disease of millions"
1964	"No Truce for Tuberculosis"
1965	"Smallpox: constant alert"
1966	"Man and his Cities"
1967	"Partners in Health"
1968	"Health in the World of Tomorrow"
1969	"Health, Labor and Productivity"
1970	"Early Detection of Cancer Saves Life"
1971	"A Full Life Despite Diabetes"
1972	"Your Heart is your Health"
1973	"Health begins at Home"
1974	"Better Food for a Healthier World"
1975	"Smallpox: Point of No Return"
1976	"Foresight Prevents Blindness"
1977	"Immunize and Protects your Child"
1978	"Down with High Blood pressure"
1979	"A healthy Child: A sure future"
1980	"Smoking or Health: Choice is yours"
1981	"Health for all by year 2000 AD"

Contd…

Themes of World Health Day

1982	"Add life to years"
1983	"Health for all by year 2000 AD: Countdown has begun"
1984	"Children's Health: Tomorrow's Wealth"
1985	"Healthy Youth: Our best Resource"
1986	"Healthy living: Everyone a winner"
1987	"Immunization: A chance for every Child"
1988	"Health for All: All for Health"
1989	"Let's talk Health"
1990	"Our Planet Our Earth: Think Globally Act Locally"
1991	"Should Disaster Strike, be prepared"
1992	"Heart beat: A rhythm of Health"
1993	"Handle life with care: Prevent Violence and Negligence"
1994	"Oral Health for a Healthy Life"
1995	"Global Polio Eradication"
1996	"Healthy Cities for better life"
1997	"Emerging infectious diseases"
1998	"Safe motherhood"
1999	"Active aging makes the difference"
2000	"Safe Blood starts with me"
2001	"Mental Health: Stop exclusion, dare to care"
2002	"Move for health"
2003	"Shape the future of life: Healthy environments for children"
2004	"Road safety"
2005	"Make every mother and child count"
2006	"Working together for health"
2007	"International health security"
2008	"Protecting health from the adverse effects of climate change"
2009	"Save lives, make hospitals safe in emergencies"
2010	"Urbanization and health: make cities healthier"
2011	"Anti-microbial resistance: No action today, no cure tomorrow"
2012	"Good health adds life to years"
2013	"Healthy heart beat, Healthy blood pressure"
2014	"Vector-borne diseases"
2015	"Food safety" (with 5 keys; Key 1: Keep clean, Key 2: Separate raw and cooked food, Key 3: Cook food thoroughly, Key 4: Keep food at safe temperatures, Key 5: Use safe water and raw materials)
2016	"Diabetes: Scale up prevention, strengthen care, and enhance surveillance"
2017	"Depression"
2018 & 2019	"Universal health coverage: Everyone, everywhere"
2020	"Year of the Nurse and Midwife"
2021	"Protecting health from climate change"

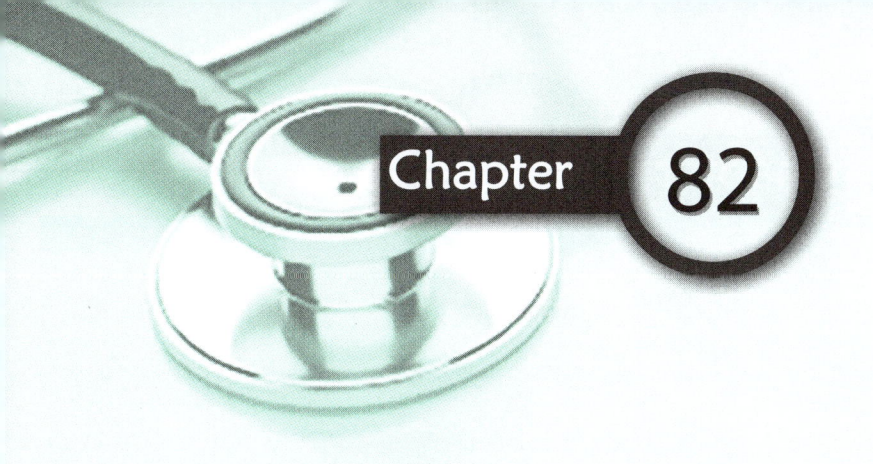

Chapter 82

World Hemophilia Day

INTRODUCTION

World Hemophilia Day is observed every year on 17th April to create awareness regarding hemophilia and other bleeding disorders. For the year 2016, the theme of the day was "Treatment for all is the vision of all".

The theme of World Hemophilia Day in 2020 was "Get+involved". It's a call to action for everyone to help drive the WFH vision of "Treatment for All" at the community and global level.

World Hemophilia Day is an international observance held on April 17, by the World Federation of Hemophilia (WFH). It is an awareness day for hemophilia and other bleeding disorders, which also serves to raise funds and attract volunteers for the WFH. It was started in 1989 and is held annually. April 17 was chosen in honor of Frank Schnabel's birthday. Frank Schnabel established the WFH in 1963.

The WFH is pleased to take the opportunity on world hemophilia day to bring attention toward the women and girls in our community who live with a bleeding disease or has some one in their lives who does.

THEMES

Themes of World Hemophilia Day	
2007	"Improve Your Life!"
2008	"Count Me In"
2009	"Together, We Care"
2010	"The Many Faces of Bleeding Disorders – United to Achieve Treatment for All"
2016	"Treatment for All, The Vision of All"
2017	"Hear Their Voices"

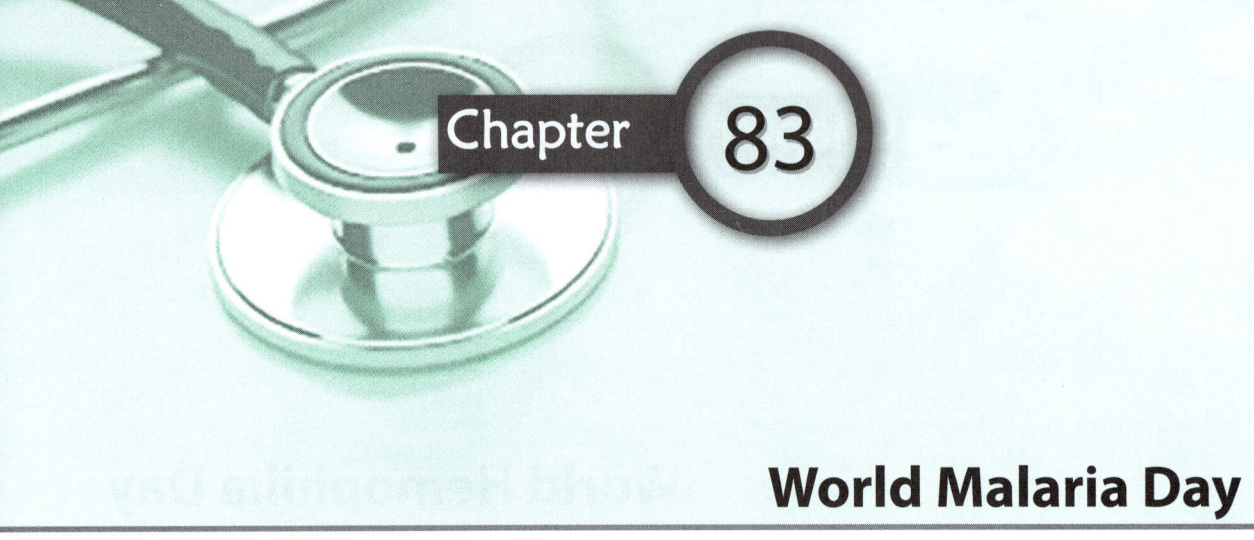

Chapter 83

World Malaria Day

INTRODUCTION

World Malaria Day is observed every year on 25th April to create awareness regarding Malaria. This year theme was "End malaria for good" Which set the vision of a malaria-free world set out in the "Global technical strategy for malaria 2016–2030".

World Malaria Day theme in 2019 was "Zero malaria starts with me".

The theme of World Malaria Day 2020—"Zero Malaria Starts with Me"—is a movement dedicated to driving action and making change, and this starts with YOU!

WHO joins partner organizations in promoting this year's World Malaria Day theme, Ready to beat malaria. The theme of 2021 underscores the collective energy and commitment of the global malaria community in uniting around the common goal of a world free of malaria.

Adopted in May 2015 by the World Health Assembly, the strategy aims to dramatically lower the global malaria burden over the next 15 years. The goal of strategy is:

- To reduce the rate of new malaria cases by at least 90%.
- To reduce malaria death rates by at least 90%.
- To eliminate malaria in at least 35 countries.
- To prevent revival of malaria in all countries that are malaria-free.

World Malaria Day, developed from Africa Malaria Day, an event that had been observed since 2001 by African governments. The observance served as a time to assess progress toward goals aimed at controlling malaria and reducing its mortality in African countries. In 2007, at the 60th session of the World Health Assembly [a meeting sponsored by the World Health Organization (WHO)], it was proposed that Africa Malaria Day be changed to World Malaria Day to recognize the existence of malaria in countries worldwide and to bring greater awareness to the global fight against the disease. Since 2008, the global community comes together to commemorate World Malaria Day on April 25. World Malaria Day was established by WHO Member States as an occasion to highlight the need for continued investment and sustained political commitment for malaria prevention and control. World Malaria Day is a chance to shine a spotlight on the global effort to control malaria. Each year, Roll Back Malaria (RBM) partner organizations unite around a common World Malaria Day theme.

World Malaria Day is a chance to highlight the advances that have already been made in malaria prevention and control, and to commit to continued investment and action to accelerate progress against this deadly disease.

Chapter 84

World Immunization Week

INTRODUCTION

World Immunization Week is observed every year during the last week of April (April 24–30) to raise awareness about the importance of immunization. The theme of 2015 and 2016 was "Close the Immunization Gap".

The World Health Assembly endorsed World Immunization Week during its May 2012 meeting. Previously, immunization week activities were observed on different dates in different regions of the world. Immunization week was observed simultaneously for the first time in 2012, with the participation of more than 180 countries and territories worldwide.

Immunization is a process in which a person is given vaccine to make him/her immune or resistant to an infectious disease. Vaccine stimulates immune system to protect the person against the disease or infection. Immunization is one of the most cost-effective public health investments. Almost one third of deaths among children under five are preventable by a vaccine shot.

According to World Health Organization (WHO), one out of five children worldwide is missing out on vital immunization. There are 25 diseases that can be prevented by vaccines including diphtheria, measles, pertussis, pneumonia, polio, rotavirus diarrhea, rubella and tetanus.

THEMES

Each World Immunization Week focuses on a theme. The themes have included the following:

Themes of World Immunization Week	
2012	"Immunization saves lives"
2013	"Protect your world—get vaccinated"
2014	"Are you up-to-date?"
2015–2016	"Close the immunization gap"
2017	"Vaccines Work"
2018	"Protected Together"
2019	"Protected Together: Vaccines Work"
2020	"Vaccines Work for all"
2021	"Vaccines bring us closer"

Chapter 85

World Asthma Day

INTRODUCTION

World Asthma Day is a day dedicated towards creating awareness about asthma across the world. It is observed every year on first Tuesday of May. The theme of 2015 was, "You can control your asthma." On this day, activities are carried out throughout the world to motivate asthma patients to keep their asthma under control.

OBJECTIVES

World Asthma Day is celebrated every year by organizing lots of programmes and events to fulfill the following objectives:

- The HSE National Asthma Programme (NAP) was established in the year 2010 by the Asthma Society, Ireland aiming to improve the asthma care.
- To identify the patient for accurate treatment of primary or secondary level based on the standard guidelines.
- Maximize the number of people without asthma and minimize the number of people with asthma to get proper control.
- Reduce death rates caused by asthma.
- Enroll all the asthma patients to ensure that all patients are diagnosed and getting treatment.
- To reduce emergency department visits because of the asthma and number of days spent by the asthmatic patients in the hospital.

World Asthma Day is a big event celebrated all over the world by the people to increase the awareness among public worldwide about the precautions and prevention of the asthma. This event is annually organized on international level by the Global Initiative for Asthma (GINA) in order to increase the asthma awareness all around the world. It is celebrated on annual basis on the first Tuesday of May. World Asthma Day celebration was first celebrated in the year 1998 by GINA in more than 35 countries after its first "World Asthma Meeting" in Barcelona, Spain. GINA organizes variety of programmes every year with the help of organizers and associates like health care groups and asthma educators to encourage and motivate common public using the sub-theme called "It is Time to Control Asthma". GINA decides every year's theme of celebration as well as distributes the materials and resources to the organizers to organize programmes. Various health care professionals, members, educators, and other health care organizations take part in the celebration by showing their activities related to the asthma at many public places in order to help people reducing their burden of asthma.

Controlling the current status of asthma all around the world is very necessary and it has become the responsibility of all the medical professionals and not only the patients. Asthma management requires collaborative efforts of the patients, asthma carers, health professionals, community health groups and other health care systems globally.

World Asthma Day 2014 celebration organized symposium to bring together the key players including asthma educators, general practitioners, respiratory nurses, practicing nurses, pharmacy assistants, pharmacists, medical researchers, medical students and other health workers.

ACTIVITIES

World Asthma Day is celebrated in the month of May every year that is why May is known as the Asthma Awareness Month when the "National Asthma Education and Prevention Programme (NAEPP)" is organized to encourage the people to take care of their asthma.

Family members and the persons having asthma are encouraged for the written Asthma Action Plan (AAP) through their health care provider to fulfill the specific needs of the asthmatic patients such as accurate medications to get prevented from the airway inflammations and environmental causes of asthma like dust mites and tobacco smoke.

The AAP is a big step taken by the NAEPP to bring together the clinicians, patients and others taking care of the asthmatic patients to work together jointly in order to seize control over the asthma. Patients of persistent asthma are motivated through many activities for using inhaled corticosteroids to get successful control over the asthma. Some of the activities are:

- The AAP aims highlighting the daily basis control over asthma and handling its symptoms or asthma attacks.
- Free checkup camps are organized to assess the severity of asthma among people to start best treatment.
- Patients are motivated for their scheduled follow-up visits at the periodic intervals of six months and controlling the environmental exposures to get prevented from allergens or irritants.
- Asthma societies in many countries celebrate World Asthma Day on national level.
- New asthma clinics and pharmacy clinics are opened in the required areas.
- TV channels and news channels distribute messages like "fighting asthma with every breath" and other awareness messages to reach to the public.
- Quiz competitions, debate, symposium, etc. on the subject of asthma are organized in the schools, colleges and pharmacies throughout the country.
- Classes are taken by the teachers on the subjects of asthma prevention and precaution methods.
- Asthma awareness posters and banners are distributed and applied in the most vulnerable areas to increase public awareness.

THEMES

Themes of World Asthma Day	
1998	"To Help Our Children Breathe"
2000	"Everyone Normal Breathing"
2001	"Unite to Overcome Asthma"
2002	"Understanding Asthma"

Contd…

Themes of World Asthma Day

Year	Theme
2003	"Reducing the Asthma Burden"
2004	"Emphasis on Asthma, Reduce the Burden of Asthma"
2005–2006	"The Unmet Needs of Asthma"
2007–2014	"You Can Control Your Asthma"
2015	"You Can Control Your Asthma" and Sub-Theme was "It is Time to Control Asthma"
2016	"Uncovering Asthma Misconceptions"
2017	"Better air better breathing"
2018	"Never too early, never too late. It's always the right time to address airways disease."
2019	"STOP for asthma"
2020	"Enough Asthma Deaths"
2021	"Uncovering Asthma Misconceptions"

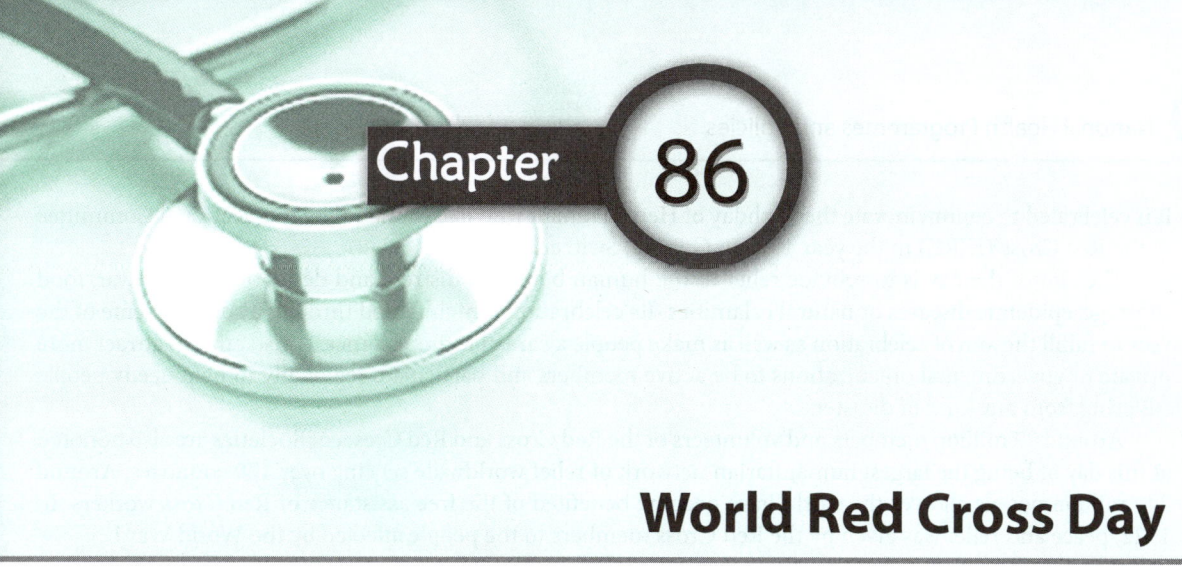

Chapter 86

World Red Cross Day

INTRODUCTION

World Red Cross Day is celebrated every year on 8th May. The date 8th of May is the birthday anniversary of the founder of the Red Cross, Henry Dunant. He was the founder of the Red Cross as well as the founder of International Committee of the Red Cross (ICRC), born in Geneva in the year 1828. He was the most famous person and the first person to receive Noble Peace prize. This day is an annual event which celebrates the principles of "International Red Cross and Red Crescent Movement." It is celebrated every year to pay tribute to the volunteers for their unprecedented contribution to the people in need.

HISTORY

Red Cross was introduced as a major contribution to the peace after the World War I by an international commission at 14th International Conference of the Red Cross. The principles of the Red Cross Truce was presented and approved on 15th International Conference at Tokyo in the year 1934 to get applicable all across the world in different regions. The possibility of its annual celebration was asked to the "League of the Red Cross Societies (LORCS)" by the International Federation of the Red Cross Societies (IFRC) General Assembly and just two years later the proposal of celebrating this day annually was adopted and was first celebrated as the Red Cross Day on 8th of May in 1948. Later, it was officially named as the "World Red Cross and Red Crescent Day" in the year 1984.

World Red Cross Day is celebrated by the people on international level to alleviate people's suffering, enhancing their dignity, protecting their life from emergencies and lots of natural disasters including epidemic diseases, flood and earthquakes. It is celebrated by all the sections of the Red Cross organizations to help people by keeping in front all fundamental principles which are humanity, independence, impartiality, neutrality, universality, voluntary and unity.

International Committee of the Red Cross and its members (National Societies) organize lots of programmes and events in order to encourage volunteers as well as facilitate and promote their humanitarian activities. International Red Cross movement members assist the people suffering from any problem. People are motivated to protect their own lives and take care of the dignity of other victims.

AIMS AND OBJECTIVES

World Red Cross Day has become an important day in the history of world which is being celebrated annually to play big role in the life-saving events as well as assisting the vulnerable social people all around the world.

It is celebrated to commemorate the birthday of Henri Dunant who had founded the International Committee of the Red Cross (ICRC) in the year 1863 in Geneva, Switzerland.

The aim of the day is to provide relief to the human beings in distress and desolation due to war, food shortage, epidemic diseases or natural calamities. Its celebration is highlighted through a special theme of the year to fulfill the aim of celebration as well as make people aware of its importance. It also aims to attract more private or governmental organizations to be active members and participate regionally to help needy people suffering from any kind of disaster.

Around 97 million members and volunteers of the Red Cross and Red Crescent Societies are also honored at this day of being the largest humanitarian network of relief worldwide serving over 170 countries. Around 240 million people all over the world have become benefited of the free assistance of Red Cross workers. In 1922, peace and relief was given by the Red Cross members to the people affected by the World War I. Following are the objectives of the World Red Cross Day celebration:

- It is celebrated to provide relief and peace to the injured people to prevent death rate due to the disasters of any kind.
- It helps in initiating active efforts all over the world to reduce casual death rate because of epidemic illnesses.
- It helps people living in the vulnerable areas to manage the public health emergencies.
- It empowers its members, civil societies and other involved local communities to provide immediate response to the health disasters in the vulnerable situations.
- It helps in reinstating the human dignity.
- Geneva conventions help in monitoring the compliance of warring parties.
- It helps the wounded people on the battlefield by organizing the nursing care.
- It avails the treatment for prisoners of war and help in searching the missing persons during conflict.
- It avails protection and nursing care to the people in civil populations.

THEMES

World Red Cross Day is celebrated every year using a particular theme of the year to run this campaign very effectively all over the world. Some of the themes are mentioned below:

Themes for World Red Cross Day	
2009	"Climate Change and its Humanitarian Consequences Serving as a Solferino of Today
2010	"Urbanization"
2011	"Find the Volunteer Inside You"
2012	"Youth on the Move"
2015–2013	"Together for Humanity"
2016	"Everywhere for everyone"
2017	"Less known Red Cross stories"
2018	"Memorable smiles from around the world"
2019 & 2020	"Love"
2021	"Keep clapping for the volunteers, staff and everyone responding to Covid-19

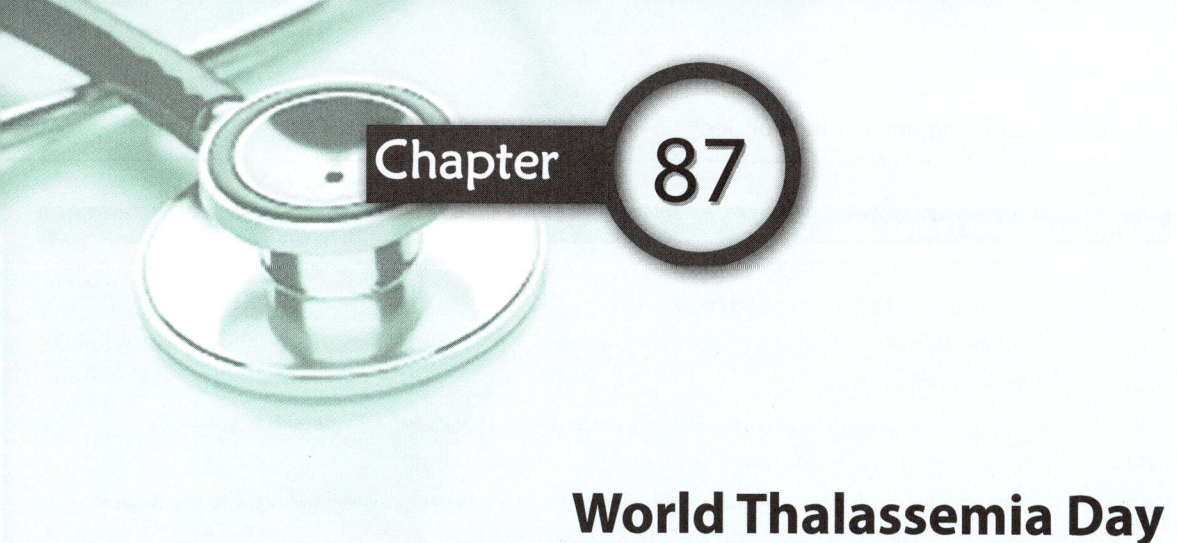

Chapter 87

World Thalassemia Day

INTRODUCTION

World Thalassemia Day is observed every year on 8th of May to spread awareness amongst people about this deadly disease and to focus on prevention to avoid its transmission. May 8 has become a very special day for the people suffering from thalassemia as it brings a chance for them to get diagnosed earlier. The day is dedicated to commemorate the thalassemia patients and give them a special chance to live like a normal person as well as prevent this disease to spread in the community, society, state, country and finally world.

OBJECTIVES

- It is celebrated to increase the awareness about the disease among common public.
- To develop the most effective prevention measure to have control on the disease.
- To motivate and encourage the common public especially youths for the blood donation in order to prevent the people suffering from thalassemia.
- To motivate doctors and other health professionals to take care of the patients especially when they need.
- To promote the people suffering from it to come to the hospital for the early detection, prevention and cure.
- To motivate the youths for the pre-marriage test to get diagnosed about this problem and prevent this disease to get inherited among new generations.
- To make the community, society, nation and world free of thalassemia and other inheritable diseases.
- To give them (people having thalassemia) equal chance of living like a normal and well-being person.
- To encourage government organizations to develop more health care facilities in the vulnerable areas.
- To reduce the death rate of people all over the world on international level because of thalassemia.
- To increase the number of healthy people without thalassemia or other fatal diseases in the country and world.

WORLD THALASSEMIA DAY THEMES

This special day is celebrated every year using a particular theme to make it very effective and encourage patients to get appropriate treatment to enhance their quality of life. Themes of some previous years are as follows:

Themes of World Thalassemia Day	
2009	"We care the industry together"
2010	"Thalassemia: Knowledge is Strength"
2011	"Equal Chance to Life"
2012	"Patient's Rights Revisited"
2013	"The right for quality health care of every patient with Thalassemia: major and beyond"
2014	"Economic Recession: Observe—Joint Forces—Safeguard Health"
2015	"Enhancing partnership towards patient-centered health systems: good health adds life to years!"
2016	"Access to Safe and Effective Drugs in Thalassemia"
2017	"Get connected! Share knowledge and experience and fight for a better tomorrow in thalassemia"
2018	"Thalassemia past, present and future: Documenting progress and patients' need worldwide."
2019	"Universal access to quality thalassemia healthcare services: Building bridges with and for patients"
2020	"The dawning of a new era for thalassemia"
2021	"Addressing Health Inequalities Across the Global Thalassemia Community"

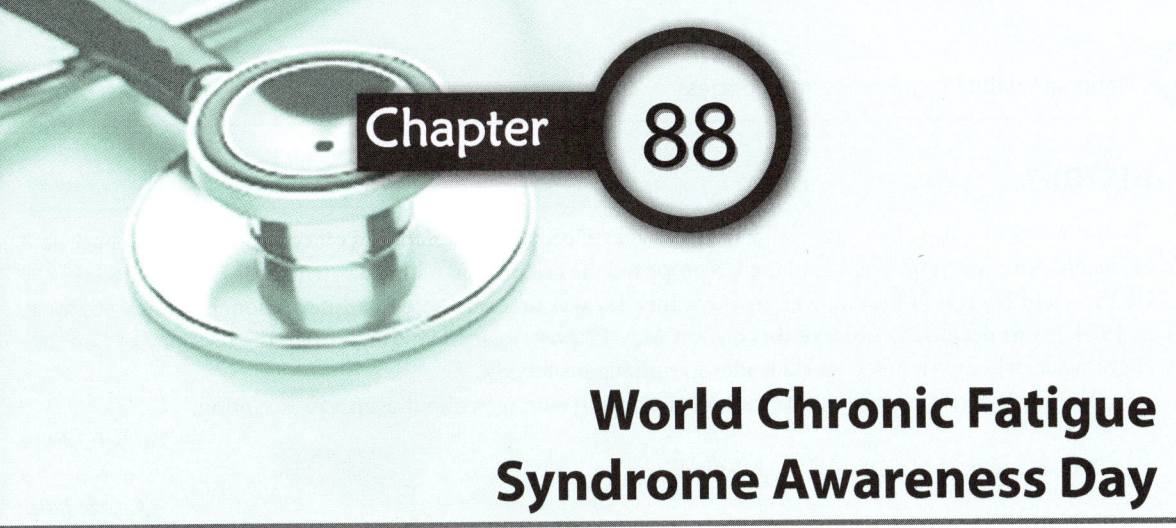

Chapter 88

World Chronic Fatigue Syndrome Awareness Day

INTRODUCTION

The 12th May, the birthday of Florence Nightingale, founder of modern nursing has been designated as World Chronic Fatigue Syndrome Awareness Day. She probably suffered from fatiguing illness resembling Chronic Fatigue Syndrome (CFS) or fibromyalgia.

The aim of the day is to spread awareness about this medical condition and its causes, symptoms and cure.

May 12th was chosen as it is the birthday of Florence Nightingale. She was believed to have suffered from encephalomyelitis (ME)/CFS.

Every year a number of events are held to mark May 12. The events are either held on May 12th or sometime during the month of May.

If love cannot cure it, Nurse can, this is a perfect saying about nurses because they care a patient with love. May 12, every year is being celebrated as **"International Nurse Day"**, in the memory of Florence Nightingale, the founder of modern nursing. The day signifies the contribution of nurses towards people's health. The theme of year 2016 was "Nurses: A Force for Change: Improving health systems' resilience". The theme signifies that the nurses play an important role to strengthen the flexibility of our medical system. The resilience of a health system is its capacity to respond, adapt and strengthen in any emergency such as a disease outbreak, natural disaster or in war.

SIGNIFICANCE

Nursing is considered as the largest health care profession in the world. Nurses are well-trained, educated and experienced for taking care of the patient through all aspects like physical, psychological and social. While the doctors are busy professionals with little encounter with the patients, the nurses are accessible and available to the patients round the clock to take care of them. The nurses are expected to be friendly, helpful and supportive to the patients in overcoming their illness and in boosting their morale.

International Nurse Day is celebrated:
- To acknowledge nurses' contribution to health services
- To educate and train nurses for patients' welfare
- To discuss about various issues related to nurses
- To appreciate their work and dedication

HISTORY

The beginning of "Nurse Day" goes back to 1953, when Dorothy Sutherland, an officer from the US Department of Health, Education and Welfare in the US proposed the celebration of this day which was further declared by US President Dwight D Eisenhower. In 1965, this day was first celebrated by International Council of Nurse. In 1974, it was decided to observe this day on May 12 every year to commemorate the birthday of Florence Nightingale, who was a noted world leader in nursing profession.

- "Nurses dispense, comfort, compassion, and caring with or without even a prescription."

  —*Val Saintsbury*

- "Nurses are the hospitality of the hospital."

  — *Carrie Lafet*

CELEBRATION

International Nurse Day is celebrated all over the world in various ways. In US and Canada, this is a whole week celebration. A complete week is dedicated to nurses and their significant role in caring patients and their contribution in health services. Various activities are held throughout the week such as educational seminars, debates, various competitions and discussions on nursing related issues. Nurses are also honored on this day by distributing gifts, flowers and organizing dinners.

In London, a candle is handed over to nurses in chain to symbolize their contribution to the health service. The main celebration usually takes place in St. Margaret's Church, the burial place of Florence Nightingale.

In India, Nursing day is organized by holding activities such as educational seminars and discussions on nursing issues. Certificates and prizes are also distributed to the nurses for their best contribution to health services.

The International Council of Nurses celebrates this important day each year with the distribution of the International Nurses' Day (IND) Kit. The IND kit pertaining to this year contains educational and public information materials including poster.

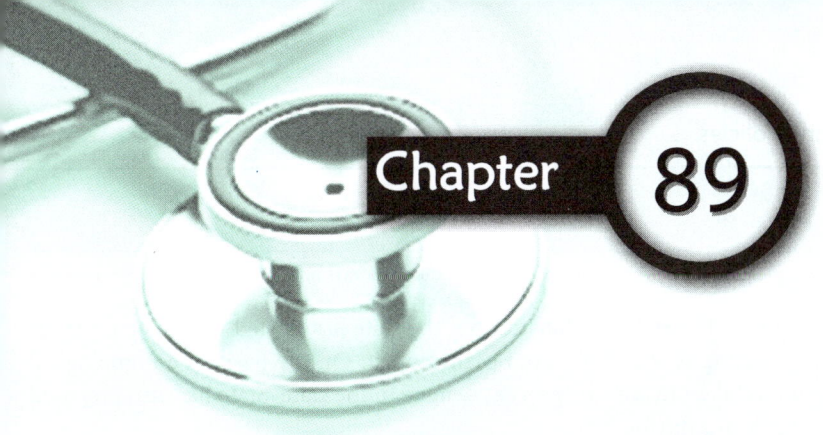

Chapter 89

National Dengue Day

INTRODUCTION

D engue prevention and control is everyone's responsibility; together we can make a difference. National Dengue Day has been observed on 16th of May, 2016 by Ministry of Health and Family Welfare (MoHFW), Government of India. The aim of this day is to control the Dengue through creating awareness, initiating preventive actions and continuing till transmission season is over.

The Government of India has recently declared May 16 as National Dengue Day to mark the toll the deadly disease has been taking in terms of lives and to reaffirm nationwide efforts to tackle the scourge by using both education and medical intervention.

OBJECTIVE

To reduce morbidity and mortality due to dengue by at least 50% in next five years.

SERVICES TO COMMON PEOPLE

All government hospitals have been instructed to provide free treatment and laboratory facilities to the suspected dengue patients.

SERVICE CENTERS AVAILABLE IN EACH DISTRICT

Treatment for dengue is available at all government hospitals at taluka and district level and medical college hospitals.

ROLE OF OTHER SECTORS

Involvement and cooperation of other related sectors are obtained through the umbrella societies at district levels.

Impact

Non-availability of separate infrastructure for dengue control and water scarcity lead to increase in number of dengue cases and deaths due to dengue day by day.

STRATEGY

Implementation of Strategies

Considering major outbreaks of dengue in the State of Maharashtra, the state has started vector surveillance from 1999 in all districts by giving training to 2 MPWs from each district. On the basis of entomological findings, following measures were undertaken to control/prevent dengue in the state. State has also prepared action plan for controlling dengue outbreaks during 2003–04.

a.	**Fever Survey:** • Collection of Blood Smears to rule out malaria • Presumptive treatment with Chloroquine • Collection of Serum samples for isolation of dengue virus if there are no malaria positive cases • Collection of Aedes Aegypti mosquitoes for isolation • The State has prepared district action plan for dengue control during the year 2003
b.	Indoor/outdoor fogging with pyrethrum extract/synthetic pyrethroid ultra low volume (ULV)
c.	To empty all domestic and peridomestic water containers to eliminate the Aedes breeding.
d.	The indoor residual spraying with synthetic pyrethroid.
e.	The State has also supplied rapid diagnostic dengue kits (Panbio) to selected districts.
f	**IEC:** Health Education regarding seriousness of dengue disease, its spread and measures to be undertaken is given at the time of house visits. Posters, pamphlets are also distributed.

ACTIVITIES

- Regular surveillance
  - Active.
  - Passive.
- Rapid fever survey.
- Collection and examination of blood smears for malaria.
- Collection of 5% serum samples of dengue suspected cases for viral isolation.
- Fogging.
- Entomological survey for search of dengue vector, i.e., Aedes aegypti.
- Container survey: House Index (HI), Brautaeu's Index (BI)
- Workshop for all district level officers regarding dengue prevention and control.
- Arrangement for platelet count and treatment of dengue cases in government institutions.
- Guidelines issued to all district level officers.
- Health education to community through different media.
- Visits of health authorities from various levels.

Chapter 90

International Day of Action for Women's Health

INTRODUCTION

In the year 1987, May 28 was declared as International Day of Action for Women's Health or International Women's Health Day. Since then each year, this day is celebrated by women's and health groups. Latin American and Caribbean Women's Health Network (LACWHN) and Women's Global Network for Reproductive Rights (WGNRR) are working together to make this campaign successful. May 28 is a special day on which the women's health takes a center stage. It is therefore an occasion to celebrate the gains for women's health as well as remind to the government, international agencies of their commitments to women's health and rights. Also it has been the platform for campaigning for advocating and advancing for the recognition of the concepts of sexuality, fiscal right and reproductive rights and health frameworks at national, and international level.

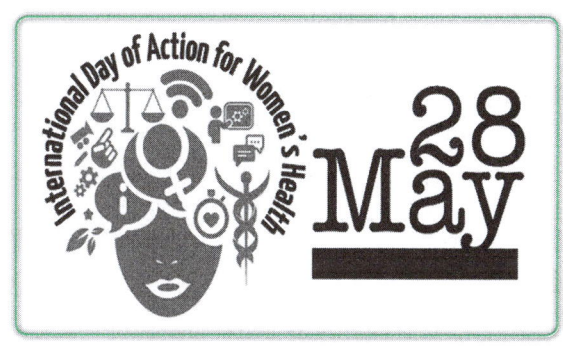

OBJECTIVE

To raise awareness on the issues related to women's health and well-being such as sexual and reproductive health and rights (SRHR). It is one of the best platforms to remind everyone specially the government leaders and parliamentarians that the women's health matters.

THEMES

Themes of International Women's Day of Action for Women's Health	
1996	"Celebrating the Past, Planning for the Future"
1997	"Women and the Peace Table"
1998	"Women and Human Rights"
1999	"World Free of Violence Against Women"
2000	"Women Uniting for Peace"

Contd...

Themes of International Women's Day of Action for Women's Health	
2001	"Women and Peace: Women Managing Conflicts"
2002	"Afghan Women Today: Realities and Opportunities"
2003	"Gender Equality and the Millennium Development Goals"
2004	Women and HIV/AIDS
2005	"Gender Equality Beyond 2005; Building a More Secure Future"
2006	"Women in Decision-making"
2007	"Ending Impunity for Violence Against Women and Girls"
2008	"Investing in Women and Girls"
2009	"Women and Men United to End Violence Against Women and Girls"
2010	"Equal Rights, Equal Opportunities: Progress for All"
2011	"Equal Access to Education, Training, and Science and Technology: Pathway to Decent Work for Women"
2012	"Empower Rural Women, End Poverty and Hunger"
2013	"A Promise is a Promise: Time for Action to End Violence Against Women"
2014	"Equality for Women is Progress for All"
2015	"Empowering Women, Empowering Humanity: Picture it!"
2016	"Planet 50-50 by 2030: Step It Up for Gender Equality"
2017	"Women in the Changing World of Work: Planet 50-50 by 2030"
2018	"Press for Progress"
2019	"Balance for better"
2020	"An equal world is an enabled world"
2021	"Empowered and connected"

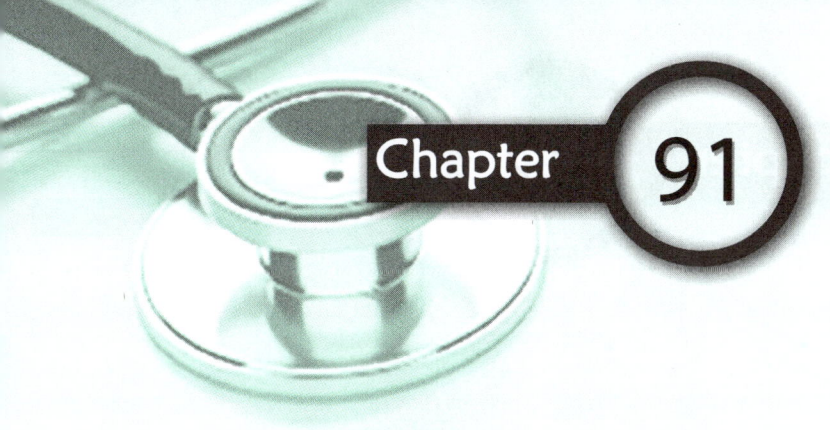

Chapter 91

World Multiple Sclerosis Day

INTRODUCTION

World Multiple Sclerosis Day is observed every year on the last Wednesday of May, worldwide. In year 2016, it was celebrated on 25th of May with the aim to create public awareness on multiple sclerosis and to make life less difficult for people affected by multiple sclerosis (MS). The theme for 2016 World MS Day was 'Independence'. This theme explored how people with MS can be independent, acknowledging that independence can mean different things to different people. It focuses on access not only to diagnosis, treatment and support but also to travel, education and employment for the people suffering from MS.

Every year, thousands of people are diagnosed with multiple sclerosis worldwide. Multiple sclerosis is a disease in which the protective sheath that covers the nerves gets destroyed which disrupts the communication between brain and the rest of the body. This leads to difficulty in speech, sight and ability to move.

In 2009, the Multiple Sclerosis International Federation (MSIF) and its members initiated the first World MS Day. Together we have reached hundreds of thousands of people around the world, with a campaign focusing on a different theme each year.

The central campaign message and theme for World MS Day is developed by staff at the MS International Federation together with an international working group. The working group is drawn from our network of MS organizations and currently has representatives from India, UK, Egypt, Ireland, Spain, and the USA.

THEME OF 2020–2022

The World MS day 2020 - 2022 theme is "Connections" as in self-connection, building community connection, and connections for quality care. The tagline 'I Connect, We Connect' is used to spread awareness. This campaign was started to address the social barriers that leave an MS patient lonely and socially isolated.

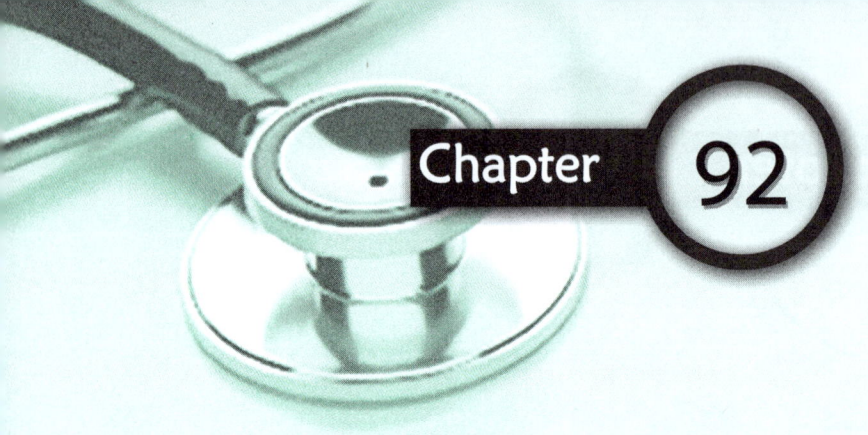

Chapter 92

World No Tobacco Day

INTRODUCTION

World No Tobacco Day is observed every year on 31st May. The theme of 2016 was 'Get Ready for Plain Packaging'. The aim of plain packaging of tobacco products was to reduce the attractiveness of these products as well as to restrict misleading packaging and labeling. It will also be helpful in eliminating tobacco advertising and promotions. Moreover, graphic health warnings will be used in plain packaging.

GOAL

To make people aware about the ill effects of tobacco and to encourage people to give up this bad habit.

It is celebrated intending to aware and encourage people to reduce or completely stop the tobacco consumption in any form all across the globe. The celebration of this day aims to draw public attention globally to spread the message of harmful effects of tobacco use as well as its complications to others. Variety of global organizations involved in this campaign such as state governments, public health organizations, etc. organize various public awareness programmes locally.

World No Tobacco Day celebration is organized on annual basis by the WHO and its member states including non-governmental and governmental organizations for the people to get aware of all the health issues caused by the tobacco use. Some of the activities which are organized for celebrating the day are public marches, demonstration programmes, big banners, advertising campaigns through educational programmes, direct oral communication with common public to encourage and promote them to stop smoking, organize meetings for involved campaigners, marches, public debates, anti-tobacco activities, public art, health camps, rallies and parades, implementing new laws to restrict the smoking in particular areas and so many effective activities. It has not been declared as a public holiday or official holiday, however, it is celebrated with lots of effective campaigns.

According to the increasing demand of "ban the tobacco use", a resolution was passed by the WHO on 15th of May in 1987 to celebrate an annual event called World No Smoking Day on 7th of April in 1988 which was later changed to be celebrated as World No Tobacco Day on 31st of May in 1989 and further according to another resolution on 17th of May in 1989.

Common people including nongovernmental and governmental organizations become actively involved in the celebration of World No Tobacco Day to draw other people's attention to make them aware of health problems of tobacco use. People use different types of symbols to attract people's mind towards the celebration to actively take part in. Some of the symbols are clean ashtrays with flowers, symbolizing major body organs (like heart, lungs, kidney, etc.) damage from tobacco use, demonstrating no smoking signs, symbolizing death of brain due to smoking, posters display directly or indirectly using internet sites, blogs and other means.

WHO is a main organization which acts as a central hub for organizing World No Tobacco Day all around the world. Award ceremonies are also organized since 1988 by the WHO to encourage organizations or individuals who actively and amazingly contribute to the event in reducing the tobacco consumption. During this award ceremony, special awards and recognition certificates are distributed to the organizations and individuals of any region or country.

OBJECTIVES

- To promote and encourage the common public to reduce or stop the use and consumption of tobacco or its products as it may lead to some lethal diseases.
- To keep constant watch on the companies involved in the sell, purchase or advertisements of tobacco or its products to enhance the consumption of their products.

TIMELINE

WHO has taken many steps in reducing or banning the use of tobacco or its products by establishing an event called World No Tobacco Day and various other health awareness campaigns on world level. Some of the special steps taken by the WHO towards no tobacco use are mentioned below:

- WHO had passed a resolution called WHA40.38 in 1987 to celebrate an event called "World No-smoking Day" on 7th of April in 1988 on its 40th anniversary aiming to request and aware tobacco users all over the world to reduce or quit the use of tobacco.
- WHO had passed another resolution called WHA42.19 in 1988 to celebrate an event called World No Tobacco Day yearly on every 31st of May. It also supports the celebration by organizing various events and tobacco-related themes.
- WHO had established another event called Tobacco Free Initiative (TFI) in 1998 aiming to focus on international resources as well as draw people's attention towards the global health issue of tobacco use. It helps in creating the public health policies globally, encouraging people across societies, etc. for effective tobacco control.
- WHO FCTC is another public health treaty adopted globally in 2003 as an agreement of implementing policies for tobacco cessation.
- WHO had declared ban on tobacco advertisement, sponsorship and promotion on the eve of World No Tobacco Day celebration in 2008 by creating the theme "Tobacco-free youth."

THEMES

Themes of World No Tobacco Day	
1987	"1st Smoke-free Olympics (1988 Olympic Winter Games—Calgary)"
1988	"Tobacco or Health: Choose health"
1989	"Women and tobacco: The female smoker: At added risk"
1990	"Childhood and youth without tobacco: Growing up without tobacco"
1991	"Public places and transport: Better be tobacco free"

Contd...

Themes of World No Tobacco Day

Year	Theme
1992	"Tobacco free workplaces: Safer and healthier"
1993	"Health services: Our windows to a tobacco free world"
1994	"Media and tobacco: Get the message across"
1995	"Tobacco costs more than you think"
1997	"United for a tobacco free world"
1996	"Sport and art without tobacco: Play it tobacco free"
1998	"Growing up without tobacco"
1999	"Leave the pack behind"
2000	"Tobacco kills, do not be duped"
2001	"Second-hand smoke kills"
2002	"Tobacco free sports"
2003	"Tobacco free film, tobacco free fashion"
2004	"Tobacco and poverty, a vicious circle"
2005	"Health professionals against tobacco"
2006	"Tobacco: Deadly in any form or disguise"
2007	"Smoke free inside"
2008	"Tobacco-free youth"
2009	"Tobacco health warnings"
2010	"Gender and tobacco with an emphasis on marketing to women"
2011	"The WHO Framework Convention on Tobacco Control"
2012	"Tobacco industry interference"
2013	"Ban tobacco advertising, promotion and sponsorship"
2014	"Raise taxes on tobacco"
2015	"Stop illicit trade of tobacco products"
2016	"Get ready for plain packaging"
2017	"Tobacco – a threat to development"
2018	"Tobacco breaks heart"
2019	"Tobacco and Lung Health"
2020	"Tobacco and heart disease"

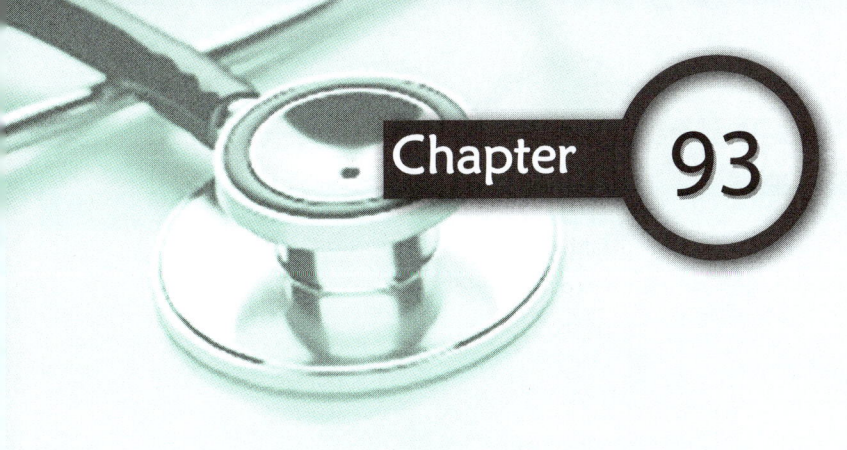

Chapter 93

World Brain Tumor Day

INTRODUCTION

World Brain Tumor Day is observed on 8th of June every year since 2000. This day was first observed by German Brain Tumor Association (Deutsche Hirntumorhilfe eV). This is a non-profit organization which raises public awareness and educates people about brain tumor.

The association created this day to be celebrated so that it would draw attention to the public and this includes the businessmen, politicians, medical and research institutions in the importance of funding the research that is done on brain tumor and the collaboration of interdisciplinary. The aim of doing this is to come up with ways of treatment that are effective and affordable.

ACTIVITIES

- Creating awareness on the type of cancer and this includes the causes, management and the treatment. Awareness will also be made on the signs and symptoms of brain tumor, its facts and advocacy issues that are vital to the brain tumor.
- The people who are suffering from brain tumor are encouraged to join support groups to reduce the stress associated with the illness. The support groups will help in sharing the challenges faced during treatment and provide hope for other people who are suffering from the condition.
- Encourage the patients who are suffering from brain tumor to research on the condition and get to know how to cope with it.
- The day is celebrated in United Kingdom by wearing a hat to show support for the cancer survivors and the ones who have been recently diagnosed with brain tumors.
- There is formation of fund raising campaigns where the money collected is channeled to paying the hospital bills of brain tumor patients as the treatment is very expensive.
- Government of India has introduced National Cancer Control Programme with the objectives of prevention, screening, early detection, diagnosis and treatment including palliative care in end stage.

Chapter 94

World Blood Donor Day

INTRODUCTION

World Blood Donor Day (sometimes referred to as World Blood Donation Day) is observed every year on 14th June. On this day, the countries around the world celebrate World Blood Donor Day as homage to Karl Landsteiner, the Nobel Prize winner, who discovered the ABO blood group. This day is observed to raise the awareness about the need for donating blood. The theme for year 2016 was **"Blood connects us all."** The theme focused on thanking blood donor and highlights the dimension of **"sharing"** and connection between blood donors and patients. The main aim of the campaign to highlight stories of people whose lives have been saved through blood donation, to motivate regular blood donors to continue donating blood, and encourage people in good health who have never given blood to begin doing so, particularly young people. The slogan for year 2016 was adopted as, **"Share life, give blood"** to draw attention to the roles that voluntary donation system plays in encouraging people to care for one another and promote community cohesion.

It was first initiated and established to be celebrated annually on 14th of June by "the World Health Organization, the International Federation of Red Cross and Red Crescent Societies" in the year 2004. World Blood Donor Day was officially established by the WHO with its 192 Member States in the month of May in 2005 at the 58th World Health Assembly in order to motivate all the countries worldwide to thank the blood donors for their precious step, promote voluntary, safe and unpaid blood donations to ensure the sufficient blood supplies.

World Blood Donor Day celebration brings a precious opportunity to all donors for celebrating it on national and global level as well as to commemorate the birth anniversary of the Karl Landsteiner (a great scientist who won the Nobel Prize for his great discovery of the ABO blood group system).

OBJECTIVES

- World Health Organization is aimed to obtain the sufficient blood supplies from the voluntary and unpaid blood donors all over the world by 2020.
- According to the statistics, it has been noted that only 62 countries are getting sufficient blood supplies from the voluntary and unpaid blood donors whereas 40 countries are still dependent for the blood donations on the patient's family member or paid donors. It is celebrated to motivate voluntary blood donors in rest of the countries worldwide.
- To make the blood donation as a precious gift to the receivers and get new life.
- WHO runs this campaign by organizing many activities in all countries highlighting people's stories who need immediate blood donation to continue their heartbeat.

- It is celebrated to thank the voluntary and unpaid blood donors all around the world for saving millions of lives.
- It is celebrated to fulfill the 100% voluntary and unpaid blood donation need worldwide.
- It is celebrated to motivate blood donors for safe blood donation for saving the life of mothers and babies (country's future).
- It is celebrated to reduce the death rates (mortality rate) because of insufficient blood supply. Approximately 800 women are dying off due to malnourished pregnancy, childbirth-related complications, severe bleeding during or after delivery, etc.
- To motivate voluntary blood donors through educational programmes and campaigns in order to strengthen the blood transfusion services.

THEMES

Themes of World Blood Donor Day	
2004	"Safe Blood Starts With Me: Blood Saves Lives"
2005	"Celebrating your gift of blood"
2006	"Commitment to Ensure Universal Access to Safe Blood"
2007	"Safe Blood for Safe Motherhood"
2008	"Giving blood regularly"
2009	"Achieving 100 percent non-remunerated donation of blood and blood components"
2010	"New blood for the World"
2011	"More blood, more life"
2012	"Every blood donor is a hero"
2013	"Give the gift of life: Donate blood"
2014	"Safe blood for saving mothers"
2015	"Thank you for saving my life"
2016	"Blood connects us all"
2017	"Give Blood. Give Now. Give Often"
2018	"Be there for someone else. Give blood"
2019	"Safe blood for all"
2020	"Safe Blood Saves Lives"

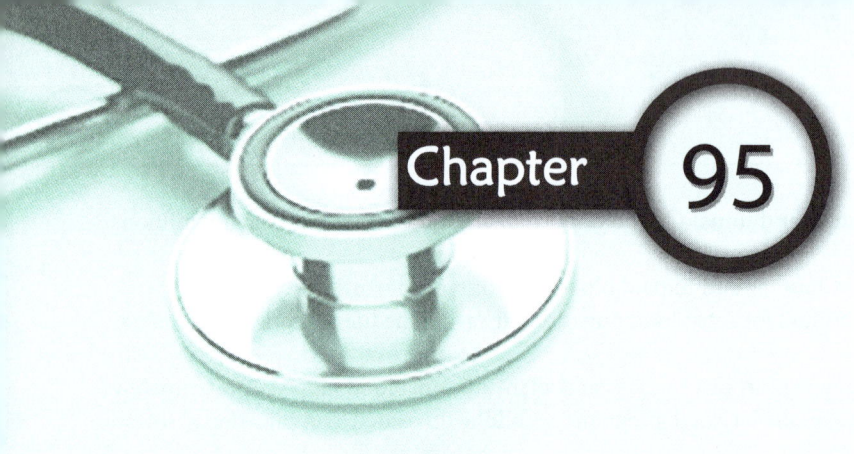

Chapter 95

Autistic Pride Day

INTRODUCTION

Autistic Pride Day is celebrated every year on 18th of June across the world. Autistic pride stands for pride in autism, which spreads the message that people suffering from autism are not diseased but different. Thus, this day acknowledges that autistic people are not sick rather they have a unique set of characteristics.

Autistic Pride Day was first celebrated in 2005 by Aspies for Freedom (AFF), and it quickly became a global event which is still celebrated widely online. AFF modelled the celebration on the gay pride movement. According to Kabie Brook, the co-founder of Autism Rights Group Highland (ARGH), "the most important thing to note about the day is that it is an autistic community event it originated from and is still led by autistic people ourselves."

Autistic pride asserts that autistic people have a unique set of characteristics that provide them many rewards and challenges. Although autism is an expression of neurodiversity, some people promoting autistic pride believe that some of the difficulties that they experience are as the result of societal issues. For instance, according to Gareth Nelson, campaigns to gain funding for autism related organizations promote feelings of pity. Researchers and autistic activists have contributed to a shift in attitudes away from the notion that autism is a deviation from the norm that must be treated or cured, and towards the view that autism is a difference rather than a disability. New Scientist magazine released an article entitled "Autistic and proud" on the first Autistic Pride Day that discussed the idea.

THEMES

Themes of Autistic Pride Day	
2005	Acceptance not cure—main event of 2005 was in Brasília, capital of Brazil.
2006	Celebrate Neurodiversity—main events of 2006 were an Autistic Pride Summer Camp in Germany and an event at the Science works Museum in Melbourne, Australia.
2007	Autistics Speak. It is time to listen
2008–2009	Without a theme
2010	Perspectives, not fear
2011	Recognize, Respect, Include
2012	No theme—main event of 2012 was in Herzliya Park in Israel.

Contd...

Themes of Autistic Pride Day	
2013	No theme—main event of 2013 was in Sacher Park in Jerusalem, Israel.
2015	No theme—main events were in Reading, UK and Hyde Park in London, UK
2016	No theme—main events were in Reading, UK and Hyde Park in London, UK, and Manchester UK
2017	"What color is your pride?"
2018	"The Transition to Adulthood"
2019	"Diversity with infinite variations and infinite possibilities"
2020	"The Transition to Adulthood"

Chapter 96

International Yoga Day

INTRODUCTION

Yoga is an invaluable gift of ancient Indian tradition. It is a spiritual discipline which focuses on bringing harmony between mind and body. The importance of Yoga has been acknowledged by the global community. **June 21** was declared as the International Day of Yoga by the United Nations General Assembly on December 11, 2014. This was declared following an appeal made by Hon'ble Prime Minister of India Shri Narendra Modi in the United Nations General Assembly (UNGA) wherein a resolution was adopted to observe 21st June as the International Day of Yoga (IDY). The Prime Minister stressed the importance of Yoga and its role in disease prevention, health promotion and management of many lifestyle-related disorders. He also announced that there will be an official website (mea.gov.in/idy.htm) to be maintained by the Ministry of External Affairs, Government of India. Further, he inaugurated the Yoga Portal of UNESCO in Paris.

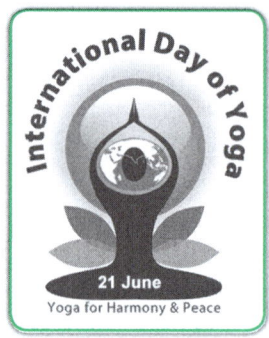

In order to create a great level of consciousness and positive change in the lifestyle of worldwide human population Indian Prime Minister, Mr Narendra Modi has put his views for adopting a day especially for Yoga while addressing to the United Nations General Assembly. He asked the world leaders to adopt International Yoga Day to deal with the declining health because of negative climate changes. Especially, he suggested 21st of June for the adoption of International Day of Yoga as this day is the longest day in Northern Hemisphere regions as well as of great significance for people in many parts of the world.

OBJECTIVES

International Day of Yoga has been adopted to fulfill the following objectives:
- To let people know the amazing and natural benefits of Yoga.
- To connect people to the nature by practicing Yoga.
- To make people get used to of meditation through Yoga.
- To draw attention of people worldwide towards the holistic benefits of Yoga.
- To reduce the rate of health challenging diseases all over the world.
- To bring communities much close together to spend a day for health from busy schedule.
- To enhance growth, development and spread peace all around the world.

- To help people in their bad situations themselves by getting relief from stress through Yoga.
- To strengthen the global coordination among people through Yoga.
- To make people aware of physical and mental diseases and their solutions through practicing Yoga.
- To protect unhealthy practices and promote and respect the good practices to make health better.
- To let people know their rights of good health and healthy lifestyle to completely enjoy the highest standard of physical and mental health.
- To link between protection of health and sustainable health development.
- To win over all the health challenges through regular Yoga practice.
- To promote better mental and physical health of people through Yoga practice.

WORLD YOGA DAY CELEBRATION

The celebration of the event International Day of Yoga is supported by various global leaders. It is celebrated by the people of more than 170 countries including USA, China, Canada, etc. It is celebrated on international level by organizing the activities like Yoga training camps, Yoga competitions and so many activities to enhance the awareness about Yoga benefits among common public all over the world. It is celebrated to let people know that regular Yoga practice leads to the better mental, physical and intellectual health. It positively changes the lifestyle of the people and increases the level of well-being.

All members, observer states, United Nations system organizations, other international organizations, regional organizations, civil society, governmental organizations, non-governmental organizations, and individuals get together to celebrate the International Day of Yoga in suitable manner according to the national priorities to raise the awareness about Yoga.

THEMES

Themes of International Yoga Day	
2015	"Yoga For Harmony And Peace"
2016	"Connect the Youth"
2017	"Yoga health"
2018	"Yoga for peace"
2019	"Yoga with Gurus"
2020	"Yoga for Health - Yoga at Home"

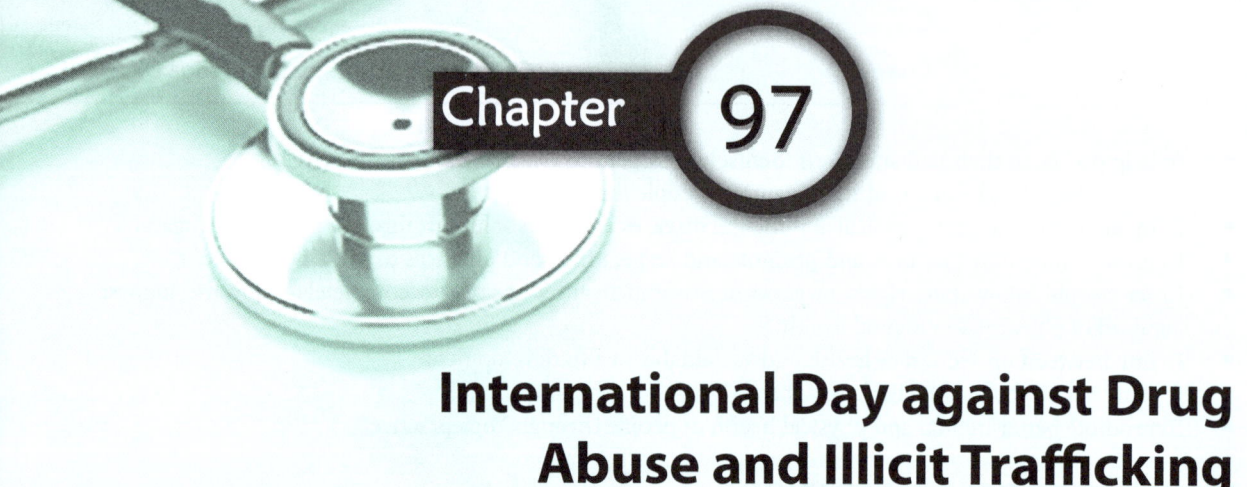

Chapter 97

International Day against Drug Abuse and Illicit Trafficking

INTRODUCTION

International Day against Drug Abuse and Illicit Trafficking is observed on 26th June every year to raise awareness about illicit drug abuse and trafficking. This day was first observed by the UN General Assembly in 1987. According to United Nations statistics, 230 million people worldwide are using drugs. The UN World Drug report 2007 stated that drugs worth around 322 billion US$ are being traded around the world every year. The theme of year 2016 was "Listen first."

'Listen First' is an initiative to increase support for prevention of drug use that is based on science and is thus an effective investment in the well-being of children and youth, their families and their communities. Listening to children and youth is the first step to help them so that they will grow healthy and safe.

According to the United Nations Office on Drugs and Crime (UNODC), nearly 200 million people are using illicit drugs such as cocaine, cannabis, hallucinogens, opiates and sedative hypnotics worldwide. In December 1987, the UN General Assembly decided to observe June 26 as the International Day against Drug Abuse and Illicit Trafficking. The UN was determined to help create an international society free of drug abuse. This resolution recommended further action with regard to the report and conclusions of the 1987 International Conference on Drug Abuse and Illicit Trafficking.

Following the resolution, the years 1991 to 2000 were heralded as the "United Nations Decade Against Drug Abuse." In 1998, the UN General Assembly adopted a political declaration to address the global drug problem. The declaration expresses UN members' commitment to fighting the problem.

Governments, organizations and individuals in many countries, including Vietnam, Borneo and Thailand, have actively participated in promotional events and larger scale activities, such as public rallies and mass media involvement, to promote the awareness of dangers associated with illicit drugs.

The Government of India passed a law in 1988 to prevent Illicit Trafficking in Narcotic Drugs and Psychotropic Substances as a measure to curb the drug haul. But still the drug menace continues widely. It is believed that in Punjab, about 75% of youth are addicted from one or the other form of drug. The use of drugs appears to be increasing in the metros along with alcohol use amongst youth and even women population. The influence of Westernization, changing family structure and peer pressure are some of the reasons behind drug abuse.

THEMES

Themes of International Day against Drug Abuse and Illicit Trafficking	
2000	"Facing reality: Denial, corruption and violence"
2001	"Sports against drugs"
2002	"Substance abuse and HIV/AIDS"
2003	"Let us talk about drugs"
2004	"Drugs: Treatment walks"
2006	"Value yourself make healthy choices"
2007–2009	"Do drugs control your life? Your life Your community No place for drugs"
2010	"Think health not drugs"
2011	"Say no"
2012	"Global action for healthy community without drugs"
2013	"Make health your new high in life not drugs"
2014	"A message of hope: Drug use disorders are preventable and treatable"
2015	"Let's Develop: Our Lives—Our Communities—Our Identities—Without Drugs"
2016	Listen first
2017–2018	"Listening to children and youth is the first step to support and help them so that they grow safe and healthy"
2019	"Health for Justice. Justice for Health"
2020	"Better Knowledge for Better Care"

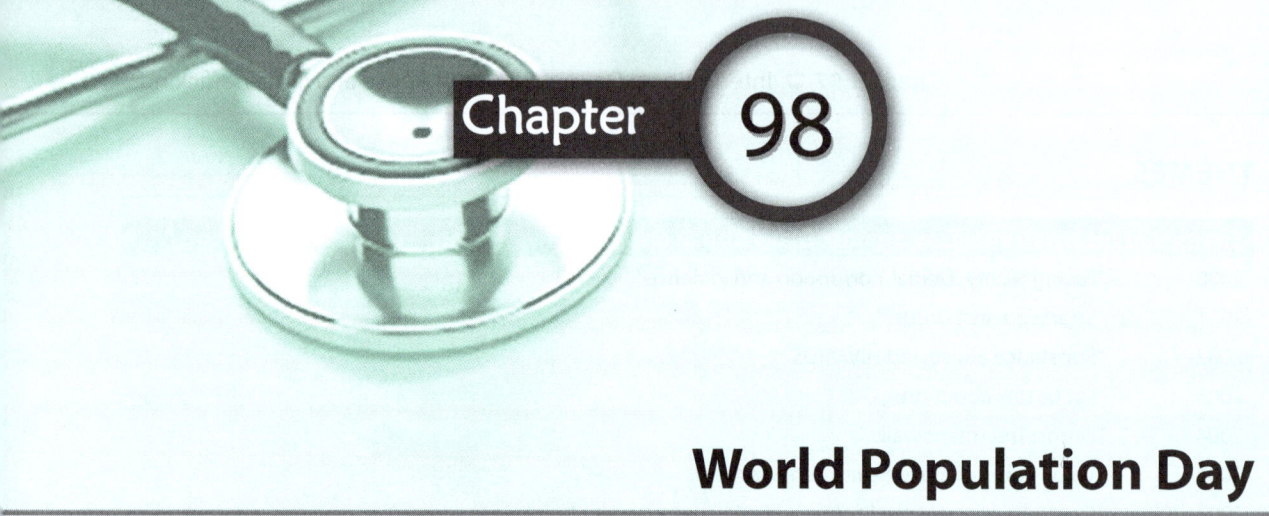

Chapter 98

World Population Day

INTRODUCTION

World Population day is celebrated every year on 11th July to raise awareness about population growth and related issues.

In 1989, the Governing Council of the United Nations Development Programme recommended that 11th July be observed as World Population Day by the international community. Main aim of this day is to focus attention on the urgency and importance of population issues. The theme of 2016 was 'Investing in teenage girls.'

World Population Day is a great event being celebrated all through the world annually on 11th of July. It is celebrated to increase the awareness of the people towards the worldwide population issues. It was first started in the year 1989 by the Governing Council of the United Nations Development Programme (UNDP). It was exalted by the interest of the public when the global population became near about five billion at 11th of July in the year 1987.

The following message "Universal Access to Reproductive Health Services" was distributed worldwide by the theme of 2012th World Population Day celebration when the worldwide population was approximately 7,025,071,966. The big step was taken by the authority for a small and healthy society as well as sustainable future of the people. A crucial investment is made to fulfill the reproductive health care demands and supply. The step was taken for increasing the reproductive health as well as reducing the social poverty by reducing the population.

OBJECTIVES

Objectives of celebrating the world population day are mentioned below:
- It is celebrated to protect and empower youths of both gender like girls and boys.
- To offer them detailed knowledge about the sexuality and delay marriages till they become able to understand their responsibilities.
- Educate youths to avoid unwanted pregnancies by using reasonable and youth-friendly measures.
- Educate people to remove the gender stereotypes from society.
- Educate them about the pregnancy related illnesses to raise the public awareness about dangers of early childbirth.
- Educate them about sexually transmitted diseases (STD) to get prevented from various infections.

- Demand for some effective laws and policies and their implementation in order to protect girl child rights.
- Make sure about the access of equal primary education to both girls and boys.
- Make sure the easy access of reproductive health services everywhere as part of the basic primary health for each couple.

THEMES

Themes of World Population Day	
1996	"Reproductive Health and AIDS"
1997	"Adolescent Reproductive Health Care"
1998	"Approaching the Six Billion"
1999	"Start the Count-up to the Day of Six Billion"
2000	"Saving Women's Lives"
2001	"Population, Environment and Development"
2002	"Poverty, Population and Development"
2003	"1,000,000,000 adolescents"
2004	"ICPD at 10"
2005	"Equality Empowers"
2006	"Being Young is Tough"
2007	"Men at Work"
2008	"Plan Your Family, Plan Your Future"
2009	"Fight Poverty: Educate Girls"
2010	"Be Counted: Say What You Need"
2011	"7 Billion Actions"
2012	"Universal Access to Reproductive Health Services"
2013	"Focus is on Adolescent Pregnancy"
2014	"A time to reflect on population trends and related issues" and "Investing in Young People"
2015	"Vulnerable Populations in Emergencies"
2016	"Investing in teenage girls"
2017	"Family Planning: Empowering People, Developing Nations"
2018	"Family Planning is a Human Right"
2019	"No specific theme
2020	"How to safeguard the health and rights of women and girls now" amid the pandemic

Chapter 99

World Hepatitis Day

INTRODUCTION

World Hepatitis Day is observed on 28th of July every year to spread awareness about hepatitis and encourage people about early diagnosis, prevention and treatment of hepatitis. Hepatitis is a group of infectious diseases known as Hepatitis A, B, C, D and E.

The theme for year 2016 was the global campaign "Elimination."

It is the world level awareness programme launched as a global public health campaign by the World Health Organization to make the world a hepatitis free world.

Earlier it was being celebrated as an International Hepatitis C Awareness day by the patient groups of European and Middle Eastern regions on 1st of October in 2004, however, in some regions it was marked as hepatitis day on different dates. In order to make this the best awareness campaign in 2008, the World Hepatitis Alliance declared 19th of May as the first World Hepatitis Day in association with the patient groups.

However, the date was changed to 28th of July after the adoption of earlier declaration in the 63rd World Health Assembly in the month of May 2010. It was titled as the World Hepatitis Day focusing to raise the awareness on national and international level through great efforts. 28th of July was declared as the final date for the celebration of World Hepatitis Day globally to honor the "Nobel Laureate Baruch Samuel Blumberg" on his birth anniversary (28th of July) as he discovered the hepatitis B virus.

World Hepatitis Day was established to be celebrated on 28th of July in order to expand the educational areas as well as provide opportunities to new generations to get better understandings about viral hepatitis to enhance global public health by solving problems. It is being celebrated very actively in more than 100 countries worldwide by organizing lots of effective activities.

OBJECTIVES

- To provide an opportunity to all focusing together on this issue.
- To raise common public awareness about various forms of the hepatitis including means of transmission.
- To strengthen people by letting them know about different measures like prevention, early diagnosis, screening, control, etc.
- To increase the awareness about hepatitis A and B vaccines.
- To get global response of the people in order to implement some solid steps towards the hepatitis.
- To expand the educational areas for immunization, prevention, diagnosis and control.
- To enhance the awareness about comprehensive care and treatment of people suffering from hepatitis.

- To increase public awareness about the risk factors, remove social stigma and promote for early testing.
- To implement new training methods and number of skilled medical professionals in order to enhance the quality care.
- To promote various health and government organizations worldwide for their active involvement in the event to create new strategies against hepatitis.
- To promote professional staff members to actively participate in the event.

THEMES

Themes of World Hepatitis Day	
2008–2009	"Am I Number 12?"
2010	"This is hepatitis"
2011	"Hepatitis affects everyone, everywhere. Know it. Confront it"
2012	"It's closer than you think"
2013	"More must be done to stop this silent killer"
2014	"Hepatitis: Think Again"
2015	"Prevention of Viral Hepatitis. Act now"
2016	"Prevent Hepatitis: It's up to you"
2017	"Eliminate Hepatitis"
2018	"Find the Missing Millions"
2019	"Invest in eliminating hepatitis"
2020	"Hepatitis Free Future"

2016 was an important year for viral hepatitis. In May, at the World Health Assembly, WHO Member States set to adopt the first ever Elimination Strategy for Viral Hepatitis, with ambitious targets and a goal to eliminate hepatitis as a public health threat by 2030. This was the first time when national governments signed up and commited to the goal of eliminating viral hepatitis.

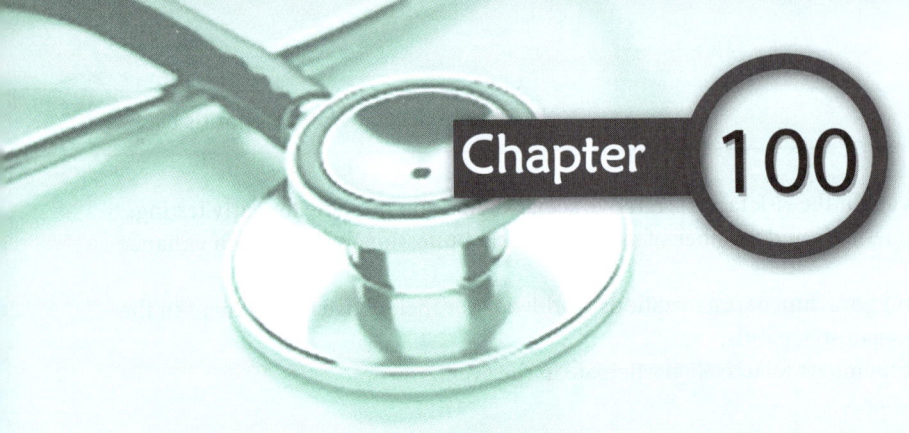

Chapter 100

Oral Rehydration Solution Day

INTRODUCTION

Oral Rehydration Solution (ORS) Day is celebrated every year on 29th July to highlight the importance of ORS as a cost-effective method of health intervention.

Annually July 29 is ORS day. Recognized in 2002 with the award of the Pollen Pediatric Research Prize to Dr Dilip Mahalanabis, Norbert Hirschhorn, David R Nalin, and Nathaniel F Pierce, the day is set aside to raise awareness. When marking the day, people are educated about and encouraged to:

- Recognize symptoms of dehydration.
- Ensure that enough water is taken to prevent dehydration.
- Urinate constantly to rid the body of unwanted waste, toxins and fat.
- Stay healthy by drinking plenty of water, as water is mostly free and good for the body.

According to WHO, diarrheal disease is the second leading cause of death in children under five years old. Diarrhea, which is frequently caused by poor sanitation and hygiene, can have serious, even deadly results, typically as a result of diarrhea-related dehydration. It particularly affects infants, children and old people.

THEMES

Themes of Oral Rehydration Solution Day	
2018	"ORS-ORS all the day keeps Dehydration at Bay"
2019	"The Amrut in Dehydration"

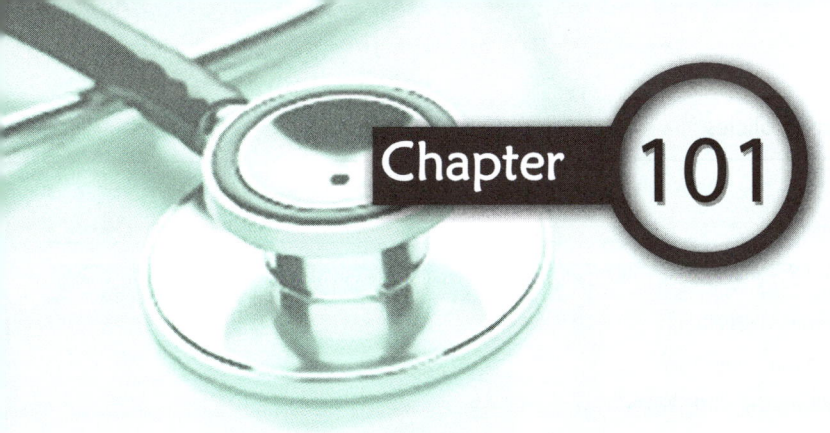

Chapter 101

World Breastfeeding Week

INTRODUCTION

World Breastfeeding Week is celebrated every year in August in more than 170 countries to encourage breastfeeding and improve the health of babies around the world. The theme for the World Breastfeeding Week 2016 was "Breastfeeding: A key to Sustainable Development."

Breastfeeding is organized and promoted worldwide by the World Alliance for Breastfeeding Action (WABA), World Health Organization (WHO) and United Nations International Children's Emergency Fund (UNICEF) to get the goal of elite breastfeeding by mothers for their baby of first 6 months in order to get the incredible health benefits, to fulfill the need of all vital nutrients, to encourage mothers for the healthy growth and development of their child, to guard them from the lethal health problems and diseases including neonatal jaundice, pneumonia, cholera and many more.

It was first started and celebrated by the World Alliance for Breastfeeding Action in the year 1992. And later it is being celebrated in more than 120 countries by the UNICEF, WHO and their participants such as individuals, associations and governments. World Alliance for Breastfeeding Action was also established in the year 1991 on 14th of February to promote the comprehensive breastfeeding culture worldwide by providing the support and achieve the real goal.

AIMS

- To make aware the peer group to support mothers in order to establish and carry on breastfeeding.
- To initiate the breastfeeding supporters to be trained to provide support to mothers and babies in more effective ways.
- To make aware the people to attend and expand the Peer Counseling programmes by letting them know the effective and efficient benefits of the Peer Counseling.
- To call on the governments to get more and worldwide maternity facilities in order to increase the rate and duration of elite breastfeeding.
- To discover the contacts of the neighboring community support so that the breastfeeding mothers can visit them to get help and support after delivery.

THEMES

Themes of World Breastfeeding Day	
1992	"Baby-Friendly Hospital Initiative (BFHI)"
1993	"Mother-Friendly Workplace Initiative (MFWI)"
1994	"Protect Breastfeeding: Making the Code Work"
1995	"Breastfeeding: Empowering Women"
1996	"Breastfeeding: A Community Responsibility"
1997	"Breastfeeding: Nature's Way"
1998	"Breastfeeding: The Best Investment"
1999	"Breastfeeding: Education for Life"
2000	"Breastfeeding: It is Your Right"
2001	"Breastfeeding in the Information Age"
2002	"Breastfeeding: Healthy Mothers and Healthy Babies"
2003	"Breastfeeding in a Globalized World for Peace and Justice"
2004	"Exclusive Breastfeeding: The Gold Standard—Safe, Sound, Sustainable"
2005	"Breastfeeding and Family Foods: Loving and Healthy—Feeding Other Foods While Breastfeeding is Continued"
2006	"Code Watch: 25 Years of Protecting Breastfeeding"
2007	"Breastfeeding: The 1st Hour—Save ONE million babies!"
2008	"Mother Support: Going for the Gold Everyone Wins!"
2009	"Breastfeeding: A Vital Emergency Response"
2010	"Breastfeeding, Just 10 Steps! : The baby friendly way"
2011	"Talk To Me! Breastfeeding: A 3D Experience"
2012	"Understanding the Past, Planning for the Future"
2013	"Breastfeeding Support: Close To Mothers"
2014	"Breastfeeding: A Winning Goal – For Life!"
2015	"Breastfeeding and Work: Let's Make it Work!"
2016	"Breastfeeding"
2017	"Sustaining breastfeeding"
2018	"Breastfeeding foundation of life. Breastfeeding nourishment for life"
2019	"Empower parents, enable breastfeeding: Now and for the future!"
2020	"Support Breastfeeding for a healthier planet"

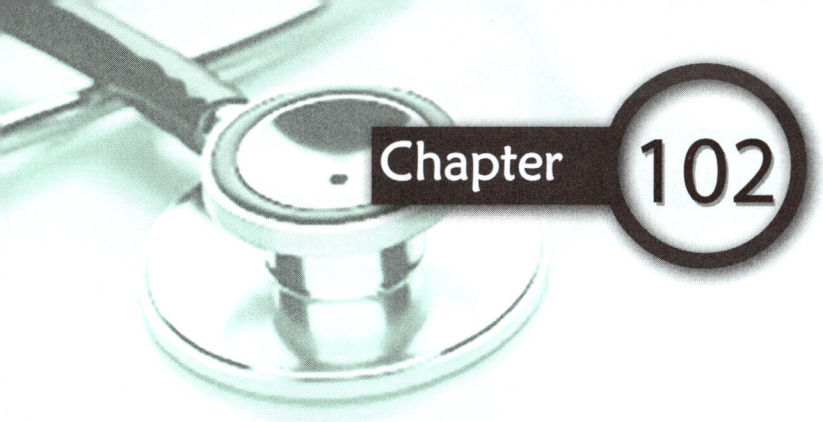

Chapter 102

World Mosquito Day

INTRODUCTION

World Mosquito Day is observed on 20th August every year globally. This day is in commemoration of Sir Ronald Ross, a doctor by profession, who discovered in 1897 that the female mosquitoes transmit malaria amongst humans.

This discovery had laid foundation for scientists across the world to better understand the deadly role of mosquitoes in disease transmission and come up with effective innovative interventions.

World Mosquito Day is celebrated in all parts of the world at a big scale in very innovative specific ways. The doctors and professionals from the domain organize health awareness campaigns in the society. They impart unique ways of handling the malarial infection that can be applied on the patients. Many open free health check-ups and awareness workshops are being organized. People visit them to seek the expert advice and suggestions. Many governments and private hospitals also give their support in the celebrations to make the events grand and successful. They promote it on the internet and get a lot of enquiries. The theme for the year 2020 was "Zero malaria starts with me."

IMPORTANCE OF THE DAY

This day is very important in the life of all human beings. With this World Mosquito Day, we try to achieve a healthy society which is very clean and beautiful. On this day, doctors can come up with new ways of handling the diseases related to the mosquitoes which can be used in more productive ways. It also creates a healthy environment in the society and people get aware of various tools and methods through which they can make them healthy. Therefore, if we celebrate this special day in the most productive way, a better and healthy environment can be achieved.

ACTIVITIES

There are many activities organized on the special World Mosquito Day in all countries and continents. Many hospitals and social agencies come up with health check-up camps. Doctors and practitioners participate in the events to help the patients. Government is also organizing big events where they call different delegates and give them certificates, accolades, prizes, memento, etc. They visit the down-trodden areas and talk to the people about the benefits of cleanliness. College students organize road shows to make people understand the dire effects of malarial parasites on the human body. People consider this as cleaning day and remove all the things from their home that can cause transmission of the disease.

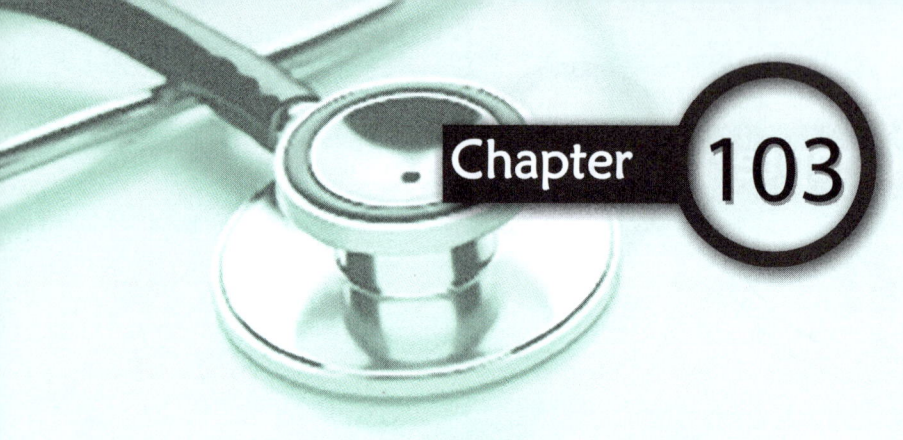

Chapter 103

National Eye Donation Fortnight

INTRODUCTION

The National Eye Donation Fortnight is observed every year from 25th August to 8th September. It is a campaign, which aims to create mass public awareness about the importance of eye donation and to motivate people to pledge their eyes for donation after death.

The day is celebrated in order to promote the eye donation process as well as to put forth the significant message to the people for being a special part of eye donation or eye pledging and giving normal life to the common public. It is organized by the Tiruvallur District Education Department which gets started through the human chain and school children's rally begins from the government school named Perunthalaivar Kamarajar Government Girls High School to the TV Nagar Educational Society School. The children of the school march on the Ambattur roads holding a poster in their hands and stating the benefits of eye donation. They cover a highly crowded area for drawing more attention and interest as well as fine media coverage to distribute their message to all over the world.

The campaign is greatly initiated by Dr Rama Rajagopal (a Deputy Director of Corneal Services from Sankara Nethralaya) through the Suryan FM radio channel on the day of National Eye Donation (8th of September). He spread a real message to the people to drive out the myths of eye donation from their mind and make people aware about the decisive need of eyes to the general public. The message was also published in the popular Tamil periodicals such as the Kumudham Snehidhi, Otunar Osai, etc.

To send the message of campaign to the mass public, members of the CU Shah Eye bank distributed the message (by the help of the popular weekly Tamil magazine named Ananda Vikatan) to the Corporates to increase awareness to a large number of people. Creating the awareness of eye donation to a large number of people may fulfill the critical needs of the eye pledge.

The National Fortnight on Eye Donation is celebrated nationally under the National Programme for Control of Blindness. According to the medical history, it is observed that about 20,000 new cases of blindness are added every year. The majority of blind people are young (due to injuries, infections, deficiency of Vitamin 'A', malnutrition, congenital or other factors) and their eyesight can be restored through corneal transplantation only. So it has become very necessary to educate the people of the society including both young and old to fill the gap between demand and supply of the cornea.

To increase the mass education and awareness, the Regional Institute of Ophthalmology has established a control room where doctors and paramedical staffs provide the detailed information concerning the eye bank.

THEMES

Themes of National Eye Donation Fortnight	
2013	"Motivation for Eye Donation"
2014	"Eye Donation—A Gift of Sight"
2015	"Mission to Vision"
2016	Not declared
2017	"Joy in giving – Donate Eyes"
2018	"Don't Leave a Will, Leave a Vision"
2019	"Light up a Life – Donate Your Eyes"
2020	"Accelerated Laksha Laqshya"

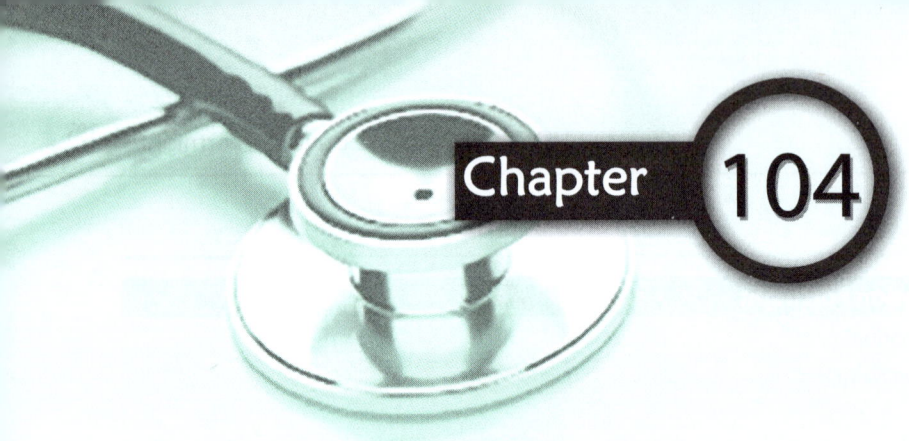

Chapter 104

National Nutrition Week

INTRODUCTION

National Nutrition Week is celebrated every year from 1st September to 7th September. The theme of the National Nutrition Week for 2016 was "Life cycle approach for better Nutrition." The main objective of this campaign is to create awareness on the importance of nutrition for health which has far reaching implications on development, productivity, economic growth and ultimately national development.

AIM

To enhance the nutritional practice awareness among people of the community through the adoptable training, timely education, seminars, different competitions, road shows and many other campaigns towards making a healthy Nation.

The one-week campaign involves one day training, preparing nutritious food with the healthy stuff, an exhibition by the students of Home Science, comment on wheat and soy bean to let them know about their nutritious value, various competitions, nutrition lecture to mothers, road shows and seminars. The National Nutrition Week campaign has a Nutrition Week Kit which is filled with the resources to aid the family to prepare healthy food. The campaign includes the World Food Day and has also added the Nude Food Day since 2010.

The Department of Food Science and Nutrition Management has established a one-day occasion for people to state the nutrition awareness on 8th of September in the year 2010. The campaign includes poster competition, a cooking contest for healthy heart food, counseling for diet, measuring the BMI, lecture on diseases and prevention of the heart and many more.

OBJECTIVES

- To review the frequency of problems through various diets and nutrition in the communities.
- To evaluate the appropriate techniques to prevent and control the nutritional problems through deep research.
- To monitor the condition of the country in terms of diet and nutrition.
- To perform the operational research in order to plan and implement the national nutrition programmes.
- To make aware people through the orientation training about health and nutrition.

HISTORY

The campaign was first started by the central government in the year 1982 in order to encourage the good health and healthy living through the nutrition education as malnutrition is the main obstruction to the National Development. To encourage the people for the same, the Food and Nutrition Board including 43 units (departments of women and child development, health and NGOs) is working all over the country to maneuver the activities.

Lactating mothers are greatly encouraged to feed their newborn baby the first milk known as the colostrum and mother milk for 6 months to provide the newborns a great level of immunity and healthy living. The Indian Dietetic Association from Bengaluru conducts an awareness programme for Nutrition and Diet at Bhagwan Mahaveer Jain Hospital, Millers Road, Bengaluru where the diet for heart disease, diabetes, children and women will also be covered.

ACTIVITIES

- Through the whole week celebration of the National Nutrition Week people are promoted by various nutritional education and training programmes.
- Mass nutrition awareness campaigns are run by the governmental and non-governmental health organizations.
- People are motivated through the distribution of nutrition related educational and training materials.
- People are given proper training for the preservation of nutritious materials like fruits, vegetables and other foods at home.
- Proper training is given to the people about food analysis and standardization.
- Various other National Nutrition Policies are run by the government in order to achieve the goal of National Nutrition Week celebration.

THEMES

Themes of National Nutrition Week	
2011	"Feeding smart from the start"
2012	"Nutrition Awareness – Key to Healthy Nation"
2013	"Project Dinnertime – Cook. Eat. Enjoy"
2014	"Poshak Aahar Desh ka Aadhar"
2015	"Better Nutrition: Key to Development"
2016	"Life cycle approach for better Nutrition"
2017	"Optimal Infant & Young Child Feeding Practices: Better Child Health"
2018	"Go Further with Food"
2019	"Har Ghar Poshan Vyavahar"
2020	"Eat Right, Bite by Bite"

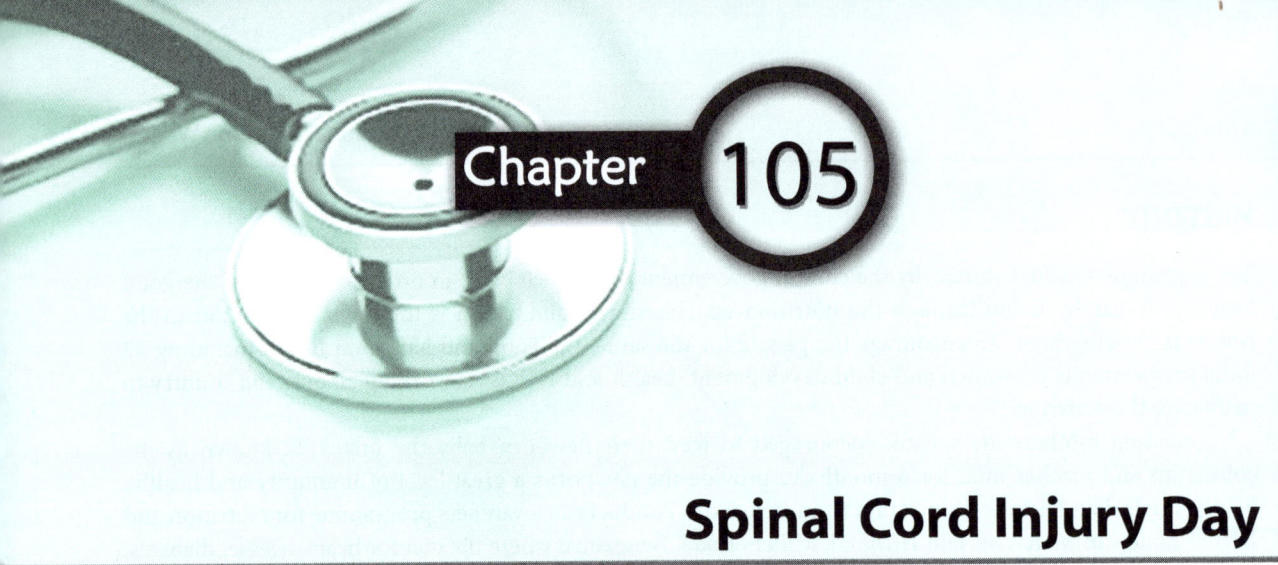

Chapter 105

Spinal Cord Injury Day

INTRODUCTION

International Spinal Cord Society had taken a big step to observe 'Spinal Cord Injury Day' from 2016 onwards. The day is observed every year on 5th September.

OBJECTIVE

To spread awareness on spinal cord injury (SCI)

AIM

To enhance the knowledge on SCI and to make it a matter of attention and effort.

On this day, organizations around the world undertake activities to promote access and inclusion, and eliminate obstacles that people face every day in their efforts to pursue their goals.

International Spinal Cord Society (ISCoS) had decided to observe 5th September as Spinal Cord Injury (SCI) Day, with the intention of increasing awareness amongst general public. The awareness facilitates an inclusive life for persons with disability and ensure success of prevention programmes.

On the 'Spinal Cord Injury Day', Spinal Cord Society (SCS) along with Association of Spine Surgeons of India (ASSI), Indian Orthopedic Association (IOA), Indian Association of Physical Medicine and Rehabilitation (IAPMR), Indian Academy of Neurology (IAN), Asian Spinal Cord Network (ASCoN), Indian Spinal Injuries Center (ISIC) and The Spinal Foundation (TSF) carry out the different activities.

ACTIVITIES

- A press release was issued by ISCoS and all affiliated as well as related Societies at least two weeks before the SCI day. ISCoS circulated a draft press release which various societies modified and translated to suit regional requirements. A press conference was held by the societies before 5th September (one week before the day).
- A slogan along with a logo for the SCI Day has been adopted by ISCoS and affiliated societies. The slogan and logo appear prominently on the website of ISCoS and all societies as well as on all correspondences of the officials and members including the press release. The slogan is translated by various societies in the local language.

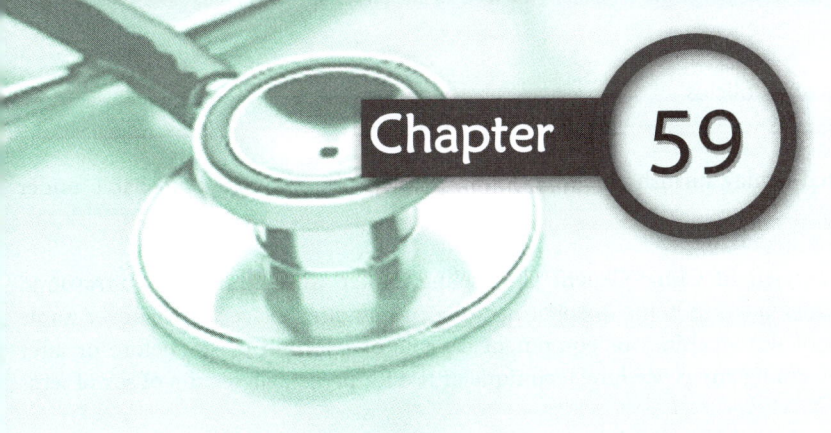

Chapter 59

National Blood Policy

INTRODUCTION

The policy aims to ensure easily accessible and adequate supply of safe and quality blood and blood components collected/procured from a voluntary, non-remunerated regular blood donor in well-equipped premises, which is free from transfusion transmitted infections, and is stored and transported under optimum conditions. Transfusion under supervision of trained personnel for all who need it irrespective of their economic or social status through comprehensive, efficient and a total quality management approach will be ensured under the policy.

OBJECTIVES

To achieve the above aim, the following objectives are drawn:

- To reiterate firmly the government commitment to provide safe and adequate quantity of blood, blood components and blood products.
- To make available adequate resources to develop and reorganize the blood transfusion services in the entire country.
- To make latest technology available for operating the blood transfusion services and ensure its functioning in an updated manner.
- To launch extensive awareness programmes for donor information, education, motivation, recruitment and retention in order to ensure adequate availability of safe blood.
- To encourage appropriate clinical use of blood and blood products.
- To strengthen the manpower through human resource development.
- To encourage research and development in the field of transfusion medicine and related technology.
- To take adequate regulatory and legislative steps for monitoring and evaluation of blood transfusion services and to take steps to eliminate profiteering in blood banks.

STRATEGIES

To reiterate firmly the government commitment to provide safe and adequate quantity of blood, blood components and blood products.

- A national blood transfusion programme shall be developed to ensure establishment of non-profit integrated national and state blood transfusion services in the country.

is reason to believe that it may furnish evidence of commission of an offence punishable under the Act.

Explanation—In these Rules—'

- 'Genetic Laboratory/Genetic Clinic/Genetic Counseling Center' would include an ultrasound center/imaging center/nursing home/hospital/institute or any other place, by whatever name called, where any of the machines or equipment capable of selection of sex before or after conception or performing any procedure, technique or test for prenatal detection of sex of fetus is used
- 'material object' would include records, machines and equipment
- 'seize' and 'seizure' would include 'seal' and 'sealing' respectively.

(2) A list of any document, record, register, book, pamphlet, advertisement or any other material object found in the Genetic Counseling Center, Genetic Laboratory, Genetic Clinic, Ultrasound Clinic or Imaging Center and seized shall be prepared in duplicate at the place of effecting the seizure. Both copies of such list shall be signed on every page by the Appropriate Authority or the officer authorized in this behalf and by the witnesses to the seizure:

Provided that the list may be prepared, in the presence of the witnesses, at a place other than the place of seizure if, for reasons to be recorded in writing, it is not practicable to make the list at the place of effecting the seizure.

(3) One copy of the list referred to in sub-rule (2) shall be handed over, under acknowledgement, to the person from whose custody the document, record, register, book, pamphlet, advertisement or any other material object have been seized:

Provided that a copy of the list of such document, record, register, book, pamphlet, advertisement or other material object seized may be delivered under acknowledgement, or sent by registered post to the owner or manager of the Genetic Counseling Center, Genetic Laboratory, Genetic Clinic, Ultrasound Clinic or Imaging Center, if no person acknowledging custody of the document, record, register, book, pamphlet, advertisement or other material object seized is available at the place of effecting the seizure.

(4) If any material object seized is perishable in nature, the Appropriate Authority, or the officer authorized in this behalf shall make arrangements promptly for sealing, identification and preservation of the material object and also convey it to a facility for analysis or test, if analysis or test be required:

Provided that the refrigerator or other equipment used by the Genetic Counseling Center, Genetic Laboratory, Genetic Clinic, Ultrasound Clinic and Imaging Center for preserving such perishable material object may be sealed until such time as arrangements can be made for safe removal of such perishable material object and in such eventuality, mention of keeping the material object seized, on the premises of the Genetic Counseling Center, Genetic Laboratory, Genetic Clinic, Ultrasound Clinic or Imaging Center shall be made in the list of seizure.

(5) In the case of noncompletion of search and seizure operation, the Appropriate Authority or the officer authorized in this behalf may make arrangement, by way of mounting a guard or sealing of the premises of the Genetic Counseling Center, Genetic Laboratory, Genetic Clinic Ultrasound Clinic or Imaging Center, for safe keeping, listing and removal of documents, records, book or any other material object to be seized, and to prevent any tampering with such documents, records, books or any other material object.

13. **Intimation of changes in employees, place or equipment**—Every Genetic Counseling Center, Genetic Laboratory, Genetic Clinic, Ultrasound Clinic and Imaging Center shall intimate every change of employee, place, address and equipment installed, to the Appropriate Authority within a period of 30 days of such change.

14. Conditions for analysis or test and prenatal diagnostic procedures—
  (1) No Genetic Laboratory shall accept for analysis or test any sample, unless referred to it by a Genetic Clinic.
  (2) Every prenatal diagnostic procedure shall invariably be immediately preceded by locating the fetus and placenta through ultrasonography, and the prenatal diagnostic procedure shall be done under direct ultrasonography monitoring so as to prevent any damage to the fetus and placenta.

15. Meetings of the Advisory Committees—The intervening period between any two meetings of Advisory Committees constituted under sub-section (5) of Section 17 to advise the Appropriate Authority shall not exceed 60 days.

16. Allowances to members of the Central Supervisory Board—
  (1) The ex-officio members, and other Central and State Government officers appointed to the Board will be entitled to Travelling Allowance and Daily Allowance for attending the meetings of the Board as per the Travelling Allowance rules applicable to them.
  (2) The nonofficial members appointed to, and Members of Parliament elected to the Board will be entitled to Travelling Allowance and Daily Allowance for attending the meetings of the Board as admissible to non-official and Members of Parliament as the case may be, under the Travelling Allowances rules of the Central Government.

17. Public Information—
  (1) Every Genetic Counseling Center, Genetic Laboratory, Genetic Clinic, Ultrasound Clinic and Imaging Center shall prominently display on its premises a notice in English and in the local language or languages for the information of the public, to effect that disclosure of the sex of the fetus is prohibited under law.
  (2) At least one copy each of the Act and these rules shall be available on the premises of every Genetic Counseling Center, Genetic Laboratory, Genetic Clinic, Ultrasound Clinic and Imaging Center, and shall be made available to the clientele on demand for perusal.
  (3) The Appropriate Authority, the Central Government, the State Government, and the Government/Administration of the Union Territory may publish periodically lists of registered Genetic Counseling Centers, Genetic Laboratories, Genetic Clinics, Ultrasound Clinics and Imaging Centers and findings from the reports and other information in their possession, for the information of the public and for use by the experts in the field.

18. Code of Conduct to be observed by persons working at Genetic Counseling Centers, Genetic Laboratories, Genetic Clinics, Ultrasound Clinics, Imaging Centers, etc.—All persons including the owner, employee or any other person associated with Genetic Counseling Centers, Genetic Laboratories, Genetic Clinics, Ultrasound Clinics, Imaging Centers registered under the Act/these Rules shall:
  (i) not conduct or associate with, or help in carrying out detection or disclosure of sex of fetus in any manner
  (ii) not employ or cause to be employed any person not possessing qualifications necessary for carrying out prenatal diagnostic techniques/procedures and tests including ultrasonography
  (iii) not conduct or cause to be conducted or aid in conducting by himself or through any other person any techniques or procedure for selection of sex before or after conception or for detection of sex of fetus except for the purposes specified in sub-section (2) of Section 4 of the Act
  (iv) not conduct or cause to be conducted or aid in conducting by himself or through any other person any techniques or test or procedure under the Act at a place other than a place registered under the Act/the Rules
  (v) ensure that no provision of the Act and these Rules are violated in any manner

- To take appropriate decisions and/or introduction of policy initiatives on the basis of factual information, operational research on various aspects such as various aspects of transfusion transmissible diseases, knowledge, attitude and practices (KAP) among donors, clinical use of blood, need assessment, etc. shall be promoted.
- Computer-based information and management systems shall be developed which can be used by all the centers regularly to facilitate networking.

To take adequate regulatory and legislative steps for monitoring and evaluation of blood transfusion services and to take steps to eliminate profiteering in blood banks.

- For grant/renewal of blood bank licenses including plan of a blood bank, a committee, comprising members from State/UT Blood Transfusion Councils including transfusion medicine expert, central and State/UT FDAs shall be constituted which will scrutinize all applications as per the guidelines provided by Drugs Controller General (India).
- Fresh licenses to stand-alone blood banks in private sector shall not be granted. Renewal of such blood banks shall be subjected to thorough scrutiny and shall not be renewed in case of noncompliance of any condition of license.
- A separate blood bank cell shall be created under a senior officer not below the rank of DDC(I) in the office of the DC(I) at the headquarter.
- As a deterrent to paid blood donors who operate in the disguise of replacement donors, institutions who prescribe blood for transfusion shall be made responsible for procurement of blood for their patients through their affiliation with licensed blood centers.
- States/UTs shall enact rules for registration of nursing homes wherein provisions for affiliation with a licensed blood bank for procurement of blood for their patients shall be incorporated.

AVAILABILITY OF DRUGS AND MEDICAL DEVICES

The policy accords special focus on production of Active Pharmaceutical Ingredient (API) which is the backbone of the generic formulations industry. Recognizing that over 70% of the medical devices and equipment are imported in India, the policy advocates the need to incentivize local manufacturing to provide customized indigenous products for Indian population in the long run. The goal with respect to medical devices shall be to encourage domestic production in consonance with the 'Make in India' national agenda. Medical technology and medical devices have a multiplier effect in the costing of healthcare delivery. The policy recognizes the need to regulate the use of medical devices so as to ensure safety and quality compliance as per the standard norms.

ALIGNING OTHER POLICIES FOR MEDICAL DEVICES AND EQUIPMENT WITH PUBLIC HEALTH GOALS

For medical devices and equipment, the policy recommends and prioritizes establishing sufficient labeling and packaging requirements on part of industry, adequate medical devices, testing facility and effective port—clearance mechanisms for medical products.

IMPROVING PUBLIC SECTOR CAPACITY FOR MANUFACTURING ESSENTIAL DRUGS AND VACCINES

Public sector capacity in manufacture of certain essential drugs and vaccines is also essential in the long-term for the health security of the country and to address some needs which are not attractive commercial propositions. These public institutions need more investment, appropriate HR policies and governance initiatives to enable them to become comparable with their benchmarks in the developed world.

ANTIMICROBIAL RESISTANCE

The problem of antimicrobial resistance calls for a rapid standardization of guidelines, regarding antibiotic use, limiting the use of antibiotics as Over-the-Counter medication, banning or restricting the use of antibiotics as growth promoters in animal livestock. Pharmacovigilance including prescription audit inclusive of antibiotic usage, in the hospital and community, is a must in order to enforce change in existing practices.

HEALTH TECHNOLOGY ASSESSMENT

Health Technology assessment is required to ensure that technology choice is participatory and is guided by considerations of scientific evidence, safety, consideration on cost-effectiveness and social values. The National Health Policy commits to the development of institutional framework and capacity for Health Technology Assessment and adoption.

DIGITAL HEALTH TECHNOLOGY ECOSYSTEM

Recognizing the integral role of technology (eHealth, mHealth, Cloud, Internet of things, wearable, etc.) in the healthcare delivery, a National Digital Health Authority (NDHA) will be set up to regulate, develop and deploy digital health across the continuum of care. The policy advocates extensive deployment of digital tools for improving the efficiency and outcome of the healthcare system. The policy aims at an integrated health

    (f)   Equipment for dry and wet sterilization.

    (g)   Equipment for carrying out emergency procedures such as evacuation of uterus or resuscitation in case of need.

    (h)   Genetic works station.

3A. **Sale of ultrasound machines/imaging machines—**

(1) No organization including a commercial organization or a person, including manufacturer, importer, dealer or supplier of ultrasound machines/imaging machines or any other equipment, capable of detecting sex of fetus, shall sell, distribute, supply, rent, allow or authorize the use of any such machine or equipment in any manner, whether on payment or otherwise, to any Genetic Counseling Center, Genetic Laboratory, Genetic Clinic, Ultrasound Clinic, Imaging Center or any other body or person unless such Center, Laboratory, Clinic, body or person is registered under the Act.

(2) The provider of such machine/equipment to any person/body registered under the Act shall send to the concerned State/UT Appropriate Authority and to the Central Government, once in three months a list of those to whom the machine/equipment has been provided.

(3) Any organization or person, including manufacturer, importer, dealer or supplier of ultrasound machines/imaging machines or any other equipment capable of detecting sex of fetus selling, distributing, supplying or authorizing in any manner, the use of any such machine or equipment to any Genetic Counseling Center, Genetic Laboratory, Genetic Clinic, Ultrasound Clinic, Imaging Center or any other body or person registered under the Act shall take an affidavit from such body or person purchasing or getting authorization for using such machine/equipment that the machine/equipment shall not be used for detection of sex of fetus or selection of sex before or after conception.

4.   **Registration of Genetic Counseling Center, Genetic Laboratory and Genetic Clinic—**

(1) An application for registration shall be made to the Appropriate Authority, in duplicate, in Form A, duly accompanied by an Affidavit containing—

    (i)   an undertaking to the effect that the *Genetic Center/Laboratory/Clinic/Ultrasound Clinic/Imaging Center*/combination thereof, as the case may be, shall not conduct any test or procedure, by whatever name called, for selection of sex before or after conception or for detection of sex of fetus except for diseases specified in Section 4(2) nor shall the sex of fetus be disclosed to anybody; and

    (ii) an undertaking to the effect that the *Genetic Center/Laboratory/Clinic*/combination thereof, as the case may be, shall display prominently a notice that they do not conduct any technique, test or procedure, etc. By whatever name called, for detection of sex of fetus or for selection of sex before or after conception.

(2) The Appropriate Authority, or any person in his office authorized in this behalf, shall acknowledge receipt of the application for registration, in the acknowledgement slip provided at the bottom of Form A, immediately if delivered at the office of the Appropriate Authority, or not later than the next working day if received by post.

5.   **Application Fee—**

(1) Every application for registration under rule 4 shall be accompanied by an application fee of:

    (a)   ₹3000/- for Genetic Counseling Center, Genetic Laboratory, Genetic Clinic, Ultrasound Clinic or Imaging Center.

    (b)   ₹4000/- for an institute, hospital, nursing home, or any place providing jointly the service of a Genetic Counseling Center, Genetic Laboratory and Genetic Clinic, Ultrasound Clinic or Imaging Center or any combination thereof.

Provided that if an application for registration of any Genetic Clinic/Laboratory/Center, etc. has been rejected by the Appropriate Authority, no fee shall be required to be paid on re-submission of the application by the applicant for the same body within 90 days of rejection. Provided further that any subsequent application shall be accompanied with the prescribed fee. Application fee once paid will not be refunded.

(2) The application fee shall be paid by a demand draft drawn in favor of the Appropriate Authority, on any scheduled bank payable at the headquarters of the Appropriate Authority concerned. The fees collected by the Appropriate Authority for registration of Genetic Counseling Center, Genetic Laboratory, Genetic Clinic, Ultrasound Clinic and Imaging Center or any other body or person under sub-rule (1), shall be deposited by the Appropriate Authority concerned in a bank account opened in the name of the official designation of the Appropriate Authority concerned and shall be utilized by the Appropriate Authority in connection with the activities connected with implementation of the provisions of the Act and these rules.

6.   **Certificate of registration—**

(1) The Appropriate Authority shall, after making such enquiry and after satisfying itself that the applicant has complied with all the requirements, place the application before the Advisory Committee for its advice.

(2) Having regard to the advice of the Advisory Committee the Appropriate Authority shall grant a certificate of registration, in duplicate, in Form B to the applicant. One copy of the certificate of registration shall be displayed by the registered Genetic Counseling Center, Genetic Laboratory, Genetic Clinic, Ultrasound Clinic or Imaging Center at a conspicuous place at its place of business: Provided that the Appropriate Authority may grant a certificate of registration to a Genetic Laboratory or a Genetic Clinic, Ultrasound Clinic or Imaging Center to conduct one or more specified prenatal diagnostic tests or procedures, depending on the availability of place, equipment and qualified employees, and standards maintained by such laboratory or clinic.

(3) If, after enquiry and after giving an opportunity of being heard to the applicant and having regard to the advice of the Advisory Committee, the Appropriate Authority is satisfied that the applicant has not complied with the requirements of the Act and these rules, it shall, for the reasons to be recorded in writing, reject the application for registration and communicate such rejection to the applicant as specified in Form C.

(4) An enquiry under sub-rule (1), including inspection at the premises of the Genetic Counseling Center, Genetic Laboratory, Genetic Clinic, Ultrasound Clinic or Imaging Center, shall, be carried out only after due notice is given to the applicant by the Appropriate Authority.

(5) Grant of certificate of registration or rejection of application for registration shall be communicated to the applicant as specified in Form B or Form C, as the case may be, within a period of 90 days from the date of receipt of application for registration.

(6) The certificate of registration shall be non-transferable. In the event of change of ownership or change of management or on ceasing to function as a Genetic Counseling Center, Genetic Laboratory, Genetic Clinic, Ultrasound Clinic or Imaging Center, both copies, of the certificate of registration shall be surrendered to the Appropriate Authority.

(7) In the event of change of ownership or change of management of the Genetic Counseling Center, Genetic Laboratory, Genetic Clinic, Ultrasound Clinic or Imaging Center, the new owner or manager of such Center, Laboratory or Clinic shall apply afresh for grant of certificate of registration.

7.   **Validity of registration—**Every certificate of registration shall be valid for a period of 5 years from the date of its issue.

Role of Panchayati Raj Institutions

Panchayati Raj Institutions would be strengthened to play an enhanced role at different levels for health governance, including the social determinants of health. There is need to make Community-Based Monitoring and Planning (CBMP) mandatory, so as to place people at the center of the health system and development process for effective monitoring of quality of services and for better accountability in management and delivery of health care services.

Improving Accountability

The policy would be to increase both horizontal and vertical accountability of the health system by providing a greater role and participation of local bodies and encouraging community monitoring, programme evaluations along with ensuring grievance redressal systems.

LEGAL FRAMEWORK FOR HEALTH CARE AND HEALTH PATHWAY

One of the fundamental policy questions being raised in recent years is whether to pass a health rights bill making health a fundamental right—in the way that was done for education. The policy question is whether we have reached the level of economic and health systems development so as to make this a justiciable right—implying that its denial is an offense. Questions that need to be addressed are manifold, namely, (a) whether when health care is a State subject, is it desirable or useful to make a Central law, (b) whether such a law should mainly focus on the enforcement of public health standards on water, sanitation, food safety, air pollution, etc., or whether it should focus on health rights—access to health care and quality of health care—i.e., whether focus should be on what the State enforces on citizens or on what the citizen demands of the State? Right to healthcare covers a wide canvas, encompassing issues of preventive, curative, rehabilitative and palliative healthcare across rural and urban areas, infrastructure availability, health human resource availability, as also issues extending beyond health sector into the domain of poverty, equity, literacy, sanitation, nutrition, drinking water availability, etc. Excellent health care system needs to be in place to ensure effective implementation of the health rights at the grassroots level. Right to health cannot be perceived unless the basic health infrastructure like doctor-patient ratio, patient-bed ratio, nurses-patient ratio, etc. are near or above threshold levels and uniformly spread-out across the geographical frontiers of the country. Further, the procedural guidelines, common regulatory platform for public and private sector, standard treatment protocols, etc. need to be put in place. Accordingly, the management, administrative and overall governance structure in the health system needs to be overhauled. Additionally, the responsibilities and liabilities of the providers, insurers, clients, regulators and Government in administering the right to health need to be clearly spelt out. The policy while supporting the need for moving in the direction of a rights-based approach to healthcare is conscious of the fact that threshold levels of finances and infrastructure is a precondition for an enabling environment, to ensure that the poorest of the poor stand to gain the maximum and are not embroiled in legalities. The policy therefore advocates a progressively incremental assurance-based approach, with assured funding to create an enabling environment for realizing health care as a right in the future.

IMPLEMENTATION OF FRAMEWORK AND WAY FORWARD

A policy is only as good as its implementation. The National Health Policy envisages that an implementation framework be put in place to deliver on these policy commitments. Such an implementation framework would provide a roadmap with clear deliverables and milestones to achieve the goals of the policy.

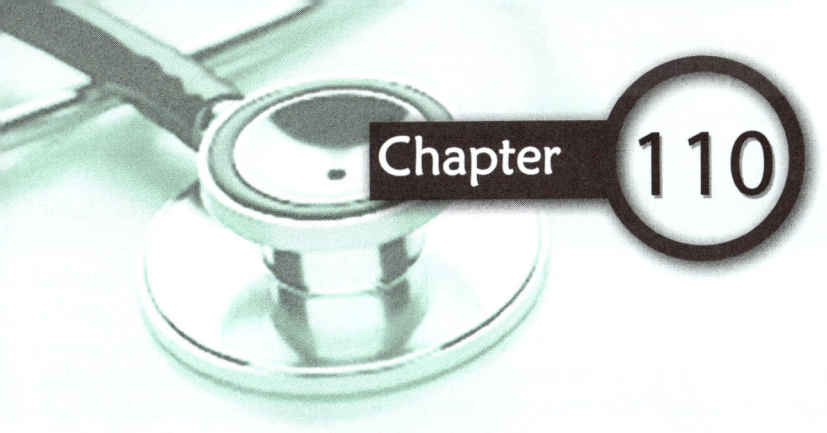

Chapter 110

World Heart Day

INTRODUCTION

- The World Heart Day is observed on 29th September, annually to create healthy heart environment.
- The theme of the World Heart Day 2016 was "Power Your Life".

  World Heart Day is a campaign established to spread awareness about the health of heart among common people throughout the world. This initiative was founded in the year 2000 to inform people to take care of their heart. A huge percentage of common public in the society is suffering from the heart diseases like stroke, heart attack, heart failure, etc. Heart problems are the leading causes of death in the world.

  A particular theme is decided for each year celebration in order to focus on the main subject and make it effective. The theme is prepared by keeping in mind the key issues of heart health. According to the World Heart Federation, at least 80% of the premature deaths (because of cardiovascular diseases) can be protected by controlling four main risk factors such as unhealthy diet, tobacco use, lack of physical activity and use of alcohol.

  The heart related problems and deaths can be solved by the active involvement of the common public through the campaign of World Heart Day. Various governmental and private organizations including NGOs all around the world are working to spread the awareness of CVD (cardiovascular disease—the world's number one killer).

HISTORY

World Heart Day was celebrated every year on the last Sunday of September since the year it was established till 2010. It is an effective event established in 2000 and organized every year by the World Heart Federation since 2000. Since the year 2011, the day is celebrated annually on 29th of September (means no longer on last Sunday of the month). World Heart Federation and its members actively involve in the celebration in order to spread the news about premature deaths from heart diseases and its risk factors (tobacco intake, lack of physical exercise, unhealthy diet and alcohol intake) to the common public. There are many collaborators of the World Heart Federation in this campaign including several major international non-profits (Indian Heart Association). Through this campaign, several effective preventative measures are promoted in order to reduce the risk of cardiovascular diseases.

World Heart Day is celebrated all across the world to reduce the number of deaths because of cardiovascular diseases worldwide. It is an international campaign to spread awareness among common public to save them and motivate to live with healthy heart. According to the WHO, cardiovascular diseases are the reason of around 30% deaths of all global deaths. Some of the most dangerous risk factors leading to the heart disease and stroke are high blood pressure, high level of bad cholesterol, increased glucose level, smoking habit, inadequate intake of healthy diet and fruit and vegetables, increased weight, and obesity.

World Heart Day is an effective way established by the World Heart Federation to aware people around the globe that heart ailments are the leading cause of death. World Heart Federation, in collaboration with the WHO, spreads important news about heart diseases and main risk factors to the public worldwide. It motivates people to get participated and take some knowledge, go through the proper heart check-ups, and follow other control measures all through the life. It is a perfect day when many people do promises to themselves to quit smoking, get involved in daily physical activities, start eating healthy diet, etc. in order to keep their heart in good working order.

It is a day when people realize about overeating, unhealthy diets, lack of exercises, bad lifestyle, etc. causing heart ailments. It brings some hope to people that heart problems can be prevented and controlled for whole life by following healthy lifestyle.

AIM

To improve global heart health by encouraging people for lifestyle changes and gain knowledge about ways to be good to the heart.

There is a target by WHO to reduce noncommunicable disease mortality rate by 2025 by reducing the premature deaths because of cardiovascular disease.

THEMES

Themes of World Heart Day	
2000	"I Love my Heart: Let it beat!"
2001	"A Heart for Life"
2002	"What Shape are you in?"
2003	"Women, Heart Disease and Stroke"
2004	"Children, Adolescents and Heart Disease"
2005	"Healthy Weight, Healthy Shape"
2006	"How Young is Your Heart?"
2007	"Team Up for Healthy Hearts!"
2008	"Know Your Risk"
2010–2009	"I Work with Heart"
2012–2011	"One World, One Heart, One Home"
2013	"Take the road to a healthy heart"
2014	"Heart Choices NOT Hard Choices"
2015	"Creating Heart-Healthy Environments"
2016	"Power your life"
2017	"Share the power"
2018	"My Heart, Your Heart"
2019	"Power your Life"
2020	"Use Heart To Beat Cardiovascular Disease"

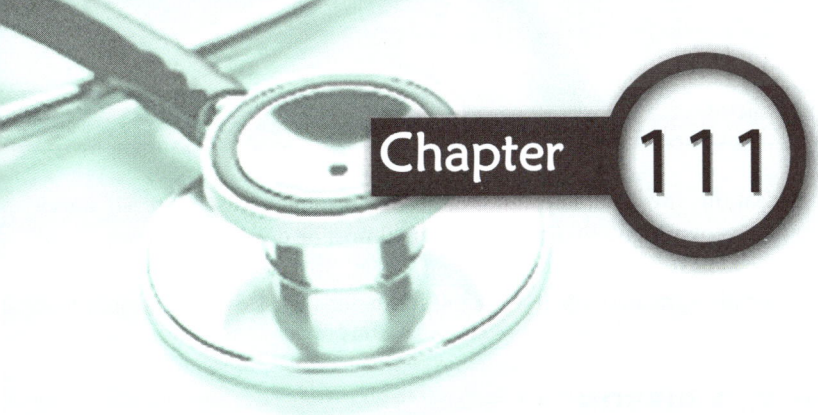

Chapter 111

Breast Cancer Awareness Month

INTRODUCTION

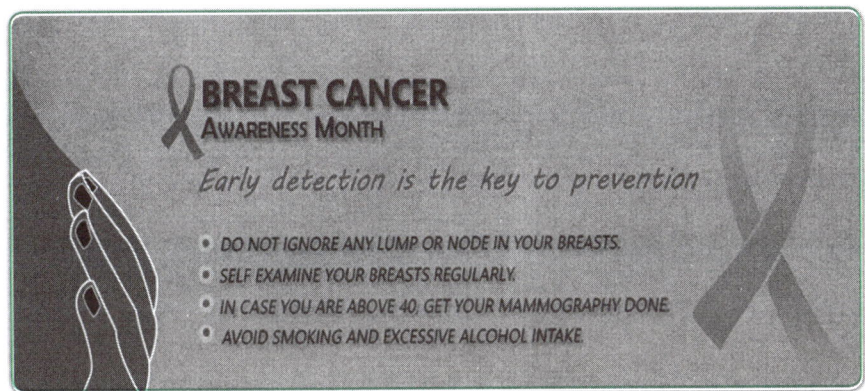

October is breast cancer awareness month, an annual campaign, to educate people about breast cancer. Breast cancer is the most prevalent form of cancer. This disease has become a major problem all across the world including India. Breast Cancer Awareness Month 2020 had the theme "Early detection can save lives." In 2019 it was celebrated under the theme 'Give Hope. Save Lives' and 2021 there is "Together, all our actions matter."

AIM

To get as many people as possible involved in raising awareness and funds for breast cancer research.

THE FIRST EVENT

In 1985, the first Breast Cancer Awareness Month (BCAM) was observed in the United States. In the US, this event is referred to as National Breast Cancer Awareness Month (NBCAM).

The US National Breast Cancer Awareness Month Website went online in 1998, and lists the organizations which are on the board of sponsors for this event. Over the years, the focus of this event has widened. A number of organizations based in the US and in other countries now support this international health awareness event.

Given the large number of organizations involved, and the huge sums of money raised, breast cancer awareness has grown into an industry in its own right; this campaign can almost be described as a year-long event.

Today, Breast Cancer Awareness Month is as much about raising funds for breast cancer research and support, as it is about raising awareness.

THE COLOR PINK AND THE PINK RIBBON

With the founding of The Breast Cancer Research Foundation in 1993, the pink ribbon, which had previously been used to symbolize breast cancer, was chosen as the symbol for breast cancer awareness.

The color pink itself, at times, has been used to striking effect in raising breast cancer awareness. Many famous buildings and landmarks across the globe have been illuminated in pink light during this event; Sydney's Harbor Bridge, Japan's Tokyo Tower and Canada's Niagara Falls to name a few.

Due to the success of this awareness event, for many people, the color pink and breast cancer awareness ribbons are now associated with breast cancer awareness.

ACTIVITIES

To sustain momentum of this awareness campaign and gather maximum support, daily events and activities are often held throughout the month of October. For example, a company may designate a day as 'Pink Day' in which employees wear pink at work.

The numerous awareness activities which take place may include sponsored walks, golf events, seminars and breast cancer screening days.

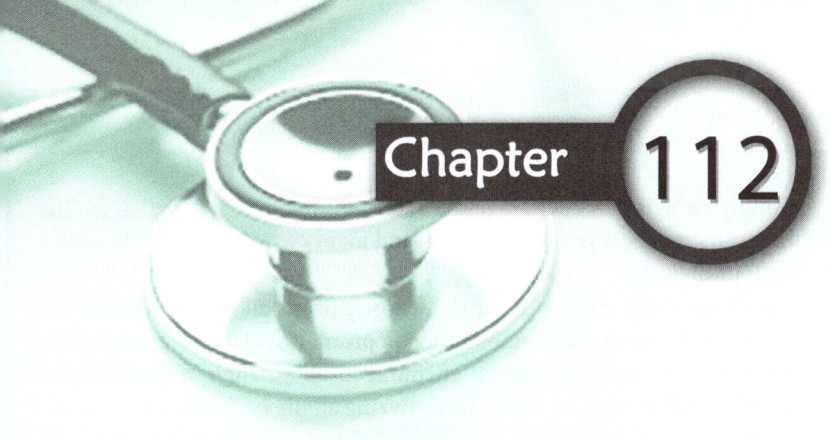

Chapter 112

International Day for the Elderly

INTRODUCTION

International Day for Elderly is celebrated every year on 1st October. This day is observed to focus on the importance of senior citizens who sometimes are neglected in our society. This day emphasizes on our responsibilities towards our elder in order to make their lives happier. The theme for year 2016 was, "Sustainability and Age Inclusiveness in the Urban Environment." The year 2015 marked the 25th anniversary of International Day of Older Persons and it will focus on the impact older people have on the new urban environment. The main aim is to generate awareness amongst people about issues which affect the elders, as well as to appreciate their contribution toward the society.

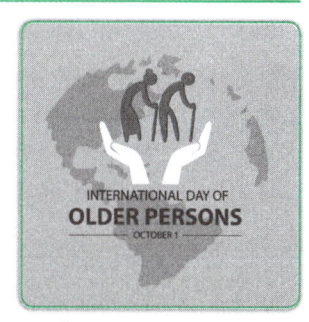

As part of commitment toward the elderly, Government of India (GoI) provides various preventive, curative and rehabilitative services for the people who are above 60 years under its National Programme of Health Care for the Elderly (NPHCE). The basic objective of the NPHCE programme is to provide separate, specialized and comprehensive health care to the senior citizens at various levels of state health care delivery system including outreach services. GoI also provides benefits like health insurance schemes, tax exemptions, and concessions in rail and air fares to the senior citizens.

HISTORY

It was celebrated for the first time on October 1st in the year 1991 to make the people aware about issues which affect the elders as well as to appreciate their contribution towards the society.

On December 14, 1990, the UN General Assembly made October 1 as the International Day of Older Persons, following up on initiatives such as the Vienna International Plan of Action on Aging, which was adopted by the 1982 World Assembly on Aging and endorsed later that year by the assembly. The International Day of Older Persons was observed for the first time throughout the world on October 1, 1991.

In 1991, the UN General Assembly adopted the United Nations Principles for Older Persons. In 2002, the second World Assembly on Aging adopted the Madrid International Plan of Action on Aging to respond to the opportunities and challenges of population aging in the 21st century and to promote the development of a society for all ages.

The day is celebrated every year to make certain the welfare of elder persons as well as to enroll their significant involvement in the society to get promoted with their knowledge and ability. The Plan of Action on

Aging was adopted by the World Assembly on aging to encourage the society development for all ages. The day is celebrated worldwide to examine issues, promote public awareness and focus on which type of behavior can help older men and women throughout their life.

International Day for Older Persons is specially celebrated for the senior citizens all across the world to focus on the responsibilities towards their lives through the demonstration of promotional material in schools, institutions, offices and public notice boards. People are getting encouraged about their responsibilities towards the lives of elder people to make their life better and happy by analyzing all the problems affecting the life of older people.

THEMES

Themes of International Day for Elderly People	
2011	"The Growing Opportunities and Challenges of Global Aging"
2012	"Longevity: Shaping the Future"
2013	"The future we want: what older persons are saying"
2014	"Leaving No One Behind: Promoting a Society for All"
2015	"Sustainability and Age Inclusiveness in the Urban Environment"
2016	"Take a Stand Against Agism"
2017	"Stepping into the Future: Tapping the Talents, Contributions and Participation of Older Persons in Society"
2018	"Celebrating Older Human Rights Champions"
2019	"The Journey to Age Equality"
2020	"Pandemics: Do They Change How We Address Age and Aging?"

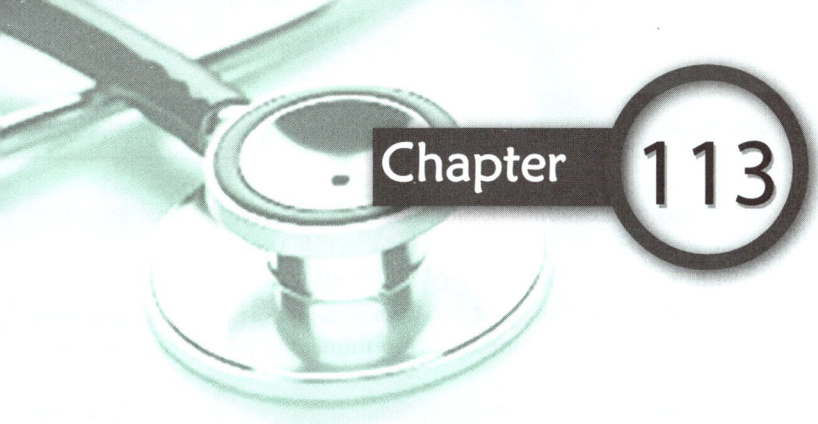

Chapter 113

World Sight Day

INTRODUCTION

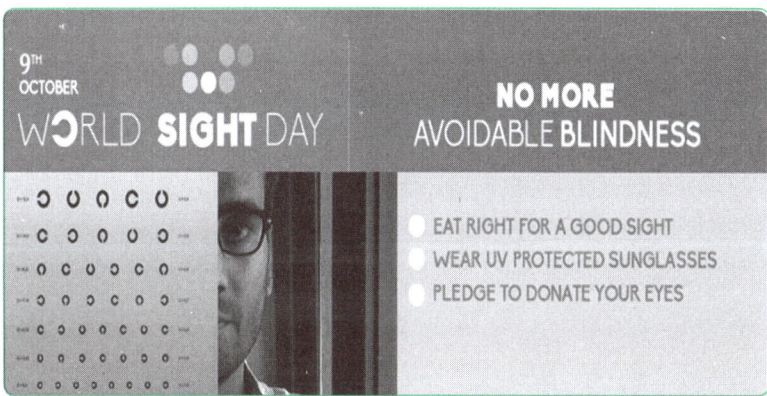

Worldsight Day is celebrated every year on the second Thursday of October. This day is celebrated to create awareness about vision impairment, blindness as well as sight related problems. World Sight Day in 2020 had the theme: "Hope In Sight."

World Sight Day highlights the importance of good vision for all people. In 2016, the 'Call to Action' for World Sight Day was: "No More Avoidable Blindness" to promote everyone's right to sight.

According to World Health Organization (WHO) estimates, approximately 285 million people worldwide suffer from low vision and blindness. Of these, 39 million are blind and 246 million have low vision. The major causes of visual impairment are uncorrected refractive errors (43%) and cataract (33%). Most of the blindness (approx 80%) is avoidable, i.e. curable or preventable.

Prevention of blindness is the most cost-effective and successful of all the health interventions. "VISION 2020: The Right to Sight" is a global initiative by WHO and International Agency for the Prevention of Blindness (IAPB) launched in 1999. Since then it has been adopted in more than 40 countries.

IAPB supports World Sight Day activities across the globe by sending promotional material like posters, bookmarks, reports and advocacy material free of cost to over 500 addresses, including ministries of health, WHO country offices, numerous organizations who work with local communities and NGOs working across geographies to mark World Sight Day.

"World Sight Day is a powerful platform to draw attention and support to blindness prevention activities globally. It is also important that we discuss the rights and issues of those with permanent sight loss. We welcome all stakeholders—NGOs, Corporations, professional bodies, hospitals and training institutes—to mark World Sight Day," said Bob McMullan, President, IAPB.

"As the global leader in eye care, Alcon is delighted to partner with IAPB to drive awareness of the importance of eye health," said Bettina Maunz, President of the Alcon Foundation. "It is a great way to support the work of organizations around the world, and underscore our joint commitment to preserve, restore and enhance vision."

The World Sight Day Challenge is the largest annual global fundraising campaign to address avoidable blindness caused by uncorrected refractive error.

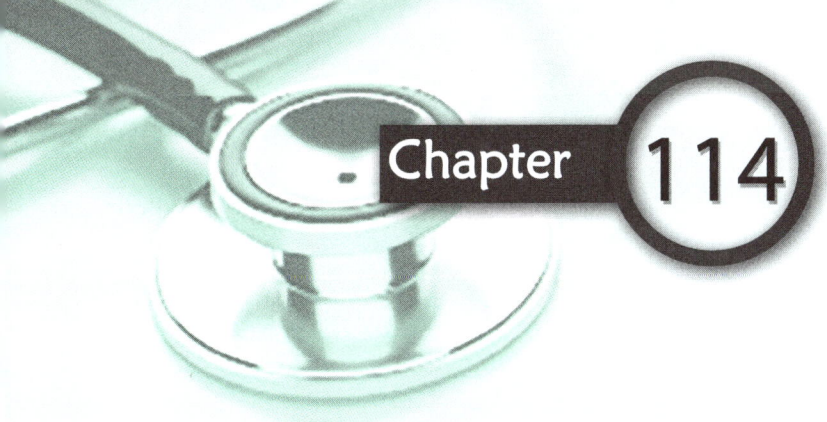

Chapter 114

World Mental Health Day

INTRODUCTION

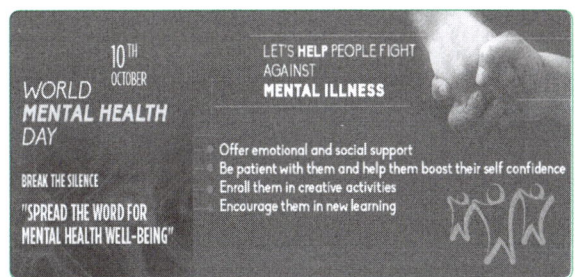

World Mental Health Day is celebrated on 10th of October annually across the world to create awareness on mental health issues. The theme for year 2016 of World Mental Health Day was "Dignity in mental health." This year, WHO will be raising awareness of that how people with mental health conditions can continue to live with dignity, through human rights oriented policy and law, training of health professionals, respect for informed consent to treatment, inclusion in decision-making processes, and public information campaigns.

The Day provides an opportunity for all stakeholders working on mental health issues to talk about their work, and what more needs to be done to make mental health care a reality for people worldwide.

It was first celebrated in 1992 at the initiative of the World Federation for Mental Health, a global mental health organization with members and contacts in more than 150 countries.

THEMES

Themes of World Mental Health Day	
2014	Living with is schizophrenia
2015	Dignity is mental health
2016	Psychological first aid
2017	"Mental health in the Workplace"
2018	"Young people and mental health in a changing world"
2019	"Suicide Prevention"
2020	"Move for mental health: Let´s invest!"

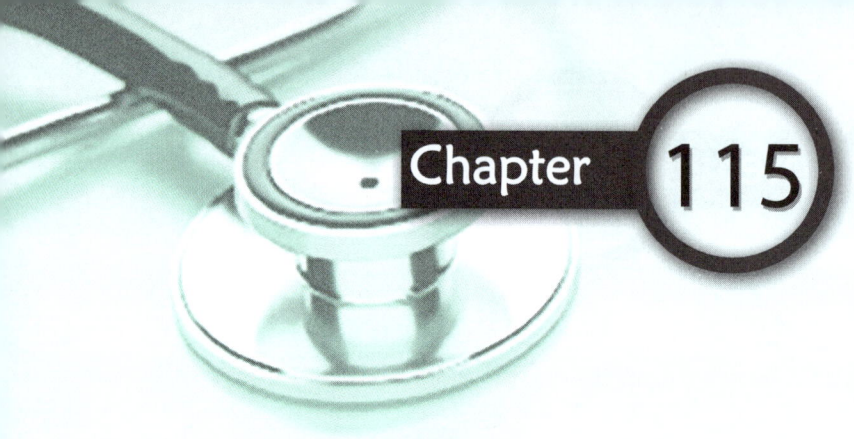

Chapter 115

World Arthritis Day

INTRODUCTION

World **Arthritis Day** is a day dedicated towards creating awareness regarding musculoskeletal diseases and is celebrated every year on 12th October. Theme for year 2016 was, "Living Better Aging Well."

World Arthritis Day (WAD) is a global initiative bringing people together to raise awareness of the issues affecting people with Rheumatic and musculoskeletal diseases (RMDs). WAD is recognized every year on 12th October and is supported by a year-round global campaign.

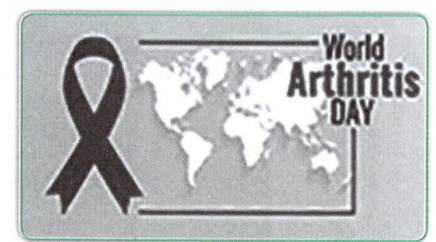

AIMS

The aims of WAD are:

- To raise awareness of RMDs amongst the medical community, people with RMDs and the general public
- To influence public policy by making decision-makers aware of the burden of RMDs and the steps which can be taken to ease them
- To ensure that all people with RMDs and their caregivers are aware of the vast support network available to them.

OBJECTIVES

Objectives for the 2016 WAD campaign were to:

- Educate people with RMDs and carers to understand available treatment options and utilize support networks.
- Educate health care teams on the importance of early diagnosis, the treatment outcomes valued by patients in addition to clinical outcomes, and how care can be optimized to meet individual patient needs.
- Ensure policy makers to understand the full extent of RMD impact on people and society, and solutions that are needed to lessen that impact.

THEMES

Themes of World Arthritis Day	
2017	"Don't delay. Connect today"
2018	"It's in your hands, take action"
2019 & 2020	"Time 2 Work"

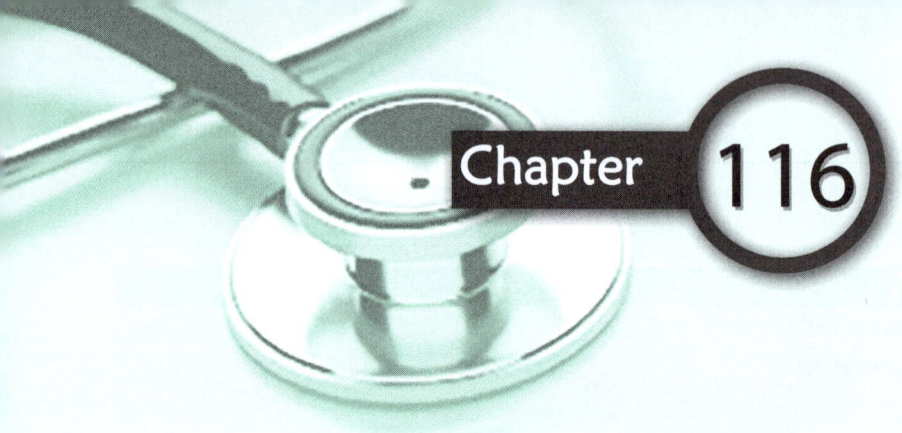

Chapter 116

Global Handwashing Day

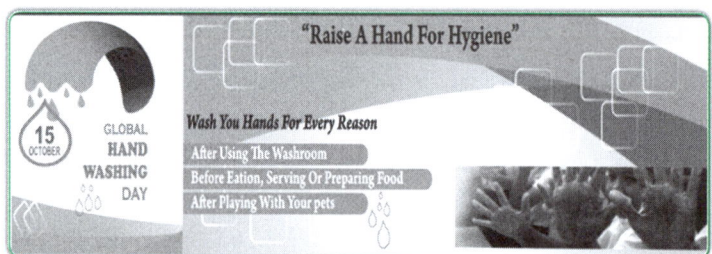

INTRODUCTION

Global Handwashing Day is observed every year on 15th October. The theme of this day is, "Choose handwashing, choose health." This campaign is initiated to motivate people around the world to wash their hands with soap.

Global Handwashing Day is designed to:

- Foster and support a global and local culture of handwashing with soap.
- Shine a spotlight on handwashing around the world.
- Raise awareness about the benefits of handwashing with soap.

The first Global Handwashing Day was held in 2008, when over 120 million children around the world washed their hands with soap in more than 70 countries. Since 2008, community and national leaders have used Global Handwashing Day to spread the word about handwashing, build sinks and tippy taps, and demonstrate the simplicity and value of clean hands. Each year, over 200 million people are involved in celebrations in over 100 countries around the world. Global Handwashing Day is endorsed by a wide array of governments, international institutions, civil society organizations, NGOs, private companies, and individuals.

The 2016 Global Handwashing Day theme was **"Make Handwashing a Habit!"** For handwashing to be effective, it must be practised consistently at key times, such as after using the toilet or before contact with food. While habits must be developed over time, this theme emphasizes the importance of handwashing as a ritual behavior for long-term sustainability. Habit formation is currently a hot topic in behavior change and the water, sanitation, and hygiene sector. This theme taps into that interest and is also a gateway to discussing what the sector knows about how habits are formed.

The campaign was initiated to reduce childhood mortality rates related respiratory and diarrheal diseases by introducing simple behavioral changes, such as handwashing with soap. This simple, accessible action can, according to research, reduce the rate of mortality from these diseases by almost 25% and 50% respectively.

The focus for Global Handwashing Day's inaugural year in 2008 was school children. In that year, the members pledged to get the maximum number of school children to handwash with soap in more than 70 countries. In India in 2008, cricket legend Sachin Tendulkar and his teammates joined an estimated 100 million school children around the country in lathering up for better health and hygiene as part of the first Global Handwashing Day.

In 2014, Global Handwashing Day was used as an opportunity to fight Ebola.

WHO declared 2020 as the Year of the Nurse and the Midwife, to recognize their crucial contribution in strengthening quality health systems.

Nurses: "Clean and safe care starts with you."

Midwives: "Your hands make all the difference for mothers and babies."

Policy Makers: "Increase nurse staffing levels to prevent infections and improve quality of care. Create the means to empower nurses and midwives."

IPC Leaders: "Empower nurses and midwives in providing clean care."

Patients and Families: "Safer care for you, with you."

THEMES

Themes of Global Handwashing Day	
2015	"Raise a hand for hygiene"
2016	"Make handwashing a habit!"
2017	"Our Hands, Our Future!"
2018	"Clean Hands—a recipe for health"
2019	"Clean Hands for All"
2020	"Hand Hygiene for All"

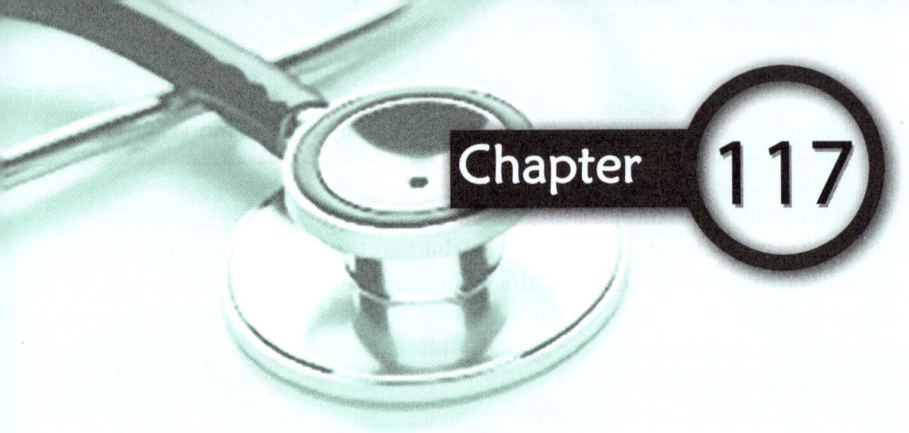

Chapter 117

World Food Day

INTRODUCTION

World Food Day is celebrated every year on 16th October. It is the foundation day of Food and Agriculture Organization (FAO). FAO was established in the year 1945 as an agency of the United Nations.

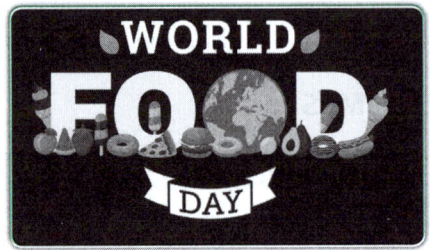

The aim of celebrating this day is to spread public awareness about hunger challenges as well as to encourage people to take action in the fight against hunger.

The theme of 2015 was "Social Protection and Agriculture: Breaking the Cycle of Rural Poverty."

OBJECTIVES

Main objectives of World Food Day:
- Encourage agricultural food production
- Encourage cooperation among developing countries in economic and technical fields
- Encourage the contribution of rural people, mainly women and the least privileged
- Promote technology transfer to the developing countries
- Spread awareness and encourage all nations to fight against hunger, malnutrition and poverty
- Draw attention to agricultural development.

THEMES

Themes of World Food Day	
2016	"Climate is changing. Food and agriculture must too"
2017	"Change the future of migration"
2018	"Our actions are our future. A #Zero Hunger world by 2030 is possible"
2019	"Healthy diets for a zero hunger world"
2020	"Grow, nourish, sustain. Together. Our actions are our future"

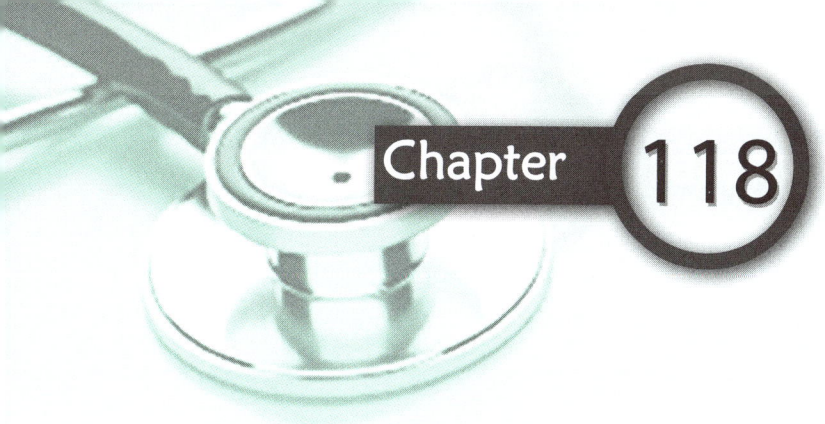

Chapter 118

World Trauma Day

INTRODUCTION

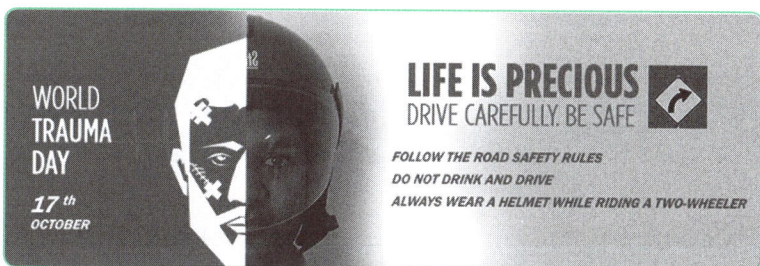

Every year, 17th October is celebrated as World Trauma Day. This day highlights the increasing rate of accidents and injuries causing death and disability across the world and the need to prevent them. The objective is to sensitize the public on the need to provide assistance to accident victims and immediate care.

THEMES

Themes of World Trauma Day	
2009	From global remembrance to global action
2010	Remembering lives last and brokers, the injured
2011	Let's make 2011–2020 a decade to remember
2012	Now is the time to learn from the post
2013	Let's have road that are safe for all
2014	Speed kills—design out speeding
2015	It is time to remember—say no to road crime
2016	Vital postcrash action: Medical care investigation justice
2017	2020 Target: Reduce road fatalities serious injustice by 50%
2019	"Support nurses and midwives for their vital role in keeping the world healthy"
2020	2020 "Trauma care in COVID-19"

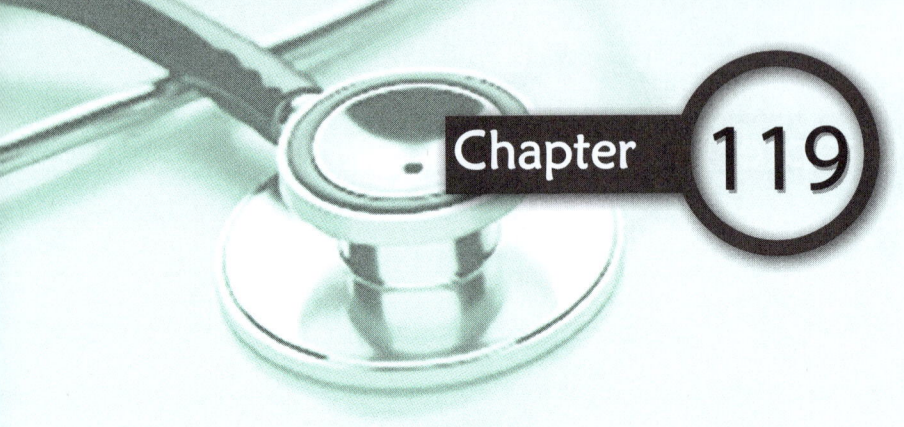

Chapter 119

World Osteoporosis Day

INTRODUCTION

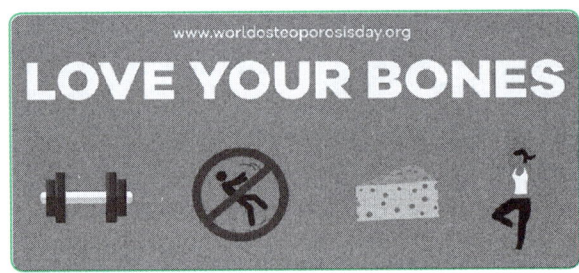

World Osteoporosis Day is observed every year on 20th October across the world, dedicated to create global awareness for prevention, diagnosis and treatment of osteoporosis. The year 2016 theme was 'Serve up bone strength' which aims to raise awareness for the right nutrients to keep the bones healthy and strong as a well-balanced diet with regular exercise that helps in reducing the risk of osteoporosis.

Organized by the International Osteoporosis Foundation (IOF) every year, World Osteoporosis Day involves campaigns by national osteoporosis patient societies from around the world with activities in over 90 countries.

The concept for World Osteoporosis Day started with a campaign launched by the United Kingdom's National Osteoporosis Society and supported by European Commission on October 20, 1996. Since 1997, the day has been organized by IOF. In 1998 and 1999, the World Health Organization acted as co-sponsor of World Osteoporosis Day. Since 1999, World Osteoporosis Day campaigns have featured a specific theme.

THEMES

Themes of World Osteoporosis Day	
1999	Early Detection
2000	Building Bone Health
2001	Invest in Your Bones: Bone Development in Youth
2002	Invest in Your Bones: Prevent the First Fracture

Contd…

- The State shall undertake measures to ensure that children without families are either placed for adoption, preferably intra-country adoption, or foster care or any other family substitute services.
- The State shall ensure that appropriate rules with respect to the implementation of such services are drafted in a manner that are in the best interest of the child and that regulatory bodies are set up to ensure the strict enforcement of these rules.
- All children shall have the right to meet their parents and other family members who may be in custody.

Responsibilities of Both Parents

The State recognizes the common responsibilities of both parents in rearing their children.

Protection of Children with Disabilities

- The State and community recognize that all children with disabilities must be helped to lead a life with dignity and respect. All measures would be undertaken to ensure that children with disabilities are encouraged to be integrated into the mainstream society and actively participate in all walks of life.
- State and community shall also provide for their education, training, health care, rehabilitation, recreation in a manner that will contribute to their overall growth and development.
- State and community shall launch preventive programmes against disabilities and early detection of disabilities so as to ensure that the families with disabled children receive adequate support and assistance in bringing up their children.
- The State shall encourage research and development in the field of prevention, treatment and rehabilitation of various forms of disabilities.

Care, protection, and welfare of children of marginalized and disadvantaged communities.

- The State and community shall provide care, protect and ensure the welfare of children from marginalized and disadvantaged communities, support them in preserving their identity, and encourage them to adopt practices that promote their best interest. The State recognizes that children from disadvantaged communities and weaker/vulnerable sections of the society are in need of special interventions and support in all matters pertaining to education, health, recreation and supportive services. It shall make adequate provisions for providing such groups with special attention in all its policies and programmes.

Ensuring Child-Friendly Procedures

- All matters and procedures relating to children, viz. judicial, administrative, educational or social, should be child-friendly. All procedures laid down under the juvenile justice system for children in conflict with law and for children in need of special care and protection shall also be child-friendly.

    (e) review in consultation with the donor agencies their funding policies from the perspective of their impact on persons with disabilities

    (f) take such other steps to ensure barrier free environment in public places, work places, public utilities, schools and other institutions

    (g) monitor and evaluate the impact of policies and programmes designed for achieving equality and full participation of persons with disabilities

    (h) to perform such other functions as may be prescribed by the Central Government.

9. (1) The Central Government shall constitute a Committee to be known as the Central Executive Committee to perform the functions assigned to it under this Act.

  (2) The Central Executive Committee shall consist of—

    (a) The Secretary to the Government of India in the Ministry of Welfare, Chairperson, *ex officio*

    (b) The Chief Commissioner, Member, *ex officio*

    (c) The Director General for Health Services, Member, *ex officio*

    (d) The Director General, Employment and Training, Member, *ex officio*

    (e) Six persons not below the rank of a Joint Secretary to the Government of India, to represent the Ministries or Departments of Rural Development, Education, Welfare, Personnel Public Grievances and Pension and Urban Affairs and Employment, Science and Technology, Members, *ex officio*

    (f) the Financial Advisor, Ministry of Welfare in the Central Government, Member, *ex officio*

    (g) Advisor (Tariff) Railway Board, Member, *ex officio*

    (h) four members to be nominated by the Central Government, by rotation, to represent the State Governments and the Union Territories in such manner as may be prescribed by the Central Government

    (i) One person to be nominated by the Central Government to represent the interest, which in the opinion of the Central Government ought to be represented, Member

    (j) Five persons, as far as practicable, being persons with disabilities, to represent non-governmental organizations or associations which are concerned with disabilities, to be nominated by the Central Government, one from each area of disability, Members:

    Provided that while nominating persons under this clause, the Central Government shall nominate at least one woman and one person belonging to Scheduled Castes or Scheduled Tribes

    (k) Joint Secretary to the Government of India in the Ministry of Welfare dealing with the welfare of the handicapped, Member-Secretary, *ex officio*.

  (3) Members nominated under clause (i) and clause (j) of sub-section (2) shall receive such allowances as may be prescribed by the Central Government.

  (4) A Member nominated under clause (i) or clause (j) of sub-section (2) may at any time resign his office by writing under his hand addressed to the Central Government and the seat of the said Member shall thereupon become vacant.

10. (1) The Central Executive Committee shall be the executive body of the Central Coordination Committee and shall be responsible for carrying out the decisions of the Central Coordination Committee.

  (2) Without prejudice to the provisions of sub-section (1), the Central Executive Committee shall also perform such other functions as may be delegated to it by the Central Coordination Committee.

11. The Central Executive Committee shall meet at least once in three months and shall observe such rules of procedure in regard to the transaction of business at its meetings as may be prescribed by the Central Government.

12. (1) The Central Executive Committee may associate with itself in such manner and for such purposes as may be prescribed by the Central Government any person whose assistance or advice it may desire to obtain in performing any of its functions under this Act.

    (2) A person associated with the Central Executive Committee under sub-section (1) for any purpose shall have the right to take part in the discussions of the Central Executive Committee relevant to that purpose, but shall not have a right to vote at a meeting of the said Committee, and shall not be a member for any other purpose.

    (3) A person associated with the said Committee under sub-section (1) for any purpose shall be paid such fees and allowances, for attending its meetings and for attending to any other work of the said Committee, as may be prescribed by the Central Government.

CHAPTER III: THE STATE COORDINATION COMMITTEE

13. (1) Every State Government shall, by notification, constitute a body to be known as the State Coordination Committee to exercise the powers conferred on, and to perform the function assigned to it, under this Act.

    (2) The State Coordination Committee shall consist of—

    (a) The Minister in-charge of the Department of Social Welfare in the State Government, Chairperson, *ex officio*

    (b) The Minister of State in-charge of the Department of Social Welfare, if any, Vice-Chairperson, *ex officio*

    (c) Secretaries to the State Government in-charge of the Departments of Welfare, Education, Woman and Child Development, Expenditure, Personnel Training and Public Grievances, Health, Rural Development, Industrial Development, Urban Affairs and Employment, Science and Technology, Public Enterprises, by whatever name called, Members, *ex officio*

    (d) Secretary of any other Department, which the State Government considers necessary, Member, *ex officio*

    (e) Chairman Bureau of Public Enterprises (by whatever name called) Member, *ex officio*

    (f) Five persons, as far as practicable, being persons with disabilities, to represent non-governmental organizations or associations which are concerned with disabilities, to be nominated by the State Government, one from each area of disability, Members:

    Provided that while nominating persons under this clause, the State Government shall nominate at least one woman and one person belonging to Scheduled Castes or Scheduled Tribes

    (g) Three Members of State Legislature, of whom two shall be elected by the Legislative assembly and one by the Legislative Council, if any

    (h) Three persons to be nominated by that State Government to represent agriculture, industry or trade or any other interest, which in the opinion of State Government ought to be represented, Members, *ex officio*

    (i) The Commissioner, Member, *ex officio*

    (j) Secretary to the State Government dealing with the welfare of the handicapped, Member-Secretary, *ex officio*.

- States will set up homes with assisted living facilities for abandoned senior citizens in every district of the country and there will be adequate budgetary support.

AREAS OF INTERVENTION

The concerned ministries at central and state level as mentioned in the "Implementation Section" would implement the policy and take necessary steps for senior citizens as under:

Income Security in Old Age

A major intervention required in old age relates to financial insecurity as more than of the elderly live below the poverty line. It would increase with age uniformly across the country.

Indira Gandhi National Old Age Pension Scheme

- Old age pension scheme would cover all senior citizens living below the poverty line.
- Rate of monthly pension would be raised to ₹1000 per month per person and revised at intervals to prevent its deflation due to higher cost of purchasing.
- The oldest old would be covered under Indira Gandhi National Old Age Pension Scheme (IGNOAPS). They would be provided additional pension in case of disability, loss of adult children and concomitant responsibility for grandchildren and women. This would be reviewed every 5 years.

Public Distribution System

The public distribution system would reach out to cover all senior citizens living below the poverty line.

Income Tax

Taxation policies would reflect sensitivity to the financial problems of senior citizens which accelerate due to very high costs of medical and nursing care, transportation and support services needed at homes.

Microfinance

Loans at reasonable rates of interest would be offered to senior citizens to start small businesses. Microfinance for senior citizens would be supported through suitable guidelines issued by the Reserve Bank of India.

Health Care

With advancing age, senior citizens have to cope with health and associated problems some of which may be chronic, of a multiple nature, require constant attention and carry the risk of disability and consequent loss of autonomy. Some health problems, especially when accompanied by impaired functional capacity require long-term management of illness and nursing care.

- Health care needs of senior citizens will be given high priority. The goal would be good, affordable health service, heavily subsidized for the poor and a graded system of user charges for others. It would have a judicious mix of public health services, health insurance, health services provided by not-for-profit organizations including trusts and charities, and private medical care. While the first of these will need to be promoted by the State, the third category given some assistance, concessions and relief and the fourth encouraged and subjected to some degree of regulation, preferably by an association of providers of private care.
- The basic structure of public health care would be through primary health care. It would be strengthened and oriented to meet the health needs of senior citizens. Preventive, curative, restorative and rehabilitative

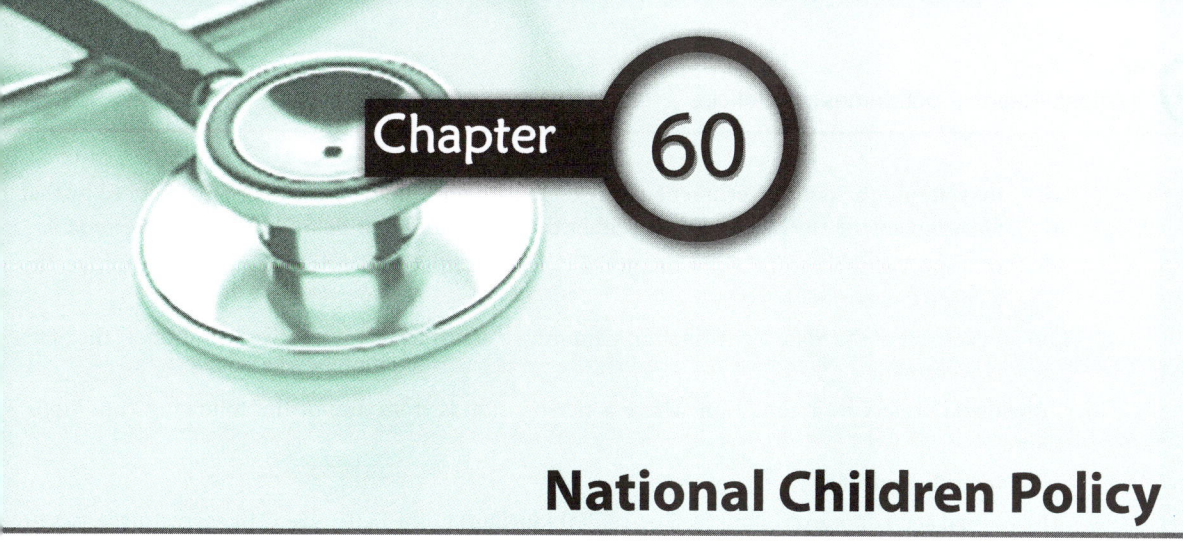

Chapter 60

National Children Policy

INTRODUCTION

The Government of India have had for consideration the question of adopting a National Charter for Children to reiterate its commitment to the cause of the children in order to see that no child remains hungry, illiterate or sick. After the consideration, it has been decided to adopt the National Charter for Children enunciated below.

NATIONAL CHARTER FOR CHILDREN, 2003

Whereas the Constitution of India enshrines both in Part III and IV the cause and the best interest of children, in so far that:

- The State can make special provisions for children [Art 15 (3)] and shall provide free and compulsory education to all children of the age of six to fourteen years, (Art 21A).
- No child below the age of 14 years shall be employed to work in a factory, mine or any other hazardous employment, (Art. 24).
- The tender age of children is not abused and that citizens are not forced by economic necessity to enter avocations unsuited to their age or strength (Art. 39 e), and that children are given opportunities and facilities to develop in a healthy manner and in conditions of freedom and dignity and that youth are protected against exploitation and against moral and material abandonment, (Art. 39 f).
- The State shall endeavor to provide early childhood care and education for all children until they complete the age of six years, (Art. 45).
- Whereas it is a fundamental duty of a parent or guardian to provide opportunities for education to his child or ward between the age of six and fourteen years (Art. 51A).
- Whereas through the National Policy for Children, 1974, we are committed to providing for adequate services to children, both before and after birth and throughout the period of growth, to ensure their full physical, mental and social development.
- Whereas we affirm that the best interest of children must be protected through combined action of the State, civil society, communities and families in their obligations in fulfilling children's basic needs.
- Whereas we also affirm that while state, society, community and family have obligations towards children, these must be viewed in the context of intrinsic and attendant duties of children and inculcating in children a sound sense of values directed towards preserving and strengthening the family, society and the Nation.

    (ii)   in relation to a State Government or any establishment wholly or substantially financed by that Government, or any local authority, other than a Cantonment Board, the State Government

    (iii)   in respect of the Central Coordination Committee and the Central Executive Committee, the Central Government

    (iv)   in respect of the State Coordination Committee and the State Executive Committee, the State Government

(b) **"Blindness"** refers to a condition where a person suffers from any of the following conditions, namely:—

    (i)   total absence of sight

    (ii)   visual acuity not exceeding 6/60 or 20/200 (Snellen) in the better eye with correcting lenses or

    (iii)   limitation of the field of vision subtending an angle of 20 degree or worse

(c) **"Central Coordination Committee"** means the Central Coordination Committee constituted under sub-section (1) of Section 3

(d) **"Central Executive Committee"** means the Central Executive Committee constituted under sub-section (1) of Section 9

(e) **"Cerebral palsy"** means a group of non-progressive conditions of a person characterized by abnormal motor control posture resulting from brain insult or injuries occurring in the pre-natal, perinatal or infant period of development

(f) **"Chief Commissioner"** means the Chief Commissioner appointed under sub-section (1) of Section 57

(g) **"Commissioner"** means the Commissioner appointed under sub-section (1) of Section 60

(h) **"Competent authority"** means the authority appointed under Section 50

(i) **"Disability"** means—

    (i)   blindness

    (ii)   low vision

    (iii)   leprosy-cured

    (iv)   hearing impairment

    (v)   loco motor disability

    (vi)   mental retardation

    (vii)   mental illness

(j) **"Employer"** means,—

    (i)   in relation to a Government, the authority notified by the Head of the Department in this behalf or where no such authority is notified, the Head of the Department and

    (ii)   in relation to an establishment, the chief executive officer of that the establishment

(k) **"Establishment"** means a corporation established by or under a Central, Provincial or State Act, or an authority or a body owned or controlled or aided by the Government or a local authority or a Government company as defined in section 617 of 'the Companies Act, 1956 and includes Departments of a Government

(l) **"Hearing impairment"** means loss of sixty decibels or more in the better year in the conversational range of frequencies

(m) **"Institution for persons with disabilities"** means an institution for the reception, care, protection, education, training, rehabilitation or any other service of persons with disabilities

(n) **"Leprosy cured person"** means any person who has been cured of leprosy but is suffering from—

    (i) loss of sensation in hands or feet as well as loss of sensation and paresis in the eye and eye-lid but with no manifest deformity

    (ii) manifest deformity and paresis but having sufficient mobility in their hands and feet to enable them to engage in normal economic activity

    (iii) extreme physical deformity as well as advanced age which prevents him from undertaking any gainful occupation, and the expression "leprosy cured" shall be construed accordingly.

(o) **"Locomotor disability"** means disability of the bones, joints muscles leading to substantial restriction of the movement of the limbs or any form of cerebral palsy

(p) **"Medical authority"** means any hospital or institution specified for the purposes of this Act by notification by the appropriate Government

(q) **"Mental illness"** means any mental disorder other than mental retardation

(r) **"Mental retardation"** means a condition of arrested or incomplete development of mind of a person which is specially characterized by subnormality of intelligence

(s) **"Notification"** means a notification published in the Official Gazette

(t) **"Person with disability"** means a person suffering from not less than forty percent of any disability as certified by a medical authority

(u) **"Person with low vision"** means a person with impairment of visual functioning even after treatment or standard refractive correction but who uses or is potentially capable of using vision for the planning or execution of a task with appropriate assistive device

(v) **"Prescribed"** means prescribed by rules made under this Act

(w) **"Rehabilitation"** refers to a process aimed at enabling persons with disabilities to reach and maintain their optimal physical, sensory, intellectual, psychiatric or social functional levels

(x) **"Special employment exchange"** means any office or place established and maintained by the Government for the collection and furnishing of information, either by keeping of registers or otherwise, respecting—

    (i) persons who seek to engage employees from amongst the persons suffering from disabilities

    (ii) persons with disability who seek employment

    (iii) vacancies to which person with disability seeking employment may be appointed

(y) **"State Coordination Committee"** means the State Coordination Committee constituted under sub-section (1) of Section 13.

(z) **"State Executive Committee"** means the State Executive Committee constituted under sub-section (l) of Section 19.

CHAPTER II: THE CENTRAL COORDINATION COMMITTEE

3. (1) The Central Government shall by notification constitute a body to be known as the Central Coordination Committee to exercise the powers conferred on, and to perform the functions assigned to it, under this Act.

    (2) The Central Coordination Committee shall consist of—

      (a) The Minister in charge of the Department of Welfare in the Central Government, Chairperson, *ex officio*

or violence. The State in partnership with the community shall ensure that such children are rescued and immediately placed under appropriate care and protection.

- The State and community shall ensure protection of children in distress for their welfare and all round development.
- The State and community shall ensure protection of children during the occurrence of natural calamities in their best interest.

Protection of the Girl Child

- The State and community shall ensure that crimes and atrocities committed against the girl child, including child marriage, discriminatory practices, forcing girls into prostitution and trafficking are speedily eradicated.
- The State shall in partnership with the community undertake measures, including social, educational and legal, to ensure that there is greater respect for the girl child in the family and society.
- The State shall take serious measures to ensure that the practice of child marriage is speedily abolished.

Empowering Adolescents

- The State and community shall take all steps to provide the necessary education and skills to adolescent children so as to equip them to become economically productive citizens. Special programmes will be undertaken to improve the health and nutritional status of the adolescent girl.

Equality, freedom of expression, freedom to seek and receive information, freedom of association and peaceful assembly.

- The State and community shall ensure that all children are treated equally without discrimination on grounds of the child's or the child's parents' or legal guardian's race, color, caste, sex, language, religion, political or other opinion, national, ethnic or social origin, disability, birth, political status, or any other consideration.
- All children shall be given every opportunity for all round development of their personality, including expression of creativity.
- Every child shall have the freedom to seek and receive information and ideas. The State and community shall provide opportunities for the child to access information that will contribute to the child's development.
- The State and community shall undertake special measures to ensure that the linguistic needs of children are taken care of and encourage the production and dissemination of child-friendly information and material in various forms.
- The State and community shall be responsible for formulating guidelines for the mass media in order to ensure that children are protected from material injuries to their well-being.
- All children shall enjoy freedom of association and peaceful assembly, subject to reasonable restrictions and in conformity with social and family values.

Strengthening family

- Every child has a right to a family. In case of separation of children from their families, the State shall ensure that priority is given to re-unifying the child with its parents. In cases where the State perceives adverse impact of such a reunification, the State shall make alternate arrangements immediately, keeping in mind the best interests and the views of the child.
- All children have a right to maintain contact with their families, even when they are within the custody of the State for various reasons.

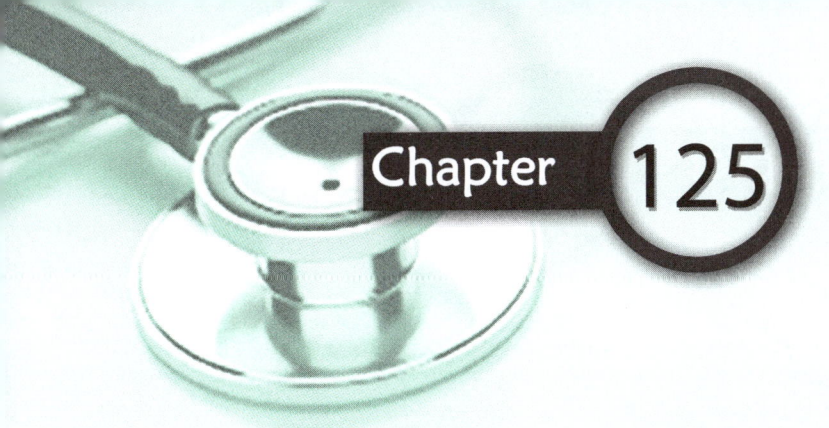

Chapter 125

National Epilepsy Day

INTRODUCTION

In India, every year November 17 is observed as National Epilepsy Day to create awareness about epilepsy. Epilepsy is a chronic disorder of brain characterized by recurrent 'seizures' or 'fits'.

National Epilepsy day in India started in 1991 with the proposal of Doctors Eddie and Piloo Barucha of the Indian Epilepsy Association as the focal point of this previous National Epilepsy week. Since then it has been celebrated annually nationwide, providing accurate and up-to-date information on epilepsy to the people of India.

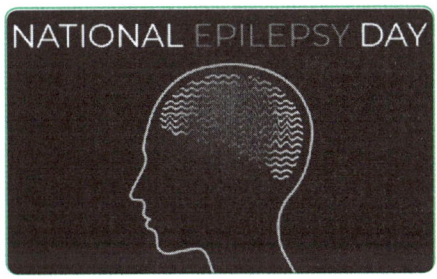

OBJECTIVE

To raise epilepsy as a new plane of acceptability in the public domain and to increase public awareness of epilepsy as a universal and treatable brain disorder.

ACTIVITIES

- On this day, the organizers are holding seminars about epilepsy. Why not join and learn new things?
- Know someone who has epilepsy? Refer them to the various specialists present in the occasion.
- Volunteer to help out on the myriad National Epilepsy Day programmes for your district. They will appreciate the help.
- Use the power of social media! Bring to the forefront of cyberspace consciousness the National Epilepsy Day.

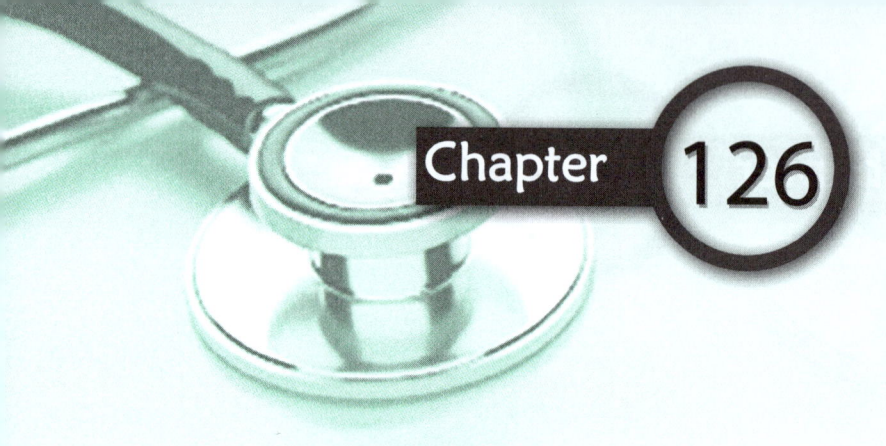

Chapter 126

World COPD Day

INTRODUCTION

World Chronic Obstructive Pulmonary Disease (COPD) Day is observed every year on the third Wednesday in November with the aim to create awareness about COPD and improve COPD care, across the world. World COPD Day 2015 was being celebrated on 18th November with the theme "It is not too late."

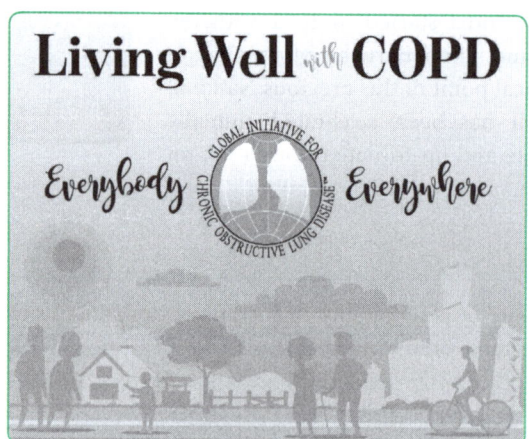

THEMES

Themes of World COPD Day	
2016	"Breathe in the knowledge"
2017	"The Many Faces of COPD"
2018	"Never too early. Never too late"
2019	"All Together to End COPD"
2020	"Living Well with COPD—Everybody, Everywhere"

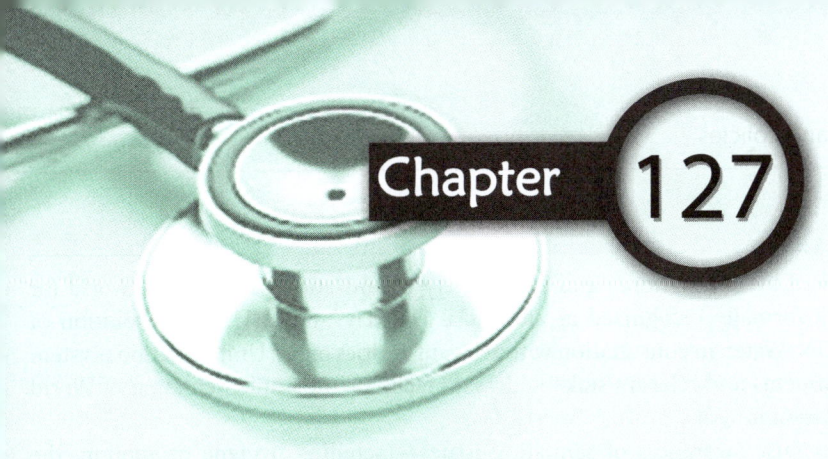

Chapter 127

World Toilet Day

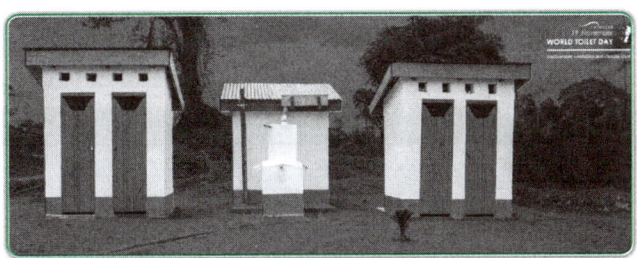

INTRODUCTION

World Toilet Day is celebrated every year on 19th November.

AIMS

- To draw global attention to the sanitation crisis.
- To raise awareness about the people in the world who do not have access to a toilet, despite the fact that it is a human right to have clean water and sanitation.

OBJECTIVES

To make sanitation for all a global development priority and urge changes in both behavior and policy on issues ranging from improving water management to ending open defecation.

In 2016, the theme of this day was "Sanitation and Nutrition." The objective of the theme was to spread awareness on poor sanitation and related nutrition problems and to do something about it.

World Toilet Day is a United Nations (UN) observance, on November 19, that highlights a serious problem—2.5 billion people in the world do not have access to proper sanitation.

International organizations, particularly the World Toilet Organization, have promoted World Toilet Day for years. In 2013, the UN officially recognized 19th November as World Toilet Day in a bid to make sanitation for all a global development priority.

HISTORY

World Toilet Day has been marked by international and civil society organizations all over the world for many years. However, it was not formally recognized as an official UN day until a UNGA resolution of 24th July 2013, which requested UN-Water, in consultation with relevant entities of the United Nation's system and in collaboration with Governments and relevant stakeholders, to facilitate the implementation of World Toilet Day in the context of Sanitation for All.

World Toilet Day intends to raise awareness of sanitation issues—including hygiene promotion, the provision of basic sanitation services, and sewerage and waste water treatment and reuse in the context of integrated water management—and make a case for sanitation for all.

It intends to encourage UN Member States and relevant stakeholders, including civil society and non-governmental organizations, to promote behavioral change and the implementation of policies in order to increase access to sanitation among the poor and end the practice of open defecation.

THEMES

Themes of World Toilet Day	
2017	"Wastewater"
2018	"When nature calls"
2019	"Leaving no one behind"
2020	"Sustainable sanitation and climate change"

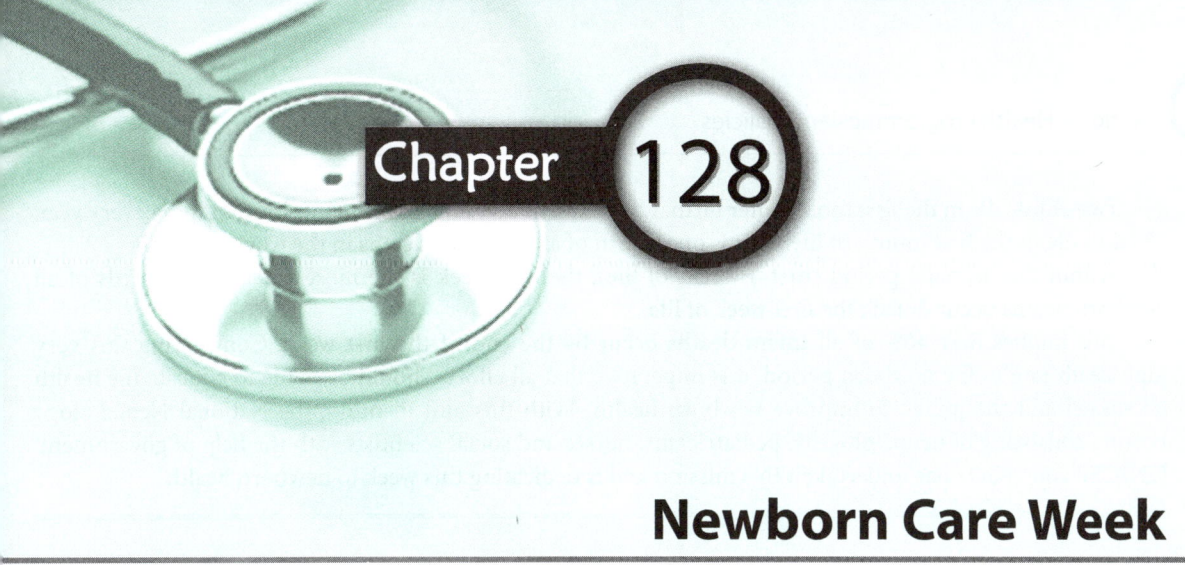

Chapter 128

Newborn Care Week

INTRODUCTION

Newborn Care Week is celebrated every year throughout the country from 15th to 21st November. The theme of year 2016 was—"Quality Improvement by Data Keeping."

National Neonatology Forum in collaboration with the Government of India, Ministry of Family Health and Welfare (MoFHW) and UNICEF is celebrating "Newborn Week" between 15th and 21st November every year.

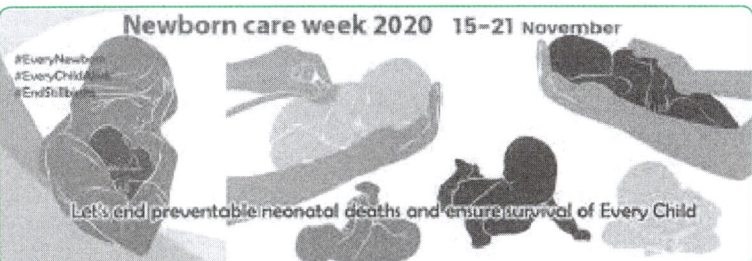

AIMS AND OBJECTIVES

November '2001' was the second year that this week was being organized all over India.

- The aim is to generate awareness and suggest measures to improve health of newborn and child survival.
- Primary objective of creating awareness amongst beneficiaries and in primary level service providers, about the importance of neonatal care in the larger context of IMR reduction at the state level.
- Theme of 2017 was "Gender gap in Neonatal Survival-Time to Act."
- The theme of 2020 was "Quality, Equity, Dignity for every newborn at every health facility and everywhere."

HISTORY

Newborn health is of paramount importance, as this contributes significantly to infant mortality in our country. Infant mortality has significantly dropped over the last one decade, but is still very high. It has reached a plateau which is mainly due to high neonatal mortality rate.

Overall, Infant Mortality Rate (IMR) in our country is 70 per 1000 live births, which means out of every 1000 newborn babies born, 70 babies die during first year of life.

Two-thirds die in the first month after birth. Of approximately 250 lakhs infants born in India every year, 12 lakhs die in the first month of life. This is one fourth of all newborn deaths in the world annually.

Within the neonatal period (first 4 weeks of life), the first week is the most crucial. Two thirds of all newborn deaths occur during the first week of life.

This implies over 40% of all infant deaths occur by the end of the first week. Considering this very high death rate in the newborn period, it is imperative that all efforts should be made to educate the health personnel and the public to improve newborn health. With this aim in mind, the National Neonatology Forum, consisting of neonatologists, pediatricians, nurses and social scientists with the help of government, UNICEF and NGO's has undertaken this mission and is dedicating this week to newborn health.

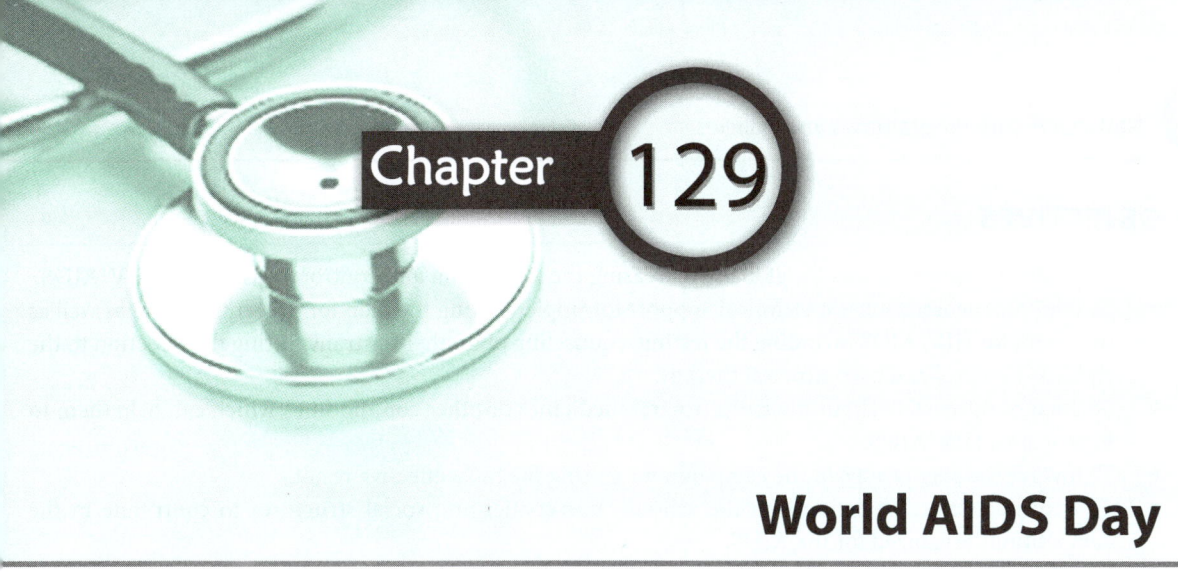

Chapter 129

World AIDS Day

INTRODUCTION

World AIDS day is celebrated every year on 1st December to generate awareness about acquired immunodeficiency syndrome (AIDS). It was celebrated in 1988 as the first ever global health day.

The day is celebrated by the government organizations, NGOs, civil society and other health officials by organizing the speeches or forums discussion related to the AIDS.

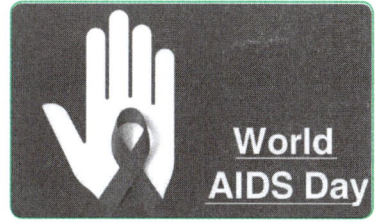

HISTORY

The President of United States declared an official announcement for World AIDS Day in the year 1995, which is followed by other countries all across the world. According to the rough estimation, around 25 million people died from 1981 to 2007 because of the HIV infection. Even after the access of antiretroviral treatment at many places, around 2 million people (at least 270,000 of total were children) in 2007 were infected with this epidemic disease.

World AIDS Day celebration has become the most recognized health day celebrations internationally. World AIDS Day celebration offers the key opportunity to the health organizations to increase the awareness among people, most possible access to the treatment as well as discussing the preventive measures.

World AIDS Day was first visualized by the Thomas Netter and James W Bunn in the month of August in 1987. Thomas Netter and James W Bunn both are the public information officers for the AIDS Global Programme at the World Health Organization (WHO) in Geneva, Switzerland. They had shared their idea about the AIDS day to Dr. Jonathan Mann (Director of the AIDS Global Programme), who had approved the idea and recommended the World AIDS Day observance on 1st of December in the year 1988.

World AIDS Day celebration was celebrated by them to be celebrated every year on 1st of December accurately. They thought that it should be celebrated far from the election time, Christmas holidays or other holidays. It should be celebrated during time when people and news media could pay more interest and attention in broadcasting the news all across the world.

The Joint United Nations Programme on HIV/AIDS, also known as the UNAIDS, came into effect in the year 1996 and started promoting worldwide. Instead of being celebrated for only one day, World AIDS Campaign was launched by the UNAIDS in the year 1997 to focus on the AIDS programmes, better communication, disease prevention and disease awareness for whole year.

OBJECTIVES

- To guide the member states for globally increasing the prevention and control measures for HIV/AIDS.
- To offer the member states a technical support for implementing the plan for prevention, care as well as treatment for HIV/AIDS including the testing, counseling of mother for transmitting the infection to the child, STI control and antiretroviral therapy.
- To make people aware about the antiretroviral medicines or other commodities which can help them to fight against HIV/AIDS.
- To involve the peer groups in the campaign for getting the most effective result.
- To encourage more students from the schools, universities and social structures to contribute in the competitions organized for the AIDS.
- To decrease and control the number of patients infected by HIV/AIDS as well as to encourage the peer groups for condom.

THEMES

In the starting years, the World AIDS Day themes were focused only on the children as well as the young people, which were later recognized as a family disease as any person of any age group can be infected with HIV. Since 2007, the World AIDS Day was started symbolizing by an iconic display of AIDS Ribbon by the White House.

Themes of World AIDS Day	
1988	"Communication"
1989	"Youth"
1990	"Women and AIDS"
1991	"Sharing the Challenge"
1992	"Community Commitment"
1993	"Act"
1994	"AIDS and the Family"
1995	"Shared Rights, Shared Responsibilities"
1996	"One World and One Hope"
1997	"Children Living in a World with AIDS"
1998	"Force for Change: World AIDS Campaign with Young People"
1999	"Listen, Learn, Live: World AIDS Campaign with Children and Young People"
2000	"AIDS: Men Make a Difference"
2001	"I care. Do you?"
2002–2003	"Stigma and Discrimination"
2004	"Women, Girls, HIV and AIDS"
2005	"Stop AIDS: Keep the Promise"
2006	"Stop AIDS: Keep the Promise-Accountability"
2007	"Stop AIDS: Keep the Promise- Leadership"

Contd...

Themes of World AIDS Day	
2008	"Stop AIDS: Keep the Promise-Lead-Empower-Deliver"
2009	"Universal Access and Human Rights"
2010	"Universal Access and Human Rights"
2011–2015	"Getting to zero: zero new HIV infections. Zero discrimination. Zero AIDS related deaths"
2016	"My Health, My Right"
2017	"My Health, My Right"
2018	"Know your status"
2019	"Communities make the difference"
2020	"Ending the HIV/AIDS Epidemic: Resilience and Impact"

ACTIVITIES

Community-based individuals and organizations should be contacted to plan the World AIDS Day activities. It can be well started from the local clinics, hospitals, social service agencies, schools, AIDS advocacy groups, etc.

- A single event or sequence of independent events can be determined for better awareness by the speakers and exhibitors through the forums, rallies, health fairs, community events, faith services, parades, block parties, etc.
- A public statement can be submitted to the agency board identifying the recognition for the World AIDS Day.
- Red ribbons should be wore or distributed to the schools, work sites or community groups to mark the hope. Electronic ribbons can also be distributed to the social media outlets.
- All the activities (like DVD showings and Aids prevention seminars) of businesses, schools, health care organizations, clergy and local agencies should be encouraged for their great work.
- A candle light vigil can be held at the public park or the nearest agency where singers, musicians, dancers, poets, story tellers, etc. could distribute the message of AIDS prevention through entertaining performances.
- World AIDS Day information can be distributed by linking it to the website of your agency.
- All the planned events and activities should be already distributed through the e-mail, newsletters, mailings or electronic bulletins.
- People can be made aware by displaying the exhibitions, posters, videos, flyers, brochures for HIV/AIDS, etc.
- World AIDS Day activities can be informed to a large group of people instantly through the blogs, Facebook, Twitter or through the other social media websites.
- Actively contribute to other groups celebrating the World AIDS Day.
- A candle light celebration can be held in the memory of died person due to HIV/AIDS.
- Religious leaders are encouraged to speak something for AIDS intolerance and dishonor.
- A service can be started to provide the meals, shelter, transportation, companionship for the people with HIV/AIDS. They can also be invited in the social work, worship or other functions to increase their morality.

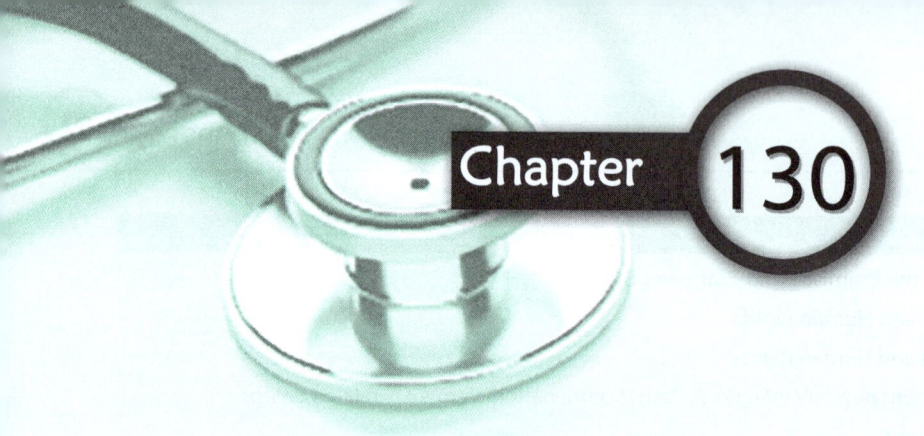

Chapter 130

National Pollution Prevention Day

INTRODUCTION

2nd December is observed as National Pollution Prevention Day in India. This day is observed in the memory of people who lost their lives in Bhopal gas calamity. Bhopal gas tragedy occurred in the year 1984 on the night of 2–3 December. Many people died due to poisonous gas Methyl Isocyanate also known as MIC. Bhopal Gas Tragedy is considered as one of the biggest industrial pollution disasters.

OBJECTIVES

- To spread awareness on managing and controlling industrial disasters
- To prevent the pollution produced by industrial processes or human negligence
- To make people and industries aware about the importance of pollution control acts.

SOME OF THE PREVENTION MEASURES TAKEN BY THE INDIAN LEGISLATION

- Water (Prevention and Control of Pollution) Act of 1974
- Water (Prevention and Control of Pollution) Cess Act of 1977
- Air (Prevention and Control of Pollution) Act of 1981
- Environment (Protection) Rules of 1986
- Environment (Protection) Act of 1986
- Manufacture, Storage and Import of Hazardous Chemical Rules of 1989
- Recycled Plastics Manufacture and Usage Rules of 1999
- Ozone Depleting Substances (Regulation) Rules of 2000
- Noise Pollution (Regulation and Control) Rules of 2000
- Batteries (Management and Handling) Rules of 2001
- Maharashtra Biodegradable Garbage (Control) Ordinance of 2006
- Environment Impact Assessment Notification of 2006

Chapter 131

International Day of Persons with Disabilities

INTRODUCTION

International Day of Persons with Disabilities is a day dedicated towards creating awareness regarding challenges faced by disabled persons in their everyday lives. Every year, it is observed on 3rd December. This day aims to mobilize people to extend support to disabled people and thus create enabling environment around them.

The day was greatly emphasized to celebrate it yearly in order to promote the awareness about the people with disabilities as well as to encourage them by implementing a lot of assistance in their real life to enhance their way of life and remove the social stigma towards them. Since 1992, it has been celebrated continuously every year with a lot of success all over the world. The vital purpose of celebration of this day is to improve the understandings of the people worldwide towards the people with disability issues as well as get together to support them to improve their self-esteem, well-being and rights in the society. It also looks for to involve all the persons with disabilities in the society in each facet of life such as the political, economic, social and cultural. That is why it is celebrated by the title of "International Day of Disabled Persons". Every year celebration of the international day of disabled persons focuses on the different issues of the disabled persons all across the world.

HISTORY

The year 1981 was announced as the "International Year of Disabled Persons" by the United Nations General Assembly in the year 1976. It was planned to emphasize the rehabilitation, prevention, promotion and equalization of opportunities for the persons with disabilities at the international, regional and national levels.

The theme decided for the celebration of international year of disabled persons was "full participation and equality," to make the people aware about the rights of disabled persons for their equal development in the societies, to emphasize the normal living standards for them as equal to normal citizens, and to improve their socioeconomic condition.

The years 1983–1992 were declared as the "United Nations Decade of Disabled Persons" by the United Nations General Assembly in order to offer the time frame to the Governments and other organizations so that they could properly implement all the recommended activities.

THEMES

Themes of International Day of Persons with Disabilities	
1998	"Arts, Culture and Independent Living"
1999	"Accessibility for all for the new Millennium"
2000	"Making information technologies work for all"
2001	"Full participation and equality: The call for new approaches to assess progress and evaluate outcome"
2002	"Independent Living and Sustainable Livelihoods"
2003	"A Voice of our Own"
2004	"Nothing about Us, Without Us"
2005	"Rights of Persons with Disabilities: Action in Development"
2006	"E-Accessibility"
2007	"Decent Work for Persons with Disabilities"
2008	"Convention on the Rights of Persons with Disabilities: Dignity and justice for all of us"
2009	"Making the MDGs Inclusive: Empowerment of persons with disabilities and their communities around the world"
2010	"Keeping the promise: Mainstreaming disability in the Millennium Development Goals towards 2015 and beyond"
2011	"Together for a better world for all: Including persons with disabilities in development"
2012	"Removing barriers to create an inclusive and accessible society for all"
2013	"Break Barriers, Open Doors: for an inclusive society and development for all"
2014	"Sustainable Development: The Promise of Technology"
2015	"Inclusion matters: access and empowerment for people of all abilities." This theme provides a frame for considering how people with disability are excluded from society by promoting the removal of all types of barriers, including those relating to the physical environment, information and communications technology (ICT), or attitudinal barriers.
2016	"Achieving 17 Goals for the Future We Want"
2017	"Transformation towards sustainable and resilient society for all"
2018	"Empowering persons with disabilities and ensuring inclusiveness and equality"
2019	"Promoting the participation of persons with disabilities and their leadership: taking action on the 2030 Development Agenda"
2020	"Building back better: towards an inclusive, accessible and sustainable post COVID-19 world by, for and with persons with disabilities"

There were also three sub-themes of that year:
- Making cities inclusive and accessible for all
- Improving disability data and statistics
- Including persons with invisible disabilities in society and development.

As per World Health Organization (WHO), "There are over one billion people in this world with some form of disability."

Chapter 132

World Patient Safety Day

INTRODUCTION

World Patient Safety day is celebrated every year on 9th December to raise awareness about the safety of patients. Patient safety is a global public health concern and is a fundamental principle of health care. The main aim of this day is to raise awareness about patient safety issues in all parts of the world.

Patient Safety Day was launched by the WHO in 2005 for increasing awareness of unsafe health care.

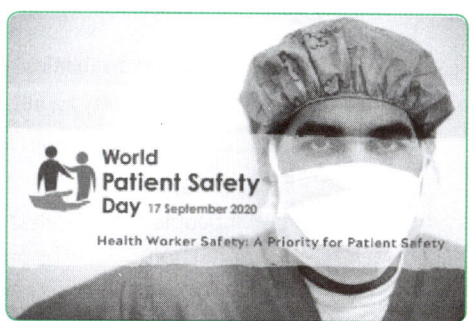

PURPOSE

The purpose of Patient Safety Day is to provide high level support and commitment for the improvement of patient safety and service issues all over the world. Its main goal is to reduce medical errors that can worsen the condition of patients and sometimes even lead to their death. The annual event also aims to improve public education about patient safety and the other issues connected to it. The WHO initiative also emphasizes the awareness of unsafe health care. It is when patients are asked to observe and adopt certain means and methods to improve health care processes and standards all over the world.

ACTIVITIES

- Use social media to help inform the public about World Patient Safety Day.
- Organize an event in your community for the initiative.
- Distribute informative materials regarding patient safety.
- Start a group in your community for advocating patient safety.

- Contact your local newspaper to create an informative article for the awareness campaign.
- Organize a World Patient Safety Day essay working with your local school or newspaper.
- Urge your local officials to create an event for the initiative.
- Encourage your local television and radio stations to make a public service announcement.
- The theme for World Day for Safety and Health at Work 2020 was "Stop the pandemic: Safety and health at work can save lives".
- In 2019, the theme was "Safety and Health and the Future of Work."
- In 2018, the theme was "Occupational Safety and Health (OSH) vulnerability of young workers."
- In 2017, the theme was "Optimize the collection and use of OSH data."

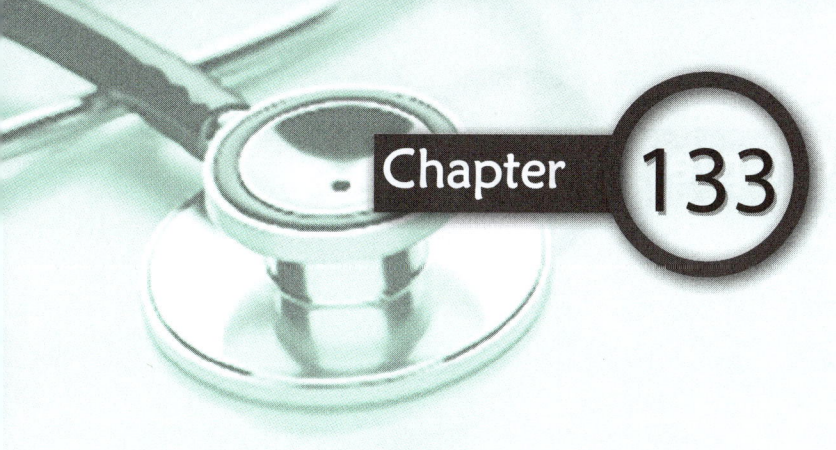

Chapter 133

Universal Health Coverage Day

INTRODUCTION

Universal Health Coverage Day is being observed every year, on 12th December as a global initiative by United Nations to ensure that every individual has access to health care without suffering from financial hardship. On 12th December 2015, a global coalition focused on universal health coverage to be an important issue for the sustainable development and a priority for all nations.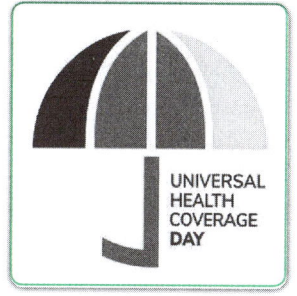

Universal Health Coverage (UHC) means ensuring equitable access to all the citizens in any part of the country, regardless of income level, social status, gender, caste or religion. It aims to provide affordable, accountable, appropriate health service of assured quality including preventive, curative and rehabilitative care.

Universal coverage is firmly based on the 1948 WHO Constitution, which declares health as a fundamental human right and commits to ensuring the highest attainable level of health for all.

600+ global partners including founding leaders The Rockefeller Foundation, World Bank Group and World Health Organization are standing for "Health for all."

The theme of UHC Day 2020 was "Health for all: protect everyone. To end this crisis and build a safer and healthier future, we must invest in health systems that protect us all—now" UHC Day Campaign on 12th December 2020 marked one year since the first case of COVID-19 were reported.

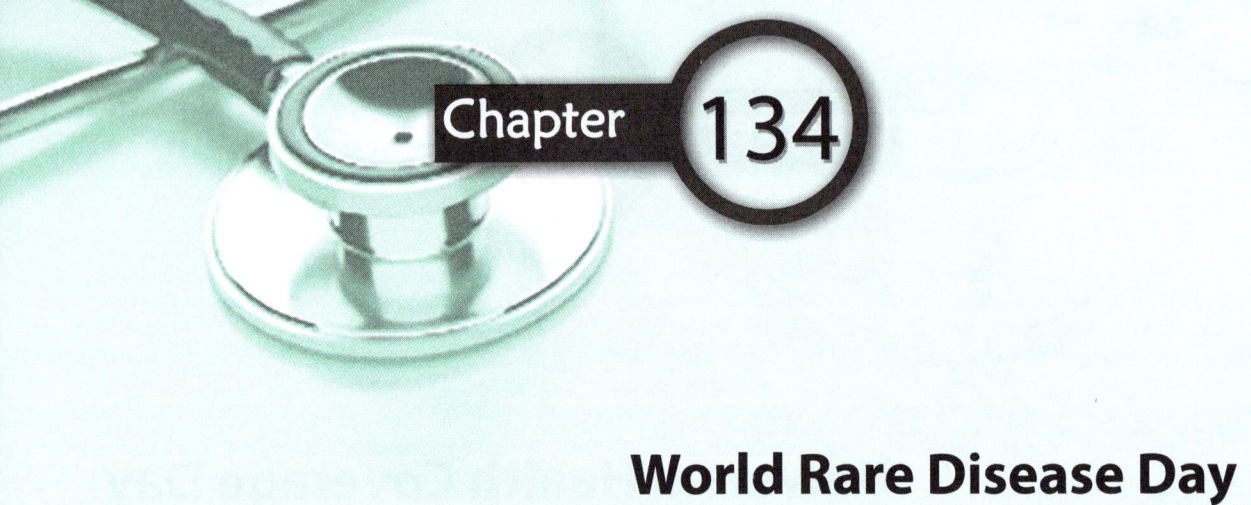

Chapter 134

World Rare Disease Day

INTRODUCTION

Rare Disease Day is an observance held on the last day of February to raise awareness about rare diseases and improve access to treatment and medical representation for individuals with rare diseases and their families. The European Organization for Rare Diseases (EURORDIS) established the day in 2008 to raise awareness for unknown or overlooked illnesses. According to EURORDIS, treatments for many rare diseases are insufficient, as are the social networks to support individuals with rare diseases and their families; furthermore, while there were already numerous days dedicated to sufferers of individual diseases (such as AIDS, cancer, etc.), there had previously not been a day for representing sufferers of rare diseases. In 2009, Rare Disease Day went global as the National Organization for Rare Disorders (NORD) and mobilized 200 rare disease patient support organizations in the United States while various organizations in China, Australia, Taiwan, and Latin America also lead efforts in their respective countries to coordinate activities and promote the day.

The first Rare Disease Day was coordinated by the European Organization for Rare Diseases (EURORDIS) and held on February 29, 2008 in many European nations and in Canada through the Canadian Organization for Rare Disorders. The date was chosen because February 29 is a 'rare day', and 2008 was the 25th anniversary of the passing of the Orphan Drug Act in the United States.

Individuals observing Rare Disease Day took part in walks and press conferences to raise public awareness of rare diseases, organized fundraisers, and wrote en masse to government representatives; health-related nonprofit organizations across several countries also held events, gatherings, and campaigns. The day also included an open session of the European Parliament specifically dedicated to discussing policy issues relating to rare diseases. The days leading up to Rare Disease Day included other policy-related events in numerous locations, such as a reception in the British Parliament where policymakers met with individuals with rare diseases to discuss issues such as "equal access and availability of prevention, diagnosis, treatment and rehabilitation."

In 2009, Rare Disease Day was observed for the first time in Panama, Colombia, Argentina, Australia, Serbia, Russia, the People's Republic of China, and the United States. In the United States, the National Organization for Rare Disorders signed on to coordinate Rare Disease Day and collaborated with The Discovery Channel and the show Mystery Diagnosis, and about 180 other partners. They committed to organize activities across the country for the observance of Rare Disease Day. Several United States state governments issued proclamations regarding Rare Disease Day. In Europe, over 600 patient advocacy and support organizations, again coordinated by EURORDIS, also planned events.

In 2010 and 2011, 46 countries participated. Latvia, Lithuania, Slovenia, Georgia, and three African countries joined the event for the first time. By 2012, thousands of patient support organizations had gotten involved, including more than 600 partners working with NORD in the US to promote Rare Disease Day.

By 2014, 84 countries were participating, with over 400 events worldwide. Nine new countries participated in 2014, Cuba, Ecuador, Egypt, Guinea, Jordan, Kazakhstan, Kenya, Oman, and Paraguay. In 2018, Cape Verde, Ghana, Syria, Togo, and Trinidad and Tobago participated for the first time, with 80 nations participating in that year's events.

WHY

Building awareness of rare diseases is so important because one in 20 people will live with a rare disease at some point in their life. Despite this, there is no cure for most of the rare diseases and many of them go undiagnosed. Rare Disease Day improves knowledge amongst the general public about the rare diseases and encourage researchers and decision makers to address the needs of those living with rare diseases.

The first Rare Disease Day was celebrated in 2008 on 29 February, a 'rare' date that occurs only once every four years. Ever since then, Rare Disease Day has taken place on the last day of February, a month known for having a 'rare' number of days.

In India, patient organizations first became involved in Rare Disease Day in 2010. Since then, they have focused on raising awareness and compassion for people living with a rare disease all across India through poster campaigns, school visits, competitions, a film festival, counseling sessions, and more. In 2012, the day attracted mass media attention when Indian star singer Shaan performed at an event.

India marked the occasion of Rare Disease Day 2020 with events across the country including India's annual 'Race for 7' event. More than 7000 participants ran a 7 km race to represent that more than 7000 rare diseases are documented so far. The Indian Organization for Rare Diseases (IORD) also hosted a meeting bringing together all stakeholders, creating a platform to brainstorm and analyze the latest rare disease policy released by the Indian Health Ministry.

Themes of Past World Rare Disease Days

Year	Theme	Slogan
2008	Rare Diseases as a Public Health Priority	A Rare Day for Very Special People
2009	Rare Diseases: A Public Health Priority	Patient Care: A Public Affair!
2010	Bridging Patients and Researchers	Patients and Researchers: Partners for Life!
2011	Rare Diseases and Health Inequalities	Rare but Equal
2012	Solidarity	Rare but Strong Together!
2013	Solidarity	Rare Disorders without Borders
2014	Care	Join Together for Better Care!
2015	Living with a Rare Disease	Day-by-day, hand-in-hand
2016	Patient Voice	Join Us in Making the Voice of Rare Diseases Heard
2017	Research	With Research, Possibilities are Limitless
2018	Research	Show your Rare. Show you Care
2019	Bridging Health and Social Care	Show your Rare. Show you Care
2020	Equity	Rare is Many. Rare is Strong. Rare is Proud!
2021	Reframe	

Notes

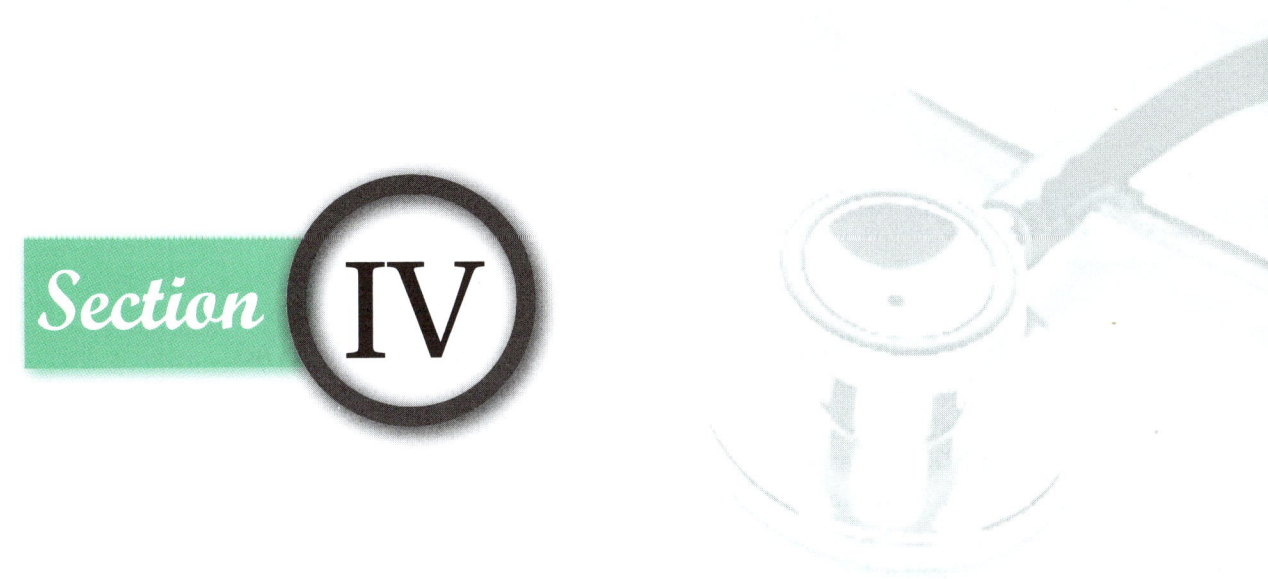

Section **IV**

HEALTH-RELATED ACTS

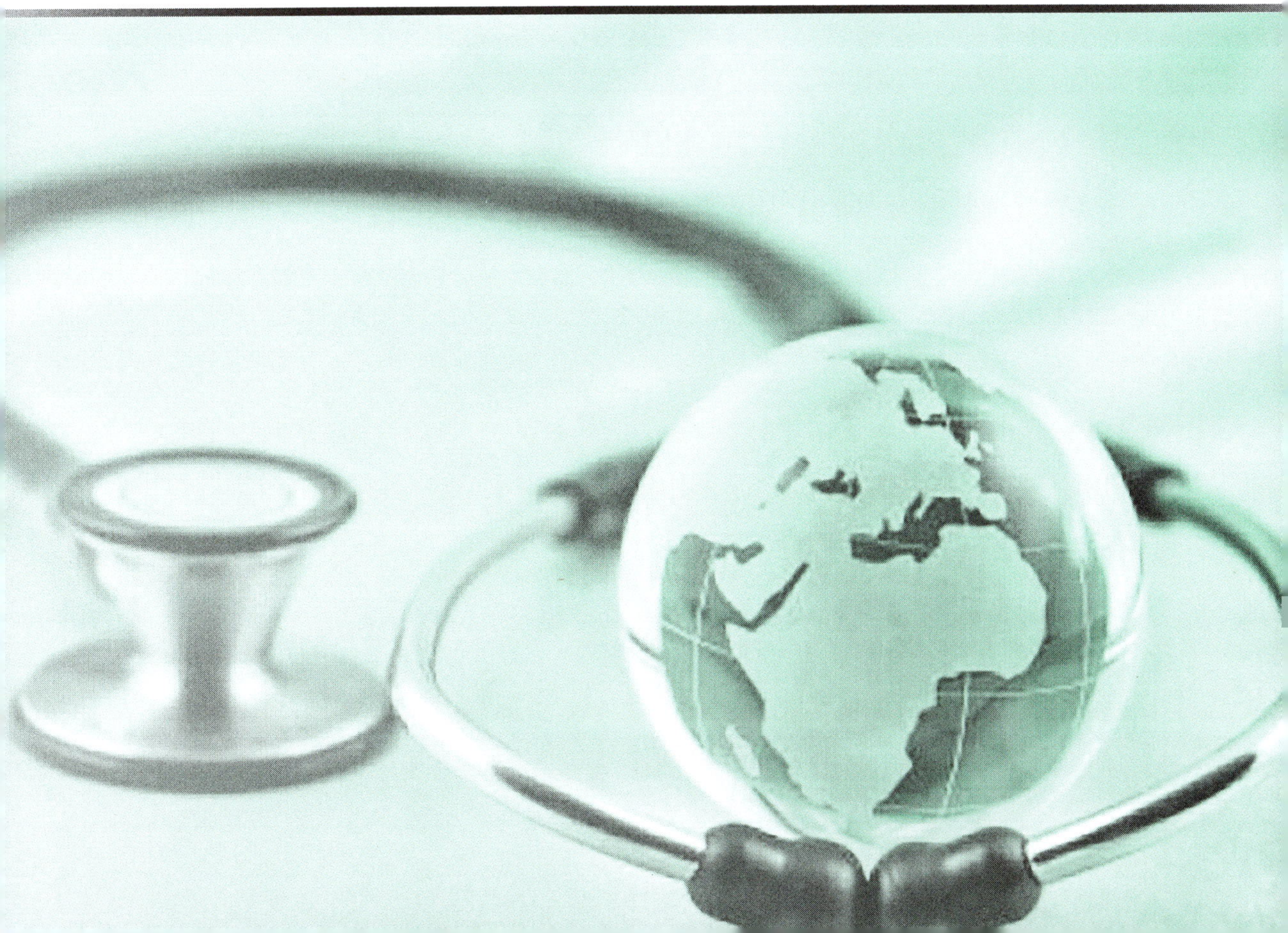

Contents

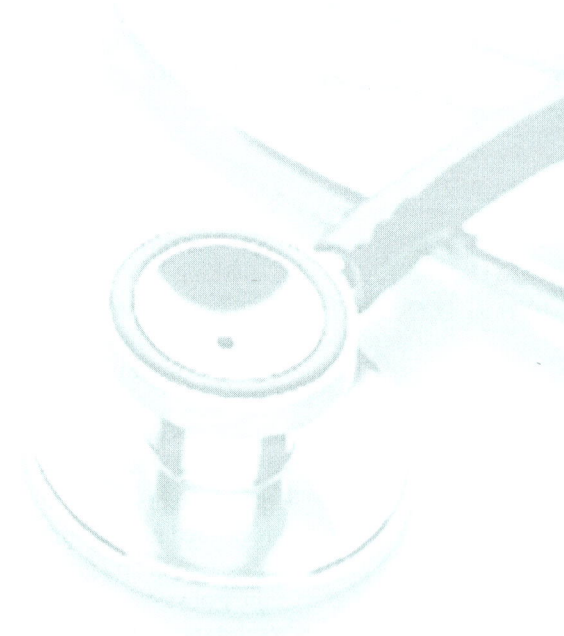

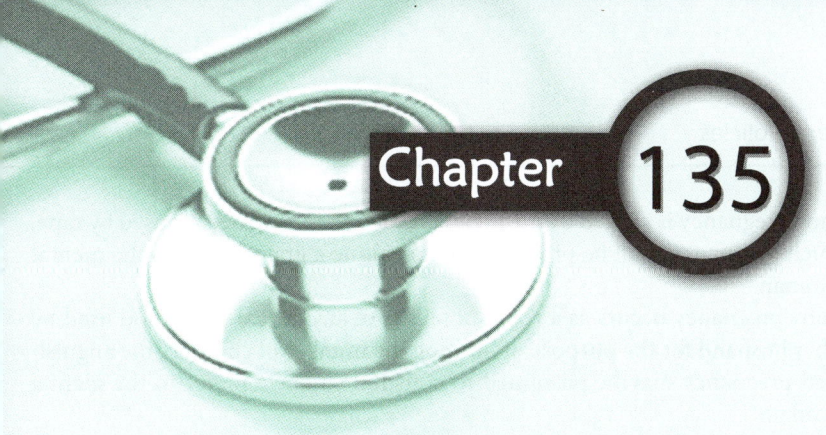

Chapter 135

Medical Termination of Pregnancy Act

INTRODUCTION

An Act to provide for the termination of certain pregnancies by registered medical practitioners and for matters connected therewith or incidental thereto.

Be it enacted by Parliament in the Twenty-second Year of the Republic of India as follows:

1. **Short title, extent, and commencement—**
   (1) This Act may be called the Medical Termination of Pregnancy Act, 1971.
   (2) It extends to the whole of India except the State of Jammu and Kashmir.
   (3) It shall come into force on such date as the Central Government may, by notification in the Official Gazette, appoint.

2. **Definitions—**In this Act, unless the context otherwise requires,—
   (a) **"guardian"** means a person having the care of the person of a minor or a lunatic;
   (b) **"lunatic"** has the meaning assigned to it in Section 3 of the Indian Lunacy Act, 1912 (4 of 1912);
   (c) **"minor"** means a person who, under the provisions of the Indian Majority Act, 1875 (9 of 1875), is to be deemed not to have attained his majority,
   (d) **"registered medical practitioner"** means a medical practitioner who possesses any recognized medical qualification as defined in Cl. (h) of Section 2 of the Indian Medical Council Act, 1956 (102 of 1956), whose name has been entered in a State Medical Register and who has such experience or training in gynecology and obstetrics as may be prescribed by rules made under this Act.

3. **When pregnancies may be terminated by registered medical practitioners—**
   (1) Notwithstanding anything contained in the Indian Penal Code (45 of 1860), a registered medical practitioner shall not be guilty of any offence under that Code or under any other law for the time being in force, if any pregnancy is terminated by him in accordance with the provisions of this Act.
   (2) Subject to the provisions of sub-section (4), a pregnancy may be terminated by a registered medical practitioner,—
      (a) where the length of the pregnancy does not exceed twelve weeks if such medical practitioner is,
      or
      (b) where the length of the pregnancy exceeds twelve weeks but does not exceed twenty weeks if not less than two registered medical practitioners are of opinion, formed in good faith, that,—
         (i) the continuance of the pregnancy would involve a risk to the life of the pregnant woman or of grave injury physical or mental health; or
         (ii) there is a substantial risk that if the child were born, it would suffer from such physical or mental abnormalities as to be seriously handicapped.

Explanation 1—Where any pregnancy is alleged by the pregnant woman to have been caused by rape, the anguish caused by such pregnancy shall be presumed to constitute a grave injury to the mental health of the pregnant woman.

Explanation 2—Where any pregnancy occurs as a result of failure of any device or method used by any married woman or her husband for the purpose of limiting the number of children, the anguish caused by such unwanted pregnancy may be presumed to constitute a grave injury to the mental health of the pregnant woman.

(3) In determining whether the continuance of pregnancy would involve such risk of injury to the health as is mentioned in sub-section (2), account may be taken of the pregnant woman's actual or reasonable foreseeable environment.

(4) (a) No pregnancy of a woman, who has not attained the age of 18 years, or, who, having attained the age of 18 years, is a lunatic, shall be terminated except with the consent in writing of her guardian.

(b) Save as otherwise provided in Cl. (a), no pregnancy shall be terminated except with the consent of the pregnant woman.

4. **Place where pregnancy may be terminated—No termination of pregnancy shall be made in accordance with this Act at any place other than,—**

(a) a hospital established or maintained by Government, or

(b) a place for the time being approved for the purpose of this Act by Government.

5. **Sections 3 and 4 when not to apply—**

(1) The provisions of Section 4 and so much of the provisions of sub-section (2) of Section 3 as relate to the length of the pregnancy and the opinion of not less than two registered medical practitioner, shall not apply to the termination of a pregnancy by the registered medical practitioner in case where he is of opinion, formed in good faith, that the termination of such pregnancy is immediately necessary to save the life of the pregnant woman.

(2) Notwithstanding anything contained in the Indian Penal Code (45 of 1860), the termination of a pregnancy by a person who is not a registered medical practitioner shall be an offence and punishable under that Code, and that Code shall, to this extent, stand modified.

6. **Power to make rules—**

(1) The Central Government may, by notification in the Official Gazette, make rules to carry out the provisions of this Act.

(2) In particular, and without prejudice to the generality of the foregoing power, such rules may provide for all or any of the following matters, namely:

(a) the experience or training, or both, which a registered medical practitioner shall have if he intends to terminate any pregnancy under this Act; and

(b) such other matters as are required to be or may be, provided by rules made under this Act.

(3) Every rule made by the Central Government under this Act shall be laid, as soon as may be after it is made, before each House of Parliament while it is in session for a total period of 30 days which may be comprised in one session or in two successive sessions, and if, before the expiry of the session which it is so laid or the session immediately following, both Houses agree in making any modification in the rule or both.

Houses agree that the rule should not be made, the rule shall thereafter have effect only in such modified form or be of no effect, as the case may be; so, however, that any such modification or annulment shall be without prejudice to the validity of anything previously done under that rule.

7. **Power to make regulations—**
   (1) The State Government may, by regulations,—
       (a) require any such opinion as is referred to in sub-section (2) of Section 3 to be certified by a registered medical practitioner or practitioners concerned in such form and at such time as be specified in such regulations, and the preservation or disposal of such certificates;
       (b) require any registered medical practitioner, who terminates a pregnancy to give intimation of such termination and such other information relating to the termination as maybe specified in such regulations;
       (c) prohibit the disclosure, except to such persons and for such purposes as may be specified in such regulations, of intimations given or information furnished in pursuance of such regulations.
   (2) The intimation given and the information furnished in pursuance of regulations made by virtue of Cl. (b) of sub-section (1) shall be given or furnished, as the case may be, to the Chief Medical Officer of the State.
   (3) Any person who willfully contravenes or willfully fails to comply with the requirements of any regulation made under sub-section (1) shall be liable to be punished with fine which may extend to one thousand rupees.

8. **Protection of action taken in good faith—**No suit for other legal proceedings shall lie against any registered medical practitioner for any damage caused likely to be caused by anything which is in good faith done or intended to be done under this Act.

THE MEDICAL TERMINATION OF PREGNANCY (AMENDMENT) BILL, 2020

According to Section 3 (2) of the Medical Termination of Pregnancy (MTP) Act, 1971, a pregnancy may be terminated by a registered medical practitioner:

Where the length of the pregnancy does not exceed twelve weeks, or

Where the length of the pregnancy exceeds twelve weeks but does not exceed twenty weeks. In this case, the abortion will take place, if not less than two registered medical practitioners are of opinion, that the continuance of the pregnancy would involve a risk to the life of the pregnant woman (her physical or mental health); or there is a substantial risk that if the child were born, it would suffer from some physical or mental abnormalities to be seriously handicapped.

The proposed amendments introduce the following provisions:

- For termination of pregnancy up to 20 weeks of gestation the opinion of one registered medical practitioner will be required, and for termination of pregnancy of 20–24 weeks of gestation opinion of two registered medical practitioners will be required.
- Extending the upper gestation limit from 20 to 24 weeks for special categories of women which includes vulnerable women including survivors of rape, victims of incest and other vulnerable women (like differently abled women, minors), etc.
- Upper gestation limit not to apply in cases of substantial fetal abnormalities diagnosed by Medical Board. The composition, functions and other details of Medical Board to be prescribed subsequently in Rules under the Act.
- Name and other particulars of a woman whose pregnancy has been terminated shall not be revealed except to a person authorized in any law for the time being in force.

- The Medical Termination of Pregnancy (Amendment) Bill, 2020 is for expanding access of women to safe and legal abortion services on therapeutic, eugenic, humanitarian or social grounds.
- The proposed amendments to increase upper gestation limit for termination of pregnancy for women in special category aim to strengthen access to comprehensive abortion care, under strict conditions, without compromising service and quality of safe abortion.

Note: At present most countries allow elective abortions but only a few including Canada, China, the Netherlands, North Korea, Singapore, the United States, and Vietnam permit (MTP) after 20 weeks. The late termination of pregnancy is legally get conflict with the viability of the fetus (where a fetus is capable of living outside the womb) and risk of maternal mortality in case of unsafe abortion or risk related to delayed abortion.

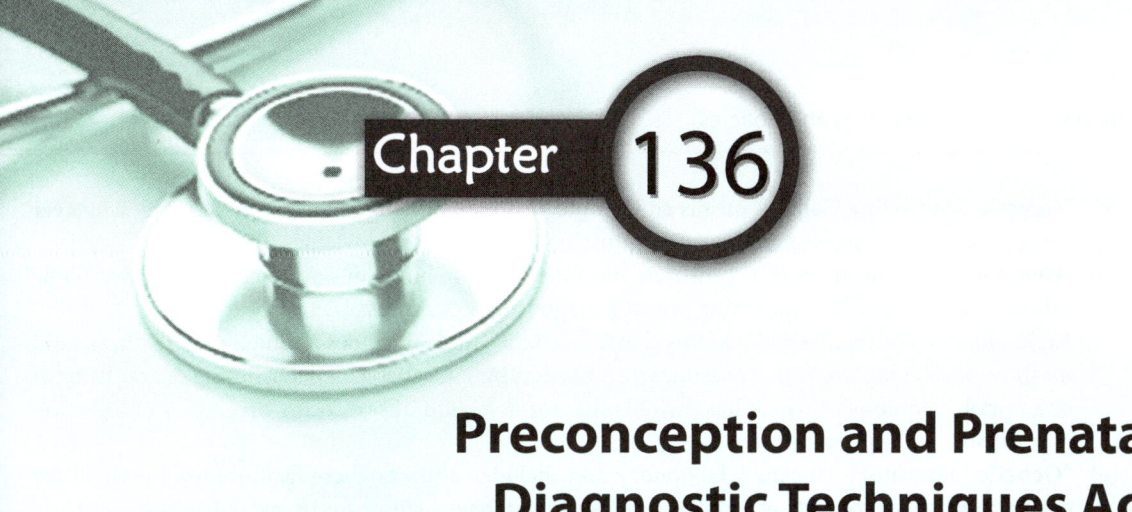

Chapter 136

Preconception and Prenatal Diagnostic Techniques Act

THE PRENATAL DIAGNOSTIC TECHNIQUES (PROHIBITION OF SEX SELECTION) ACT, 1994

[Act No. 57 of 1994]

[20th September, 1994]

An Act to provide for the prohibition of sex selection, before or after conception, and for regulation of prenatal diagnostic techniques for the purposes of detecting genetic abnormalities or metabolic disorders or chromosomal abnormalities or certain congenital malformations or sex-linked disorders and for the prevention of their misuse for sex determination leading to female feticide; and, for matters connected therewith or incidental thereto.

Be it enacted by Parliament in the Forty-fifth Year of the Republic of India as follows:

CHAPTER I: PRELIMINARY

1. **Short title, extent and commencement—**
   (a) This Act may be called the Preconception and Pre-natal Diagnostic Techniques (Prohibition of Sex Selection) Act, 1994.
   (b) It shall extend to the whole of India except the State of Jammu and Kashmir.
   (c) It shall come into force on such date as the Central Government may, by notification in the Official Gazette, appoint.
2. **Definitions—**In this Act, unless the context otherwise requires,—
   (a) **"Appropriate Authority"** means the Appropriate Authority appointed under section 17.
   (b) **"Board"** means the Central Supervisory Board constituted under section 7.
   (ba)**"Conceptus"** means any product of conception at any stage of development from fertilization until birth including extra embryonic membranes as well as the embryo or fetus.
   (bb) **"Embryo"** means a developing human organism after fertilization till the end of eight weeks (56 days).
   (bc) **"Fetus"** means a human organism during the period of its development beginning on the fifty-seventh day following fertilization or creation (excluding any time in which its development has been suspended) and ending at the birth.

(c) **"Genetic Counseling Center"** means an institute, hospital, nursing home or any place, by whatever name called, which provides for genetic counseling to patients.

(d) **"Genetic Clinic"** means a clinic, institute, hospital, nursing home or any place, by whatever name called, which is used for conducting prenatal diagnostic procedures.

   Explanation— For the purposes of this clause, 'Genetic Clinic' includes a vehicle, where ultrasound machine or imaging machine or scanner or other equipment capable of determining sex of the fetus or a portable equipment which has the potential for detection of sex during pregnancy or selection of sex before conception, is used.

(e) **"Genetic Laboratory"** means a laboratory and includes a place where facilities are provided for conducting analysis or tests of samples received from Genetic Clinic for prenatal diagnostic test.

   Explanation—For the purposes of this clause, 'Genetic Laboratory' includes a place where ultrasound machine or imaging machine or scanner or other equipment capable of determining sex of the fetus or a portable equipment which has the potential for detection of sex during pregnancy or selection of sex before conception, is used.

(f) **"Gynecologist"** means a person who possesses a postgraduate qualification in gynecology and obstetrics.

(g) **"Medical geneticist"** includes a person who possesses a degree or diploma in genetic science in the fields of sex selection and prenatal diagnostic techniques or has experience of not less than 2 years in such field after obtaining—

   (i)   any one of the medical qualifications recognized under the Indian Medical Council Act, 1956 (102 of 1956); or

   (ii) A postgraduate degree in biological sciences.

(h) **"Pediatrician"** means a person who possesses a postgraduate qualification in pediatrics.

(i) **"Prenatal diagnostic procedures"** means all gynecological or obstetrical or medical procedures such as ultrasonography, fetoscopy, taking or removing samples of amniotic fluid, chorionic villi, blood or any other tissue or fluid of a man, or of a woman for being sent to a Genetic Laboratory or Genetic Clinic for conducting any type of analysis or prenatal diagnostic tests for selection of sex before or after conception.

(j) **"Prenatal Diagnostic Techniques"** includes all prenatal diagnostic procedures and prenatal diagnostic tests.

(k) **"Prenatal Diagnostic Test"** means ultrasonography or any test or analysis of amniotic fluid, chorionic villi, blood or any tissue or fluid of a pregnant woman or conceptus conducted to detect genetic or metabolic disorders or chromosomal abnormalities or congenital anomalies or hemoglobinopathies or sex-linked diseases.

(l) **"Prescribed"** means prescribed by rules made under this Act.

(m) **"Registered Medical Practitioner"** means a medical practitioner who possesses any recognized medical qualification as defined in clause (h) of Section 2 of the Indian Medical Council Act, 1956, (102 of 1956) and whose name has been entered in a State Medical Register.

(n) **"Regulations"** means regulations framed by the Board under this Act.

(o) **"Sex selection"** includes any procedure, technique, test or administration or prescription or provision of anything for the purpose of ensuring or increasing the probability that an embryo will be of a particular sex.

(p) **"Sonologist or imaging specialist"** means a person who possesses any one of the medical qualifications recognized under the Indian Medical Council Act, 1956 or who possesses a postgraduate qualification in ultrasonography or imaging techniques or radiology.

(q) **"State Board"** means a State Supervisory Board or a Union Territory Supervisory Board constituted under Section 16A.

(r) "State Government" in relation to Union Territory with Legislature means the Administrator of that Union Territory appointed by the President under article 239 of Constitution.

CHAPTER II: REGULATION OF GENETIC COUNSELING CENTERS, GENETIC LABORATORIES AND GENETIC CLINICS

3. **Regulation of genetic counseling centers, genetic laboratories and genetic clinics**—On and from the commencement of this Act,—

    (1) No Genetic Counseling Center, Genetic Laboratory or Genetic Clinic unless registered under this Act, shall conduct or associate with, or help in, conducting activities relating to prenatal diagnostic techniques.

    (2) No Genetic Counseling Center or Genetic Laboratory or Genetic Clinic shall employ or cause to be employed or take services of any person, whether on honorary basis or on payment who does not possess qualifications as may be prescribed.

    (3) No medical geneticist, gynecologist, pediatrician, registered medical practitioner or any other person shall conduct or cause to be conducted or aid in conducting by himself or through any other person, any prenatal diagnostic techniques at a place other than a place registered under this Act.

3A. **Prohibition of sex selection**—No person, including a specialist or a team of specialists in the field of infertility, shall conduct or cause to be conducted or aid in conducting by himself or by any other person, sex selection on a woman or a man or on both or on any tissue, embryo, conceptus, fluid or gametes derived from either or both of them.

3B. **Prohibition on sale of ultrasound machines, etc., to persons, laboratories, clinics, etc. not registered under the Act**—No person shall sell any ultrasound machine or imaging machine or scanner or any other equipment capable of detecting sex of fetus to any Genetic Counseling Center, Genetic Laboratory, Genetic Clinic or any other person not registered under the Act.

CHAPTER III: REGULATION OF PRENATAL DIAGNOSTIC TECHNIQUES

4. **Regulation of prenatal diagnostic techniques**—On and from the commencement of this Act,—

    (1) No place including a registered Genetic Counseling Center or Genetic Laboratory or Genetic Clinic shall be used or caused to be used by any person for conducting prenatal diagnostic techniques except for the purposes specified in clause (2) and after satisfying any of the conditions specified in clause (3).

    (2) No prenatal diagnostic techniques shall be conducted except for the purposes of detection of any of the following abnormalities, namely

       (i)   Chromosomal abnormalities

      (ii)   Genetic metabolic diseases

     (iii)   Hemoglobinopathies

     (iv)   Sex-linked genetic diseases

      (v)   Congenital anomalies

     (vi)   Any other abnormalities or diseases as may be specified by the Central Supervisory Board.

(3) No prenatal diagnostic techniques shall be used or conducted unless the person qualified to do so is satisfied for reasons to be recorded in writing that any of the following conditions are fulfilled, namely:

   (i)   Age of the pregnant woman is above 35 years

   (ii)   The pregnant woman has undergone of two or more spontaneous abortions or fetal loss

   (iii)   The pregnant woman had been exposed to potentially teratogenic agents such as drugs, radiation, infection or chemicals

   (iv)   The pregnant woman or her spouse has a family history of mental retardation or physical deformities such as, spasticity or any other genetic disease

   (v)   Any other condition as may be specified by the Central Supervisory Board; provided that the person conducting ultrasonography on a pregnant woman shall keep complete record thereof in the clinic in such manner, as may be prescribed, and any deficiency or inaccuracy found therein shall amount to contravention of provisions of section 5 or section 6 unless contrary is proved by the person conducting such ultrasonography.

(4) No person including a relative or husband of the pregnant woman shall seek or encourage the conduct of any prenatal diagnostic techniques on her except for the purposes specified in clause (2).

(5) No person including a relative or husband of a woman shall seek or encourage the conduct of any sex-selection technique on her or him or both.

5.   **Written consent of pregnant woman and prohibition of communicating the sex of fetus—**

   (1)   No person referred to in clause (2) of Section 3 shall conduct the prenatal diagnostic procedures unless—

      (a)   He has explained all known side and after effects of such procedures to the pregnant woman concerned

      (b)   He has obtained in the prescribed form her written consent to undergo such procedures in the language which she understands; and

      (c)   A copy of her written consent obtained under clause (b) is given to the pregnant woman.

   (2)   No person including the person conducting prenatal diagnostic procedures shall communicate to the pregnant woman concerned or her relatives or any other person the sex of the fetus by words, signs or in any other manner.

6.   **Determination of sex prohibited**—On and from the commencement of this Act,—

   (a)   No Genetic Counseling Center or Genetic Laboratory or Genetic Clinic shall conduct or cause to be conducted in its Center, Laboratory or Clinic, prenatal diagnostic techniques including ultrasonography, for the purpose of determining the sex of a fetus

   (b)   No person shall conduct or cause to be conducted any prenatal diagnostic techniques including ultrasonography for the purpose of determining the sex of a fetus

   (c)   No person shall, by whatever means, cause or allow to be caused selection of sex before or after conception.

CHAPTER IV: CENTRAL SUPERVISORY BOARD

7.   **Constitution of Central Supervisory Board—**

   (1)   The Central Government shall constitute a Board to be known as the Central Supervisory Board to exercise the powers and perform the functions conferred on the Board under this Act.

   (2)   The Board shall consist of—

      (a)   The Minister in charge of the Ministry or Department of Family Welfare, who shall be the Chairman, *ex officio*

(b) The Secretary to the Government of India in charge of the Department of Family Welfare, who shall be the Vice-Chairman, *ex-officio*

(c) Three members to be appointed by the Central Government to represent the Ministries of Central Government in charge of Women and Child Development, Department of Legal Affairs or Legislative Department in the Ministry of Law and Justice, and Indian System of Medicine and Homoeopathy, *ex-officio*

(d) The Director General of Health Services of the Central Government, *ex-officio*

(e) Ten members to be appointed by the Central Government, two each from amongst—

    (i) Eminent medical geneticists

    (ii) Eminent gynecologist and obstetrician or expert of *stri-roga or prasuti-tantra*

    (iii) Eminent pediatricians

    (iv) Eminent social scientists

    (v) Representatives of women welfare organizations

(f) three women Members of Parliament, of whom two shall be elected by the House of the People and one by the Council of States

(g) four members to be appointed by the Central Government by rotation to represent the States and the Union territories, two in the alphabetical order and two in the reverse alphabetical order: Provided that no appointment under this clause shall be made except on the recommendation of the State Government or, as the case may be, the Union Territory

(h) an officer, not below the rank of a Joint Secretary or equivalent of the Central Government, in charge of Family Welfare, who shall be the Member-Secretary, *ex officio*.

8. **Term of office of members—**

(1) The term of office of a member, other than an ex officio member, shall be,—

    (a) In case of appointment under clause (e) or clause (f) of sub-section (2) of Section 7, 3 years

    (b) In case of appointment under clause (g) of the said subsection, one year.

(2) If a casual vacancy occurs in the office of any other members, whether by reason of his death, resignation or inability to discharge his functions owing to illness or other incapacity, such vacancy shall be filled by the Central Government by making a fresh appointment and the member so appointed shall hold office for the remainder of the term of office of the person in whose place he is so appointed.

(3) The Vice-Chairman shall perform such functions as may be assigned to him by the Chairman from time to time.

(4) The procedure to be followed by the members in the discharge of their functions shall be such as may be prescribed.

9. **Meetings of the Board—**

(1) The Board shall meet at such time and place, and shall observe such rules of procedure in regard to the transaction of business at its meetings (including the quorum at such meetings) as may be provided by regulations: Provided that the Board shall meet at least once in six months.

(2) The Chairman and in his absence the Vice-Chairman shall preside at the meetings of the Board.

(3) If for any reason the Chairman or the Vice-Chairman is unable to attend any meeting of the Board, any other member chosen by the members present at the meeting shall preside at the meeting.

(4) All questions which come up before any meeting of the Board shall be decided by a majority of the votes of the members present and voting, and in the event of an equality of votes, the Chairman, or in his absence, the person presiding, shall have and exercise a second or casting vote.

(5) Members other than ex officio members shall receive such allowances, if any, from the Board as may be prescribed.

10. **Vacancies, etc., not to invalidate proceedings of the Board**—No act or proceeding of the Board shall be invalid merely by reason of—
   (a) Any vacancy in, or any defect in the Constitution of, the Board.
   (b) Any defect in the appointment of a person acting as a member of the Board.
   (c) Any irregularity in the procedure of the Board not affecting the merits of the case.

11. **Temporary association of persons with the Board for particular purposes.**
   (1) The Board may associate with itself, in such manner and for such purposes as may be determined by regulations, any person whose assistance or advice it may desire in carrying out any of the provisions of this Act.
   (2) A person associated with it by the Board under sub-section (1) for any purpose shall have a right to take part in the discussions relevant to that purpose, but shall not have a right to vote at a meeting of the Board and shall not be a member for any other purpose.

12. **Appointment or officers and other employees of the Board**—
   (1) For the purpose of enabling it efficiently to discharge its functions under this Act, the Board may, subject to such regulations as may be made in this behalf, appoint (whether on deputation or otherwise) such number of officers and other employees as it may consider necessary: Provided that the appointment of such category of officers, as may be specified in such regulations, shall be subject to the approval of the Central Government.
   (2) Every officer or other employee appointed by the Board shall be subject to such conditions of service and shall be entitled to such remuneration as may be specified in the regulations.

13. **Authentication of orders and other instruments of the Board**—All orders and decisions of the Board shall be authenticated by the signature of the Chairman or any other member authorized by the Board in this behalf, and all other instruments issued by the Board shall be authenticated by the signature of the Member-Secretary or any other officer of the Board authorized in like manner in this behalf.

14. **Disqualifications for appointment as member**—A person shall be disqualified for being appointed as a member if, he—
   (a) has been convicted and sentenced to imprisonment for an offence which, in the opinion of the Central Government, involves moral turpitude
   (b) is an undischarged insolvent
   (c) is of unsound mind and stands so declared by a competent court
   (d) has been removed or dismissed from the service of the Government or a Corporation owned or controlled by the Government
   (e) has, in the opinion of the Central Government, such financial or other interest in the Board as is likely to affect prejudicially the discharge by him of his functions as a member
   (f) has, in the opinion of the Central Government, been associated with the use or promotion of prenatal diagnostic technique for determination of sex or with any sex selection technique.

15. **Eligibility of member for reappointment**—Subject to the other terms and conditions of service as may be prescribed, any person ceasing to be a member shall be eligible for reappointment as such member. Provided that no member other than an *ex officio* member shall be appointed for more than two consecutive terms.

16. **Functions of the Board**—The Board shall have the following functions, namely:
   (i) To advise the Central Government on policy matters relating to use of prenatal diagnostic techniques, sex selection techniques are against their misuse
   (ii) To review and monitor implementation of the Act and rules made there under and recommend to the Central Government changes in the said Act and rules

(iii) To create public awareness against the practice of preconception sex selection and prenatal determination of sex of fetus leading to female feticide

(iv) To lay down code of conduct to be observed by persons working at Genetic Counseling Centers, Genetic Laboratories and Genetic Clinics

(v) To oversee the performance of various bodies constituted under the Act and take appropriate steps to ensure its proper and effective implementation

(vi) Any other functions as may be prescribed under the Act.

16A. Constitution of State Supervisory Board and Union Territory Supervisory Board—

(1) Each State and Union Territory having Legislature shall constitute a Board to be known as the State Supervisory Board or the Union Territory Supervisory Board, as the case may be, which shall have the following functions:

    (i) To create public awareness against the practice of preconception sex selection and prenatal determination of sex of fetus leading to female feticide in the State

    (ii) To review the activities of the Appropriate Authorities functioning in the State and recommend appropriate action against them

    (iii) To monitor the implementation of provisions of the Act and the rules and make suitable recommendations relating thereto, to the Board

    (iv) To send such consolidated reports as may be prescribed in respect of the various activities undertaken in the State under the Act to the Board and the Central Government

    (v) Any other functions as may be prescribed under the Act.

(2) The State Board shall consist of:

    (a) The Minister in charge of Health and Family Welfare in the State, who shall be the Chairperson, *ex officio*

    (b) The Secretary in charge of the Department of Health and Family Welfare who shall be the Vice-Chairperson, *ex officio*

    (c) Secretaries or Commissioners in charge of Departments of Women and Child Development, Social Welfare, Law and Indian System of Medicines and Homoeopathy, *ex officio*, or their representatives

    (d) Director of Health and Family Welfare or Indian System of Medicines and Homoeopathy of the State Government, *ex officio*

    (e) Three women members of Legislative Assembly or Legislative Council

    (f) Ten members to be appointed by the State Government out of which two each shall be from the following categories:

        (i) Eminent social scientists and legal experts

        (ii) Eminent women activists from non-governmental organizations or otherwise

        (iii) Eminent gynecologists and obstetricians or experts of *stri-roga or prasuti tantra*

        (iv) Eminent pediatricians or medical geneticists

        (v) Eminent radiologists or sonologists

    (g) An officer not below the rank of Joint Director in charge of Family Welfare, who shall be the Member Secretary, *ex officio*.

(3) The State Board shall meet at least once in four months.

(4) The term of office of a member, other than an *ex officio* member, shall be 3 years.

(5) If a vacancy occurs in the office of any member other than an *ex officio* member, it shall be filled by making fresh appointment.

(6) If a member of the Legislative Assembly or member of the Legislative Council who is a member of the State Board, becomes Minister or Speaker or Deputy Speaker of the Legislative Assembly or Chairperson or Deputy Chairperson of the Legislative Council, she shall cease to be a member of the State Board.

(7) One-third of the total number of members of the State Board shall constitute the quorum.

(8) The State Board may co-opt a member as and when required, provided that the number of co-opted members does not exceed one-third of the total strength of the State Board.

(9) The co-opted members shall have the same powers and functions as other members, except the right to vote and shall abide by the rules and regulations.

(10) In respect of matters not specified in this section, the State Board shall follow procedures and conditions as are applicable to the Board.

CHAPTER V: APPROPRIATE AUTHORITY AND ADVISORY COMMITTEE

17. Appropriate Authority and Advisory Committee—

(1) The Central Government shall appoint, by notification in the Official Gazette, one or more Appropriate Authorities for each of the Union territories for the purposes of this Act.

(2) The State Government shall appoint, by notification in the Official Gazette, one or more Appropriate Authorities for the whole or part of the State for the purposes of this Act having regard to the intensity of the problem of prenatal sex determination leading to female feticide.

(3) The officers appointed as Appropriate Authorities under sub-section (1) or sub-section (2) shall be,—

(a) When appointed for the whole of the State or the Union Territory, consisting of the following three members

(i) An officer of or above the rank of the Joint Director of Health and Family Welfare-Chairperson

(ii) An eminent woman representing women's organization

(iii) An officer of Law Department of the State or the Union Territory concerned: Provided that it shall be the duty of the State or the Union Territory concerned to constitute multi-member State or Union Territory Level Appropriate Authority within three months of the coming into force of the Prenatal Diagnostic Techniques (Regulation and Prevention of Misuse) Amendment Act, 2002: Provided further that any vacancy occurring therein shall be filled within three months of that occurrence.

(b) When appointed for any part of the State or the Union territory, of such other rank as the State Government or the Central Government, as the case may be, may deem fit.

(4) The Appropriate Authority shall have the following functions, namely:

(a) To grant, suspend or cancel registration of a Genetic Counseling Center, Genetic Laboratory or Genetic Clinic

(b) To enforce standards prescribed for the Genetic Counseling Center, Genetic Laboratory and Genetic Clinic

(c) To investigate complaints of breach of the provisions of this Act or the rules made there under and take immediate action

(d) To seek and consider the advice of the Advisory Committee, constituted under sub-section (5), on application for registration and on complaints for suspension or cancellation of registration

(e) To take appropriate legal action against the use of any sex selection technique by any person at any place, *suo-motu* or brought to its notice and also to initiate independent investigations in such matter

(f) To create public awareness against the practice of sex selection or prenatal determination of sex

(g) To supervise the implementation of the provisions of the Act and rules

(h) To recommend to the CSB and State Boards modifications required in the rules in accordance with changes in technology or social conditions

(i) To take action on the recommendations of the Advisory Committee made after investigation of complaint for suspension or cancellation of registration.

(5) The Central Government or the State Government, as the case may be, shall constitute an Advisory Committee for each Appropriate Authority to aid and advise the Appropriate Authority in the discharge of its functions, and shall appoint one of the members of the Advisory Committee to be its Chairman.

(6) The Advisory Committee shall consist of—

(a) Three medical experts from amongst gynecologists, obstetricians, pediatricians and medical geneticists

(b) One legal expert

(c) One officer to represent the department dealing with information and publicity of the State Government or the Union Territory, as the case may be

(d) Three eminent social workers of whom not less than one shall be from amongst representatives of women's organizations.

(7) No person who has been associated with the use or promotion of prenatal diagnostic technique for determination of sex or sex selection shall be appointed as a member of the Advisory Committee.

(8) The Advisory Committee may meet as and when it thinks fit or on the request of the Appropriate Authority for consideration of any application for registration or any complaint for suspension or cancellation of registration and to give advice thereon: Provided that the period intervening between any two meetings shall not exceed the prescribed period.

(9) The terms and conditions subject to which a person may be appointed to the Advisory Committee and the procedure to be followed by such Committee in the discharge of its functions shall be such as may be prescribed.

17A. Powers of Appropriate Authorities—The Appropriate Authority shall have the powers in respect of the following matters, namely:

(a) Summoning of any person who is in possession of any information relating to violation of the provisions of this Act or the rules made thereunder

(b) Production of any document or material object relating to clause (a)

(c) Issuing search warrant for any place suspected to be indulging in sex selection techniques or prenatal sex determination

(d) Any other matter which may be prescribed.

CHAPTER VI: REGISTRATION OF GENETIC COUNSELING CENTERS, GENETIC LABORATORIES AND GENETIC CLINICS

18. **Registration of Genetic Counseling Centers, Genetic Laboratories or Genetic Clinics—**

   (1) No person shall open any Genetic Counseling Center, Genetic Laboratory or Genetic Clinic, including clinic, laboratory or center having ultrasound or imaging machine or scanner or any other technology capable of undertaking determination of sex of fetus and sex selection, or render services to any of them, after the commencement of the Prenatal Diagnostic Techniques (Regulation and Prevention of Misuse) Amendment Act, 2002 unless such center, laboratory or clinic is duly registered under the Act.

   (2) Every application for registration under sub-section (1), shall be made to the Appropriate Authority in such form and in such manner and shall be accompanied by such fees as may be prescribed.

   (3) Every Genetic Counseling Center, Genetic Laboratory or Genetic Clinic engaged, either partly or exclusively, in counseling or conducting prenatal diagnostic techniques for any of the purposes mentioned in section 4, immediately before the commencement of this Act, shall apply for registration within 60 days from the date of such commencement.

   (4) Subject to the provisions of section 6, every Genetic Counseling Center, Genetic Laboratory or Genetic Clinic engaged in counseling or conducting prenatal diagnostic techniques shall cease to conduct any such counseling or technique on the expiry of 6 months from the date of commencement of this Act unless such Center, Laboratory or Clinic has applied for registration and is so registered separately or jointly or till such application is disposed of, whichever is earlier.

   (5) No Genetic Counseling Center, Genetic Laboratory or Genetic Clinic shall be registered under this Act unless the Appropriate Authority is satisfied that such Center, Laboratory or Clinic is in a position to provide such facilities, maintain such equipment and standards as may be prescribed.

19. **Certificate of registration:**

   (1) The Appropriate Authority shall, after holding an inquiry and after satisfying itself that the applicant has complied with all the requirements of this Act and the rules made there under and having regard to the advice of the Advisory Committee in this behalf, grant a certificate of registration in the prescribed form jointly or separately to the Genetic Counseling Center, Genetic Laboratory or Genetic Clinic, as the case may be.

   (2) If, after the inquiry and after giving an opportunity of being heard to the applicant and having regard to the advice of the Advisory Committee, the Appropriate Authority is satisfied that the applicant has not complied with the requirements of this Act or the rules, it shall, for reasons to be recorded in writing, reject the application for registration.

   (3) Every certificate of registration shall be renewed in such manner and after such period and on payment of such fees as may be prescribed.

   (4) The certificate of registration shall be displayed by the registered Genetic Counseling Center, Genetic Laboratory or Genetic Clinic in a conspicuous place at its place of business.

20. **Cancellation or suspension of registration—**

   (1) The Appropriate Authority may *suo-motu*, or on complaint, issue a notice to the Genetic Counseling Center, Genetic Laboratory or Genetic Clinic to show cause why its registration should not be suspended or cancelled for the reasons mentioned in the notice.

   (2) If, after giving a reasonable opportunity of being heard to the Genetic Counseling Center, Genetic Laboratory or Genetic Clinic and having regard to the advice of the Advisory Committee, the Appropriate Authority is satisfied that there has been a breach of the provisions of this Act or the

rules, it may, without prejudice to any criminal action that it may take against such Center, Laboratory or Clinic, suspend its registration for such period as it may think fit or cancel its registration, as the case may be.

(3) Notwithstanding anything contained in sub-sections (1) and (2), if the Appropriate Authority is, of the opinion that it is necessary or expedient so to do in the public interest, it may, for reasons to be recorded in writing, suspend the registration of any Genetic Counseling Center, Genetic Laboratory or Genetic Clinic without issuing any such notice referred to in sub-section (1).

21. **Appeal**—The Genetic Counseling Center, Genetic Laboratory or Genetic Clinic may, within 30 days from the date of receipt of the order of suspension or cancellation of registration passed by the Appropriate Authority under Section 20, prefer an appeal against such order to—

(i) The Central Government, where the appeal is against the order of the Central Appropriate Authority; and

(ii) The State Government, where the appeal is against the order of the State Appropriate Authority, in the prescribed manner.

CHAPTER VII: OFFENCES AND PENALTIES

22. **Prohibition of advertisement relating to prenatal determination of sex and punishment for contravention**—

(1) No person, organization, Genetic Counseling Center, Genetic Laboratory or Genetic Clinic, including clinic, laboratory or center having ultrasound machine or imaging machine or scanner or any other technology capable of undertaking determination of sex of fetus or sex selection shall issue, publish, distribute, communicate or cause to be issued, published, distributed or communicated any advertisement, in any form, including internet, regarding facilities of prenatal determination of sex or sex selection before conception available at such center, laboratory, clinic or at any other place.

(2) No person or organization including Genetic Counseling Center, Genetic Laboratory or Genetic Clinic shall issue, publish, distribute, communicate or cause to be issued, published, distributed or communicated any advertisement in any manner regarding prenatal determination or preconception selection of sex by any means whatsoever, scientific or otherwise.

(3) Any person who contravenes the provisions of sub-section (1) or sub-section (2) shall be punishable with imprisonment for a term which may extend to 3 years and with fine which may extend to ten thousand rupees.

Explanation—For the purposes of this section, "advertisement" includes any notice, circular, label, wrapper or any other document including advertisement through internet or any other media in electronic or print form and also includes any visible representation made by means of any hoarding, wall-painting, signal, light, sound, smoke or gas.

23. **Offences and Penalties**—

(1) Any medical geneticist, gynecologist, registered medical practitioner or any person who owns a Genetic Counseling Center, a Genetic Laboratory or a Genetic Clinic or is employed in such a Center, Laboratory or Clinic and renders his professional or technical services to or at such a Center, Laboratory or Clinic, whether on an honorary basis or otherwise, and who contravenes any of the provisions of this Act or rules made there under shall be punishable with imprisonment for a term which may extend to 3 years and with fine which may extend to ten thousand rupees and on any subsequent conviction, with imprisonment which may extend to 5 years and with fine which may extend to fifty thousand rupees.

(2) The name of the registered medical practitioner shall be reported by the Appropriate Authority to the State Medical Council concerned for taking necessary action including suspension of the registration if the charges are framed by the court and till the case is disposed of and on conviction for removal of his name from the register of the Council for a period of 5 years for the first offence and permanently for the subsequent offence.

(3) Any person who seeks the aid of a Genetic Counseling Center, Genetic Laboratory, Genetic Clinic or ultrasound clinic or imaging clinic or of a medical geneticist, gynecologist, sonologist or imaging specialist or registered medical practitioner or any other person for sex selection or for conducting prenatal diagnostic techniques on any pregnant women for the purposes other than those specified in sub-section (2) of Section 4, he shall, be punishable with imprisonment for a term which may extend to 3 years and with fine which may extend to fifty thousand rupees for the first offence and for any subsequent offence with imprisonment which may extend to 5 years and with fine which may extend to 1 lakh rupees.

(4) For the removal of doubts, it is hereby provided, that the provisions of sub-section (3) shall not apply to the woman who was compelled to undergo such diagnostic techniques or such selection.

24. **Presumption in the case of conduct of prenatal diagnostic techniques**—Notwithstanding anything contained in the Indian Evidence Act, 1872, the court shall presume unless the contrary is proved that the pregnant woman was compelled by her husband or any other relative, as the case may be, to undergo prenatal diagnostic technique for the purposes other than those specified in sub-section (2) of Section 4 and such person shall be liable for abetment of offence under sub-section (3) of Section 23 and shall be punishable for the offence specified under that section.

25. **Penalty for contravention of the provisions of the Act or rules for which no specific punishment is provided**—Whoever contravenes any of the provisions of this Act or any rules made thereunder, for which no penalty has been elsewhere provided in this Act, shall be punishable with imprisonment for a term which may extend to three months or with fine, which may extend to one thousand rupees or with both and in the case of continuing contravention with an additional fine which may extend to five hundred rupees for every day during which such contravention continues after conviction for the first such contravention.

26. **Offences by companies—**

(1) Where any offence, punishable under this Act has been committed by a company, every person who, at the time the offence was committed was in charge of, and was responsible to the company for the conduct of the business of the company, as well as the company, shall be deemed to be guilty of the offence and shall be liable to be proceeded against and punished accordingly: Provided that nothing contained in this sub-section shall render any such person liable to any punishment, if he proves that the offence was committed without his knowledge or that he had exercised all due diligence to prevent the commission of such offence.

(2) Notwithstanding anything contained in sub-section (1), where any offence punishable under this Act has been committed by a company and it is proved that the offence has been committed with the consent or connivance of, or is attributable to any neglect on the part of, any director, manager, secretary or other officer of the company, such director, manager, secretary or other officer shall also be deemed to be guilty of that offence and shall be liable to be proceeded against and punished accordingly.

Explanation—For the purposes of this section,—

(a) "Company" means anybody corporate and includes a firm or other association of individuals, and

(b) "Director", in relation to a firm, means a partner in the firm.

27. **Offence to be cognizable, nonbailable and noncompoundable**—Every offence under this Act shall be cognizable, nonbailable and noncompoundable.

28. **Cognizance of offences**—

(1) No court shall take cognizance of an offence under this Act except on a complaint made by—

(a) The Appropriate Authority concerned, or any officer authorized in this behalf by the Central Government or State Government, as the case may be, or the Appropriate Authority

(b) A person who has given notice of not less than 15 days in the manner prescribed, to the Appropriate Authority, of the alleged offence and of his intention to make a complaint to the court.

Explanation—For the purpose of this clause, "person" includes a social organization.

(2) No court other than that of a Metropolitan Magistrate or a Judicial Magistrate of the first class shall try any offence punishable under this Act.

(3) Where a complaint has been made under clause (b) of subsection (1), the court may, on demand by such person, direct the Appropriate Authority to make available copies of the relevant records in its possession to such person.

CHAPTER VIII: MISCELLANEOUS

29. **Maintenance of records**—

(1) All records, charts, forms, reports, consent letters and all other documents required to be maintained under this Act and the rules shall be preserved for a period of 2 years or for such period as may be prescribed: Provided that, if any criminal or other proceedings are instituted against any Genetic Counseling Center, Genetic Laboratory or Genetic Clinic, the records and all other documents of such Center, Laboratory or Clinic shall be preserved till the final disposal of such proceedings.

(2) All such records shall, at all reasonable times, be made available for inspection to the Appropriate Authority or to any other person authorized by the Appropriate Authority in this behalf.

30. **Power to search and seize records, etc.:**

(1) If the Appropriate Authority has reason to believe that an offence under this Act has been or is being committed at any Genetic Counseling Center, Genetic Laboratory or Genetic Clinic or any other place, such Authority or any officer authorized thereof in this behalf may, subject to such rules as may be prescribed, enter and search at all reasonable times with such assistance, if any, as such authority or officer considers necessary, such Genetic Counseling Center, Genetic Laboratory or Genetic Clinic or any other place and examine any record, register, document, book, pamphlet, advertisement or any other material object found therein and seize and seal the same if such Authority or officer has reason to believe that it may furnish evidence of the commission of an office punishable under this Act.

(2) The provisions of the Code of Criminal Procedure, 1973 (2 of 1974) relating to searches and seizures shall, so far as may be, apply to every search or seizure made under this Act.

31. **Protection of action taken in good faith**—No suit, prosecution or other legal proceeding shall lie against the Central or the State Government or the Appropriate Authority or any officer authorized by the Central or State Government or by the Authority for anything which is in good faith done or intended to be done in pursuance of the provisions of this Act.

31A. Removal of difficulties—

(1) If any difficulty arises in giving effect to the provisions of the Prenatal Diagnostic Techniques (Regulation and Prevention of Misuse) Amendment Act, 2002, the Central Government may, by order published in the Official Gazette, make such provisions not inconsistent with the provisions of the said Act as appear to it to be necessary or expedient for removing the difficulty. Provided that no order shall be made under this section after the expiry of a period of 3 years from the date of commencement of the Prenatal Diagnostic Techniques (Regulation and Prevention of Misuse) Amendment Act, 2002.

(2) Every order made under this section shall be laid, as soon as may be after it is made, before each House of Parliament.

32. Power to make rules—

(1) The Central Government may make rules for carrying out the provisions of this Act.

(2) In particular and without prejudice to the generality of the foregoing power, such rules may provide for—

    (i) The minimum qualifications for persons employed at a registered Genetic Counseling Center, Genetic Laboratory or Genetic Clinic under clause (2) of Section 3

    (i-a) The manner in which the person conducting ultrasonography on a pregnant woman shall keep record thereof in the clinic under the proviso to sub-section (3) of Section 4

    (ii) The form in which consent of a pregnant woman has to be obtained under Section 5

    (iii) The procedure to be followed by the members of the Central Supervisory Board in the discharge of their functions under sub-section (4) of Section 8

    (iv) Allowances for members other than ex officio members admissible under sub-section (5) of Section 9

    (iv-a) Code of conduct to be observed by persons working at Genetic Counseling Centers, Genetic Laboratories and Genetic Clinics to be laid down by the Central Supervisory Board under clause (iv) of Section 16

    (iv-b) The manner in which reports shall be furnished by the State and Union territory Supervisory Boards to the Board and the Central Government in respect of various activities undertaken in the State under the Act under clause (iv) of sub-section (1) of Section 16A

    (iv-c) Empowering the Appropriate Authority in any other matter under clause (d) of Section 17A

    (v) The period intervening between any two meetings of the Advisory Committee under the proviso to sub-section (8) of Section 17

    (vi) The terms and conditions subject to which a person may be appointed to the Advisory Committee and the procedure to be followed by such Committee under sub-section (9) of Section 17

    (vii) The form and manner in which an application shall be made for registration and the fee payable thereof under sub-section (2) of Section 18

    (viii) The facilities to be provided, equipment and other standards to be maintained by the Genetic Counseling Center, Genetic Laboratory or Genetic Clinic under sub-section (5) of Section 18

    (ix) The form in which a certificate of registration shall be issued under subsection (1) of Section 19

    (x) The manner in which and the period after which a certificate of registration shall be renewed and the fee payable for such renewal under sub-section (3) of Section 19

    (xi) The manner in which an appeal may be preferred under section 21

(xii) The period up to which records, charts, etc., shall be preserved under sub-section (1) of Section 29

(xiii) The manner in which the seizure of documents, records, objects, etc., shall be made and the manner in which seizure list shall be prepared and delivered to the person from whose custody such documents, records or objects were seized under sub-section (1) of Section 30

(xiv) Any other matter that is required to be, or may be, prescribed.

33. **Power to make regulations—**The Board may, with the previous sanction of the Central Government, by notification in the Official Gazette, make regulations not inconsistent with the provisions of this Act and the rules made there under to provide for—

(a) The time and place of the meetings of the Board and the procedure to be followed for the transaction of business at such meetings and the number of members which shall form the quorum under sub-section (1) of Section 9

(b) The manner in which a person may be temporarily associated with the Board under sub-section (1) of Section 11

(c) The method of appointment, the conditions of service and the scales of pay and allowances of the officer and other employees of the Board appointed under Section 12

(d) Generally for the efficient conduct of the affairs of the Board.

34. **Rules and regulations to be laid before Parliament—**Every rule and every regulation made under this Act shall be laid, as soon as may be after it is made, before each House of Parliament, while it is in session, for a total period of 30 days which may be comprised in one session or in two or more successive sessions, and if, before the expiry of the session immediately following the session or the successive sessions aforesaid, both Houses agree in making any modification in the rule or regulation or both Houses agree that the rule or regulation should not be made, the rule or regulation shall thereafter have effect only in such modified form or be of no effect, as the case may be; so, however, that any such modification or annulment shall be without prejudice to the validity of anything previously done under that rule or regulation.

THE PRENATAL DIAGNOSTIC TECHNIQUES (PROHIBITION OF SEX SELECTION) RULES, 1996

1. **Short title and commencement—**

(1) These rules may be called the Preconception and Prenatal Diagnostic Techniques (Prohibition of Sex Selection) Rules, 1996.

(2) They shall come into force on the date of their publication in the Official Gazette.

2. **Definitions—**In these rules, unless the context otherwise requires:-

(a) "Act" means The Prenatal Diagnostic Techniques (Regulation and Prevention of Misuse) Act, 1994 (57 of 1994)

(b) "Employee" means a person working in or employed by a Genetic Counseling Center, a Genetic Laboratory or a Genetic Clinic, and includes those working on part-time, contractual, consultancy, honorary or on any other basis

(c) "Form" means a Form appended to these rules

(d) "Section" means a section of the Act

(e) Words and expressions used herein and not defined in these rules but defined in the Act, shall have the meanings, respectively, assigned to them in the Act.

3. **The qualifications of the employees, the requirement of equipment, etc. For a genetic counseling center, genetic laboratory, genetic clinic, ultrasound clinic and imaging center shall be as under—**

(1) Any person being or employing

    (i) a gynecologist or a pediatrician, having six months experience or four weeks training in genetic counseling.

    (ii) a medical geneticist, having adequate space and educational charts/models/equipment for carrying out genetic counseling may set up a genetic counseling center and get it registered as a genetic counseling center.

(2) (a) Any person having adequate space and being or employing

    (i) a Medical Geneticist and

    (ii) a laboratory technician having a B.Sc. degree in Biological Sciences or a degree or diploma in medical laboratory course with at least one year experience in conducting appropriate prenatal diagnostic techniques, tests or procedures may set up a genetic laboratory.

    (b) Such laboratory should have or acquire such of the following equipment as may be necessary for carrying out chromosomal studies, bio-chemical studies and molecular studies:

    (i) Chromosomal studies

        (1) Laminar flow hood with ultraviolet and fluorescent light or other suitable culture hood

        (2) Photomicroscope with fluorescent source of light

        (3) Inverted microscope

        (4) Incubator and oven

        (5) Carbon dioxide incubator or closed system with 5% CO_2 atmosphere

        (6) Autoclave

        (7) Refrigerator

        (8) Water bath

        (9) Centrifuge

        (10) Vortex mixer

        (11) Magnetic stirrer

        (12) pH meter

        (13) A sensitive balance (preferable electronic) with sensitivity of 0.1 milligram

        (14) Double distillation apparatus (glass)

        (15) Such other equipment as may be necessary

    (ii) Biochemical studies: (requirements according to tests to be carried out)

        (1) Laminar flow hood with ultraviolet and fluorescent light or other suitable culture hood

        (2) Inverted microscope

        (3) Incubator and oven

        (4) Carbon dioxide incubator or closed system with 5% CO_2 atmosphere

        (5) Autoclave

        (6) Refrigerator

        (7) Water bath

        (8) Centrifuge

        (9) Electrophoresis apparatus and power supply

        (10) Chromatography chamber

        (11) Spectrophotometer and Elisa reader or radioimmunoassay system (with gamma beta counter) or fluorometer for various biochemical test

        (12) Vortex mixer

(13) Magnetic stirrer

(14) pH meter

(15) A sensitive balance (preferable electronic) with sensitivity of 0.1 milligram

(16) Double distillation apparatus (glass)

(17) Liquid nitrogen tank

(18) Such other equipment as may be necessary

(iii) Molecular studies

(1) Inverted microscope

(2) Incubator

(3) Oven

(4) Autoclave

(5) Refrigerators (4 degrees and minus 20°C)

(6) Water bath

(7) Microcentrifuge

(8) Electrophoresis apparatus and power supply

(9) Vortex mixer

(10) Magnetic stirrer

(11) pH meter

(12) A sensitive balance (preferable electronic) with sensitivity of 0.1 milligram

(13) Double distillation apparatus (glass)

(14) PCR machine

(15) Refrigerated centrifuge

(16) UV illuminator with photographic attachment or other documentation system

(17) Precision micropipettes.

(18) Such other equipment as may be necessary.

(3) (1) Any person having adequate space and being or employing—

(a) Gynecologist having experience of performing at least 20 procedures in chorionic villi aspirations per vagina or per abdomen, chorionic villi biopsy, amniocentesis, Cordocentesis fetoscopy, fetal skin or organ biopsy or fetal blood sampling, etc. under supervision of an experienced gynecologist in these fields.

(b) A Sonologist, Imaging Specialist, Radiologist or Registered Medical Practitioner having Postgraduate degree or diploma or six months training or one year experience in sonography or image scanning.

(c) A medical geneticist may set up a genetic clinic/ultrasound clinic/imaging center.

(2) The Genetic Clinic/Ultrasound clinic/Imaging center should have or acquire such of the following equipment as may be necessary for carrying out the tests or procedures—

(a) Equipment and accessories necessary for carrying out clinical examination by an obstetrician or gynecologist.

(b) An ultrasonography machine including mobile ultrasound machine, imaging machine or any other equipment capable of conducting fetal ultrasonography.

(c) Appropriate catheters and equipment for carrying out chorionic villi aspirations per vagina or per abdomen.

(d) Appropriate sterile needles for amniocentesis or cordocentesis.

(e) A suitable fetoscopy with appropriate accessories for fetoscopy, fetal skin or organ biopsy or fetal blood sampling shall be optional.

(f) Equipment for dry and wet sterilization.

(g) Equipment for carrying out emergency procedures such as evacuation of uterus or resuscitation in case of need.

(h) Genetic works station.

3A. Sale of ultrasound machines/imaging machines—

(1) No organization including a commercial organization or a person, including manufacturer, importer, dealer or supplier of ultrasound machines/imaging machines or any other equipment, capable of detecting sex of fetus, shall sell, distribute, supply, rent, allow or authorize the use of any such machine or equipment in any manner, whether on payment or otherwise, to any Genetic Counseling Center, Genetic Laboratory, Genetic Clinic, Ultrasound Clinic, Imaging Center or any other body or person unless such Center, Laboratory, Clinic, body or person is registered under the Act.

(2) The provider of such machine/equipment to any person/body registered under the Act shall send to the concerned State/UT Appropriate Authority and to the Central Government, once in three months a list of those to whom the machine/equipment has been provided.

(3) Any organization or person, including manufacturer, importer, dealer or supplier of ultrasound machines/imaging machines or any other equipment capable of detecting sex of fetus selling, distributing, supplying or authorizing in any manner, the use of any such machine or equipment to any Genetic Counseling Center, Genetic Laboratory, Genetic Clinic, Ultrasound Clinic, Imaging Center or any other body or person registered under the Act shall take an affidavit from such body or person purchasing or getting authorization for using such machine/equipment that the machine/equipment shall not be used for detection of sex of fetus or selection of sex before or after conception.

4. Registration of Genetic Counseling Center, Genetic Laboratory and Genetic Clinic—

(1) An application for registration shall be made to the Appropriate Authority, in duplicate, in Form A, duly accompanied by an Affidavit containing—

(i) an undertaking to the effect that the *Genetic Center/Laboratory/Clinic/Ultrasound Clinic/ Imaging Center*/combination thereof, as the case may be, shall not conduct any test or procedure, by whatever name called, for selection of sex before or after conception or for detection of sex of fetus except for diseases specified in Section 4(2) nor shall the sex of fetus be disclosed to anybody; and

(ii) an undertaking to the effect that the *Genetic Center/Laboratory/Clinic*/combination thereof, as the case may be, shall display prominently a notice that they do not conduct any technique, test or procedure, etc. By whatever name called, for detection of sex of fetus or for selection of sex before or after conception.

(2) The Appropriate Authority, or any person in his office authorized in this behalf, shall acknowledge receipt of the application for registration, in the acknowledgement slip provided at the bottom of Form A, immediately if delivered at the office of the Appropriate Authority, or not later than the next working day if received by post.

5. Application Fee—

(1) Every application for registration under rule 4 shall be accompanied by an application fee of:

(a) ₹3000/- for Genetic Counseling Center, Genetic Laboratory, Genetic Clinic, Ultrasound Clinic or Imaging Center.

(b) ₹4000/- for an institute, hospital, nursing home, or any place providing jointly the service of a Genetic Counseling Center, Genetic Laboratory and Genetic Clinic, Ultrasound Clinic or Imaging Center or any combination thereof.

Provided that if an application for registration of any Genetic Clinic/Laboratory/Center, etc. has been rejected by the Appropriate Authority, no fee shall be required to be paid on re-submission of the application by the applicant for the same body within 90 days of rejection. Provided further that any subsequent application shall be accompanied with the prescribed fee. Application fee once paid will not be refunded.

(2) The application fee shall be paid by a demand draft drawn in favor of the Appropriate Authority, on any scheduled bank payable at the headquarters of the Appropriate Authority concerned. The fees collected by the Appropriate Authority for registration of Genetic Counseling Center, Genetic Laboratory, Genetic Clinic, Ultrasound Clinic and Imaging Center or any other body or person under sub-rule (1), shall be deposited by the Appropriate Authority concerned in a bank account opened in the name of the official designation of the Appropriate Authority concerned and shall be utilized by the Appropriate Authority in connection with the activities connected with implementation of the provisions of the Act and these rules.

6. **Certificate of registration—**

(1) The Appropriate Authority shall, after making such enquiry and after satisfying itself that the applicant has complied with all the requirements, place the application before the Advisory Committee for its advice.

(2) Having regard to the advice of the Advisory Committee the Appropriate Authority shall grant a certificate of registration, in duplicate, in Form B to the applicant. One copy of the certificate of registration shall be displayed by the registered Genetic Counseling Center, Genetic Laboratory, Genetic Clinic, Ultrasound Clinic or Imaging Center at a conspicuous place at its place of business: Provided that the Appropriate Authority may grant a certificate of registration to a Genetic Laboratory or a Genetic Clinic, Ultrasound Clinic or Imaging Center to conduct one or more specified prenatal diagnostic tests or procedures, depending on the availability of place, equipment and qualified employees, and standards maintained by such laboratory or clinic.

(3) If, after enquiry and after giving an opportunity of being heard to the applicant and having regard to the advice of the Advisory Committee, the Appropriate Authority is satisfied that the applicant has not complied with the requirements of the Act and these rules, it shall, for the reasons to be recorded in writing, reject the application for registration and communicate such rejection to the applicant as specified in Form C.

(4) An enquiry under sub-rule (1), including inspection at the premises of the Genetic Counseling Center, Genetic Laboratory, Genetic Clinic, Ultrasound Clinic or Imaging Center, shall, be carried out only after due notice is given to the applicant by the Appropriate Authority.

(5) Grant of certificate of registration or rejection of application for registration shall be communicated to the applicant as specified in Form B or Form C, as the case may be, within a period of 90 days from the date of receipt of application for registration.

(6) The certificate of registration shall be non-transferable. In the event of change of ownership or change of management or on ceasing to function as a Genetic Counseling Center, Genetic Laboratory, Genetic Clinic, Ultrasound Clinic or Imaging Center, both copies, of the certificate of registration shall be surrendered to the Appropriate Authority.

(7) In the event of change of ownership or change of management of the Genetic Counseling Center, Genetic Laboratory, Genetic Clinic, Ultrasound Clinic or Imaging Center, the new owner or manager of such Center, Laboratory or Clinic shall apply afresh for grant of certificate of registration.

7. **Validity of registration—**Every certificate of registration shall be valid for a period of 5 years from the date of its issue.

8. **Renewal of registration—**

(1) An application for renewal of certificate of registration shall be made in duplicate in Form A, to the Appropriate Authority 30 days before the date of expiry of the certificate of registration. Acknowledgement of receipt of such application shall be issued by the Appropriate Authority in the manner specified in sub-rule (2) of Rule 4.

(2) The Appropriate Authority shall, after holding an enquiry and after satisfying itself that the applicant has complied with all the requirements of the Act and these rules and having regard to the advice of the Advisory Committee in this behalf, renew the certificate of registration, as specified in Form B, for a further period of 5 years from the date of expiry of the certificate of registration earlier granted.

(3) If, after enquiry and after giving an opportunity of being heard to the applicant and having regard to the advice of the Advisory Committee, the Appropriate Authority is satisfied that the applicant has not complied with the requirements of the Act and these rules, it shall, for reasons to be recorded in writing, reject the application for renewal of certificate of registration and communicate such rejection to the applicant as specified in Form C.

(4) The fees payable for renewal of certificate of registration shall be one half of the fees provided in sub-rule (1) of Rule 5.

(5) On receipt of the renewed certificate of registration in duplicate or on receipt of communication of rejection of application for renewal, both copies of the earlier certificate of registration shall be surrendered immediately to the Appropriate Authority by the Genetic Counseling Center, Genetic Laboratory, Genetic Clinic, Ultrasound Clinic or Imaging Center.

(6) In the event of failure of the Appropriate Authority to renew the certificate of registration or to communicate rejection of application for renewal of registration within a period of 90 days from the date of receipt of application for renewal of registration, the certificate of registration shall be deemed to have been renewed.

9. **Maintenance and preservation of records—**

(1) Every Genetic Counseling Center, Genetic Laboratory, Genetic Clinic, Ultrasound Clinic and Imaging Center shall maintain a register showing, in serial order, the names and addresses of the men or women given genetic counseling, subjected to prenatal diagnostic procedures or prenatal diagnostic tests, the names of their spouses or fathers and the date on which they first reported for such counseling, procedure or test.

(2) The record to be maintained by every Genetic Counseling Center, in respect of each woman counselled shall be as specified in Form D.

(3) The record to be maintained by every Genetic Laboratory, in respect of each man or woman subjected to any prenatal diagnostic procedure/technique/test, shall be as specified in Form E.

(4) The record to be maintained by every Genetic Clinic, in respect of each man or woman subjected to any prenatal diagnostic procedure/technique/test, shall be as specified in Form F.

(5) The Appropriate Authority shall maintain a permanent record of applications for grant or renewal of certificate of registration as specified in Form H. Letters of intimation of every change of employee, place, address and equipment installed shall also be preserved as permanent records.

(6) All case related records, forms of consent, laboratory results, microscopic pictures, sonographic plates or slides, recommendations and letters shall be preserved by the Genetic Counseling Center, Genetic Laboratory, Genetic Clinic, Ultrasound Clinic or Imaging Center for a period of 2 years from the date of completion of counseling, prenatal diagnostic procedure or prenatal diagnostic test, as the case may be. In the event of any legal proceedings, the records shall be preserved till the final disposal of legal proceedings, or till the expiry of the said period of 2 years, whichever is later.

(7) In case the Genetic Counseling Center or Genetic Laboratory, Genetic Clinic, Ultrasound Clinic or Imaging Center maintains records on computer or other electronic equipment, a printed copy of the record shall be taken and preserved after authentication by a person responsible for such record.

(8) Every Genetic Counseling Center, Genetic Laboratory, Genetic Clinic, Ultrasound Clinic and Imaging Center shall send a complete report in respect of all preconception or pregnancy related procedures/techniques/tests conducted by them in respect of each month by 5th day of the following month to the concerned Appropriate Authority.

10. Conditions for conducting prenatal diagnostic procedures—

(1) Before conducting pre-implantation genetic diagnosis, or any prenatal diagnostic technique/test/procedure such as amniocentesis, chorionic villi biopsy, fetal skin or organ biopsy or cordocentesis, a written consent, as specified in Form G, in a language the person undergoing such procedure understands, shall be obtained from her/him: Provided that where a Genetic Clinic has taken a sample of any body tissue or body fluid and sent it to a Genetic Laboratory for analysis or test, it shall not be necessary for the Genetic Laboratory to obtain a fresh consent in Form G.

(1A) Any person conducting ultrasonography/image scanning on a pregnant woman shall give a declaration on each report on ultrasonography/image scanning that he/she has neither detected nor disclosed the sex of fetus of the pregnant woman to anybody. The pregnant woman shall before undergoing ultrasonography/image scanning declare that she does not want to know the sex of her fetus.

(2) All the State Governments and Union Territories may issue translation of Form G in languages used in the State or Union Territory and where no official translation in a language understood by the pregnant woman is available, the Genetic Clinic may translate Form G into a language she understands.

11. Facilities for inspection—

(1) Every Genetic Counseling Center, Genetic Laboratory and Genetic Clinic, Ultrasound Clinic, Imaging Center, nursing home, hospital, institute or any other place where any of the machines or equipment capable of performing any procedure, technique or prenatal determination of sex or selection of sex before or after conception is used, shall afford all reasonable facilities for inspection of the place, equipment and records to the Appropriate Authority or to any other person authorized by the Appropriate Authority in this behalf for registration of such institutions, by whatever name called, under the Act, or for detection of misuse of such facilities or advertisement therefore or for selection of sex before or after conception or for detection/disclosure of sex of fetus or for detection of cases of violation of the provisions of the Act in any other manner.

(2) The Appropriate Authority or the officer authorized by it may seal and seize any ultrasound machine, scanner or any other equipment, capable of detecting sex of fetus, used by any organization if the organization has not got itself registered under the Act. These machines of the organizations may be released if such organization pays penalty equal to five times of the registration fee to the Appropriate Authority concerned and gives an undertaking that it shall not undertake detection of sex of fetus or selection of sex before or after conception.

12. Procedure for search and seizure—

(1) The Appropriate Authority or any officer authorized in this behalf may enter and search at all reasonable times any Genetic Counseling Center, Genetic Laboratory, Genetic Clinic, Imaging Center or Ultrasound Clinic in the presence of two or more independent witnesses for the purposes of search and examination of any record, register, document, book, pamphlet, advertisement, or any other material object found therein and seal and seize the same if there

is reason to believe that it may furnish evidence of commission of an offence punishable under the Act.

Explanation—In these Rules—

- 'Genetic Laboratory/Genetic Clinic/Genetic Counseling Center' would include an ultrasound center/imaging center/nursing home/hospital/institute or any other place, by whatever name called, where any of the machines or equipment capable of selection of sex before or after conception or performing any procedure, technique or test for prenatal detection of sex of fetus is used
- 'material object' would include records, machines and equipment
- 'seize' and 'seizure' would include 'seal' and 'sealing' respectively.

(2) A list of any document, record, register, book, pamphlet, advertisement or any other material object found in the Genetic Counseling Center, Genetic Laboratory, Genetic Clinic, Ultrasound Clinic or Imaging Center and seized shall be prepared in duplicate at the place of effecting the seizure. Both copies of such list shall be signed on every page by the Appropriate Authority or the officer authorized in this behalf and by the witnesses to the seizure:

Provided that the list may be prepared, in the presence of the witnesses, at a place other than the place of seizure if, for reasons to be recorded in writing, it is not practicable to make the list at the place of effecting the seizure.

(3) One copy of the list referred to in sub-rule (2) shall be handed over, under acknowledgement, to the person from whose custody the document, record, register, book, pamphlet, advertisement or any other material object have been seized:

Provided that a copy of the list of such document, record, register, book, pamphlet, advertisement or other material object seized may be delivered under acknowledgement, or sent by registered post to the owner or manager of the Genetic Counseling Center, Genetic Laboratory, Genetic Clinic, Ultrasound Clinic or Imaging Center, if no person acknowledging custody of the document, record, register, book, pamphlet, advertisement or other material object seized is available at the place of effecting the seizure.

(4) If any material object seized is perishable in nature, the Appropriate Authority, or the officer authorized in this behalf shall make arrangements promptly for sealing, identification and preservation of the material object and also convey it to a facility for analysis or test, if analysis or test be required:

Provided that the refrigerator or other equipment used by the Genetic Counseling Center, Genetic Laboratory, Genetic Clinic, Ultrasound Clinic and Imaging Center for preserving such perishable material object may be sealed until such time as arrangements can be made for safe removal of such perishable material object and in such eventuality, mention of keeping the material object seized, on the premises of the Genetic Counseling Center, Genetic Laboratory, Genetic Clinic, Ultrasound Clinic or Imaging Center shall be made in the list of seizure.

(5) In the case of noncompletion of search and seizure operation, the Appropriate Authority or the officer authorized in this behalf may make arrangement, by way of mounting a guard or sealing of the premises of the Genetic Counseling Center, Genetic Laboratory, Genetic Clinic Ultrasound Clinic or Imaging Center, for safe keeping, listing and removal of documents, records, book or any other material object to be seized, and to prevent any tampering with such documents, records, books or any other material object.

13. **Intimation of changes in employees, place or equipment**—Every Genetic Counseling Center, Genetic Laboratory, Genetic Clinic, Ultrasound Clinic and Imaging Center shall intimate every change of employee, place, address and equipment installed, to the Appropriate Authority within a period of 30 days of such change.

14. **Conditions for analysis or test and prenatal diagnostic procedures—**
    (1) No Genetic Laboratory shall accept for analysis or test any sample, unless referred to it by a Genetic Clinic.
    (2) Every prenatal diagnostic procedure shall invariably be immediately preceded by locating the fetus and placenta through ultrasonography, and the prenatal diagnostic procedure shall be done under direct ultrasonography monitoring so as to prevent any damage to the fetus and placenta.

15. **Meetings of the Advisory Committees—**The intervening period between any two meetings of Advisory Committees constituted under sub-section (5) of Section 17 to advise the Appropriate Authority shall not exceed 60 days.

16. **Allowances to members of the Central Supervisory Board—**
    (1) The ex-officio members, and other Central and State Government officers appointed to the Board will be entitled to Travelling Allowance and Daily Allowance for attending the meetings of the Board as per the Travelling Allowance rules applicable to them.
    (2) The nonofficial members appointed to, and Members of Parliament elected to the Board will be entitled to Travelling Allowance and Daily Allowance for attending the meetings of the Board as admissible to non-official and Members of Parliament as the case may be, under the Travelling Allowances rules of the Central Government.

17. **Public Information—**
    (1) Every Genetic Counseling Center, Genetic Laboratory, Genetic Clinic, Ultrasound Clinic and Imaging Center shall prominently display on its premises a notice in English and in the local language or languages for the information of the public, to effect that disclosure of the sex of the fetus is prohibited under law.
    (2) At least one copy each of the Act and these rules shall be available on the premises of every Genetic Counseling Center, Genetic Laboratory, Genetic Clinic, Ultrasound Clinic and Imaging Center, and shall be made available to the clientele on demand for perusal.
    (3) The Appropriate Authority, the Central Government, the State Government, and the Government/Administration of the Union Territory may publish periodically lists of registered Genetic Counseling Centers, Genetic Laboratories, Genetic Clinics, Ultrasound Clinics and Imaging Centers and findings from the reports and other information in their possession, for the information of the public and for use by the experts in the field.

18. **Code of Conduct to be observed by persons working at Genetic Counseling Centers, Genetic Laboratories, Genetic Clinics, Ultrasound Clinics, Imaging Centers, etc.—**All persons including the owner, employee or any other person associated with Genetic Counseling Centers, Genetic Laboratories, Genetic Clinics, Ultrasound Clinics, Imaging Centers registered under the Act/these Rules shall:
    (i) not conduct or associate with, or help in carrying out detection or disclosure of sex of fetus in any manner
    (ii) not employ or cause to be employed any person not possessing qualifications necessary for carrying out prenatal diagnostic techniques/procedures and tests including ultrasonography
    (iii) not conduct or cause to be conducted or aid in conducting by himself or through any other person any techniques or procedure for selection of sex before or after conception or for detection of sex of fetus except for the purposes specified in sub-section (2) of Section 4 of the Act
    (iv) not conduct or cause to be conducted or aid in conducting by himself or through any other person any techniques or test or procedure under the Act at a place other than a place registered under the Act/the Rules
    (v) ensure that no provision of the Act and these Rules are violated in any manner

(vi) ensure that the person conducting any techniques, test or procedure leading to detection of sex of fetus for purposes not covered under Section 4 (2) of the Act or selection of sex before or after conception, is informed that such procedures lead to violation of the Act and the Rules which are punishable offences

(vii) help the law enforcing agencies in bringing to book the violators of the provisions of the Act and the Rules

(viii) display his/her name and designation prominently on the dress worn by him/her

(ix) write his/her name and designation in full under his/her signature

(x) on no account conduct or allow/cause to be conducted female feticide

(xi) not commit any other act of professional misconduct.

19. Appeals—

(1) Anybody aggrieved by the decision of the Appropriate Authority at sub-district level may appeal to the Appropriate Authority at district level within 30 days of the order of the sub-district level Appropriate Authority.

(2) Anybody aggrieved by the decision of the Appropriate Authority at district level may appeal to the Appropriate Authority at State/UT level within 30 days of the order of the District Level Appropriate Authority.

(3) Each appeal shall be disposed of by the District Appropriate Authority or by the State/Union Territory Appropriate Authority, as the case may be, within 60 days of its receipt.

AMENDMENTS

The act was amended in 2003 to improve the regulation of the technology used in sex selection. The Act was amended to bring the technique of preconception sex selection and ultrasound technique within the ambit of the act.

The amendment also empowered the central supervisory board and state level supervisory board was constituted. In 1988, the State of Maharashtra became the first in the country to ban prenatal sex determination through enacting the Maharashtra Regulation of Prenatal Diagnostic Techniques Act.

Prenatal Diagnostic Techniques (Regulation and Prevention of Misuse) Act, 1994 (PNDT), was amended in 2003 to The Preconception and Prenatal Diagnostic Techniques (Prohibition of Sex Selection) Act (PCPNDT Act) to improve the regulation of the technology used in sex selection. The Act was amended to bring the technique of preconception sex selection and ultrasound technique within the ambit of the act. The amendment also empowered the central supervisory board and state level supervisory board was constituted.

Persons with Disabilities (Equal Opportunities, Protection of Rights and Full Participation) Act, 1995

PUBLISHED IN PART II, SECTION 1 OF THE EXTRAORDINARY GAZETTE OF INDIA

MINISTRY OF LAW, JUSTICE AND COMPANY AFFAIRS
(Legislative Department)
New Delhi, the 1st January, 1996/Pausa 11, 1917 (Saka)

The following Act of Parliament received the assent of the President on the 1st January, 1996, and is hereby published for general information: No. 1 of 1996 *[1st January 1996]*

An Act to give effect to the Proclamation on the Full Participation and Equality of the People with Disabilities in the Asian and Pacific Region.

Whereas the Meeting to Launch the Asian and Pacific Decade of Disabled Persons 1993–2002 convened by the Economic and Social Commission for Asia and Pacific held at Beijing on 1st to 5th December, 1992, adopted the Proclamation on the Full Participation and Equality of People with Disabilities in the Asian and Pacific Region

And whereas India is a signatory to the said Proclamation and whereas it is considered necessary to implement the Proclamation aforesaid.

Be it enacted by Parliament in the Forty-sixth Year of the Republic of India as follows:

CHAPTER I: PRELIMINARY

1. (1) This Act may be called the Persons with Disabilities (Equal Opportunities, Protection of Rights and Full Participation) Act, 1995.
   (2) It extends to the whole of India except the State of Jammu and Kashmir.
   (3) It shall come into force on such date as the Central Government may, by notification, appoint.
2. **In this Act, unless the context otherwise requires,—**
   (a) **"Appropriate Government"** means,—
      (i) in relation to the Central Government or any establishment wholly or substantially financed by that Government, or a Cantonment Board constituted under the Cantonment Act, 1924, the Central Government

(ii)   in relation to a State Government or any establishment wholly or substantially financed by that Government, or any local authority, other than a Cantonment Board, the State Government

(iii) in respect of the Central Coordination Committee and the Central Executive Committee, the Central Government

(iv)   in respect of the State Coordination Committee and the State Executive Committee, the State Government

(b) **"Blindness"** refers to a condition where a person suffers from any of the following conditions, namely:—

(i)   total absence of sight

(ii)   visual acuity not exceeding 6/60 or 20/200 (Snellen) in the better eye with correcting lenses or

(iii) limitation of the field of vision subtending an angle of 20 degree or worse

(c) **"Central Coordination Committee"** means the Central Coordination Committee constituted under sub-section (1) of Section 3

(d) **"Central Executive Committee"** means the Central Executive Committee constituted under sub-section (1) of Section 9

(e) **"Cerebral palsy"** means a group of non-progressive conditions of a person characterized by abnormal motor control posture resulting from brain insult or injuries occurring in the pre-natal, perinatal or infant period of development

(f) **"Chief Commissioner"** means the Chief Commissioner appointed under sub-section (1) of Section 57

(g) **"Commissioner"** means the Commissioner appointed under sub-section (1) of Section 60

(h) **"Competent authority"** means the authority appointed under Section 50

(i) **"Disability"** means—

(i)   blindness

(ii)   low vision

(iii) leprosy-cured

(iv)   hearing impairment

(v)   loco motor disability

(vi)   mental retardation

(vii) mental illness

(j) **"Employer"** means,—

(i)   in relation to a Government, the authority notified by the Head of the Department in this behalf or where no such authority is notified, the Head of the Department and

(ii)   in relation to an establishment, the chief executive officer of that the establishment

(k) **"Establishment"** means a corporation established by or under a Central, Provincial or State Act, or an authority or a body owned or controlled or aided by the Government or a local authority or a Government company as defined in section 617 of 'the Companies Act, 1956 and includes Departments of a Government

(l) **"Hearing impairment"** means loss of sixty decibels or more in the better year in the conversational range of frequencies

(m) **"Institution for persons with disabilities"** means an institution for the reception, care, protection, education, training, rehabilitation or any other service of persons with disabilities

(n) **"Leprosy cured person"** means any person who has been cured of leprosy but is suffering from—

   (i) loss of sensation in hands or feet as well as loss of sensation and paresis in the eye and eye-lid but with no manifest deformity

   (ii) manifest deformity and paresis but having sufficient mobility in their hands and feet to enable them to engage in normal economic activity

   (iii) extreme physical deformity as well as advanced age which prevents him from undertaking any gainful occupation, and the expression "leprosy cured" shall be construed accordingly.

(o) **"Locomotor disability"** means disability of the bones, joints muscles leading to substantial restriction of the movement of the limbs or any form of cerebral palsy

(p) **"Medical authority"** means any hospital or institution specified for the purposes of this Act by notification by the appropriate Government

(q) **"Mental illness"** means any mental disorder other than mental retardation

(r) **"Mental retardation"** means a condition of arrested or incomplete development of mind of a person which is specially characterized by subnormality of intelligence

(s) **"Notification"** means a notification published in the Official Gazette

(t) **"Person with disability"** means a person suffering from not less than forty percent of any disability as certified by a medical authority

(u) **"Person with low vision"** means a person with impairment of visual functioning even after treatment or standard refractive correction but who uses or is potentially capable of using vision for the planning or execution of a task with appropriate assistive device

(v) **"Prescribed"** means prescribed by rules made under this Act

(w) **"Rehabilitation"** refers to a process aimed at enabling persons with disabilities to reach and maintain their optimal physical, sensory, intellectual, psychiatric or social functional levels

(x) **"Special employment exchange"** means any office or place established and maintained by the Government for the collection and furnishing of information, either by keeping of registers or otherwise, respecting—

   (i) persons who seek to engage employees from amongst the persons suffering from disabilities

   (ii) persons with disability who seek employment

   (iii) vacancies to which person with disability seeking employment may be appointed

(y) **"State Coordination Committee"** means the State Coordination Committee constituted under sub-section (1) of Section 13.

(z) **"State Executive Committee"** means the State Executive Committee constituted under sub-section (l) of Section 19.

CHAPTER II: THE CENTRAL COORDINATION COMMITTEE

3. (1) The Central Government shall by notification constitute a body to be known as the Central Coordination Committee to exercise the powers conferred on, and to perform the functions assigned to it, under this Act.

   (2) The Central Coordination Committee shall consist of—

     (a) The Minister in charge of the Department of Welfare in the Central Government, Chairperson, *ex officio*

(b) The Minister of State incharge of the Department of Welfare in the Central Government, Vice-Chairperson, *ex officio*

(c) Secretaries to the Government of India in-charge of the Departments of Welfare, Education, Woman and Child Development, Expenditure, Personnel, Training and Public Grievances, Health, Rural Development, Industrial Development, Urban Affairs and Employment, Science and Technology, Legal Affairs, Public Enterprises, Members, *ex officio*

(d) Chief Commissioner, Member, *ex officio*

(e) Chairman Railway Board, Member, *ex officio*

(f) Director General of Labor, Employment and Training, Member, *ex officio*

(g) Director, National Council for Educational Research and Training, Member, *ex officio*

(h) Three Members of Parliament of whom two shall be elected by the House of the People and one by the Council of States, Members

(i) Three persons to be nominated by the Central Government to represent the interests, which in the opinion of that Government ought to be represented, Members

(j) Directors of the—
   (i) National Institute for the Visually Handicapped, Dehradun
   (ii) National Institute for the Mentally Handicapped, Secunderabad
   (iii) National Institute for the Orthopedically Handicapped, Kolkata
   (iv) Ali Yavar Jung National Institute for the Hearing Handicapped, Mumbai, Members, *ex officio*

(k) Four Members to be nominated by the Central Government by rotation to represent the States and the Union territories in such manner as may be prescribed by the Central Government:

Provided that no appointment under this clause shall be made except on the recommendation of the State Government or, as the case may be, the Union territory

(l) Five persons as far as practicable, being persons with disabilities. to represent non-governmental organizations or associations which are concerned with disabilities, to be nominated by the Central Government, one from each area of disability, Members provided that while nominating persons under this clause, the Central Government shall nominate at least one woman and one person belonging to Scheduled Castes or Scheduled Tribes

(m) Joint Secretary to the Government of India in the Ministry of Welfare dealing with the welfare of the handicapped, Member Secretary, *ex officio*.

(3) The office of the Member of the Central Coordination Committee shall not disqualify its holder for being chosen as or for being a Member of either House of Parliament.

4. (1) Save as otherwise provided by or under this Act a Member of Central Coordination Committee nominated under clause (i) or clause (l) of sub-section (2) of Section 3 shall hold office for a term of 3 years from the date of his nomination: Provided that such a Member shall, notwithstanding the expiration of his term, continue to hold office until his successor enters upon his office.

(2) The term of office of an *ex officio* Member shall come to an end as soon as he ceases to hold the office by virtue of which he was so nominated.

(3) The Central Government may if it thinks fit remove any Member nominated under clause (i) or clause (l) of sub-section (2) of Section 3, before the expiry of his term of office after giving him a reasonable opportunity of showing cause against the same.

(4) A Member nominated under clause (i) or clause (l) of sub-section (2) of Section 3 may at any time resign his office by writing under his hand addressed to the Central Government and the seat of the said Member shall thereupon become vacant.

(5) A casual vacancy in the Central Coordination Committee shall be filled by a fresh nomination and the person nominated to fill the vacancy shall hold office only for the remainder of the term for which the Member in whose place he was so dominated.

(6) A Member nominated under clause (i) or clause (l) of sub-section (2) of Section 3 shall be eligible for renomination (7) Members nominated under clause (i) and clause (l) of sub-section (2) of Section 3 shall receive such allowances as may be prescribed by the Central Government.

5. (1) No person shall be a Member of the Central Coordination Committee, who—

    (a) is, or at any time has been, adjudged insolvent or has suspended payment of his debts or has compounded with his creditors, or

    (b) is of unsound mind and stands so declared by a competent court, or

    (c) is or has been convicted of an offence which, in the opinion of the Central Government, involves moral turpitude, or

    (d) is or at any time has been convicted of an offence under this Act, or

    (e) has so abused in the opinion of the Central Government his position as a Member as to render his continuance in the Central Coordination Committee detrimental to the interests of the general public.

(2) No order of removal shall be made by the Central Government under this section unless the Member concerned has been given a reasonable opportunity of showing cause against the same.

(3) Notwithstanding anything contained in sub-section (1) or sub-section (6) of Section 4, a Member who has been removed under this Section shall not be eligible for renomination as a Member.

6. If a Member of the Central Coordination Committee becomes subject to any of the disqualifications specified in Section 5, his seat shall become vacant.

7. The Central Coordination Committee shall meet at least once in every six months and shall observe such rules of procedure in regard to the transaction of business at its meetings as may be prescribed by the Central Government.

8. (1) Subject to the provisions of this Act, the function of the Central Coordination Committee shall be to serve as the national focal point on disability matters and facilitate the continuous evolution of a comprehensive policy towards solving the problems faced by persons with disabilities.

(2) In particular and without prejudice to the generality of the foregoing, the Central Coordination Committee may perform all or any of the following functions, namely:

    (a) review and coordinate the activities of all the Departments of Government and other Governmental and Nongovernmental Organizations which are dealing with matters relating to persons with disabilities

    (b) develop a national policy to address issues faced by persons with disabilities

    (c) advise the Central Government on the formulation of policies, programmes, legislation and projects with respect to disability

    (d) take up the cause of persons with disabilities with the concerned authorities and the international organizations with a view to provide for schemes and projects for the disabled in the national plans and other programmes and policies evolved by the international agencies

    (e) review in consultation with the donor agencies their funding policies from the perspective of their impact on persons with disabilities

    (f) take such other steps to ensure barrier free environment in public places, work places, public utilities, schools and other institutions

    (g) monitor and evaluate the impact of policies and programmes designed for achieving equality and full participation of persons with disabilities

    (h) to perform such other functions as may be prescribed by the Central Government.

9. (1) The Central Government shall constitute a Committee to be known as the Central Executive Committee to perform the functions assigned to it under this Act.

  (2) The Central Executive Committee shall consist of—

    (a) The Secretary to the Government of India in the Ministry of Welfare, Chairperson, *ex officio*

    (b) The Chief Commissioner, Member, *ex officio*

    (c) The Director General for Health Services, Member, *ex officio*

    (d) The Director General, Employment and Training, Member, *ex officio*

    (e) Six persons not below the rank of a Joint Secretary to the Government of India, to represent the Ministries or Departments of Rural Development, Education, Welfare, Personnel Public Grievances and Pension and Urban Affairs and Employment, Science and Technology, Members, *ex officio*

    (f) the Financial Advisor, Ministry of Welfare in the Central Government, Member, *ex officio*

    (g) Advisor (Tariff) Railway Board, Member, *ex officio*

    (h) four members to be nominated by the Central Government, by rotation, to represent the State Governments and the Union Territories in such manner as may be prescribed by the Central Government

    (i) One person to be nominated by the Central Government to represent the interest, which in the opinion of the Central Government ought to be represented, Member

    (j) Five persons, as far as practicable, being persons with disabilities, to represent non-governmental organizations or associations which are concerned with disabilities, to be nominated by the Central Government, one from each area of disability, Members:

      Provided that while nominating persons under this clause, the Central Government shall nominate at least one woman and one person belonging to Scheduled Castes or Scheduled Tribes

    (k) Joint Secretary to the Government of India in the Ministry of Welfare dealing with the welfare of the handicapped, Member-Secretary, *ex officio*.

  (3) Members nominated under clause (i) and clause (j) of sub-section (2) shall receive such allowances as may be prescribed by the Central Government.

  (4) A Member nominated under clause (i) or clause (j) of sub-section (2) may at any time resign his office by writing under his hand addressed to the Central Government and the seat of the said Member shall thereupon become vacant.

10. (1) The Central Executive Committee shall be the executive body of the Central Coordination Committee and shall be responsible for carrying out the decisions of the Central Coordination Committee.

  (2) Without prejudice to the provisions of sub-section (1), the Central Executive Committee shall also perform such other functions as may be delegated to it by the Central Coordination Committee.

11. The Central Executive Committee shall meet at least once in three months and shall observe such rules of procedure in regard to the transaction of business at its meetings as may be prescribed by the Central Government.

12. (1) The Central Executive Committee may associate with itself in such manner and for such purposes as may be prescribed by the Central Government any person whose assistance or advice it may desire to obtain in performing any of its functions under this Act.

   (2) A person associated with the Central Executive Committee under sub-section (1) for any purpose shall have the right to take part in the discussions of the Central Executive Committee relevant to that purpose, but shall not have a right to vote at a meeting of the said Committee, and shall not be a member for any other purpose.

   (3) A person associated with the said Committee under sub-section (1) for any purpose shall be paid such fees and allowances, for attending its meetings and for attending to any other work of the said Committee, as may be prescribed by the Central Government.

CHAPTER III: THE STATE COORDINATION COMMITTEE

13. (1) Every State Government shall, by notification, constitute a body to be known as the State Coordination Committee to exercise the powers conferred on, and to perform the function assigned to it, under this Act.

   (2) The State Coordination Committee shall consist of—

   (a) The Minister in-charge of the Department of Social Welfare in the State Government, Chairperson, *ex officio*

   (b) The Minister of State in-charge of the Department of Social Welfare, if any, Vice-Chairperson, *ex officio*

   (c) Secretaries to the State Government in-charge of the Departments of Welfare, Education, Woman and Child Development, Expenditure, Personnel Training and Public Grievances, Health, Rural Development, Industrial Development, Urban Affairs and Employment, Science and Technology, Public Enterprises, by whatever name called, Members, *ex officio*

   (d) Secretary of any other Department, which the State Government considers necessary, Member, *ex officio*

   (e) Chairman Bureau of Public Enterprises (by whatever name called) Member, *ex officio*

   (f) Five persons, as far as practicable, being persons with disabilities, to represent non-governmental organizations or associations which are concerned with disabilities, to be nominated by the State Government, one from each area of disability, Members:

   Provided that while nominating persons under this clause, the State Government shall nominate at least one woman and one person belonging to Scheduled Castes or Scheduled Tribes

   (g) Three Members of State Legislature, of whom two shall be elected by the Legislative assembly and one by the Legislative Council, if any

   (h) Three persons to be nominated by that State Government to represent agriculture, industry or trade or any other interest, which in the opinion of State Government ought to be represented, Members, *ex officio*

   (i) The Commissioner, Member, *ex officio*

   (j) Secretary to the State Government dealing with the welfare of the handicapped, Member-Secretary, *ex officio*.

(3) Notwithstanding anything contained in this section, no State Coordination Committee shall be constituted for a Union Territory and in relation to a Union Territory the Central Coordination Committee shall exercise the functions and perform the functions of a State Coordination Committee for the Union Territory, provided that in relation to a Union Territory, the Central Coordination Committee may delegate all or any of its powers and functions under this sub-section to such person or body of persons as the Central Government may specify.

14. (1) Save as otherwise provided by or under this Act, a Member of a State Coordination Committee nominated under clause (f) or clause (h) of sub-section (2) of Section 13 shall hold office for a term of 3 years from the date of his nomination:

Provided that such a Member shall, notwithstanding the expiration of his term, continue to hold office until his successor enters upon his office.

(2) The term of office of an *ex officio* Member shall come to an end as soon as he ceases to hold the office by virtue of which he was so nominated.

(3) The State Government may, if it thinks fit, remove any Member nominated under clause (f) or clause (h) of sub-section (2) of Section 13, before the expiry of his term of office after giving him a reasonable opportunity of showing cause against the same.

(4) A Member nominated under clause (f) or clause (h) of sub-section (2) of Section 13 may, at any time, resign his office by writing under his hand addressed to the State Government and the seat of the said Member shall thereupon become vacant.

(5) A casual vacancy in the State Coordination Committee shall be filled by a fresh nomination and the person nominated to fill the vacancy shall hold office only for the remainder of the term for which the Member in whose place he was so nominated.

(6) A Member nominated under clause (f) and clause (h) of sub-section (2) of Section 13 shall be eligible for renomination.

(7) Members nominated under clause (f) and clause (h) of sub-section (2) of Section 13 shall receive such allowances as may he prescribed by the State Government.

15. (1) No person shall be a Member of the State Coordination Committee, who—
   (a) is, or at any time, has been adjudged insolvent or has suspended payment of his debts or has compounded with his creditors, or
   (b) is of unsound mind and stands so declared by a competent court, or
   (c) is or has been convicted of an offence which in the opinion of the State Government involves moral turpitude, or
   (d) is or at any time has been convicted of an offence under this Act, or
   (e) has so abused, in the opinion of the State Government, his position as a member as to render his continuance in the State Coordination Committee detrimental to the interests of the general public.

(2) No order of removal shall be made by the State Government under this section unless the Member concerned has been given a reasonable opportunity of showing cause against the same.

(3) Notwithstanding anything contained in sub-section (1) or sub-section (6) of Section 14, a Member who has been removed under this section shall net be eligible for renomination as a Member.

16. If a Member of the State Coordination Committee becomes subject to any of the disqualifications specified in Section 15, his seat shall become vacant.

17. The State Coordination Committee shall meet at least once in every six months and shall observe such rules of procedure in regard to the transaction of business at its meetings as may be prescribed.

18. (1) Subject to the provisions of this Act, the function of the State Coordination Committee shall be to serve as the state focal point on disability matters and facilitate the continuous evolution of a comprehensive policy towards solving the problems faced by persons with disabilities.

    (2) In particular and without prejudice to the generality of the foregoing function the State Coordination Committee may, within the State perform all or any of the following functions, namely.

    (a) Review and coordinate the activities of all the Departments of Government and other Governmental and Nongovernmental Organizations which are dealing with matters relating to persons with disabilities

    (b) Develop a State policy to address issues faced by persons with disabilities

    (c) Advise the State Government on the formulation of policies, programmes, legislation and projects with respect to disability

    (d) Review, in consultation with the donor agencies, their funding from the perspective of their impact on persons with disabilities

    (e) Take such other steps to ensure barrier free environment in public places, work places, public utilities, schools and other institutions

    (f) Monitor and evaluate the impact of policies and programmes designed for achieving equality and full participation of persons with disabilities

    (g) To perform other functions as may be prescribed by the State Government.

19. (1) The State Government shall constitute a committee to be known as the State Executive Committee to perform the functions assigned to it under this Act.

    (2) The State Executive Committee shall consist of—

    (a) The Secretary, Department of Social Welfare, Chairperson, *ex officio*

    (b) The Commissioner, Member, *ex officio*

    (c) Nine persons not below the rank of a Joint Secretary to the State Government, to represent the Departments of Health, Finance, Rural Development, Education, Welfare, Personnel Public Grievances, Urban Affairs Labor and Employment, Science and Technology, Members, *ex officio*

    (d) One person to be nominated by the State Government to represent the interest, which in the opinion of the State Government ought to be represented, Member

    (e) Five persons, as far as practicable being persons with disabilities, to represent Nongovernmental organizations or associations which are concerned with disabilities, to be nominated by the State Government, one from each area of disability, Members, provided that while nominating persons under this clause, the State Government shall nominate at least one woman and one person belonging to Scheduled Castes or Scheduled Tribes

    (f) Joint Secretary dealing with the disability division in the Department of Welfare, Member-Secretary, *ex officio*.

    (3) Members nominated under clause (d) and clause (e) of sub-section (2) shall receive such allowances as may be prescribed by the State Government.

    (4) A Member nominated under clause (d) or clause (e) may at any time resign his office by writing under his hand addressed to the State Government and the seat of the said Member shall thereupon become vacant.

20. (1) The State Executive Committee shall be the executive body of the State Coordination Committee and shall be responsible for carrying out the decisions of the State Coordination Committee.

    (2) Without prejudice to the provisions of sub-section (1), the State Executive Committee shall also perform such other functions as may be delegated to it by the State Coordination Committee.

21. The State Executive Committee shall meet at least once in three months and shall observe such rules of procedure in regard to the transaction of business at its meetings as may be prescribed by the State Government.

22. (1) The State Executive Committee may associate with itself in such manner and for such purposes as may be prescribed by the State Government any person whose assistance or advice it may desire to obtain in performing any of its functions under this Act.

    (2) A person associated with the State Executive Committee under sub-section (1) for any purpose shall have the right to take part in the discussions of the State Executive Committee relevant to that purpose, but shall not have a right to vote at a meeting of the said Committee, and shall not be a member for any other purpose.

    (3) A person associated with the said Committee under sub-section (1) for any purpose shall be paid such fees and allowances, for attending its meetings and for attending to any other work of the said Committee, as may be prescribed by the State Government.

23. In the performance of its functions under this Act—

    (a) The Central Coordination Committee shall be bound by such directions in writing, as the Central Government may give to it and

    (b) The State Coordination Committee shall be bound by such directions in writing, as the Central Coordination Committee or the State Government may give to it:

    Provided that where a direction given by the State Government is inconsistent with any direction given by the Central Coordination Committee, the matter shall be referred to the Central Government for its decision.

24. No act or proceeding of the Central Coordination Committee, the Central Executive Committee, a State Coordination Committee or a State Executive Committee shall be called in question on the ground merely on the existence of any vacancy in or any defect in the constitution of such Committees.

CHAPTER IV: PREVENTION AND EARLY DETECTION OF DISABILITIES

25. Within the limits of their economic capacity and development, the appropriate Governments and the local authorities, with a view to preventing the occurrence of disabilities, shall—

    (a) undertake or cause to be undertaken surveys, investigations and research concerning the cause of occurrence of disabilities

    (b) promote various methods of preventing disabilities

    (c) screen all the children at least once in a year for the purpose of identifying "at-risk" cases

    (d) provide facilities for training to the staff at the primary health centers

    (e) sponsor or cause to be sponsored awareness campaigns and disseminated or cause to be disseminated information for general hygiene, health and sanitation

    (f) take measures for pre-natal, parental and post-natal care of mother and child

(g) educate the public through the pre-schools, schools, primary health centers, village level workers and anganwadi workers

(h) create awareness amongst the masses through television, radio and other mass media on the causes of disabilities and the preventive measures to be adopted.

CHAPTER V: EDUCATION

26. The appropriate Governments and the local authorities shall—
    (a) ensure that every child with a disability has access to free education in an appropriate environment till he attains the age of 18 years
    (b) endeavor to promote the integration of students with disabilities in the normal schools
    (c) promote setting up of special schools in Government and private sector for those in need of special education, in such a manner that children with disabilities living in any part of the country have access to such schools
    (d) endeavor to equip the special schools for children with disabilities with vocational training facilities.

27. The appropriate Governments and the local authorities shall by notification make schemes for—
    (a) conducting part-time classes in respect of children with disabilities who having completed education up to class fifth and could not continue their studies on a whole-time basis
    (b) conducting special part-time classes for providing functional literacy for children in the age group of sixteen and above
    (c) imparting non-formal education by utilizing the available manpower in rural areas after giving them appropriate orientation
    (d) imparting education through open schools or open universities
    (e) conducting class and discussions through interactive electronic or other media
    (f) providing every child with disability free of cost special books and equipment needed for his education.

28. The appropriate Governments shall initiate or cause to be initiated research by official and non-governmental agencies for the purpose of designing and developing new assistive devices, teaching aids, special teaching materials or such other items as are necessary to give a child with disability equal opportunities in education.

29. The appropriate Governments shall set up adequate number of teachers' training institutions and assist the national institutes and other voluntary organizations to develop teachers' training programmes specializing in disabilities so that requisite trained manpower is available for special schools and integrated schools for children with disabilities.

30. Without prejudice to the foregoing provisions, the appropriate Governments shall by notification prepare a comprehensive education scheme which shall make provision for—
    (a) transport facilities to the children with disabilities or in the alternative financial incentives to parents or guardians to enable their children with disabilities to attend schools.
    (b) the removal of architectural barriers from schools, colleges or other institution, imparting vocational and professional training
    (c) the supply of books, uniforms and other materials to children with disabilities attending school.
    (d) the grant of scholarship to students with disabilities
    (e) setting up of appropriate fora for the redressal of grievances of parent, regarding the placement of their children with disabilities

(f) suitable modification in the examination system to eliminate purely mathematical questions for the benefit of blind students and students with low vision

(g) restructuring of curriculum for the benefit of children with disabilities

(h) restructuring the curriculum for benefit of students with hearing impairment to facilitate them to take only one language as part of their curriculum.

31. All educational institutions shall provide or cause to be provided amanuensis to blind students and students with or low vision.

CHAPTER VI: EMPLOYMENT

32. Appropriate Governments shall—
    (a) identify posts, in the establishments, which can be reserved for the persons with disability
    (b) at periodical intervals not exceeding 3 years, review the list of posts identified and up-date the list taking into consideration the developments in technology.

33. Every appropriate Government shall appoint in every establishment such percentage of vacancies not less than three percent, for persons or class of persons with disability of which one percent, each shall be reserved for persons suffering from—
    (i) blindness or low vision
    (ii) bearing impairment
    (iii) locomotor disability or cerebral palsy in the posts identified for each disability, provided that the appropriate Government may, having regard to the type of work carried on in any department or establishment, by notification subject to such conditions, if any, as may be specified in such notification, exempt any establishment from the provisions of this section.

34. (1) The appropriate Government may, by notification, require that from such date as may be specified, by notification, the employer in every establishment shall furnish such information or return as may be prescribed in relation to vacancies appointed for person with disability that have occurred or are about to occur in that establishment to such Special Employment Exchange as may be prescribed and the establishment shall thereupon comply with such requisition.

    (2) The form in which and the intervals of time for which information or returns shall be furnished and the particulars, they shall contain shall be such as may be prescribed.

35. Any person authorized by the Special Employment Exchange in writing, shall have access to any relevant record or document in the possession of any establishment and may enter at any reasonable time and premises where he believes such record or document to be, and inspect or take copies of relevant records or documents or ask any question necessary for obtaining any information.

36. Where in any recruitment year any vacancy under Section 33, cannot be filled up due to non- availability of a suitable person with disability or, for any other sufficient reason, such vacancy shall be carried forward in the succeeding recruitment year and if in the succeeding recruitment year also suitable person with disability is not available, it may first be filled by interchange among the three categories and only when there is no parson with disability available for the post in that year, the employer shall fill up the vacancy by appointment of a person, other than a person with disability:

    Provided that if the nature of vacancies in an establishment is such that a given category of person cannot be employed, the vacancies may be interchanged among the three categories with the prior approval of the appropriate Government.

37. (1) Every employer shall maintain such record in relation to the person with disability employed in his establishment in such form and in such manner as may be prescribed by the appropriate Government.

   (2) The records maintained under sub-section (1) shall be open to inspection at all reasonable hours by such persons as may be authorized in this behalf by general or special order by the appropriate Government.

38. (1) The appropriate Governments and local authorities shall by notification formulate schemes for ensuring employment of persons with disabilities, and such schemes may provide for—

   (a) the training and welfare of persons with disabilities

   (b) the relaxation of upper age limit

   (c) regulating the employment

   (d) health and safety measures and creation of a non-handicapping environment in places where persons with disabilities are employed

   (e) the manner in which and the person by whom the cost of operating the schemes is to be defrayed and

   (f) constituting the authority responsible for the administration of the scheme.

39. All Government educational institutions and other educational institutions receiving aid from the Government, shall reserve not less than three percent seats for persons with disabilities.

40. The appropriate Governments and local authorities shall reserve not less than 3% in all poverty alleviation schemes for the benefit of persons with disabilities.

41. The appropriate Governments and the local authorities shall, within the limits of their economic capacity and development, provide incentives to employers both in public and private sectors to ensure that at least five percent of their work force is composed of persons with disabilities.

CHAPTER VII: AFFIRMATIVE ACTION

42. The appropriate Governments shall by notification make schemes to provide aids and appliances to persons with disabilities.

43. The appropriate Governments and local authorities shall by notification frame schemes in favor of persons with disabilities, for the preferential allotment of land at concession] rates for—

   (a) house

   (b) setting up business

   (c) setting up of special recreation centers

   (d) establishment of special schools

   (e) establishment of research centers

   (f) establishment of factories by entrepreneurs with disabilities.

CHAPTER VIII: NONDISCRIMINATION

44. Establishments in the transport sector shall, within the limits of their economic capacity and development for the benefit of persons with disabilities, take special measures to—

   (a) adapt rail compartments, buses, vessels and aircrafts in such a way as to permit easy access to such persons

(b) adapt toilets in rail compartments, vessels, aircrafts and waiting rooms in such a way as to permit the wheel chair users to use them conveniently.

45. The appropriate Governments and the local authorities shall, within the limits of their economic capacity and development, provide for—

(a) installation of auditory signals at red lights in the public roads for the benefit of persons with visually handicap

(b) causing curb cuts and slopes to be made in pavements for the easy access of wheelchair users

(c) engraving on the surface of the zebra crossing for the blind or for persons with low vision

(d) engraving on the edges of railway platforms for the blind or for persons with low vision

(e) devising appropriate symbols of disability

(f) warning signals at appropriate places.

46. The appropriate Governments and the local authorities shall, within the limits of their economic capacity and development, provide for—

(a) ramps in public buildings

(b) adaptation of toilets for wheelchair users

(c) braille symbols and auditory signals in elevators or lifts

(d) ramps in hospitals, primary health centers and other medical care and rehabilitation institutions.

47. (1) No establishment shall dispense with, or reduce in rank, an employee who acquires a disability during his service:

Provided that, if an employee, after acquiring disability is not suitable for the post he was holding, could be shifted to some other post with the same pay scale and service benefits.

Provided further that if it is not possible to adjust the employee against any post, he may be kept on a supernumerary post until a suitable post is available or he attains the age of superannuation, whichever is earlier.

(2) No promotion shall be denied to a person merely on the ground of his disability:

Provided that the appropriate Government may, having regard to the type of work carried on in any establishment, by notification and subject to such conditions, if any, as may be specified in such notification, exempt any establishment from the provisions of this section.

CHAPTER IX: RESEARCH AND MANPOWER DEVELOPMENT

48. The appropriate Governments and local authorities shall promote and sponsor research, *inter alia*, in the following areas—

(a) prevention of disability

(b) rehabilitation including community based rehabilitation

(c) development of assistive devices including their psychosocial aspects

(d) job identification

(e) on site modifications in offices and factories.

49. The appropriate Governments shall provide financial assistance to universities, other institutions of higher learning, professional bodies and non-governmental research-units or institutions, for undertaking research for special education, rehabilitation and manpower development.

CHAPTER X: RECOGNITION OF INSTITUTIONS FOR PERSONS WITH DISABILITIES

50. The State Government shall appoint any authority, as it deems fit to be a competent authority for the purposes of this Act.

51. Save as otherwise provided under this Act, no person shall establish or maintain any institution for persons with disabilities except under and in accordance with a certificate of registration issued in this behalf by the competent authority:

Provided that a person maintaining an institution for persons with disabilities immediately before the commencement of this Act may continue to maintain such institution for a period of six months from such commencement and if he has made an application for such certificate under this section within the said period of six months, till the disposal of such application.

52. (1) Every application for a certificate of registration shall be made to the competent authority in such form and in such manner as may be prescribed by the State Government.

(2) On receipt of an application under sub-section (1), the competent authority shall make such enquiries as it may deem fit and where it is satisfied that the applicant has complied with the requirements of this Act and the rules made thereunder it shall grant a certificate of registration to the applicant and where it is not so satisfied the competent authority shall, by order, refuse to grant the certificate applied for:

Provided that before making any order refusing to grant a certificate the competent authority shall give to the applicant a reasonable opportunity of being heard and every order of refusal to grant a certificate shall be communicated to the applicant in such manner as may be prescribed by the State Government.

(3) No certificate of registration shall be granted under sub-section (2) unless the institution with respect to which an application has been made is in a position to provide such facilities and maintain such standards as may be prescribed by the State Government.

(4) A certificate of registration granted under this section,—

(a) shall, unless revoked under Section 53, remain in force for such period as may be prescribed by the State Government.

(b) may be renewed from time to time for a like period and

(c) shall be in such form and shall be subject to such conditions as may be prescribed by the State Government.

(5) An application for renewal of a certificate of registration shall be made not less than 60 days before the period of validity.

(6) The certificate of registration shall be displayed by the institution in a conspicuous place.

53. (1) The competent authority may, if it has reasonable cause to believe that the holder of the certificate of registration granted under sub-section (2) of Section 52 has—

(a) made a statement in relation to any application for the issue of renewal of the certificate which is incorrect or false in material particulars or

(b) committed or has caused to be committed any breach of rules or any conditions subject to which the certificate was granted,

it may after making such inquiry, as it deems fit, by order, revoke the certificate:

    Provided that no such order shall he made until an opportunity is given to the holder of the certificate to show cause as to why the certificate should not be revoked.

(2) Where a certificate in respect of an institution has been revoked under sub-section (1), such institution shall cease to function from the date of such revocation:

    Provided that where an appeal lies under Section 54 against the order of revocation, such institution shall cease to function—

    (a) where no appeal has been preferred immediately on the expiry of the period prescribed for the filing of such appeal, or

    (b) where such appeal has been preferred, but the order of revocation has been upheld, from the date of the order of appeal.

(3) On the revocation of a certificate in respect of an institution, the competent authority may direct that any person with disability who is an inmate of such institution on the date of such revocation, shall be—

    (a) restored to the custody of her or his parent, spouse or lawful guardian, as the case may be, or

    (b) transferred to any other institution specified by the competent authority.

(4) Every institution, which holds a certificate of registration, which is revoked, under this section shall, immediately after such revocation, surrender such certificate to the competent authority.

54. (1) Any person aggrieved by the order of the competent authority refusing to grant a certificate or revoking a certificate may, within such period as may be prescribed by the State Government, prefer an appeal to that Government against such refusal or revocation.

(2) The order of the State Government on such appeal shall he final.

55. Nothing contained in this Chapter shall apply to an institution for persons with disabilities established or maintained by the Central Government or State Government.

CHAPTER XI: INSTITUTION FOR PERSONS WITH SEVERE DISABILITIES

56. (1) The appropriate Government may establish and maintain institutions for persons with severe disabilities at such places as it thinks fit.

(2) Where, the appropriate Government is of opinion that any institution other than an institution, established under sub-section (1), is fit for the rehabilitation of the persons with severe disabilities, the Government may recognize such institution as an institution for persons with severe disabilities for the purposes of this Act:

    Provided that no institution shall be recognized under this section unless such institution has complied with the requirements of this Act and the rules made there under.

(3) Every institution established under sub-section (1) shall be maintained in such manner and satisfy such conditions as may be prescribed by, the appropriate Government.

(4) For the purposes of this section "person with severe disability" means a person with eighty percent or more of one or more disabilities.

CHAPTER XII: THE CHIEF COMMISSIONER AND COMMISSIONERS FOR PERSONS WITH DISABILITIES

57. (1) The Central Government may, by notification appoint a Chief Commissioner for persons with disabilities for the purposes of this Act.

(2) A person shall not be qualified for appointment as the Chief Commissioner unless he has special knowledge or practical experience in respect of matters relating to rehabilitation.

(3) The salary and allowances payable to and other terms and conditions of service (including pension, gratuity and other retirement benefits of the Chief Commissioner shall be such as may be prescribed by the Central Government.

(4) The Central Government shall determine the nature and categories of officers and other employees required to assist the Chief Commissioner in the discharge of his functions and provide the Chief Commissioner with such officers and other employees as it thinks fit.

(5) The officers and employees provided to the Chief Commissioner shall discharge their functions under the general superintendence of the Chief Commissioner.

(6) The salaries and allowances and other conditions of service of officers and employees provided to the Chief Commissioner shall be such as may be prescribed by the Central Government.

58. The Chief Commissioner shall—

(a) coordinate the work of the Commissioners

(b) monitor the utilization of funds disbursed by the Central Government

(c) take steps to safeguard the rights and facilities made available to persons with disabilities

(d) submit reports to the Central Government on the implementation of the Act at such intervals as that Government may prescribe.

59. Without prejudice to the provisions of Section 58 the Chief Commissioner may of his own motion or on the application of any aggrieved person or otherwise look into complaints with respect to matters relating to—

(a) deprivation of rights of persons with disabilities.

(b) non-implementation of laws, rules, bye-laws, regulations, executive orders, guidelines or instructions made or issued by the appropriate Governments and the local authorities for the welfare and protection of rights or persons with disabilities,

and take up the matter with the appropriate authorities.

60. (1) Every State Government may, by notification appoint a Commissioner for persons with disabilities for the purpose of this Act.

(2) A person shall not be qualified for appointment as a Commissioner unless he has special knowledge or practical experience in respect of matters relating to rehabilitation.

(3) The salary and allowances payable to and other terms and conditions of service (including pension gratuity and other retirement benefits) of the Commissioner shall be such as may be prescribed by the State Government.

(4) The State Government shall determine the nature and categories of officers and other employees required to assist the Commissioner in the discharge of his functions and provide the Commissioner with such officers and other employees as it thinks fit.

(5) The officers and employees provided to the Commissioner shall discharge their functions under the general superintendence of the Commissioner.

(6) The salaries and allowances and other conditions of service of officers and employees provided to the Commissioner shall be such as may he prescribed by the State Government.

61. The Commissioner within the State shall—

(a) coordinate with the departments of the State Government for the programmes and schemes, for the benefit of persons with disabilities

(b) monitor the utilization of funds disbursed by the State Government

(c) take steps to safeguard the rights and facilities made available to persons with disabilities.

(d) submit reports to the State Government on the implementation of the Act at such intervals as that Government may prescribe and forward a copy thereof to the Chief Commissioner.

62. Without prejudice to the provisions of Section 61 the Commissioner may of his own motion or on the application of any aggrieved person or otherwise look into complaints with respect to matters relating to—

(a) deprivation of rights of persons with disabilities

(b) nonimplementation of laws, rules, bye-laws, regulations, executive orders, guidelines or instructions made or issued by the appropriate Governments and the local authorities for the welfare and protection of rights of persons with disabilities, and take up the matter with the appropriate authorities.

63. The Chief Commissioner and the Commissioners shall, for the purpose of discharging their functions under this Act, have the same powers as are vested in a court under the Code of Civil Procedure, 1908 while trying a suit, in respect of the following matters, namely:-

(a) summoning and enforcing the attendance of witnesses

(b) requiring the discovery and production of any documents

(c) requisitioning any public record or copy thereof from any court or office

(d) receiving evidence on affidavits

(e) issuing commissions for the examination of witnesses or documents.

(f) every proceeding before the Chief Commissioner and Commissioners shall be a judicial proceeding within the meaning of Sections 193 and 228 of the Indian Penal Code and the Chief Commissioner, the Commissioner, the competent authority, shall be deemed to be a civil court for the purposes of Section 195 and Chapter XXVI of the Code of Criminal Procedure, 1973.

64. (1) The Chief Commissioner shall prepare in such form and at such time for each financial year as may be prescribed by the Central Government an annual report giving a full account of his activities during the previous financial year and forward a copy thereof to the Central Government.

(2) The Central Government shall cause the annual report to be laid before each House of Parliament along with the recommendations explaining the action taken or proposed to be taken on the recommendation made therein in so far as they relate to the Central Government and the reasons for non-acceptance, if any, of any such recommendation or part.

65. (1) The Commissioner shall prepare in such form and at such time for each financial year as may be prescribed by the State Government an annual report giving a full account of his activities during the previous financial year and forward a copy thereof to the State Government.

(2) The State Government shall cause the annual report to be laid before each State Legislature along with the recommendations explaining the action taken or proposed to be taken on the recommendation made therein in so far as they relate to the State Government and the reasons for non-acceptance, if any, of any such recommendation or part.

CHAPTER XIII: SOCIAL SECURITY

66. (1) The appropriate Governments and the local authorities shall within the limits of their economic capacity and development undertake or cause to be undertaken rehabilitation of all persons with disabilities.

(2) For purposes of sub-section (1), the appropriate Governments and local authorities shall grant financial assistance to non-governmental organizations.

(3) The appropriate Governments and local authorities while formulating rehabilitation policies shall consult the non-governmental organizations working for the cause of persons with disabilities.

67. (1) The appropriate Government shall by notification frame an insurance scheme for the benefit of its employees with disabilities.

(2) Notwithstanding anything contained in this section, the appropriate Government may instead of framing an insurance scheme frame an alternative security scheme for its employees with disabilities.

68. The appropriate Governments shall within the limits of their economic capacity and development shall by notification frame a scheme for payment of an unemployment allowance to persons with disabilities registered with the Special Employment Exchange for more than 2 years and who could not he placed in any gainful occupation.

CHAPTER XIV: MISCELLANEOUS

69. Whoever fraudulently avails or attempts to avail, any benefit meant for persons with disabilities, shall be punishable with imprisonment for a term which may extend to 2 years or with fine which may extend to twenty thousand rupees or with both.

70. The Chief Commissioner, the Commissioners and other officers and staff provided to them shall be deemed to be public servants within the meaning of Section 21 of the Indian Penal Code.

71. No suit, prosecution or other legal proceeding shall lie against the Central Government, the State Governments or the local authority or any officer of the Government in respect of anything which is done in good faith or intended to be done in pursuance of this Act and any rules or orders made there under.

72. The provisions of this Act, or the rules made there under shall be in addition to, and not in derogation of any other law for the time being in force or any rules, order or any instructions issued there under, enacted or issued for the benefit of persons with disabilities.

73. (1) The appropriate Government may, by notification, make rules for carrying out the provisions of this Act.

(2) In particular, and without prejudice to the generality of the foregoing powers, such rules may provide for all or any of the following matters, namely:

(a) the manner in which a State Government or a Union Territory shall be chosen under clause (k) of sub-section (2) of Section 3

(b) allowances, which members shall receive under sub-section (7) of Section 4

(c) rules of procedure, which the Central Coordination Committee shall observe in regard to the transaction of business in its meetings under Section 7

(d) such other functions, which the Central Coordination Committee may perform under clause (h) of sub-section (2) of Section 8

(e) the manner in which a State Government or a Union Territory shall be chosen under clause (h) of sub-section (2) of Section 9

(f) the allowances, which the members shall receive under sub-section (3) of Section 9

(g) rules of procedure, which the Central Executive Committee shall observe in regard to transaction of business at its meetings under Section 11

(h) the manner and purposes for which a person may be associated under sub-section (I) of Section 12

(i) fees and allowances which a person associated with the Central Executive Committee shall receive under sub-section (3) of Section 12

(j) allowances which members shall receive under sub-section (7) of Section 14

(k) rules of procedure, which a State Coordination Committee shall observe in regard to transaction of business in its meetings under Section 17

(l) such other functions, which a State Coordination Committee may perform under clause (g) of sub-section (2) of Section 18

(m) the allowances, which members shall receive under sub-section (3) of Section 19

(n) rules of procedure, which a State Executive Committee shall observe in regard to transaction of business at its meetings under Section 21

(o) the manner and purposes for which a person may be associated under sub-section (1) of Section 22

(p) fees and allowances which a person associated with the State Executive Committee may receive under sub-section (3) of Section 22

(q) information or return which the employer in every establishment should furnish and the Special Employment Exchange to which such information or return shall be furnished under sub-section (1) of Section 34

(r) the form and the manner in which record shall be maintained by an employer under sub-section (1) of Section 37

(s) the form and manner in which an application shall be made under sub-section (1) of Section 52

(t) the manner in which an order of refusal shall be communicated under sub-section (2) of Section 52

(u) facilities or standards required to be provided or maintained under sub-section (3) of Section 52

(v) the period for which a certificate of registration shall be valid under clause (a) of sub-section (4) of Section 52

(w) the form in which and conditions subject to which a certificate of registration shall be granted under clause (c) of sub-section (4) of Section 52

(x) period within which an appeal shall lie under sub-section (1) of Section 54

(y) the manner in which an institution for persons with severe disabilities shall be maintained and conditions which have to be satisfied under sub-section (3) of Section 56

(z) the salary, allowances and other terms and conditions of service of the Chief Commissioner under sub-section (6) of Section 57

(za) the salary, allowances and other conditions of service of officers and employees under sub-section (6) of Section 57

(zb) intervals at which the Chief Commissioner shall report to the Central Government under clause (d) of Section 58

(zc) the salary, allowances and other terms and conditions of service of the Commissioner under sub-section (3) of Section 60 (zd) the salary, allowances and other conditions of service of officers and employees under sub-section (6) of Section 60

(ze) intervals within which the Commissioner shall report to the State Government under clause (d) of Section 61

(zf) the form and time in which annual report shall be prepared under sub-section (1) of Section 64

(zg) the form and time in which annual report shall be prepared under sub-section (1) of Section 65

(zh) any other matter which is required to be or may be prescribed.

(3) Every notification made by the Central Government under die proviso to Section 33, proviso to sub-section (2) of Section 47, every scheme framed by it under Section 27, Section 30, sub-section (1) of Section 38, Section 42, Section 43, Section 67, Section 68 and every rule made by it under sub-section (1). shall be laid, as soon as may be after it is made, before each House of Parliament, while it is in session for a total period of 30 days which may be comprised in one session or in two or more successive sessions, and if, before the expiry of the session immediately following the session or the successive sessions aforesaid, both Houses agree in making any modification in the rule, notification or scheme, both Houses agree that the rule, notification or scheme should not be made, the rule, notification or scheme shall thereafter have effect only in such modified form or be of no effect, as the case may be so, however, that any such modification or annulment shall be without prejudice to the validity of anything previously done under that rule, notification or scheme, as the case may be.

(4) Every notification made by the State Government under the proviso to Section 33 proviso to sub-section (2) of Section 47, every scheme made by it under Section 27, Section 30, sub-section (1) of Section 38, Section 42. Section 43, Section 67, Section 68 and every rule made by it under sub-section (1), shall be laid, as soon as may be after it is made, before each House of State Legislature, where it consists of two Houses or where such legislature consists of one House before that House.

74. In Section 12 of the Legal Services Authorities Act, 1987, for clause (d), the following clause shall be substituted, namely:-

"(d) A person with disability as defined in clause (i) of Section 2 of the Persons With Disabilities (Equal Opportunities, Protection of Rights and Full Participation) Act, 1995."

KL Mohanpuria

Secretary to the Government of India

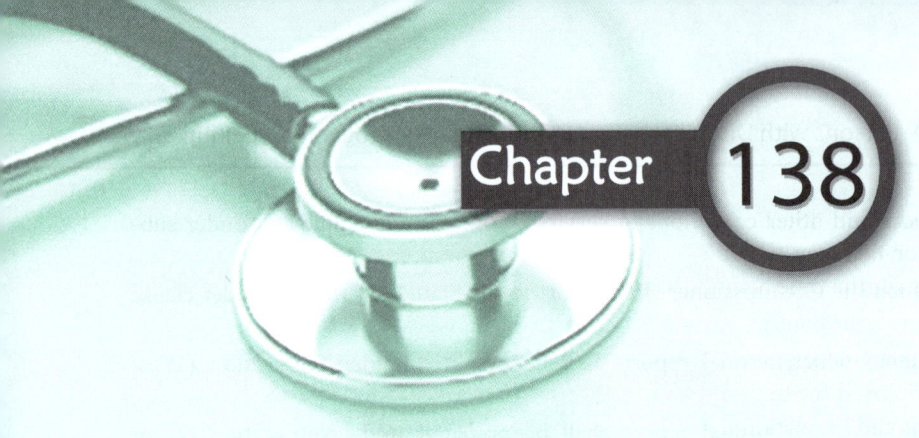

Chapter 138

Maternity Benefit Act

(ACT NO. 53 OF 1961)

[12th December, 1961]

*A*n Act to regulate the employment of women in certain establishments for certain period before and after child-birth and to provide for maternity benefit and certain other benefits.

Be it enacted by Parliament in the Twelfth Year of the Republic of India as follows:

1. **Short title, extent and commencement—**

    (1) This Act may be called the Maternity Benefit Act, 1961.

    (2) It extends to the whole of India[1].

    (3) It shall come into force on such date[2] as may be notified in this behalf in the Official Gazette,—

    [3][(a) in relation to mines and to any other establishment wherein persons are employed for the exhibition of equestrian, acrobatic and other performances, by the Central Government and]

    (b) in relation to other establishments in a State, by the State Government.

2. **Application of Act—**[4][(1) It applies, in the first instance,—

    (a) to every establishment being a factory, mine or plantation including any such establishment belonging to Government and to every establishment wherein persons are employed for the exhibition of equestrian, acrobatic and other performances

    (b) to every shop or establishment within the meaning of any law for the time being in force in relation to shops and establishments in a State, in which ten or more persons are employed, or were employed, on any day of the preceding twelve months:]

    Provided that the State Government may, with the approval of the Central Government, after giving not less than two months' notice of its intention of so doing, by notification in the Official Gazette, declare that all or any of the provisions of this Act shall apply also to any other establishment or class of establishments, industrial, commercial, agricultural or otherwise.

---

[1]The words "except the State of Jammu and Kashmir" omitted by Act 51 of 1970. Section 2 and Schedule (w.e.f. 1-9-1971).

[2]1st November, 1963: vide Notification No. S. O. 2920, dated 5th October, 1963. Gazette of India, Pt. II, Section 3, p. 3735.

[3]Subs. by Act 52 of 1973. Section 2 (w.e.f. 1-3-1975).

[4]Subs. by Act 61 of 1988. Section 2 (w.e.f. 10-1-1989).

(2) [5][Save as otherwise provided in [6][Sections 5A and 5B], nothing contained in this Act] shall apply to any factory or other establishment to which the provisions of the Employees' State Insurance Act, 1948 (34 of 1948), apply for the time being.

3. **Definitions**—In this Act, unless the context otherwise requires,—

(a) **"Appropriate Government"** means, in relation to an establishment being a mine, [7][or an establishment wherein persons are employed for the exhibition of equestrian, acrobatic and other performances] the Central Government and in relation to any other establishment, the State Government

(b) **"Child"** includes a still-born child

(c) **"Delivery"** means the birth of a child

(d) **"Employer"** means—

   (i) in relation to an establishment which is under the control of the Government, a person or authority appointed by the Government for the supervision and control of employees or where no person or authority is so appointed, the head of the department

   (ii) in relation to an establishment under any local authority, the person appointed by such authority for the supervision and control of employees or where no person is so appointed, the chief executive officer of the local authority

   (iii) in any other case, the person who, or the authority which, has the ultimate control over the affairs of the establishment and where the said affairs are entrusted to any other person whether called a manager, managing director, managing agent, or by any other name, such person

[8][(e) **"Establishment"** means—

   (i) a factory

   (ii) a mine

   (iii) a plantation

   (iv) an establishment wherein persons are employed for the exhibition of equestrian, acrobatic and other performances[9]

   [10][(iva) a shop or establishment or

   (v) an establishment to which the provisions of this Act have been declared under sub-section (1) of Section 2 to be applicable]

(f) **"Factory"** means a factory as defined in clause (m) of Section 2 of the Factories Act, 1948 (63 of 1948)

(g) **"Inspector"** means an Inspector appointed under Section 14

(h) **"Maternity benefit"** means the payment referred to in sub-section (1) of Section 5

[11][(ha) **"Medical termination of pregnancy"** means the termination permissible under the provisions of Medical Termination of Pregnancy Act, 1971.]

(i) **"Mine"** means a mine as defined in clause (j) of Section 2 of the Mines Act, 1952 (35 of 1952)

---

[5]Subs. by Act 21 of 1972. Section 2, for "Northing contained in this Act".
[6]Subs. by Act 53 of 1976. Section 2, for "Section 5A".
[7]Ins. by Act 52 of 1973, Section 4 (w.e.f. 1-3-1975).
[8]Ins. by Act 52 of 1973, Section 4 (w.e.f. 1-3-1975)
[9]Word "or" omitted by Act 61 of 1988, Section 3 (w.e.f. 10-1-1989)
[10]Ins. by Act 61 of 1988, Section 3 (w.e.f. 10-1-1989)
[11]Ins. by Act 29 of 1995, Section 2 (w.e.f 1-2-1996)

(j) **"Miscarriage"** means expulsion of the contents of a pregnant uterus at any period prior to or during the 26 weeks of pregnancy but does not include any miscarriage, the causing of which is punishable under the Indian Penal Code (45 of 1860)

(k) **"Plantation"** means a plantation as defined in clause (f) of Section 2 of the Plantations Labor Act, 1951 (69 of 1951)

(l) **"Prescribed"** means prescribed by rules made under this Act

(m) **"State Government",** in relation to a Union Territory, means the Administrator thereof

(n) **"Wages"** means all remuneration paid or payable in cash to a woman, if the terms of the contract of employment, express or implied, were fulfilled and includes—

    (1) such cash allowances (including dearness allowance and house rent allowance) as a woman is for the time being entitled to,

    (2) incentive bonus

    (3) the money value of the concessional supply of food grains and other articles, but does not include—

       (i) any bonus other than incentive bonus

       (ii) overtime earnings and any deduction or payment made on account of fines

       (iii) any contribution paid or payable by the employer to any pension fund or provident fund or for the benefit of the woman under any law for the time being in force

       (iv) any gratuity payable on the termination of service

(o) **"Woman"** means a woman employed, whether directly or through any agency, for wages in any establishment.

4. **Employment of women prohibited during certain period—**

    (1) No employer shall knowingly employ a woman in any establishment during the six weeks immediately following the day of her delivery, [12][miscarriage of medical termination of pregnancy].

    (2) No woman shall work in any establishment during the 6 weeks immediately following the day of her delivery, [13][miscarriage or medical termination of pregnancy].

    (3) Without prejudice to the provisions of section 6, no pregnant woman shall, on a request being made by her in this behalf, be required by her employer to do during the period specified in subsection (4) any work which is of an arduous nature or which involves long hours of standing, or which in any way is likely to interfere with her pregnancy or the normal development of the fetus, or is likely to cause her miscarriage or otherwise to adversely affect her health.

    (4) The period referred to in sub-section (3) shall be—

       (a) the period of one month immediately preceding the period of six weeks, before the date of her expected delivery

       (b) any period during the said period of six weeks for which the pregnant woman does not avail of leave of absence under Section 6.

5. **Right to payment of maternity benefit—**

    [14](1) Subject to the provisions of this Act, every woman shall be entitled to, and her employer shall be liable for, the payment of maternity benefit at the rate of the average daily wage for the period of her

---

[12]Subs. by Act 29 of 1995, Section 3(a), for "or her miscarriage" (w.e.f. 1-2-1996)

[13]Subs. by Act 29 of 1995, Section 3(b), for "or her miscarriage" (w.e.f. 1-2-1996)

[14]Subs. by Act 61 of 1988, Section 4 (w.e.f. 10-1-1989)

actual absence, that is to say, the period immediately preceding the day of her delivery, the actual day of her delivery and any period immediately following that day.

Explanation—For the purpose of this sub-section, the average daily wage means the average of the woman's wages payable to her for the days on which she has worked during the period of three calendar months immediately preceding the date from which she absents herself on account of maternity, [15][the minimum rate of wage fixed or revised under the Minimum Wages Act, 1948 (11 of 1948) or 10 rupees, whichever is the highest].

(2) No woman shall be entitled to maternity benefit unless she has actually worked in an establishment of the employer from whom she claims maternity benefit, for a period of not less than [16][eighty days] in the twelve months immediately preceding the date of her expected delivery:

Provided that the qualifying period of [17][eighty days] aforesaid shall not apply to a woman who has immigrated into the State of Assam and was pregnant at the time of the immigration.

Explanation—For the purpose of calculating under this sub-section the days on which a woman has actually worked in the establishment, [16][the days for which she has been laid off or was on holidays declared under any law for the time being in force to be holidays with wages] during the period of twelve months immediately preceding the date of her expected delivery shall be taken into account.

(3) The maximum period for which any woman shall be entitled to maternity benefit shall be twelve weeks of which not more than six weeks shall precede the date of her expected delivery:

Provided that where a woman dies during this period, the maternity benefit shall be payable only for the days up to and including the day of her death:

[18][Provided further that where a woman, having been delivered of a child, dies during her delivery or during the period immediately following the date of her delivery for which she is entitled for the maternity benefit, leaving behind in either case the child, the employer shall be liable for the maternity benefit for that entire period but if the child also dies during the said period, then, for the days up to and including the date of the death of the child.]

[19]**5A. Continuance of payment of maternity benefit in certain cases**—Every woman entitled to the payment of maternity benefit under this Act shall, notwithstanding the application of the Employees' State Insurance Act, 1948 (34 of 1948), to the factory or other establishment in which she is employed, continue to be so entitled until she becomes qualified to claim maternity benefit under Section 50 of that Act.

[20]**5B. Payment of maternity benefit in certain cases**—Every woman—

(a) who is employed in a factory or other establishment to which the provisions of the Employees' State Insurance Act, 1948 (34 of 1948), apply

(b) whose wages (excluding remuneration for over-time work) for a month exceed the amount specified in sub-clause (b) of clause (9) of Section 2 of that Act and

(c) who fulfils the conditions specified in sub-section (2) of section 5, shall be entitled to the payment of maternity benefit under this Act.

---

[15]Subs. by Act 61 of 1988, Section 4 (w.e.f. 10-1-1989)
[16]Subs. by Act 61 of 1988, Section 4, for "one hundred and sixty days" (w.e.f. 10-1-1989)
[17]Subs. by Act 61 of 1988, Section 4 for "one hundred and sixty days" (w.e.f. 10-1-1989)
[18]Subs. by Act 61 of 1988, Section 4 (w.e.f. 10-1-1988
[19]Ins. by Act 21 of 1972, Section 3
[20]Ins. by Act 53 of 1976, Section 3 (w.e.f. 1-5-1976)

6. **Notice of claim for maternity benefit and payment thereof—**

    (1) Any woman employed in an establishment and entitled to maternity benefit under the provisions of this Act may give notice in writing in such form may be prescribed, to her employer, stating that her maternity benefit and any other amount to which she may be entitled under this Act may be paid to her or to such person as she may nominate in the notice and that she will not work in any establishment during the period for which she receives maternity benefit.

    (2) In the case of a woman who is pregnant, such notice shall state the date from which she will be absent from work, not being a date earlier than six weeks from the date of her expected delivery.

    (3) Any woman who has not given the notice when she was pregnant may give such notice as soon as possible after the delivery.

    [21](4) On receipt of the notice, the employer shall permit such woman to absent herself from the establishment during the period for which she receives the maternity benefit.

    (5) The amount of maternity benefit for the period preceding the date of her expected delivery shall be paid in advance by the employer to the woman on production of such proof as may be prescribed that the woman is pregnant, and the amount due for the subsequent period shall be paid by the employer to the woman within forty-eight hours of production of such proof as may be prescribed that the woman has been delivered of a child.

    (6) The failure to give notice under this section shall not disentitle a woman to maternity benefit or any other amount under this Act if she is otherwise entitled to such benefit or amount and in any such case an Inspector may either of his own motion or on an application made to him by the woman, order the payment of such benefit or amount within such period as may be specified in the order.

7. **Payment of maternity benefit in case of death of a woman—**If a woman entitled to maternity benefit or any other amount under this Act, dies before receiving such maternity benefit or amount, or where the employer is liable for maternity benefit under the second proviso to sub-section (3) of Section 5, the employer shall pay such benefit or amount to the person nominated by the woman in the notice given under section 6 and in case there is no such nominee, to her legal representative.

8. **Payment of medical bonus—**Every woman entitled to maternity benefit under this Act shall also be entitled to receive from her employer a medical bonus of [22][two hundred and fifty rupees], if no pre-natal confinement and post-natal care is provided for by the employer free of charge.

9. [23]**Leave for miscarriage, etc.—**In case of miscarriage or medical termination of pregnancy, a woman shall, on production of such proof as may be prescribed, be entitled to leave with wages at the rate of maternity benefit, for a period of six weeks immediately following the day of her miscarriage or, as the case may be, her medical termination of pregnancy.

[24]**9A. Leave with wages for tubectomy operation,—**In case of tubectomy operation, a woman shall, on production of such proof as may be prescribed, be entitled to leave with wages at the rate of maternity benefit for a period of two weeks immediately following the day of her tubectomy operation.

10. **Leave for illness arising out of pregnancy, delivery, premature birth of child, [25][miscarriage, medical termination of pregnancy or tubectomy operation]—**A woman suffering from illness arising out of

---

[21]Subs. by Act 61 of 1988, Section 5 (w.e.f. 10-1-1989)

[22]Subs. by Act 61 of 1988, Section 6, for "twenty five rupees" (w.e.f. 10-1-1989)

[23]Sus. by Act 29 of 1995, Section 4 (w.e.f. 1-2-1996)

[24]Ins. by Act 29 of 1995, Section 5 (w.e.f. 1-2-1996)

[25]Subs. by Act 29 of 1995, Section 6, for "or miscarriage" (w.e.f. 1-2-1996)

pregnancy, delivery, premature birth of child [26][miscarriage, medical termination of pregnancy or tubectomy operation] shall, on production of such proof as may be prescribed, be entitled, in addition to the period of absence allowed to her under Section 6, or, as the case may be, under Section 9, to leave with wages at the rate of maternity benefit for a maximum period of one month.

11. **Nursing breaks**—Every woman delivered of a child who returns to duty after such delivery shall, in addition to the interval for rest allowed to her, be allowed in the course of her daily work two breaks of the prescribed duration for nursing the child until the child attains the age of fifteen months.

12. **Dismissal during absence of pregnancy**—

(1) When a woman absents herself from work in accordance with the provisions of this Act, it shall be unlawful for her employer to discharge or dismiss her during or on account of such absence or to give notice of discharge or dismissal on such a day that the notice will expire during such absence, or to vary to her disadvantage any of the conditions of her service.

(2) (a) The discharge or dismissal of a woman at any time during her pregnancy, if the woman but for such discharge or dismissal would have been entitled to maternity benefit or medical bonus referred to in Section 8, shall not have the effect of depriving her of the maternity benefit or medical bonus:

Provided that where the dismissal is for any prescribed gross misconduct, the employer may, by order in writing communicated to the woman, deprive her of the maternity benefit or medical bonus or both.

[27][(b) Any woman deprived of maternity benefit or medical bonus, or both, or discharged or dismissed during or on account of her absence from work in accordance with the provisions of this Act, may, within 60 days from the date on which order of such deprivation or discharge or dismissal is communicated to her, appeal to such authority as may be prescribed, and the decision of that authority on such appeal, whether the woman should or should not be deprived of maternity benefit or medical bonus, or both, or discharged or dismissed shall be final].

(c) Nothing contained in this sub-section shall affect the provisions contained in sub-section (1).

13. **No deduction of wages in certain cases**—No deduction from the normal and usual daily wages of a woman entitled to maternity benefit under the provisions of this Act shall be made by reason only of—

(a) the nature of work assigned to her by virtue of the provisions contained in sub-section (3) of Section 4

(b) breaks for nursing the child allowed to her under the provisions of Section 11.

14. **Appointment of Inspectors**—The appropriate Government may, by notification in the Official Gazette, appoint such officers as it thinks fit to be Inspectors for the purposes of this Act and may define the local limits of the jurisdiction within which they shall exercise their functions under this Act.

15. **Powers and duties of Inspectors**—An Inspector may, subject to such restrictions or conditions as may be prescribed, exercise all or any of the following powers, namely:—

(a) enter at all reasonable times with such assistants, if any, being persons in the service of the Government or any local or other public authority, as he thinks fit, any premises or place where women are employed or work is given to them in an establishment, for the purposes of examining any registers, records and notices required to be kept or exhibited by or under this Act and require their production for inspection

---

[26]Subs. by Act 29 of 1995, Section 6, for "or miscarriage" (w.e.f. 1-2-1996)
[27]Subs. by Act 61 of 1988, Section 7 (w.e.f. 10-1-1989)

(b) examine any person whom he finds in any premises or place and who, he has reasonable cause to believe, is employed in the establishment:

Provided that no person shall be compelled under this Section to answer any question or give any evidence tending to incriminate himself

(c) require the employer to give information regarding the names and addresses of women employed, payments made to them, and applications or notices received from them under this Act and

(d) take copies of any registers and records or notices or any portions thereof.

16. **Inspectors to be public servants**—Every Inspector appointed under this Act shall be deemed to be a public servant within the meaning of Section 21 of the Indian Penal Code (45 of 1860).

17. **Power of Inspector to direct payments to be made—**

[28](1) Any woman claiming that—

(a) maternity benefit or any other amount to which she is entitled under this Act and any person claiming that payment due under Section 7 has been improperly withheld

(b) her employer has discharged or dismissed her during or on account of her absence from work in accordance with the provisions of this Act, may make a complaint to the Inspector.

(2) The Inspector may, of his own motion or on receipt of a complaint referred to in sub-section (1), make an inquiry or cause an inquiry to be made and if satisfied that—

(a) payment has been wrongfully withheld, may direct the payment to be made in accordance with his orders

(b) she has been discharged or dismissed during or on account of her absence from work in accordance with the provisions of this Act, may pass such orders as are just and proper according to the circumstances of the case.]

(3) Any person aggrieved by the decision of the Inspector under sub-section (2) may, within 30 days from the date on which such decision is communicated to such person, appeal to the prescribed authority.

(4) The decision of the prescribed authority where an appeal has been preferred to it under sub-section (3) or of the Inspector where no such appeal has been preferred, shall be final.

[29][(5) Any amount payable under this section shall be recoverable by the Collector on a certificate issued for that amount by the Inspector as an arrear of land revenue.]

18. **Forfeiture of maternity benefit**—If a woman works in any establishment after she has been permitted by her employer to absent herself under the provisions of Section 6 for any period during such authorized absence, she shall forfeit her claim to the maternity benefit for such period.

19. **Abstract of Act and rules thereunder to be exhibited**—An abstract of the provisions of this Act and the rules made thereunder in the language or languages of the locality shall be exhibited in a conspicuous place by the employer in every part of the establishment in which women are employed.

20. **Registers, etc.**—Every employer shall prepare and maintain such registers, records and muster-rolls and in such manner as may be prescribed.

[30]21. **Penalty for contravention of Act by employer—**

(1) If any employer fails to pay any amount of maternity benefit to a woman entitled under this Act or discharges or dismisses such woman during or on account of her absence from work in accordance

---

[28]Subs. by Act 61 of 1988, Section 8 (w.e.f. 10-1-1989)
[29]Subs. by Act 61 of 1988, Section 8 (w.e.f. 10-1-1989)
[30]Subs. by Act 61 of 1988, Section 9 (w.e.f. 10-1-1989)

with the provisions of this Act, he shall be punishable with imprisonment which shall not be less than 3 months but which may extend to one year and with fine which shall not be less than two thousand rupees but which may extend to five thousand rupees:

Provided that the court may, for sufficient reasons to be recorded in writing, impose a sentence of imprisonment for a lesser term or fine only in lieu of imprisonment.

(2) If any employer contravenes the provisions of this Act or the rules made thereunder, he shall, if no other penalty is elsewhere provided by or under this Act for such contravention, be punishable with imprisonment which may extend to one year, or with fine which may extend to five thousand rupees, or with both:

Provided that where the contravention is of any provision regarding maternity benefit or regarding payment of any other amount and such maternity benefit or amount has not already been recovered, the court shall, in addition, recover such maternity benefit or amount as if it were a fine and pay the same to the person entitled thereto.]

22. Penalty for obstructing Inspector—Whoever fails to produce on demand by the Inspector any register or document in his custody kept in pursuance of this Act or the rules made thereunder or conceals or prevents any person from appearing before or being examined by an Inspector shall be punishable with imprisonment which may extend to [31][one year, or with fine which may extend to five thousand rupees], or with both.

[32]**23. Cognizance of offences**—

(1) Any aggrieved woman, an office-bearer of a trade union registered under the Trade Unions Act, 1926 (16 of 1926) of which such woman is a member or a voluntary organization registered under the Societies Registration Act, 1860 (21 of 1860) or an Inspector, may file a complaint regarding the commission of an offence under this Act in any court of competent jurisdiction and no such complaint shall be filed after the expiry of one year from the date on which the offence is alleged to have been committed.

(2) No court inferior to that of a Metropolitan Magistrate or a Magistrate of the first class shall try any offence under this Act.]

24. Protection of action taken in good faith—No suit, prosecution or other legal proceeding shall lie against any person for anything which is in good faith done or intended to be done in pursuance of this Act or of any rule or order made thereunder.

25. Power of Central Government to give directions—The Central Government may give such directions as it may deem necessary to a State Government regarding the carrying into execution of the provisions of this Act and the State Government shall comply with such directions.

26. Power to exempt establishments—If the appropriate Government is satisfied that having regard to an establishment or a class of establishments providing for the grant of benefits which are not less favorable than those provided in this Act, it is necessary so to do, it may, by notification in the Official Gazette, exempt, subject to such conditions and restrictions, if any, as may be specified in the notification, the establishment or class of establishments from the operation of all or any of the provisions of this Act or of any rule made thereunder.

---

[31]Subs. by Act 61 of 1988, Section 10 (w.e.f. 10-1-1989)
[32]Subs. by Act 61 of 1988, Section 11 (w.e.f. 10-1-1989)

27. **Effect of laws and agreements inconsistent with this Act—**

(1) The provisions of this Act shall have effect notwithstanding anything inconsistent therewith contained in any other law or in the terms of any award, agreement or contract of service, whether made before or after the coming into force of this Act:

Provided that where under any such award, agreement, contract of service or otherwise, a woman is entitled to benefits in respect of any matter which are more favorable to her than those to which she would be entitled under this Act, the woman shall continue to be entitled to the more favorable benefits in respect of that matter, notwithstanding that she is entitled to receive benefits in respect of other matters under this Act.

(2) Nothing contained in this Act shall be construed to preclude a woman from entering into an agreement with her employer for granting her rights or privileges in respect of any matter which are more favorable to her than those to which she would be entitled under this Act.

28. **Power to make rules—**

(1) The appropriate Government may, subject to the condition of previous publication and by notification in the Official Gazette, make rules for carrying out the purposes of this Act.

(2) In particular, and without prejudice to the generality of the foregoing power, such rules may provide for—

(a) the preparation and maintenance of registers, records and muster-rolls

(b) the exercise of powers (including the inspection of establishments) and the performance of duties by Inspectors for the purposes of this Act

(c) the method of payment of maternity benefit and other benefits under this Act in so far as provision has not been made therefor in this Act

(d) the form of notices under Section 6

(e) the nature of proof required under the provisions of this Act

(f) the duration of nursing-breaks referred to in Section 11

(g) acts which may constitute gross misconduct for purposes of Section 12

(h) the authority to which an appeal under clause (b) of sub-section (2) of Section 12 shall lie the form and manner in which such appeal may be made and the procedure to be followed in disposal thereof

(i) the authority to which an appeal shall lie against the decision of the Inspector under Section 17 the form and manner in which such appeal may be made and the procedure to be followed in disposal thereof

(j) the form and manner in which complaints may be made to Inspectors under sub-section (1) of Section 17 and the procedure to be followed by them when making inquiries or causing inquiries to be made under sub-section (2) of that section

(k) any other matter which is to be, or may be, prescribed.

[33](3) Every rule made by the Central Government under this section shall be laid as soon as may be after it is made, before each House of Parliament while it is in session for a total period of 30 days which may be comprised in one session [or in two or more successive sessions, and if, before the expiry of the session immediately following the session or the successive sessions aforesaid] both Houses agree in making any modification in the rule or both Houses agree that the rule should not be made,

---

[33]Subs. by Act 52 of 1973, Section 5 (w.e.f. 1-3-1975)

the rule shall thereafter have effect only in such modified form or be of no effect, as the case may be so however that any such modification or annulment shall be without prejudice to the validity of anything previously done under that rule.

29. **Amendment of Act 69 of 1951**—In Section 32 of the Plantations Labor Act, 1951,—

(a) in sub-section (1), the letter and brackets "(a)" before the words "in the case of sickness", the word "and" after the words "sickness allowance" and clause (b) shall be omitted

(b) in sub-section (2), the words "or maternity" shall be omitted.

30. **Repeal**—On the application of this Act—

(i) to mines, the Mines Maternity Benefit Act, 1941 (19 of 1941)

(ii) to factories situate in the Union Territory of Delhi, the Bombay Maternity Benefit Act, 1929 (Bombay Act VII of 1929); as in force in that territory, shall stand repealed.

MATERNITY BENEFIT AMENDMENT ACT, 2017

No. S-36012/03/ 2015-SS-I

Government of India

Ministry of Labor & Employment

In line with recommendations of the 44th, 45th & 46th Session of Indian Labor Conference (ILC) and demands from various quarters, the Government has recently enacted the Maternity Benefit (Amendment) Act, 2017. Through this Amendment Act, following provisions have been added to the Maternity Benefit Act, 1961:-

- Increase in the maternity leave from existing 12 to 26 weeks for working women with less than two surviving children.
- Provisions for work from home for nursing mothers.
- Mandatory provisions for establishments having fifty or more employees to have the facility of crèche.
- Extension of twelve weeks of maternity benefit to the 'commissioning mother' and the 'adopting mother' from the date the child is handed over.

Provisions of the Amendment Act have come into force w.e.f. 1st April, 2017, except those relating to crèche facility {Section 4(1)} which would come into force from 01.07.2017.

After the enactment of the said Act, the Ministry has been receiving numerous queries relating the revised provisions of the Act. The Ministry has examined such queries in consultation with Chief Labor Commissioner (Central) and the same are clarified as below:

Sl. no.	Query	Clarification
1.	Applicability of the Act to contractual or consultant women employees.	Since there is no amendment in Sec. 2 of the Act, hence the original provision prevails. The Act is applicable to all women who are employed in any capacity directly or through any agency i.e. either on contractual or as consultant.
2.	Whether enhanced maternity benefit, as modified by the Maternity Benefit (Amendment) bill, 2016 can be extended to women who are already under maternity leave at the time of enforcement of this Amendment Act?	Yes.

Contd...

Sl. no.	Query	Clarification
3.	Whether enhance maternity benefit can be extended to those women who have joined after availing 12 weeks of the maternity leave?	Those women employee who had already availed 12 weeks of maternity leave before enforcement of the Maternity Benefit (Amendment) Act, 2017 i.e. 1st April, 2017, shall not be entitled to avail the extended benefit of the 26 weeks leave.
4.	Protection of women in case she is fired by the employer after learning her pregnancy?	Under Section 12 of the M.B. Act, 1961 it is emphasized that any dismissal or discharge of a women during the pregnancy is unlawful and such employer can be punished under Section 21 of the Act.
5.	Whether benefits of this Act can be extended to the employed women in the unorganized Sector	The Maternity Benefit Act is applicable to all mines, plantations, shops and establishments and factories. Mines, plantations, shop and establishments could be either in organized sector or unorganized sector. Also, clarification at SL. No. 1 may be seen.

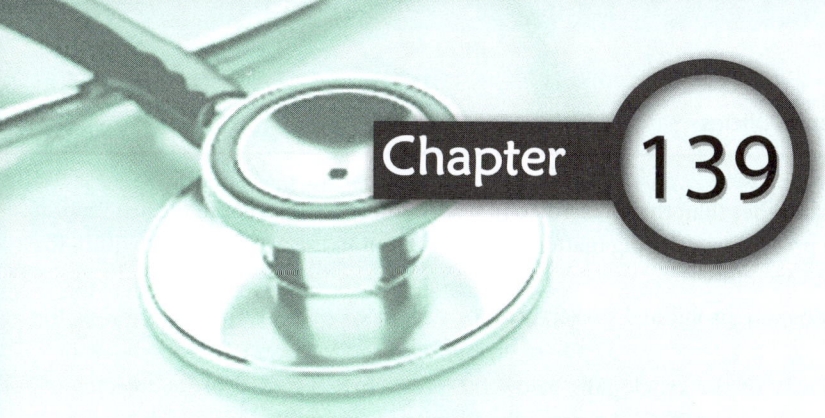

Prevention of Food Adulteration Act

[ACT NO. 37 OF 1954]

[29th September 1954]

An Act to make provision for the prevention of adulteration of food.
Be it enacted by Parliament in the fifth year of the Republic of India as follows:—

1. **Short title, extent and commencement—**

    (1) This Act may be called the Prevention of Food Adulteration Act, 1954.

    (2) It extends to the whole of India.

    (3) It shall come into force on such date as the Central Government may, by notification in the Official Gazette, appoint.

2. **Definitions—**In this Act unless the context otherwise requires,—

    [(i) **"Adulterant"** means any material which is or could be employed for the purposes of adulteration]

    [(ia)] **"Adulterated"**—an article of food shall be deemed to be adulterated—

    (a) if the article sold by a vendor is not of the nature, substance or quality demanded by the purchaser and is to his prejudice, or is not of the nature, substance or quality which it purports or is represented to be

    (b) if the article contains any other substance which affects, or if the article is so processed as to affect, injuriously the nature, substance or quality thereof

    (c) if any inferior or cheaper substance has been substituted wholly or in part for the article so as to affect injuriously the nature, substance or quality thereof

    (d) if any constituent of the article has been wholly or in part abstracted so as to affect injuriously the nature, substance or quality thereof

    (e) if the article had been prepared, packed or kept under insanitary conditions whereby it has become contaminated or injurious to health

    (f) if the article consists wholly or in part of any filthy, putrid, rotten, decomposed or diseased animal or vegetable substance or is insect-infested or is otherwise unfit for human consumption

    (g) if the article is obtained from a diseased animal

    (h) if the article contains any poisonous or other ingredient which renders it injurious to health

    (i) if the container of the article is composed, whether wholly or in part, of any poisonous or deleterious substance which renders its contents injurious to health

(j)   if any coloring matter other than that prescribed in respect thereof is present in the article, or if the amounts of the prescribed coloring matter which is present in the article are not within the prescribed limits of variability

(k)   if the article contains any prohibited preservative or permitted preservative in excess of the prescribed limits

(l)   if the quality or purity of the article falls below the prescribed standard or its constituents are present in quantities not within the prescribed limits of variability, but which renders it injurious to health

(m)   if the quality or purity of the article falls below the prescribed standard or its constituents are present in quantities not within the prescribed limits of variability but which does not render it injurious to health: Provided that, where the quality or purity of the article, being primary food, has fallen below the prescribed standards or its constituents are present in quantities not within the prescribed limits of variability in either case, solely due to natural causes and beyond the control of human agency, then, such article shall not be deemed to be adulterated within the meaning of this sub-clause.

Explanation—Where two or more articles of primary food are mixed together and the resultant article of food—

(a)   is stored, sold or distributed under a name which denotes the ingredients thereof and

(b)   is not injurious to health, then, such resultant article shall not be deemed to be adulterated within the meaning of this clause

(ii)   **"Central Food Laboratory"** means any laboratory or institute established or specified under Section 4

(iii)   **"Committee"** means the Central Committee for Food Standards constituted under Section 3

(iv)   **"Director of the Central Food Laboratory"** means the person appointed by the Central Government by notification in the Official Gazette as the Director of the Central Food Laboratory and includes any person appointed by the Central Government in like manner to perform all or any of the functions of the Director under this Act:

Provided that no person who has any financial interest in the manufacture, import or sale of any article of food shall be appointed to be a Director under this clause

(v)   **"Food"** means any article used as food or drink for human consumption other than drugs and water and includes—

(a)   any article which ordinarily enters into, or is used in the composition or preparation of, human food,

(b)   any flavoring matter or condiments, and

(c)   any other article which the Central Government may, having regard to its use, nature, substance or quality, declare, by notification in the Official Gazette, as food for the purposes of this Act

(vi)   **"Food (Health) Authority"** means the Director of Medical and Health Services or the Chief Officer in-charge of Health administration in a State, by whatever designation he is known, and includes any officer empowered by the Central Government or the State Government, by notification in the Official Gazette, to exercise the powers and perform the duties of the Food (Health) Authority under this Act with respect to such local area as may be specified in the notification

(vii)   **"Local area"** means any area, whether urban or rural, declared by [the Central Government or the State Government] by notification in the Official Gazette, to be a local area for the purposes of this Act

(viii) **"Local authority"** means in the case of:—

    (1)   a local area which is—

        (a)   a municipality, the municipal board or municipal corporation

        (b)   a cantonment, the cantonment authority

        (c)   a notified area, the notified area committee

    (2)   any other local area, such authority as may be prescribed by [the Central Government or the State Government] under this Act

(viii a) **"Local (Health) Authority"**, in relation to a local area, means the officer appointed by the Central Government or the State Government, by notification in the Official Gazette, to be in-charge of Health administration in such area with such designation as may be specified therein

(viii b) **"Manufacture"** includes any process incidental or ancillary to the manufacture of an article of food]

  (ix) **"Misbranded"**—an article of food shall be deemed to be misbranded—

    (a)   if it is an imitation of, or is a substitute for, or resembles in a manner likely to deceive, another article of food under the name of which it is sold, and is not plainly and conspicuously labelled so as to indicate its true character

    (b)   if it is falsely stated to be the product of any place or country

    (c)   if it is sold by a name which belongs to another article of food

    (d)   if it is so colored, flavored or coated, powdered or polished that the fact that the article is damaged is concealed or if the article is made to appear better or of greater value than it really is

    (e)   if false claims are made for it upon the label or otherwise

    (f)   if, when sold in packages which have been sealed or prepared by or at the instance of the manufacturer or producer and which bear his name and address, the contents of each package are not conspicuously and correctly stated on the outside thereof within the limits of variability prescribed under this Act

    (g)   if the package containing it, or the label on the package bears any statement, design or device regarding the ingredients or the substances contained therein, which is false or misleading in any material particular or if the package is otherwise deceptive with respect to its contents

    (h)   if the package containing it or the label on the package bears the name of a fictitious individual or company as the manufacturer or producer of the article

    (i)   if it purports to be, or is represented as being, for special dietary uses, unless its label bears such information as may be prescribed concerning its vitamin, mineral, or other dietary properties in order sufficiently to inform its purchaser as to its value for such uses

    (j)   if it contains any artificial flavoring, artificial coloring or chemical preservative, without a declaratory label stating that fact, or in contravention of the requirements of this Act or rules made thereunder

    (k)   if it is not labelled in accordance with the requirements of this Act or rules made thereunder

  (x) **"Package"** means a box, bottle, casket, tin, barrel, case, receptacle, sack, bag, wrapper or other thing in which an article of food is placed or packed

  (xi) **"Premises"** include any shop, stall, or place where any article of food is sold or manufactured or stored for sale

(xii) **"Prescribed"** means prescribed by rules made under this Act

(xii a) **"Primary food"** means any article of food, being a produce of agriculture or horticulture in its natural form

(xiii) **"Sale"** with its grammatical variations and cognate expressions, means the sale of any article of food, whether for cash or on credit or by way of exchange and whether by wholesale or retail, for human consumption or use, or for analysis, and includes an agreement for sale, an offer for sale, the exposing for sale or having in possession for sale of any such article, and includes also an attempt to sell any such article

(xiv) **"Sample"** means a sample of any article of food taken under the provisions of this Act or of any rules made thereunder

(xv) the word **"unwholesome"** and **"noxious"** when used in relation to an article of food mean respectively that the article is harmful to health or repugnant to human use.

2A. Rule of construction—Any reference in this Act to a law which is not in force in the State of Jammu and Kashmir shall, in relation to that State, be construed as a reference to the corresponding law, if any, in force in that State.

3. The Central Committee for Food Standards—

(1) The Central Government shall, as soon as may be after the commencement of this Act, constitute a Committee called the Central Committee for Food Standards to advise the Central Government and the State Governments on matters arising out of the administration of this Act and to carry out the other functions assigned to it under this Act.

(2) The Committee shall consist of the following members, namely:—

(a) the Director-General, Health Services, *ex-officio*, who shall be the Chairman

(b) the Director of the Central Food Laboratory or, in a case where more than one Central Food Laboratory is established, the Directors of such Laboratories, *ex-officio*

(c) two experts nominated by the Central Government

(d) one representative each of the Departments of Food and Agriculture in the Central Ministry of Food and Agriculture and one representative each of the Central Ministries of Commerce, defense, Industry and Supply and Railways, nominated by the Central Government

(e) one representative each nominated by the Government of each State

(f) two representatives nominated by the Central Government to represent the [Union Territories]

(g) one representative each, nominated by the Central Government, to represent the agricultural, commercial and industrial interests

(g i) five representatives nominated by the Central Government to represent the consumer's interests, one of whom shall be from the hotel industry

(h) one representative of the medical profession nominated by the Indian Council of Medical Research

(i) one representative nominated by the Indian Standards Institution referred to in clause (e) of Section 2 of the Indian Standards Institution (Certification Marks) Act, 1952 (36 of 1952).

(3) The members of the Committee referred to in clauses (c), (d), (e), (f), (g), (gg), (h), and (i) of sub-section (2) shall, unless their seats become vacant earlier by resignation, death or otherwise, be entitled to hold office for 3 years and shall be eligible for renomination.

(4) The functions of the Committee may be exercised notwithstanding any vacancy therein.

(5) The Committee may appoint such and so many sub-committees as it deems fit and may appoint to them persons who are not members of the Committee to exercise such powers and perform such duties as may, subject to such conditions, if any, as the Committee may impose, be delegated to them by the Committee.

(6) The Committee may, subject to the previous approval of the Central Government, make bye laws for the purpose of regulating its own procedure and the transaction of its business.

3A. Appointment of Secretary and other staff—

(1) The Central Government shall appoint a Secretary, to the Committee who shall, under the control and direction of the Committee, exercise such powers and perform such duties as may be prescribed or as may be delegated to him by the Committee.

(2) The Central Government shall provide the Committee with such clerical and other staff as that Government considers necessary.

4. Central Food Laboratory—

(1) The Central Government shall, by notification in the Official Gazette, establish one or more Central Food Laboratory or Laboratories to carry out the functions entrusted to the Central Food Laboratory by this Act or any rules made under this Act:

Provided that the Central Government may, by notification in the Official Gazette, also specify any laboratory or institute as a Central Food Laboratory for the purposes of this Act.

(2) The Central Government may, after consultation with the Committee, make rules prescribing—

   (a) the functions of a Central Food Laboratory and the local area or areas within which such functions may be carried out

   (b) the procedure for the submission to the said Laboratory of samples of articles of food for analysis or tests, the forms of the Laboratory's reports thereon and the fees payable in respect of such reports

   (c) such other matters as may be necessary or expedient to enable the said laboratory to carry out its functions.

5. Prohibition of import of certain articles of food—No person shall import into India—

(i) any adulterated food

(ii) any misbranded food

(iii) any article of food for the import of which a license is prescribed, except in accordance with the conditions of the license

(iv) any article of food in contravention of any other provision of this Act or of any rule made thereunder.

6. Application of law relating to Sea customs and Powers of Customs Officers—

(1) The law for the time being in force relating to sea customs and to goods, the import of which is prohibited by Section 18 of the Sea Customs Act, 1878 (8 of 1878), shall, subject to the provisions of Section 16 of this Act, apply in respect of articles of food, the import of which is prohibited under Section 5 of this Act, and officers of Customs and officers empowered under that Act to perform the duties imposed thereby on a [Commissioner of Customs] and other officers of Customs shall have the same powers in respect of such articles of food as they have for the time being in respect of such goods as aforesaid.

(2) Without prejudice to the provisions of sub-section (1) the [Commissioner of Customs], or any officer of the Government authorized by the Central Government in this behalf, may detain any imported package which he suspects to contain any article of food the import of which is prohibited under

Section 5 of this Act and shall forthwith report such detention to the Director of the Central Food Laboratory and, if required by him, forward the package or send samples of any suspected article of food found therein to the said Laboratory.

7. **Prohibitions of manufacture, sale, etc., of certain articles of food**—No person shall himself or by any person on his behalf manufacture for sale, or store, sell or distribute—

   (i) any adulterated food

   (ii) any misbranded food

   (iii) any article of food for the sale of which a license is prescribed, except in accordance with the conditions of the license

   (iv) any article of food the sale of which is for the time being prohibited by the Food (Health) Authority in the interest of public health

   (v) any article of food in contravention of any other provision of this Act or of any rule made thereunder [or]

   (vi) any adulterant.

   Explanation—For the purposes of this section, a person shall be deemed to store any adulterated food or misbranded food or any article of food referred to in clause (iii) or clause (iv) or clause (v) if he stores such food for the manufacture therefrom of any article of food for sale.

8. **Public Analysts**—The Central Government or the State Government may, by notification in the Official Gazette, appoint such persons as it thinks fit, having the prescribed qualifications to be public analysts for such local areas as may be assigned to them by the Central Government or the State Government, as the case may be:

   Provided that no person who has any financial interest in the manufacture, import or sale of any article or food shall be appointed to be a public analyst under this section:

   Provided further that different public analysts may be appointed for different articles of food.

9. **Food Inspectors**—

   (1) The Central Government or the State Government may, by notification in the Official Gazette, appoint such persons as it thinks fit, having the prescribed qualifications to be food inspectors for such local areas as may be assigned to them by the Central Government or the State Government, as the case may be:

   Provided that no person who has any financial interest in the manufacture, import or sale of any article of food shall be appointed to be a food inspector under this section.

   (2) Every food inspector shall be deemed to be a public servant within the meaning of Section 21 of the Indian Penal Code (45 of 1860) and shall be officially subordinate to such authority as the Government appointing him, may specify in this behalf.

10. **Powers of food inspectors**—

    (1) A food inspector shall have power—

        (a) to take samples of any article of food from—

            (i) any person selling such article

            (ii) any person who is in the course of conveying, delivering or preparing to deliver such article to a purchaser or consignee

            (iii) a consignee after delivery of any such article to him and

        (b) to send such sample for analysis to the public analyst for the local area within which such sample has been taken

(c) with the previous approval of the Local (Health) Authority having jurisdiction in the local area concerned, or with the previous approval of the Food (Health) Authority, to prohibit the sale of any article of food in the interest of public health.

Explanation—For the purposes of sub-clause (iii) of clause (a), **"consignee"** does not include a person who purchases or receives any article of food for his own consumption.]

(2) Any food inspector may enter and inspect any place where any article of food is manufactured, or stored for sale, or stored for the manufacture of any other article of food for sale, or exposed or exhibited for sale or where any adulterant is manufactured or kept, and take samples of such article of food or adulterant for analysis:

Provided that no sample of any article of food, being primary food, shall be taken under this sub-section if it is not intended for sale as such food.

(3) Where any sample is taken under clause (a) of sub-section (1) or sub-section (2), its cost calculated at the rate at which the article is usually sold to the public shall be paid to the person from whom it is taken.

(4) If any article intended for food appears to any food inspector to be adulterated or misbranded, he may seize and carry away or keep in the safe custody of the vendor such article in order that it may be dealt with as hereinafter provided [and he shall, in either case, take a sample of such article and submit the same for analysis to a public analyst]:

Provided that where the food inspector keeps such article in the safe custody of the vendor he may require the vendor to execute a bond for a sum of money equal to the value of such article with one or more sureties as the food inspector deems fit and the vendor shall execute the bond accordingly.

(4A) Where any article of food seized under sub-section (4) is of a perishable nature and the Local (Health) Authority is satisfied that such article of food is so deteriorated that it is unfit for human consumption, the said Authority may, after giving notice in writing to the vendor, cause the same to be destroyed.

(5) The power conferred by this section includes power to break open any package in which any article of food may be contained or to break open the door of any premises where any article of food may be kept for sale:

Provided that the power to break open the package or door shall be exercised only after the owner or any other person in charge of the package or, as the case may be, in occupation of the premises, if he is present therein, refuses to open the package or door on being called upon to do so, and in either case after recording the reasons for doing so:

Provided further that the food inspector shall, in exercising the powers of entry upon, and inspection of any place under this section, follow, as far as may be, the provisions of the [Code of Criminal Procedure, 1973 (2 of 1974)] relating to the search or inspection of a place by a police officer executing a search warrant issued under that Code.

(6) [Any adulterant found in the possession of a manufacturer or distributor of, or dealer in, any article of food or in any of the premises occupied by him as such] and for the possession of which he is unable to account to the satisfaction of the food inspector, [and any books of account or other documents found in his possession or control and which would be useful for, or relevant to, any investigation or proceeding under this Act, may be seized by the food inspector] and [a sample of such adulterant] submitted for analysis to a public analyst:

Provided that no such books of account or other documents shall be seized by the food inspector except with the previous approval of the authority to which he is officially subordinate.

(7) Where the food inspector takes any action under clause (a) of sub-section (1), sub-section (2), sub-section (4) or sub-section (6), he shall call one or more persons to be present at the time when such action is taken and take his or their signatures.

(7A) Where any books of account or other documents are seized under sub-section (6), the food inspector shall within a period not exceeding 30 days from the date of seizure, return the same to the person from whom they were seized after copies thereof or extracts therefrom as certified by that person in such manner as may be prescribed have been taken:

Provided that where such person refuses to so certify, and a prosecution has been instituted against him under this Act, such books of account or other documents shall be returned to him only after copies thereof or extracts therefrom as certified by the court have been taken.

(7B) When any adulterant is seized under sub-section (6), the burden of proving that such adulterant is not meant for purposes of adulteration shall be on the person from whose possession such adulterant was seized.

(8) Any food inspector may exercise the powers of a police officer [under section 42 of the Code of Criminal Procedure, 1973 (2 of 1974)] for the purpose of ascertaining the true name and residence of the person from whom a sample is taken or an article of food is seized.

(9) Any food inspector exercising powers under this Act or under the rules made thereunder who—

(a) vexatiously and without any reasonable grounds of suspicion seizes any article of food [or adulterant] or

(b) commits any other act to the injury of any person without having reason to believe that such act is necessary for the execution of his duty, shall be guilty of an offence under this Act and shall be punishable for such offence [with fine which shall not be less than five hundred rupees but which may extend to one thousand rupees].

11. Procedure to be followed by food inspectors—

(1) When a food inspector takes a sample of food for analysis, he shall—

(a) give notice in writing then and there of his intention to have it so analyzed to the person from whom he has taken the sample and to the person, if any, whose name, address and other particulars have been disclosed under section 14A

(b) except in special cases provided by rules under this Act, divide the sample then and there into three parts and mark and seal or fasten up each part in such a manner as its nature permits and take the signature or thumb impression of the person from whom the sample has been taken in such place and in such manner as may be prescribed:

Provided that where such person refuses to sign or put his thumb impression the food inspector shall call upon one or more witnesses and take his or their signatures or thumb impressions, as the case may be, in lieu of the signature or thumb impression of such person

(c) (i) send one of the parts for analysis to the public analyst under intimation to the Local (Health) Authority and

(ii) send the remaining two parts to the Local (Health) Authority for the purposes of sub-section (2) of this section and sub-sections (2A) and (2E) of Section 13.

[(2) Where the part of the sample sent to the public analyst under sub-clause (i) of clause (c) of sub-section (1) is lost or damaged, the Local (Health) Authority shall, on a requisition made to it by the public analyst or the food inspector dispatch one of the parts of the sample sent to it under sub-clause (ii) of the said clause (c) to the public analyst for analysis.]

(3) When a sample of any article of food [or adulterant] is taken under sub-section (1) or sub-section (2) of Section 10, [the food inspector shall, by the immediately succeeding working day, send a sample of the article of food or adulterant or both, as the case may be, in accordance with the rules prescribed for sampling to the public analyst for the local area concerned.

(4) An article of food seized under sub-section (4) of Section 10, unless destroyed under sub-section (4A) of that section, and any adulterant seized under sub-section (6) of that section shall be produced before a magistrate as soon as possible and in any case not later than 7 days after the receipt of the report of the public analyst:

Provided that if an application is made to the magistrate in this behalf by the person from whom any article of food has been seized, the magistrate shall by order in writing direct the food inspector to produce such article before him within such time as may be specified in the order.

(5) If it appears to the magistrate on taking such evidence as he may deem necessary—

   (a) that the article of food produced before him under sub-section (4) is adulterated or misbranded, he may order it—

      (i) to be forfeited to the Central Government, the State Government or the local authority, as the case may be or

      (ii) to be destroyed at the cost of the owner or the person from whom it was seized so as to prevent its being used as human food or

      (iii) to be so disposed of as to prevent its being again exposed for sale or used for food under its deceptive name or

      (iv) to be returned to the owner, on his executing a bond with or without sureties, for being sold under its appropriate name or, where the magistrate is satisfied that the article of food is capable of being made to conform to prescribed standards for human consumption after reprocessing, for being sold after reprocessing under the supervision or such officer as may be specified in the order

   (b) that the adulterant seized under sub-section (6) of section 10 and produced before him is apparently of a kind which may be employed for purposes of adulteration and for the possession of which the manufacturer, distributor or dealer, as the case may be, is unable to account satisfactorily, he may order it to be forfeited to the Central Government, the State Government or the local authority, as the case may be.

(6) If it appears to the magistrate that any such—

   (a) article of food is not adulterated

   (b) adulterant which is purported to be an adulterant is not an adulterant,

the person from whose possession the article of food or adulterant was taken shall be entitled to have it restored to him and it shall be in the discretion of the magistrate to award such person from such fund as the State Government may direct in this behalf, such compensation not exceeding the actual loss which he has sustained as the magistrate may think proper.

12. Purchaser may have food analyzed—Nothing contained in this Act shall be held to prevent a purchaser of any article of food other than a food inspector [or a recognized consumer association, whether the purchaser is a member of that association or not,] from having such article analyzed by the public analyst on payment of such fees as may be prescribed and from receiving from the public analyst a report of his analysis:

Provided that [such purchaser or recognized consumer association shall inform the vendor at the time of purchase of his or its intention] to have such article so analyzed:

Provided further that the provisions of sub-section (1) sub-section (2) and sub-section (3) of Section 11 shall, as far as may be, apply to a [purchaser of article of food or recognized consumer association who or which intends] to have such articles so analyzed, as they apply to a food inspector who takes a sample of food for analysis:

Provided also that if the report of the public analyst shows that the article of food is adulterated, the [purchaser or recognized consumer association shall be entitled to get refund of the fees paid by him or it] under this section.

Explanation—For the purpose of this section and Section 20, "recognized consumer association" means a voluntary consumer association registered under the Companies Act, 1956 (1 of 1956), or under any other law for the time being in force.

13. **Report of public analyst—**

(1) The public analyst shall deliver, in such form as may be prescribed, a report to the Local (Health) Authority of the result of the analysis of any article of food submitted to him for analysis.

(2) On receipt of the report of the result of the analysis under sub-section (1) to the effect that the article of food is adulterated, the Local (Health) Authority shall, after the institution of prosecution against the persons from whom the sample of the article of food was taken and the person, if any, whose name, address and other particulars have been disclosed under Section 14A, forward, in such manner as may be prescribed, a copy of the report of the result of the analysis to such person or persons, as the case may be, informing such person or persons that if it is so desired, either or both of them may make an application to the court within a period of 10 days from the date of receipt of the copy of the report to get the sample of the article of food kept by the Local (Health) Authority analyzed by the Central Food Laboratory.

(2A) When an application is made to the court under sub-section (2), the court shall require the Local (Health) Authority to forward the part or parts of the sample kept by the said Authority and upon such requisition being made, the said Authority shall forward the part or parts of the sample to the court within a period of 5 days from the date of receipt of such requisition.

(2B) On receipt of the part or parts of the sample from the Local (Health) Authority under sub-section (2A), the court shall first ascertain that the mark and seal or fastening as provided in clause (b) of sub-section (1) of Section 11 are intact and the signature or thumb impression, as the case may be, is not tampered with, and dispatch the part or, as the case may be, one of the parts of the sample under its own seal to the Director of the Central Food Laboratory who shall thereupon send a certificate to the court in the prescribed form within one month from the date of receipt of the part of the sample specifying the result of the analysis.

(2C) Where two parts of the sample have been sent to the court and only one part of the sample has been sent by the court to the Director of the Central Food Laboratory under sub-section (2B), the court shall, as soon as practicable, return the remaining part to the Local (Health) Authority and that Authority shall destroy that part after the certificate from the Director of the Central Food Laboratory has been received by the court:

Provided that where the part of the sample sent by the court to the Director of the Central Food Laboratory is lost or damaged, the court shall require the Local (Health) Authority to forward the part of the sample, if any, retained by it to the court and on receipt thereof, the court shall proceed in the manner provided in sub-section (2B).

(2D) Until the receipt of the certificate of the result of the analysis from the Director of the Central Food Laboratory, the court shall not continue with the proceedings pending before it in relation to the prosecution.

(2E) If, after considering the report, if any, of the food inspector or otherwise, the Local (Health) Authority is of the opinion that the report delivered by the public analyst under sub-section (1) is erroneous, the said Authority shall forward one of the parts of the sample kept by it to any other public analyst for analysis and if the report of the result of the analysis of that part of the sample by that other public analyst is to the effect that the article of food is adulterated, the provisions of sub-sections (2) to (2D) shall, so far as may be, apply.

(3) The certificate issued by the Director of the Central Food Laboratory [under sub-section (2B)] shall supersede the report given by the public analyst under sub-section (1).

(4) Where a certificate obtained from the Director of the Central Food Laboratory [under sub-section (2B)] is produced in any proceeding under this Act, or under sections 272 to 276 of the Indian Penal Code (45 of 1860), it shall not be necessary in such proceeding to produce any part of the sample of food taken for analysis.

(5) Any document purporting to be a report signed by a public analyst, unless it has been superseded under sub-section (3), or any document purporting to be a certificate signed by the Director of the Central Food Laboratory, may be used as evidence of the facts stated therein in any proceeding under this Act or under sections 272 to 276 of the Indian Penal Code (45 of 1860):

Provided that any document purporting to be a certificate signed by the Director of the Central Food Laboratory [not being a certificate with respect to the analysis of the part of the sample of any article of food referred to in the proviso to sub-section (1A) of Section 16] shall be final and conclusive evidence of the facts stated therein.

Explanation—In this section, and in clause (f) of sub-section (1) of Section 16, "Director of the Central Food Laboratory" shall include the officer for the time being in charge of any Food Laboratory (by whatever designation he is known) recognized by the Central Government for the purposes of this section.

14. Manufacturers, distributors and dealers to give warranty—No manufacturer or distributor of, or dealer in, any article of food shall sell such article to any vendor unless he also gives a warranty in writing in the prescribed form about the nature and quality of such article to the vendor:

Provided that a bill, cash memorandum or invoice in respect of the sale of any article of food given by a manufacturer or distributor of, or dealer in, such article to the vendor thereof shall be deemed to be a warranty given by such manufacturer, distributor or dealer under this section.

Explanation—In this section, in sub-section (2) of Section 19 and in Section 20A, the expression "distributor" shall include a commission agent.

14A Vendor to disclose the name, etc., of the person from whom the article of food was purchased—Every vendor of an article of food shall, if so required, disclose to the food inspector the name, address and other particulars of the person from whom he purchased the article of food.

15. Notification of food poisoning—The Central Government or the State Government may, by notification in the Official Gazette, require medical practitioners carrying on their profession in any local area specified in the notification to report all occurrences of food poisoning coming within their cognizance to such officer as may be specified in the notification.

16. Penalties—

(1) Subject to the provisions of sub-section (1A) if any person—

(a) whether by himself or by any other person on his behalf, imports into India or manufactures for sales or stores, sells or distributes any article of food—

(i) which is adulterated within the meaning of sub-clause (m) of clause (ia) of Section 2 or misbranded within the meaning of clause (ix) of that section or the sale of which is prohibited under any provision of this Act or any rule made thereunder or by an order of the Food (Health) Authority

(ii) other than an article of food referred to in sub-clause (i), in contravention of any of the provisions of this Act or of any rule made thereunder or

(b) whether by himself or by any other person on his behalf, imports into India or manufactures for sales or stores, sells or distributes any adulterant which is not injurious to health or

(c) prevents a food inspector from taking a sample as authorized by this Act or

(d) prevents a food inspector from exercising any other power conferred on him by or under this Act or

(e) being a manufacturer of an article of food, has in his possession, or in any of the premises occupied by him, any adulterant which is not injurious to health or

(f) uses any report or certificate of a test or analysis made by the Director of the Central Food Laboratory or by a public analyst or any extract thereof for the purpose of advertising any article of food or

(g) whether by himself or by any other person on his behalf, gives to the vendor a false warranty in writing in respect of any article of food sold by him,

he shall, in addition to the penalty to which he may be liable under the provisions of Section 6, be punishable with imprisonment for a term which shall not be less than six months but which may extend to 3 years, and with fine which shall not be less than one thousand rupees:

Provided that—

(i) if the offence is under sub-clause (i) of clause (a) and is with respect to an article of food, being primary food, which is adulterated due to human agency or is with respect to an article of food which is misbranded within the meaning of sub-clause (k) of clause (ix) of Section 2 or

(ii) if the offence is under sub-clause (ii) of clause (a), but not being an offence with respect to the contravention of any rule made under clause (a) or clause (g) of sub-section (1A) of Section 23 or under clause (b) of sub-section (2) of Section 24,

the court may, for any adequate and special reasons to be mentioned in the judgment, impose a sentence of imprisonment for a term which shall not be less than three months but which may extend to 2 years, and with fine which shall not be less than five hundred rupees:

Provided further that if the offence is under sub-clause (ii) of clause (a) and is with respect to the contravention of any rule made under clause (a) or clause (g) of sub-section (1A) of Section 23 or under clause (b) of sub-section (2) of Section 24, the court may, for any adequate and special reasons to be mentioned in the judgment, impose a sentence of imprisonment for a term which may extend to three months and with fine which may extend to five hundred rupees.

[(1A) If any person whether by himself or by any other person on his behalf, imports into India or manufactures for sale, or stores, sells or distributes,—

(i) any article of food which is adulterated within the meaning of any of the sub-clauses (e) to (l) (both inclusive) of clause (ia) of Section 2 or

(ii) any adulterant which is injurious to health, he shall, in addition to the penalty to which he may be liable under the provisions of Section 6, be punishable with imprisonment for a term which shall not be less than one year but which may extend to 6 years and with fine which shall not be less than two thousand rupees:

Provided that if such article of food or adulterant when consumed by any person is likely to cause his death or is likely to cause such harm on his body as would amount to grievous hurt within the meaning of Section 320 of the Indian Penal Code (45 of 1860), he shall be punishable with imprisonment for a term which shall not be less than 3 years but which may extend to term of life and with fine which shall not be less than five thousand rupees.

[(1AA)] if any person in whose safe custody any article of food has been kept under sub-section (4) of Section 10, tampers or in any other manner interferes with such article, he shall be punishable with imprisonment for a term which shall not be less than six months but which may extend to 2 years and with fine which shall not be less than one thousand rupees.

[(1B) if any person in whose safe custody any article of food has been kept under sub-section (4) of Section 10, sells or distributes such article which is found by the magistrate before whom it is produced to be adulterated within the meaning of sub-clause (h) of clause (ia) of Section 2 and which, when consumed by any person, is likely to cause his death or is likely to cause such harm on his body as would amount to grievous hurt within the meaning of Section 320 of the Indian Penal Code (45 of 1860), then, notwithstanding anything contained in sub-section (1AA), he shall be punishable with imprisonment for a term which shall not be less than 3 years but which may extend to term of life and with fine which shall not be less than five thousand rupees.]

(1C) if any person contravenes the provisions of Section 14 or Section 14A, he shall be punishable with imprisonment for a term which may extend to six months and with fine which shall not be less than five hundred rupees.

(1D) if any person convicted of an offence under this Act commits a like offence afterwards, then, without prejudice to the provisions of sub-section (2), the court, before which the second or subsequent conviction takes place, may order the cancellation of the license, if any, granted to him under this Act and thereupon such license shall, notwithstanding anything contained in this Act, or in the rules made thereunder, stand cancelled.

(2) if any person convicted of an offence under this Act commits a like offence afterwards it shall be lawful for the court before which the second or subsequent conviction takes place to cause the offender's name and place of residence, the offence and the penalty imposed to be published at the offender's expense in such newspapers or in such other manner as the court may direct. The expenses of such publication shall be deemed to be part of the cost attending the conviction and shall be recoverable in the same manner as a fine.

[**16A. Power of court to try cases summarily**—Notwithstanding anything contained in the Code of Criminal Procedure, 1973 (2 of 1974), all offences under sub-section

(1) of Section 16 shall be tried in a summary way by a Judicial Magistrate of the first class specially empowered in this behalf by the State Government or by a Metropolitan Magistrate and the provisions of Sections 262 to 265 (both inclusive) of the said Code shall, as far as may be, apply to such trial:

Provided that in the case of any conviction in a summary trial under this section, it shall be lawful for the Magistrate to pass a sentence of imprisonment for a term not exceeding one year:

Provided further that when at the commencement of, or in the course of, a summary trial under this section it appears to the Magistrate that the nature of the case is such that a sentence of imprisonment for a term exceeding one year may have to be passed or that it is, for any other reason, undesirable to try the case summarily, the Magistrate shall after hearing the parties, record an order to that effect and thereafter recall any witness who may have been examined and proceed to hear or rehear the case in the manner provided by the said Code.

17. **Offences by companies—**

(1) Where an offence under this Act has been committed by a company—

    (a)   (i)   the person, if any, who has been nominated under sub-section (2) to be in charge of, and responsible to, the company for the conduct of the business of the company (hereafter in this section referred to as the person responsible), or

        (ii)   where no person has been so nominated, every person who at the time the offence was committed was in charge of, and was responsible to, the company for the conduct of the business of the company and

    (b)   the company, shall be deemed to be guilty of the offence and shall be liable to be proceeded against and punished accordingly:

    Provided that nothing contained in this sub-section shall render any such person liable to any punishment provided in this Act if he proves that the offence was committed without his knowledge and that he exercised all due diligence to prevent the commission of such offence.

(2) Any company may, by order in writing, authorize any of its directors or managers (such manager being employed mainly in a managerial or supervisory capacity) to exercise all such powers and take all such steps as may be necessary or expedient to prevent the commission by the company of any offence under this Act and may give notice to the Local (Health) Authority, in such form and in such manner as may be prescribed, that it has nominated such director or manager as the person responsible, along with the written consent of such director or manager for being so nominated.

Explanation—Where a company has different establishments or branches or different units in any establishment or branch, different persons may be nominated under this sub-section in relation to different establishments or branches or units and the person nominated in relation to any establishment, branch or unit shall be deemed to be the person responsible in respect of such establishment, branch or unit.

(3) The person nominated under sub-section (2) shall, until—

    (i)   further notice cancelling such nomination is received from the company by the Local (Health) Authority or

    (ii)   he ceases to be a director or, as the case may be, manager of the company or

    (iii)   he makes a request in writing to the Local (Health) Authority, under intimation to the company, to cancel the nomination [which request shall be complied with by the Local (Health) Authority], whichever is the earliest, continue to be the person responsible:

    Provided that where such person ceases to be a director or, as the case may be, manager of the company, he shall intimate the fact of such successor to the Local (Health) Authority:

    Provided further that where such person makes a request under clause (iii), the Local (Health) Authority shall not cancel such nomination with effect from a date earlier than the date on which the request is made.

(4) Notwithstanding anything contained in the foregoing sub-sections, where an offence under this Act has been committed by a company and it is proved that the offence has been committed with the consent or connivance of, or is attributable to, any neglect on the part of, any director, manager, secretary or other officer of the company [not being a person nominated under sub-section (2)] such director, manager, secretary or other officer shall also be deemed to be guilty of that offence and shall be liable to be proceeded against and punished accordingly.

Explanation—For the purposes of this section—

(a) **"Company"** means anybody corporate and includes a firm or other association of individuals

(b) **"Director"**, in relation to a firm, means a partner in the firm and

(c) **"Manager"**, in relation to a company engaged in hotel industry, includes the person in charge of the catering department of any hotel managed or run by it.]

18. **Forfeiture of property**—Where any person has been convicted under this Act for the contravention of any of the provisions of this Act or of any rule thereunder, the article of food in respect of which the contravention has been committed may be forfeited to the Government:

Provided that where the court is satisfied that the article of food is capable of being made to conform to prescribed standards for human consumption after reprocessing, the court may order the article of food to be returned to the owner, on his executing a bond with or without sureties, for being sold, subject to the other provisions of this Act, after reprocessing under the supervision of such officer as may be specified therein.

19. **Defenses which may or may not be allowed in prosecutions under this Act**—

(1) It shall be no defense in a prosecution for an offence pertaining to the sale of any adulterated or misbranded article of food to allege merely that the vendor was ignorant of the nature, substance or quality of the food sold by him or that the purchaser having purchased any article for analysis was not prejudiced by the sale.

[(2) A vendor shall not be deemed to have committed an offence pertaining to the sale of any adulterated or misbranded article of food if he proves—

(a) that he purchased the article of food—

(i) in a case where a license is prescribed for the sale thereof, from a duly licensed manufacturer, distributor or dealer,

(ii) in any other case, from any manufacturer, distributor or dealer,

with a written warranty in the prescribed form and

(b) that the article of food while in his possession was properly stored and that he sold it in the same state as he purchased it.]

(3) Any person by whom a warranty as is referred to [in Section 14] is alleged to have been given shall be entitled to appear at the hearing and give evidence.

20. **Cognizance and trial of offences**—

(1) [No prosecution for an offence under this Act, not being an offence under Section 14 or Section 14A] shall be instituted except by, or with the written consent of, [the Central Government or the State Government or a person authorized in this behalf, by general or special order, by the Central Government or the State Government

Provided that a prosecution for an offence under this Act may be instituted by a purchaser [or recognized consumer association] referred to in Section 12, [if he or it produces] in court a copy of the report of the public analyst along with the complaint.

[(2) No court inferior to that of a Metropolitan Magistrate or a Judicial Magistrate of the first class shall try any offence under this Act.

(3) Notwithstanding anything contained in the Code of Criminal Procedure, 1973 (2 of 1974), an offence punishable under sub-section (1AA) of Section 16 shall be cognizable and nonbailable.]

[**20A. Power of court to implead manufacturer, etc.**—Where at any time during the trial of any offence under this Act alleged to have been committed by any person, not being the manufacturer, distributor or dealer of any article of food, the court is satisfied, on the evidence adduced before it, that such manufacturer, distributor or dealer is also concerned with that offence, then, the court may, notwithstanding anything contained in [sub-section (3) of Section 319 of the Code of Criminal Procedure, 1973 (2 of 1974)] or in Section 20 proceed against him as though a prosecution had been instituted against him under Section 20.]

[**20AA. Application of the Probation of Offenders Act, 1958 and Section 360 of the Code of Criminal Procedure, 1973**—Nothing contained in the Probation of Offenders Act, 1958 (20 of 1958), or Section 360 of the Code of Criminal Procedure, 1973 (2 of 1974), shall apply to a person convicted of an offence under this Act unless that person is under 18 years of age.]

[**21. Magistrate's power to impose enhanced penalties**—Notwithstanding anything contained in Section 29 of the Code of Criminal Procedure, 1973 (2 of 1974), it shall be lawful for any Metropolitan Magistrate or any Judicial Magistrate of the first class to pass any sentence authorized by this Act, except a sentence of imprisonment for life or for a term exceeding 6 years, in excess of his powers under the said section.]

22. **Protection of action taken in good faith**—No suit, prosecution or other legal proceedings shall lie against any person for anything which is in good faith done or intended to be done under this Act.

[**22A. Power of Central Government to give directions**—The Central Government may give such directions as it may deem necessary to a State Government regarding the carrying into execution of all or any of the provisions of this Act and the State Government shall comply with such directions.]

23. **Power of the Central Government to make rules**—

(1) The Central Government may, after consultation with the Committee and after previous publication by notification in the Official Gazette, make rules to carry out the provisions of this Act:

Provided that consultation with the Committee may be dispensed with if the Central Government is of the opinion that circumstances have arisen which render it necessary to make rules without such consultation, but, in such a case, the Committee shall be consulted within six months of the making of the rules and the Central Government shall take into consideration any suggestions which the Committee may make in relation to the amendment of the said rules.]

[(1A)] In particular and without prejudice to the generality of the foregoing power, such rules may provide for all or any of the following matters, namely:—

(a) specifying the articles of food or classes of food for the import of which a license is required and prescribing the form and conditions of such license, the authority empowered to issue the same [the fees payable therefor, the deposit of any sum as security for the performance of the conditions of the license and the circumstances under which such license or security may be cancelled or forfeited]

(b) defining the standards of quality for, and fixing the limits of variability permissible in respect of, any article of food

(c) laying down special provisions for imposing rigorous control over the production, distribution and sale of any article or class of articles of food which the Central Government may, by notification in the Official Gazette, specify in this behalf including registration of the premises where they are manufactured, maintenance of the premises in a sanitary condition and maintenance of the healthy state of human beings associated with the production, distribution and sale of such article or class of articles

(d) restricting the packing and labeling of any article of food and the design of any such package or label with a view to preventing the public or the purchaser being deceived or misled as to the character, quality or quantity of the article [or to preventing adulteration]

(e) defining the qualifications, powers and duties of food inspectors and public analyst

[(ee) defining the laboratories where samples of articles of food or adulterants may be analyzed by public analysts under this Act]

(f) prohibiting the sale of defining the conditions of sale of any substance which may be injurious to health when used as food or restricting in any manner its use as an ingredient in the manufacture of any article of food or regulating by the issue of licenses the manufacture or sale of any article of food

(g) defining the conditions of sale or conditions for license of sale of any article of food in the interest of public health

(h) specifying the manner in which containers for samples of food purchased for analysis shall be sealed up or fastened up

[(hh) defining the methods of analysis

(i) specifying a list of permissible preservatives, other than common salt and sugar, which alone shall be used in preserved fruits, vegetables or their products or any other article of food as well as the maximum amounts of each preservative

(j) specifying the coloring matter and the maximum quantities thereof which may be used in any article of food

(k) providing for the exemption from this Act or of any requirements contained therein and subject to such conditions, if any, as may be specified, of any article or class of articles of food

(l) prohibiting or regulating the manufacture, transport or sale of any article known to be used as an adulterant of food

(m) prohibiting or regulating—
    (i) the addition of any water, or other diluent or adulterant to any article of food
    (ii) the abstraction of any ingredient from any article of food
    (iii) the sale of any article of food to which such addition or from which such abstraction has been made or which has been otherwise artificially treated
    (iv) the mixing of two or more articles of food which are similar in nature or appearance

(n) providing for the destruction of such articles of food as are not in accordance with the provisions of this Act or of the rules made thereunder.

[(2) Every rule made by the Central Government under this Act shall be laid as soon as may be after it is made before each House of Parliament while it is in session for a total period of 30 days [which may be comprised in one session or in two or more successive sessions, and if, before the expiry of the session immediately following the session or the successive sessions aforesaid] both Houses agree in making any modification in the rule or both Houses agree that the rule should not be made, the rule shall thereafter have effect only in such modified form or be of no effect as the case may be so, however, that any such modification or annulment shall be without prejudice to the validity of anything previously done under that rule.]

24. **Power of the State Government to make rules—**

(1) The State Government may, after consultation with the Committee and subject to the condition of previous publication, make rules for the purpose of giving effect to the provisions of this Act in matters not falling within the purview of Section 23.

(2) In particular, and without prejudice to the generality of the foregoing power, such rules may—

   (a) define the powers and duties of the Food (Health) Authority, [local authority and Local (Health) Authority under this Act]

   (b) prescribe the forms of licenses for the manufacture for sale, for the storage, for the sale and for the distribution of articles of food or any specified article of food or class of articles of food, the form of application for such licenses, the conditions subject to which such licenses may be issued, the authority empowered to issue the same, [the fees payable therefore, the deposit of any sum as security for the performance of the conditions of the licenses and the circumstances under which such licenses or security (may be suspended, cancelled or forfeited)]

   (c) direct a fee to be paid for analyzing any article of food or for any matter for which a fee may be prescribed under this Act

   (d) direct that the whole or any part of the fines imposed under this Act shall be paid to a local authority on realization

   (e) provide for the delegation of the powers and functions conferred by this Act on the State Government or the Food (Health) Authority to subordinate authorities or to local authorities.

(3) All rules made by the State Governments under this Act, shall, as soon as possible after they are made, be laid before the respective State Legislatures.

25. **Repeal and saving—**

(1) If, immediately before the commencement of this Act, there is in force in any State to which this Act extends any law corresponding to this Act, that corresponding law shall upon such commencement stand repealed.

(2) Notwithstanding the repeal by this Act of any corresponding law, all rules, regulations and bye-laws relating to the prevention of adulteration of food, made under such corresponding law and in force immediately before the commencement of this Act shall except where and so far as they are inconsistent with or repugnant to the provisions of this Act, continue in force until altered, amended or repealed by rules made under this Act.

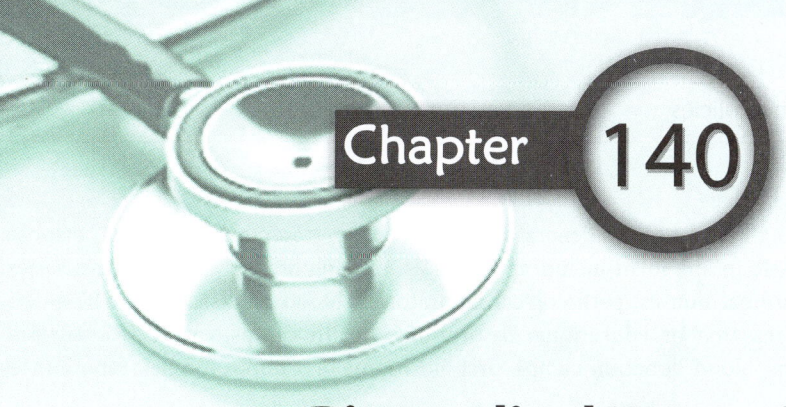

Chapter 140

Biomedical Waste (Management and Handling) Rules, 1998

[PUBLISHED IN THE GAZETTE OF INDIA, EXTRAORDINARY, PART II, SECTION 3, SUB-SECTION (I)]

GOVERNMENT OF INDIA

MINISTRY OF ENVIRONMENT, FOREST AND CLIMATE CHANGE NOTIFICATION

New Delhi, the 28th March, 2016

G.S.R. 343(E)—Whereas the Biomedical Waste (Management and Handling) Rules, 1998 was published *vide* notification number S.O. 630 (E) dated the 20th July, 1998, by the Government of India in the erstwhile Ministry of Environment and Forests, provided a regulatory frame work for management of biomedical waste generated in the country;

And whereas, to implement these rules more effectively and to improve the collection, segregation, processing, treatment and disposal of these biomedical wastes in an environmentally sound management thereby, reducing the biomedical waste generation and its impact on the environment, the Central Government reviewed the existing rules;

And whereas, in exercise of the powers conferred by Sections 6, 8 and 25 of the Environment (Protection) Act, 1986 (29 of 1986), the Central Government published the draft rules in the Gazette vide number G.S.R. 450 (E), dated the 3rd June, 2015 inviting objections or suggestions from the public within 60 days from the date on which copies of the Gazette containing the said notification were made available to the public;

And whereas, the copies of the Gazette containing the said draft rules were made available to the public on the 3rd June, 2015;

And whereas, the objections or comments received within the specified period from the public in respect of the said draft rules have been duly considered by the Central Government;

Now, therefore, in exercise of the powers conferred by Sections 6, 8 and 25 of the Environment (Protection) Act, 1986 (29 of 1986), and in supersession of the Biomedical Waste (Management and Handling) Rules, 1998, except as respects things done or omitted to be done before such suppression, the Central Government hereby makes the following rules, namely:—

1. **Short title and commencement—**

   (1) These rules may be called the Biomedical Waste Management Rules, 2016.

   (2) They shall come into force on the date of their publication in the Official Gazette.

2. **Application—**

(1) These rules shall apply to all persons who generate, collect, receive, store, transport, treat, dispose, or handle biomedical waste in any form including hospitals, nursing homes, clinics, dispensaries, veterinary institutions, animal houses, pathological laboratories, blood banks, AYUSH hospitals, clinical establishments, research or educational institutions, health camps, medical or surgical camps, vaccination camps, blood donation camps, first aid rooms of schools, forensic laboratories and research labs.

(2) These rules shall not apply to,—

   (a) radioactive wastes as covered under the provisions of the Atomic Energy Act, 1962 (33 of 1962) and the rules made there under;

   (b) hazardous chemicals covered under the Manufacture, Storage and Import of Hazardous Chemicals Rules, 1989 made under the Act;

   (c) solid wastes covered under the Municipal Solid Waste (Management and Handling) Rules, 2000 made under the Act;

   (d) the lead acid batteries covered under the Batteries (Management and Handling) Rules, 2001 made under the Act;

   (e) hazardous wastes covered under the Hazardous Wastes (Management, Handling and Transboundary Movement) Rules, 2008 made under the Act;

   (f) waste covered under the e-Waste (Management and Handling) Rules, 2011 made under the Act; and

   (g) hazardous microorganisms, genetically engineered microorganisms and cells covered under the Manufacture, Use, Import, Export and Storage of Hazardous Microorganisms, Genetically Engineered Microorganisms or Cells Rules, 1989 made under the Act.

3. **Definitions—**In these rules, unless the context otherwise requires,—

   (a) **"Act"** means the Environment (Protection) Act, 1986 (29 of 1986);

   (b) **"Animal house"** means a place where animals are reared or kept for the purpose of experiments or testing;

   (c) **"Authorization"** means permission granted by the prescribed authority for the generation, collection, reception, storage, transportation, treatment, processing, disposal or any other form of handling of biomedical waste in accordance with these rules and guidelines issued by the Central Government or Central Pollution Control Board as the case may be;

   (d) **"Authorized person"** means an occupier or operator authorized by the prescribed authority to generate, collect, receive, store, transport, treat, process, dispose or handle biomedical waste in accordance with these rules and the guidelines issued by the Central Government or the Central Pollution Control Board, as the case may be;

   (e) **"Biological"** means any preparation made from organisms or microorganisms or product of metabolism and biochemical reactions intended for use in the diagnosis, immunization or the treatment of human beings or animals or in research activities pertaining thereto;

   (f) **"Biomedical waste"** means any waste, which is generated during the diagnosis, treatment or immunization of human beings or animals or research activities pertaining thereto or in the production or testing of biological or in health camps, including the categories mentioned in Schedule I appended to these rules;

(g) **"Biomedical waste treatment and disposal facility"** means any facility wherein treatment, disposal of biomedical waste or processes incidental to such treatment and disposal is carried out, and includes common biomedical waste treatment facilities;

(h) **"Form"** means the Form appended to these rules;

(i) **"Handling"** in relation to biomedical waste includes the generation, sorting, segregation, collection, use, storage, packaging, loading, transportation, unloading, processing, treatment, destruction, conversion, or offering for sale, transfer, disposal of such waste;

(j) **"Health care facility"** means a place where diagnosis, treatment or immunization of human beings or animals is provided irrespective of type and size of health treatment system, and research activity pertaining thereto;

(k) **"Major accident"** means accident occurring while handling of biomedical waste having potential to affect large masses of public and includes toppling of the truck carrying biomedical waste, accidental release of biomedical waste in any water body but exclude accidents like needle prick injuries, mercury spills;

(l) **"Management"** includes all steps required to ensure that biomedical waste is managed in such a manner as to protect health and environment against any adverse effects due to handling of such waste;

(m) **"Occupier"** means a person having administrative control over the institution and the premises generating biomedical waste, which includes a hospital, nursing home, clinic, dispensary, veterinary institution, animal house, pathological laboratory, blood bank, health care facility and clinical establishment, irrespective of their system of medicine and by whatever name they are called;

(n) **"Operator of a common biomedical waste treatment facility"** means a person who owns or controls a Common Biomedical Waste Treatment Facility (CBMWTF) for the collection, reception, storage, transport, treatment, disposal or any other form of handling of biomedical waste;

(o) **"Prescribed authority"** means the State Pollution Control Board in respect of a State and Pollution Control Committees in respect of a Union Territory;

(p) **"Schedule"** means the Schedule appended to these rules.

4. **Duties of the Occupier**—It shall be the duty of every occupier to—

(a) take all necessary steps to ensure that biomedical waste is handled without any adverse effect to human health and the environment and in accordance with these rules;

(b) make a provision within the premises for a safe, ventilated and secured location for storage of segregated biomedical waste in colored bags or containers in the manner as specified in Schedule I, to ensure that there shall be no secondary handling, pilferage of recyclables or inadvertent scattering or spillage by animals and the biomedical waste from such place or premises shall be directly transported in the manner as prescribed in these rules to the common biomedical waste treatment facility or for the appropriate treatment and disposal, as the case may be, in the manner as prescribed in Schedule I;

(c) pre-treat the laboratory waste, microbiological waste, blood samples and blood bags through disinfection or sterilization on-site in the manner as prescribed by the World Health Organization (WHO) or National AIDs Control Organization (NACO) guidelines and then sent to the common biomedical waste treatment facility for final disposal;

(d) phase out use of chlorinated plastic bags, gloves and blood bags within 2 years from the date of notification of these rules;

(e) dispose of solid waste other than biomedical waste in accordance with the provisions of respective waste management rules made under the relevant laws and amended from time to time;

(f) not to give treated biomedical waste with municipal solid waste;

(g) provide training to all its health care workers and others, involved in handling of bio medical waste at the time of induction and thereafter at least once every year and the details of training programmes conducted, number of personnel trained and number of personnel not undergone any training shall be provided in the Annual Report;

(h) immunize all its health care workers and others, involved in handling of biomedical waste for protection against diseases including Hepatitis B and Tetanus that are likely to be transmitted by handling of biomedical waste, in the manner as prescribed in the National Immunization Policy or the guidelines of the Ministry of Health and Family Welfare issued from time to time;

(i) establish a Bar-Code System for bags or containers containing biomedical waste to be sent out of the premises or place for any purpose within one year from the date of the notification of these rules;

(j) ensure segregation of liquid chemical waste at source and ensure pre-treatment or neutralization prior to mixing with other effluent generated from health care facilities;

(k) ensure treatment and disposal of liquid waste in accordance with the Water (Prevention and Control of Pollution) Act, 1974 (6 of 1974);

(l) ensure occupational safety of all its health care workers and others involved in handling of biomedical waste by providing appropriate and adequate personal protective equipment;

(m) conduct health check up at the time of induction and at least once in a year for all its health care workers and others involved in handling of biomedical waste and maintain the records for the same;

(n) maintain and update on day to day basis the biomedical waste management register and display the monthly record on its website according to the biomedical waste generated in terms of category and color coding as specified in Schedule I;

(o) report major accidents including accidents caused by fire hazards, blasts during handling of biomedical waste and the remedial action taken and the records relevant thereto, (including nil report) in Form I to the prescribed authority and also along with the annual report;

(p) make available the annual report on its web-site and all the health care facilities shall make own website within 2 years from the date of notification of these rules;

(q) inform the prescribed authority immediately in case the operator of a facility does not collect the biomedical waste within the intended time or as per the agreed time;

(r) establish a system to review and monitor the activities related to biomedical waste management, either through an existing committee or by forming a new committee and the Committee shall meet once in every 6 months and the record of the minutes of the meetings of this committee shall be submitted along with the annual report to the prescribed authority and the healthcare establishments having less than 30 beds shall designate a qualified person to review and monitor the activities relating to biomedical waste management within that establishment and submit the annual report;

(s) maintain all record for operation of incineration, hydro or autoclaving etc., for a period of 5 years;

(t) existing incinerators to achieve the standards for treatment and disposal of biomedical waste as specified in Schedule II for retention time in secondary chamber and Dioxin and Furans within 2 years from the date of this notification.

5. **Duties of the operator of a common biomedical waste treatment and disposal facility**—It shall be the duty of every operator to—

 (a) take all necessary steps to ensure that the biomedical waste collected from the occupier is transported, handled, stored, treated and disposed of, without any adverse effect to the human health and the environment, in accordance with these rules and guidelines issued by the Central Government or, as the case may be, the central pollution control board from time to time;

 (b) ensure timely collection of biomedical waste from the occupier as prescribed under these rules;

 (c) establish bar coding and global positioning system for handling of biomedical waste within one year;

 (d) inform the prescribed authority immediately regarding the occupiers which are not handing over the segregated biomedical waste in accordance with these rules;

 (e) provide training for all its workers involved in handling of biomedical waste at the time of induction and at least once a year thereafter;

 (f) assist the occupier in training conducted by them for biomedical waste management;

 (g) undertake appropriate medical examination at the time of induction and at least once in a year and immunize all its workers involved in handling of biomedical waste for protection against diseases, including Hepatitis B and Tetanus, that are likely to be transmitted while handling biomedical waste and maintain the records for the same;

 (h) ensure occupational safety of all its workers involved in handling of biomedical waste by providing appropriate and adequate personal protective equipment;

 (i) report major accidents including accidents caused by fire hazards, blasts during handling of biomedical waste and the remedial action taken and the records relevant thereto, (including nil report) in Form I to the prescribed authority and also along with the annual report;

 (j) maintain a log book for each of its treatment equipment according to weight of batch; categories of waste treated; time, date and duration of treatment cycle and total hours of operation;

 (k) allow occupier, who are giving waste for treatment to the operator, to see whether the treatment is carried out as per the rules;

 (l) shall display details of authorization, treatment, annual report, etc. on its website;

 (m) after ensuring treatment by autoclaving or microwaving followed by mutilation or shredding, whichever is applicable, the recyclables from the treated biomedical wastes such as plastics and glass, shall be given to recyclers having valid consent or authorization or registration from the respective State Pollution Control Board or Pollution Control Committee;

 (n) supply non-chlorinated plastic colored bags to the occupier on chargeable basis, if required;

 (o) common biomedical waste treatment facility shall ensure collection of biomedical waste on holidays also;

 (p) maintain all record for operation of incineration, hydro or autoclaving for a period of 5 years; and

 (q) upgrade existing incinerators to achieve the standards for retention time in secondary chamber and Dioxin and Furans within 2 years from the date of this notification.

6. **Duties of authorities**—The Authority specified in column (2) of Schedule-III shall perform the duties as specified in column (3) thereof in accordance with the provisions of these rules.

7. **Treatment and disposal**—

 (1) Biomedical waste shall be treated and disposed of in accordance with Schedule I, and in compliance with the standards provided in Schedule II by the health care facilities and common biomedical waste treatment facility.

(2) Occupier shall hand over segregated waste as per the Schedule I to common biomedical waste treatment facility for treatment, processing and final disposal:

Provided that the lab and highly infectious biomedical waste generated shall be pre-treated by equipment like autoclave or microwave.

(3) No occupier shall establish on-site treatment and disposal facility, if a service of common biomedical waste treatment facility is available at a distance of seventy-five kilometers.

(4) In cases where service of the common biomedical waste treatment facility is not available, the occupiers shall set up requisite biomedical waste treatment equipment like incinerator, autoclave or microwave, shredder prior to commencement of its operation, as per the authorization given by the prescribed authority.

(5) Any person including an occupier or operator of a common bio medical waste treatment facility, intending to use new technologies for treatment of bio medical waste other than those listed in Schedule I shall request the Central Government for laying down the standards or operating parameters.

(6) On receipt of a request referred to in sub-rule (5), the Central Government may determine the standards and operating parameters for new technology which may be published in Gazette by the Central Government.

(7) Every operator of common biomedical waste treatment facility shall set up requisite biomedical waste treatment equipment like incinerator, autoclave or microwave, shredder and effluent treatment plant as a part of treatment, prior to commencement of its operation.

(8) Every occupier shall phase out use of non-chlorinated plastic bags within 2 years from the date of publication of these rules and after 2 years from such publication of these rules, the chlorinated plastic bags shall not be used for storing and transporting of biomedical waste and the occupier or operator of a common biomedical waste treatment facility shall not dispose of such plastics by incineration and the bags used for storing and transporting biomedical waste shall be in compliance with the Bureau of Indian Standards. Till the Standards are published, the carry bags shall be as per the Plastic Waste Management Rules, 2011.

(9) After ensuring treatment by autoclaving or microwaving followed by mutilation or shredding, whichever is applicable, the recyclables from the treated biomedical wastes such as plastics and glass shall be given to such recyclers having valid authorization or registration from the respective prescribed authority.

(10) The Occupier or Operator of a common biomedical waste treatment facility shall maintain a record of recyclable wastes referred to in sub-rule (9) which are auctioned or sold and the same shall be submitted to the prescribed authority as part of its annual report. The record shall be open for inspection by the prescribed authorities.

(11) The handling and disposal of all the mercury waste and lead waste shall be in accordance with the respective rules and regulations.

8. **Segregation, packaging, transportation and storage—**

(1) No untreated biomedical waste shall be mixed with other wastes.

(2) The biomedical waste shall be segregated into containers or bags at the point of generation in accordance with Schedule I prior to its storage, transportation, treatment and disposal.

(3) The containers or bags referred to in sub-rule (2) shall be labeled as specified in Schedule IV.

(4) Bar code and global positioning system shall be added by the Occupier and common biomedical waste treatment facility in one-year time.

(5) The operator of common biomedical waste treatment facility shall transport the biomedical waste from the premises of an occupier to any off-site biomedical waste treatment facility only in the vehicles having label as provided in part 'A' of the Schedule IV along with necessary information as specified in part 'B' of the Schedule IV.

(6) The vehicles used for transportation of biomedical waste shall comply with the conditions if any stipulated by the State Pollution Control Board or Pollution Control Committee in addition to the requirement contained in the Motor Vehicles Act, 1988 (59 of 1988), if any or the rules made there under for transportation of such infectious waste.

(7) Untreated human anatomical waste, animal anatomical waste, soiled waste and, biotechnology waste shall not be stored beyond a period of forty eight hours:

Provided that in case for any reason it becomes necessary to store such waste beyond such a period, the occupier shall take appropriate measures to ensure that the waste does not adversely affect human health and the environment and inform the prescribed authority along with the reasons for doing so.

(8) Microbiology waste and all other clinical laboratory waste shall be pre-treated by sterilization to Log 6 or disinfection to Log 4, as per the World Health Organization guidelines before packing and sending to the common biomedical waste treatment facility.

9. **Prescribed authority—**

(1) The prescribed authority for implementation of the provisions of these rules shall be the State Pollution Control Boards in respect of States and Pollution Control Committees in respect of Union Territories.

(2) The prescribed authority for enforcement of the provisions of these rules in respect of all health care establishments including hospitals, nursing homes, clinics, dispensaries, veterinary institutions, animal houses, pathological laboratories and blood banks of the Armed Forces under the Ministry of Defense shall be the Director General, Armed Forces Medical Services, who shall function under the supervision and control of the Ministry of Defense.

(3) The prescribed authorities shall comply with the responsibilities as stipulated in Schedule III of these rules.

10. **Procedure for authorization—**Every occupier or operator handling biomedical waste, irrespective of the quantity shall make an application in Form II to the prescribed authority, i.e., State Pollution Control Board and Pollution Control Committee, as the case may be, for grant of authorization and the prescribed authority shall grant the provisional authorization in Form III and the validity of such authorization for bedded health care facility and operator of a common facility shall be synchronized with the validity of the consents.

(1) The authorization shall be one time for non-bedded occupiers and the authorization in such cases shall be deemed to have been granted, if not objected by the prescribed authority within a period of 90 days from the date of receipt of duly completed application along with such necessary documents.

(2) In case of refusal of renewal, cancellation or suspension of the authorization by the prescribed authority, the reasons shall be recorded in writing:

Provided that the prescribed authority shall give an opportunity of being heard to the applicant before such refusal of the authorization.

(3) Every application for authorization shall be disposed of by the prescribed authority within a period of 90 days from the date of receipt of duly completed application along with such necessary documents, failing which it shall be deemed that the authorization is granted under these rules.

(4) In case of any change in the biomedical waste generation, handling, treatment and disposal for which authorization was earlier granted, the occupier or operator shall intimate to the prescribed authority about the change or variation in the activity and shall submit a fresh application in Form II for modification of the conditions of authorization.

11. **Advisory Committee—**

(1) Every State Government or Union Territory Administration shall constitute an Advisory Committee for the respective State or Union Territory under the chairmanship of the respective health secretary to oversee the implementation of the rules in the respective state and to advice any improvements and the Advisory Committee shall include representatives from the Departments of Health, Environment, Urban Development, Animal Husbandry and Veterinary Sciences of that State Government or Union Territory Administration, State Pollution Control Board or Pollution Control Committee, urban local bodies or local bodies or Municipal Corporation, representatives from Indian Medical Association, common biomedical waste treatment facility and nongovernmental organization.

(2) Notwithstanding anything contained in sub-rule (1), the Ministry of Defense shall constitute the Advisory Committee (Defense) under the chairmanship of Director General of Health Services of Armed Forces consisting of representatives from the Ministry of Defense, Ministry of Environment, Forest and Climate Change, Central Pollution Control Board, Ministry of Health and Family Welfare, Armed Forces Medical College or Command Hospital.

(3) The Advisory Committee constituted under sub-rule (1) and (2) shall meet at least once in six months and review all matters related to implementation of the provisions of these rules in the State and Armed Forces Health Care Facilities, as the case may be.

(4) The Ministry of Health and Defense may co-opt representatives from the other Governmental and non-governmental organizations having expertise in the field of biomedical waste management.

12. **Monitoring of implementation of the rules in health care facilities—**

(1) The Ministry of Environment, Forest and Climate Change shall review the implementation of the rules in the country once in a year through the State Health Secretaries and Chairmen or Member Secretary of State Pollution Control Boards and Central Pollution Control Board and the Ministry may also invite experts in the field of biomedical waste management, if required.

(2) The Central Pollution Control Board shall monitor the implementation of these rules in respect of all the Armed Forces health care establishments under the Ministry of Defense.

(3) The Central Pollution Control Board along with one or more representatives of the Advisory Committee constituted under sub-rule (2) of rule 11, may inspect any Armed Forces health care establishments after prior intimation to the Director General Armed Forces Medical Services.

(4) Every State Government or Union Territory Administration shall constitute District Level Monitoring Committee in the districts under the chairmanship of District Collector or District Magistrate or Deputy Commissioner or Additional District Magistrate to monitor the compliance of the provisions of these rules in the health care facilities generating biomedical waste and in the common biomedical waste treatment and disposal facilities, where the biomedical waste is treated and disposed of.

(5) The District Level Monitoring Committee constituted under sub-rule (4) shall submit its report once in six months to the State Advisory Committee and a copy thereof shall also be forwarded to State Pollution Control Board or Pollution Control Committee concerned for taking further necessary action.

(6) The District Level Monitoring Committee shall comprise of District Medical Officer or District Health Officer, representatives from State Pollution Control Board or Pollution Control Committee, Public Health Engineering Department, local bodies or municipal corporation, Indian Medical Association, common biomedical waste treatment facility and registered non-governmental organizations working in the field of biomedical waste management and the Committee may co-opt other members and experts, if necessary and the District Medical Officer shall be the Member Secretary of this Committee.

13. **Annual report—**

(1) Every occupier or operator of common biomedical waste treatment facility shall submit an annual report to the prescribed authority in Form IV, on or before the 30th June of every year.

(2) The prescribed authority shall compile, review and analyze the information received and send this information to the Central Pollution Control Board on or before the 31st July of every year.

(3) The Central Pollution Control Board shall compile, review and analyze the information received and send this information, along with its comments or suggestions or observations to the Ministry of Environment, Forest and Climate Change on or before 31st August every year.

(4) The Annual Reports shall also be available online on the websites of Occupiers, State Pollution Control Boards and Central Pollution Control Board.

14. **Maintenance of records—**

(1) Every authorized person shall maintain records related to the generation, collection, reception, storage, transportation, treatment, disposal or any other form of handling of biomedical waste, for a period of 5 years, in accordance with these rules and guidelines issued by the Central Government or the Central Pollution Control Board or the prescribed authority as the case may be.

(2) All records shall be subject to inspection and verification by the prescribed authority or the Ministry of Environment, Forest and Climate Change at any time.

15. **Accident reporting—**

(1) In case of any major accident at any institution or facility or any other site while handling biomedical waste, the authorized person shall intimate immediately to the prescribed authority about such accident and forward a report within 24 hours in writing regarding the remedial steps taken in Form I.

(2) Information regarding all other accidents and remedial steps taken shall be provided in the annual report in accordance with rule 13 by the occupier.

16. **Appeal—**

(1) Any person aggrieved by an order made by the prescribed authority under these rules may, within a period of 30 days from the date on which the order is communicated to him, prefer an appeal in Form V to the Secretary (Environment) of the State Government or Union territory administration.

(2) Any person aggrieved by an order of the Director General Armed Forces Medical Services under these rules may, within 30 days from the date on which the order is communicated to him, prefer an appeal in Form V to the Secretary, Ministry of Environment, Forest and Climate Change.

(3) The authority referred to in sub-para (1) and (2) as the case may be, may entertain the appeal after the expiry of the said period of 30 days, if it is satisfied that the appellant was prevented by sufficient cause from filing the appeal in time.

(4) The appeal shall be disposed of within a period of 90 days from the date of its filing.

17. **Site for common biomedical waste treatment and disposal facility—**
   (1) Without prejudice to rule 5 of these rules, the department in the business allocation of land assignment shall be responsible for providing suitable site for setting up of common biomedical waste treatment and disposal facility in the State Government or Union Territory Administration.
   (2) The selection of site for setting up of such facility shall be made in consultation with the prescribed authority, other stakeholders and in accordance with guidelines published by the Ministry of Environment, Forest and Climate Change or Central Pollution Control Board.

18. **Liability of the occupier, operator of a facility—**
   (1) The occupier or an operator of a common biomedical waste treatment facility shall be liable for all the damages caused to the environment or the public due to improper handling of biomedical wastes.
   (2) The occupier or operator of common biomedical waste treatment facility shall be liable for action under Section 5 and Section 15 of the Act, in case of any violation.

SCHEDULE I
[SEE RULES 3(E), 4(B), 7(1), 7(2), 7(5), 7(6) AND 8(2)]

PART-1

Biomedical wastes categories and their segregation, collection, treatment, processing and disposal options

Category	Type of waste	Type of bag or container to be used	Treatment and disposal options
Yellow	**(a) Human anatomical waste:** Human tissues, organs, body parts and fetus below the viability period (as per the Medical Termination of Pregnancy Act 1971, amended from time to time).	Yellow colored non-chlorinated plastic bags	Incineration or Plasma Pyrolysis or deep burial*
	(b) Animal anatomical waste: Experimental animal carcasses, body parts, organs, tissues, including the waste generated from animals used in experiments or testing in veterinary hospitals or colleges or animal houses.		
	(c) Soiled waste: Items contaminated with blood, body fluids like dressings, plaster casts, cotton swabs and bags containing residual or discarded blood and blood components.		Incineration or Plasma Pyrolysis or deep burial* In absence of above facilities, autoclaving or micro-waving/ hydroclaving followed by shredding or mutilation or combination of sterilization and shredding. Treated waste to be sent for energy recovery.

Contd...

Category	Type of waste	Type of bag or container to be used	Treatment and disposal options
	(d) Expired or discarded medicines: Pharmaceutical waste like antibiotics, cytotoxic drugs including all items contaminated with cytotoxic drugs along with glass or plastic ampoules, vials, etc.	Yellow colored non-chlorinated plastic bags or containers	Expired cytotoxic drugs and items contaminated with cytotoxic drugs to be returned back to the manufacturer or supplier for incineration at temperature >1200°C or to common biomedical waste treatment facility or hazardous waste treatment, storage and disposal facility for incineration at >1200°C or Encapsulation or Plasma Pyrolysis at >1200°C. All other discarded medicines shall be either sent back to manufacturer or disposed by incineration.
	(e) Chemical waste: Chemicals used in production of biological and used or discarded disinfectants.	Yellow colored containers or non-chlorinated plastic bags	Disposed of by incineration or Plasma Pyrolysis or Encapsulation in hazardous waste treatment, storage and disposal facility.
	(f) Chemical liquid waste: Liquid waste generated due to use of chemicals in production of biological and used or discarded disinfectants, Silver X-ray film developing liquid, discarded Formalin, infected secretions, aspirated body fluids, liquid from laboratories and floor washings, cleaning, house-keeping, and disinfecting activities, etc.	Separate collection system leading to effluent treatment system	After resource recovery, the chemical liquid waste shall be pretreated before mixing with other wastewater. The combined discharge shall confirm to the discharge norms given in Schedule-III.
	(g) Discarded linen, mattresses, beddings contaminated with blood or body fluid.	Non-chlorinated yellow plastic bags or suitable packing material	Non-chlorinated chemical disinfection followed by incineration or Plasma Pyrolysis or for energy recovery. In absence of above facilities, shredding or mutilation or combination of sterilization and shredding. Treated waste to be sent for energy recovery or incineration or Plasma Pyrolysis.

Contd…

Category	Type of waste	Type of bag or container to be used	Treatment and disposal options
	(h) Microbiology, biotechnology and other clinical laboratory waste: Blood bags, Laboratory cultures, stocks or specimens of microorganisms, live or attenuated vaccines, human and animal cell cultures used in research, industrial laboratories, production of biological, residual toxins, dishes and devices used for cultures.	Autoclave safe plastic bags or containers	Pre-treat to sterilize with non-chlorinated chemicals on-site as per National AIDS Control Organization or World Health Organization guidelines thereafter for Incineration.
Red	**Contaminated waste (Recyclable)** (a) Wastes generated from disposable items such as tubing, bottles, intravenous tubes and sets, catheters, urine bags, syringes (without needles and *fixed needle syringes*) and vacutainers with their needles cut) and gloves.	Red colored non-chlorinated plastic bags or containers	Autoclaving or micro-waving/ hydroclaving followed by shredding or mutilation or combination of sterilization and shredding. Treated waste to be sent to registered or authorized recyclers or for energy recovery or plastics to diesel or fuel oil or for road making, whichever is possible. Plastic waste should not be sent to landfill sites.
White (translucent)	**Waste sharps including metals:** Needles, syringes with fixed needles, needles from needle tip cutter or burner, scalpels, blades, or any other contaminated sharp object that may cause puncture and cuts. This includes both used, discarded and contaminated metal sharps.	Puncture proof, Leak proof, tamper proof containers	Autoclaving or Dry Heat Sterilization followed by shredding or mutilation or encapsulation in metal container or cement concrete; combination of shredding cum autoclaving; and sent for final disposal to iron foundries (having consent to operate from the State Pollution Control Boards or Pollution Control Committees) or sanitary landfill or designated concrete waste sharp pit.
Blue	**(a) Glassware:** Broken or discarded and contaminated glass including medicine vials and ampoules except those contaminated with cytotoxic wastes.	Cardboard boxes with blue colored marking	Disinfection (by soaking the washed glass waste after cleaning with detergent and Sodium Hypochlorite treatment) or through autoclaving or microwaving or hydroclaving and then sent for recycling.
	(b) Metallic body implants	Cardboard boxes with blue colored marking	

*Disposal by deep burial is permitted only in rural or remote areas where there is no access to common biomedical waste treatment facility. This will be carried out with prior approval from the prescribed authority and as per the Standards specified in Schedule-III. The deep burial facility shall be located as per the provisions and guidelines issued by Central Pollution Control Board from time to time.

PART–2

1. All plastic bags shall be as per BIS standards as and when published, till then the prevailing Plastic Waste Management Rules shall be applicable.

2. Chemical treatment using at least 10% Sodium Hypochlorite having 30% residual chlorine for twenty minutes or any other equivalent chemical reagent that should demonstrate $Log_{10}4$ reduction efficiency for microorganisms as given in Schedule-III.

3. Mutilation or shredding must be to an extent to prevent unauthorized reuse.

4. There will be no chemical pretreatment before incineration, except for microbiological, lab and highly infectious waste.

5. Incineration ash (ash from incineration of any biomedical waste) shall be disposed through hazardous waste treatment, storage and disposal facility, if toxic or hazardous constituents are present beyond the prescribed limits as given in the Hazardous Waste (Management, Handling and Transboundary Movement) Rules, 2008 or as revised from time to time.

6. Dead Fetus below the viability period (as per the Medical Termination of Pregnancy Act 1971, amended from time to time) can be considered as human anatomical waste. Such waste should be handed over to the operator of common biomedical waste treatment and disposal facility in yellow bag with a copy of the official Medical Termination of Pregnancy certificate from the Obstetrician or the Medical Superintendent of hospital or healthcare establishment.

7. Cytotoxic drug vials shall not be handed over to unauthorized person under any circumstances. These shall be sent back to the manufactures for necessary disposal at a single point. As a second option, these may be sent for incineration at common biomedical waste treatment and disposal facility or TSDFs or plasma pyrolys is at temperature >1200°C.

8. Residual or discarded chemical wastes, used or discarded disinfectants and chemical sludge can be disposed at hazardous waste treatment, storage and disposal facility. In such case, the waste should be sent to hazardous waste treatment, storage and disposal facility through operator of common biomedical waste treatment and disposal facility only.

9. On-site pre-treatment of laboratory waste, microbiological waste, blood samples, blood bags should be disinfected or sterilized as per the Guidelines of World Health Organization or National AIDS Control Organization and then given to the common biomedical waste treatment and disposal facility.

10. Installation of in-house incinerator is not allowed. However, in case there is no common biomedical facility nearby, the same may be installed by the occupier after taking authorization from the State Pollution Control Board.

11. Syringes should be either mutilated or needles should be cut and or stored in tamper proof, leak proof and puncture proof containers for sharps storage. Wherever the occupier is not linked to a disposal facility it shall be the responsibility of the occupier to sterilize and dispose in the manner prescribed.

12. Biomedical waste generated in households during healthcare activities shall be segregated as per these rules and handed over in separate bags or containers to municipal waste collectors. Urban Local Bodies shall have tie up with the common biomedical waste treatment and disposal facility to pick up this waste from the Material Recovery Facility (MRF) or from the household directly, for final disposal in the manner as prescribed in this Schedule.

SCHEDULE II
[SEE RULES 4(T), 7(1) AND 7(6)]
STANDARDS FOR TREATMENT AND DISPOSAL OF BIOMEDICAL WASTES

1. **Standards for incineration—**

   All incinerators shall meet the following operating and emission standards-

   A. **Operating standards:**

   1. Combustion efficiency (CE) shall be at least 99.00 %.
   2. The combustion efficiency is computed as follows:

   $$CE = \frac{\% \ CO_2}{\% \ CO_2 + \% \ CO} \times 100$$

   3. The temperature of the primary chamber shall be a minimum of 800 °C and the secondary chamber shall be minimum of 1050 °C + or –50 °C.
   4. The secondary chamber gas residence time shall be at least two seconds.

   B. **Emission standards:**

Sl. no.	Parameter	Standards	
		Limiting concentration in mg Nm^3 unless stated	Sampling Duration in minutes, unless stated
1.	Particulate matter	50	30 or 1 Nm^3 of sample volume, whichever is more
2.	Nitrogen oxides NO and NO_2 expressed as NO_2	400	30 for online sampling or grab sample
3.	HCl	50	30 or 1 Nm^3 of sample volume, whichever is more
4.	Total Dioxins and Furans	0.1 ng TEQ/Nm^3 (at 11 % O_2)	8 hours or 5 Nm^3 of sample volume, whichever is more
5.	Hg and its compounds	0.05	2 hours or 1 Nm^3 of sample volume, whichever is more

   C. **Stack height:** Minimum stack height shall be 30 meters above the ground and shall be attached with the necessary monitoring facilities as per requirement of monitoring of 'general parameters' as notified under the Environment (Protection) Act, 1986 and in accordance with the Central Pollution Control Board Guidelines of Emission Regulation Part-III.

Note:

(a) The existing incinerators shall comply with the above within a period of 2 years from the date of the notification.

(b) The existing incinerators shall comply with the standards for Dioxins and Furans of 0.1 ng TEQ/Nm^3, as given below within 2 years from the date of commencement of these rules.

(c) All upcoming common biomedical waste treatment facilities having incineration facility or captive incinerator shall comply with standards for Dioxins and Furans.

(d) The existing secondary combustion chambers of the incinerator and the pollution control devices shall be suitably retrofitted, if necessary, to achieve the emission limits.

(e) Wastes to be incinerated shall not be chemically treated with any chlorinated disinfectants.

(f) Ash from incineration of biomedical waste shall be disposed of at common hazardous waste treatment and disposal facility. However, it may be disposed of in municipal landfill, if the toxic metals in incineration ash are within the regulatory quantities as defined under the Hazardous Waste (Management and Handling and Transboundary Movement) Rules, 2008 as amended from time to time.

(g) Only low Sulphur fuel like Light Diesel Oil or Low Sulphur Heavy Stock or Diesel, Compressed Natural Gas, Liquefied Natural Gas or Liquefied Petroleum Gas shall be used as fuel in the incinerator.

(h) The occupier or operator of a common biomedical waste treatment facility shall monitor the stack gaseous emissions (under optimum capacity of the incinerator) once in three months through a laboratory approved under the Environment (Protection) Act, 1986 and record of such analysis results shall be maintained and submitted to the prescribed authority. In case of dioxins and furans, monitoring should be done once in a year.

(i) The occupier or operator of the common biomedical waste treatment facility shall install continuous emission monitoring system for the parameters as stipulated by State Pollution Control Board or Pollution Control Committees in authorization and transmit the data real time to the servers at State Pollution Control Board or Pollution Control Committees and Central Pollution Control Board.

(j) All monitored values shall be corrected to 11 % oxygen on dry basis.

(k) Incinerators (combustion chambers) shall be operated with such temperature, retention time and turbulence, as to achieve Total Organic Carbon content in the slag and bottom ashes less than 3 % or their loss on ignition shall be less than 5 % of the dry weight.

(l) The occupier or operator of a common biomedical waste incinerator shall use combustion gas analyzer to measure CO_2, CO and O_2.

2. **Operating and Emission Standards for Disposal by Plasma Pyrolysis or Gasification—**

A. **Operating standards:** All the operators of the Plasma Pyrolysis or Gasification shall meet the following operating and emission standards:

1. Combustion Efficiency (CE) shall be at least 99.99 %.

2. The Combustion Efficiency is computed as follows:

$$CE = \frac{\% \, CO_2}{\% \, CO_2 + \% \, CO} \times 100$$

3. The temperature of the combustion chamber after plasma gasification shall be 1050 ± 50 with gas residence time of at least 2 (two) second, with minimum 3% oxygen in the stack gas.

4. The Stack height should be minimum of 30 m above ground level and shall be attached with the necessary monitoring facilities as per requirement of monitoring of 'general parameters' as notified under the Environment (Protection) Act, 1986 and in accordance with the CPCB Guidelines of Emission Regulation Part-III.

B. Air emission standards and air pollution control measures:

(i) Emission standards for incinerator, notified at Sl. no. 1 above in this Schedule, and revised from time to time, shall be applicable for the Plasma Pyrolysis or Gasification also.

(ii) Suitably designed air pollution control devices shall be installed or retrofitted with the Plasma Pyrolysis or Gasification to achieve the above emission limits, if necessary.

(iii) Wastes to be treated using Plasma Pyrolysis or Gasification shall not be chemically treated with any chlorinated disinfectants and chlorinated plastics shall not be treated in the system.

C. Disposal of ash vitrified material: The ash or vitrified material generated from the 'Plasma Pyrolysis or Gasification shall be disposed of in accordance with the Hazardous Waste (Management, Handling and Transboundary Movement) Rules 2008 and revisions made thereafter in case the constituents exceed the limits prescribed under Schedule II of the said Rules or else in accordance with the provisions of the Environment (Protection) Act, 1986, whichever is applicable.

3. **Standards for autoclaving of biomedical waste—**

The autoclave should be dedicated for the purposes of disinfecting and treating biomedical waste.

(1) When operating a gravity flow autoclave, medical waste shall be subjected to:

   (i) a temperature of not less than 121 °C and pressure of 15 pounds per square inch (psi) for an autoclave residence time of not less than 60 minutes; or

   (ii) temperature of not less than 135 °C and a pressure of 31 psi for an autoclave residence time of not less than 45 minutes; or

   (iii) a temperature of not less than 149 °C and a pressure of 52 psi for an autoclave residence time of not less than 30 minutes.

(2) When operating a vacuum autoclave, medical waste shall be subjected to a minimum of three pre-vacuum pulse to purge the autoclave of all air. The air removed during the pre-vacuum, cycle should be decontaminated by means of HEPA and activated carbon filtration, steam treatment, or any other method to prevent release of pathogen. The waste shall be subjected to the following:

   (i) a temperature of not less than 121 °C and pressure of 15 psi per an autoclave residence time of not less than 45 minutes; or

   (ii) a temperature of not less than 135 °C and a pressure of 31 psi for an autoclave residence time of not less than 30 minutes;

(3) Medical waste shall not be considered as properly treated unless the time, temperature and pressure indicators indicate that the required time, temperature and pressure were reached during the autoclave process. If for any reasons, time temperature or pressure indicator indicates that the required temperature, pressure or residence time was not reached, the entire load of medical waste must be autoclaved again until the proper temperature, pressure and residence time were achieved.

(4) **Recording of operational parameters:** Each autoclave shall have graphic or computer recording devices which will automatically and continuously monitor and record dates, time of day, load identification number and operating parameters throughout the entire length of the autoclave cycle.

(5) **Validation test for autoclave:** The validation test shall use four biological indicator strips, one shall be used as a control and left at room temperature, and three shall be placed in the approximate center of three containers with the waste. Personal protective equipment (gloves, face mask and coveralls) shall be used when opening containers for the purpose of placing the biological indicators. At least one of the containers with a biological indicator should be placed in the most difficult location for steam to penetrate, generally the bottom center of the waste pile. The

occupier or operator shall conduct this test three consecutive times to define the minimum operating conditions. The temperature, pressure and residence time at which all biological indicator vials or strips for three consecutive tests show complete inactivation of the spores shall define the minimum operating conditions for the autoclave. After determining the minimum temperature, pressure and residence time, the occupier or operator of a common biomedical waste treatment facility shall conduct this test once in three months and records in this regard shall be maintained.

(6) **Routine test:** A chemical indicator strip or tape that changes color when a certain temperature is reached can be used to verify that a specific temperature has been achieved. It may be necessary to use more than one strip over the waste package at different locations to ensure that the inner content of the package has been adequately autoclaved. The occupier or operator of a common biomedical waste treatment facility shall conduct this test during autoclaving of each batch and records in this regard shall be maintained.

(7) **Spore testing:** The autoclave should completely and consistently kill the approved biological indicator at the maximum design capacity of each autoclave unit. Biological indicator for autoclave shall be Geobacillus stearothermophilus 1×10^6 spores using vials or spore Strips; with at least 1×10^6 spores. Under no circumstances will an autoclave have minimum operating parameters less than a residence time of 30 minutes, a temperature less than 121 °C or a pressure less than 15 psi. The occupier or operator of a common biomedical waste treatment and disposal facility shall conduct this test at least once in every week and records in this regard shall be maintained.

4. **Standards of microwaving—**

   (1) Microwave treatment shall not be used for cytotoxic, hazardous or radioactive wastes, contaminated animal carcasses, body parts and large metal items.

   (2) The microwave system shall comply with the efficacy test or routine tests and a performance guarantee may be provided by the supplier before operation of the limit.

   (3) The microwave should completely and consistently kill the bacteria and other pathogenic organisms that are ensured by approved biological indicator at the maximum design capacity of each microwave unit. Biological indicators for microwave shall be Bacillus atrophaeus spores using vials or spore strips with at least 1×10^4 spores per detachable strip. The biological indicator shall be placed with waste and exposed to same conditions as the waste during a normal treatment cycle.

5. **Standards for deep burial—**

   (1) A pit or trench should be dug about two meters deep. It should be half filled with waste, then covered with lime within 50 cm of the surface, before filling the rest of the pit with soil.

   (2) It must be ensured that animals do not have any access to burial sites. Covers of galvanized iron or wire meshes may be used.

   (3) On each occasion, when wastes are added to the pit, a layer of 10 cm of soil shall be added to cover the wastes.

   (4) Burial must be performed under close and dedicated supervision.

   (5) The deep burial site should be relatively impermeable and no shallow well should be close to the site.

   (6) The pits should be distant from habitation, and located so as to ensure that no contamination occurs to surface water or ground water. The area should not be prone to flooding or erosion.

   (7) The location of the deep burial site shall be authorized by the prescribed authority.

   (8) The institution shall maintain a record of all pits used for deep burial.

   (9) The ground water table level should be a minimum of six meters below the lower level of deep burial pit.

6. **Standards for efficacy of chemical disinfection—**

Microbial inactivation efficacy is equated to "Log10 kill" which is defined as the difference between the logarithms of number of test microorganisms before and after chemical treatment. Chemical disinfection methods shall demonstrate a 4 Log10 reduction or greater for Bacillus subtilis (ATCC 19659) in chemical treatment systems.

7. **Standards for dry heat sterilization**

Waste sharps can be treated by dry heat sterilization at a temperature not less than 185 °C, at least for a residence period of 150 minutes in each cycle, which sterilization period of 90 minutes. There should be automatic recording system to monitor operating parameters.

(i) **Validation test for sharps sterilization unit:** Waste sharps sterilization unit should completely and consistently kill the biological indicator Geobacillus stearothermophilus or Bacillus atrophaeus spores using vials with at least $\log_{10}6$ spores per mL. The test shall be carried out once in three months.

(ii) **Routine test:** A chemical indicator strip or tape that changes color when a certain temperature is reached can be used to verify that a specific temperature has been achieved. It may be necessary to use more than one strip over the waste to ensure that the inner content of the sharps has been adequately disinfected. This test shall be performed once in week and records in this regard shall be maintained.

8. **Standards for liquid waste—**

(1) The effluent generated or treated from the premises of occupier or operator of a common bio medical waste treatment and disposal facility, before discharge into the sewer should confirm to the following limits—

Parameters	Permissible limits
pH	6.5–9.0
Suspended solids	100 mg/L
Oil and grease	10 mg/L
BOD	30 mg/L
COD	250 mg/L
Bio-assay test	90 % survival of fish after 96 hours in 100 % effluent.

(2) Sludge from Effluent Treatment Plant shall be given to common biomedical waste treatment facility for incineration or to hazardous waste treatment, storage and disposal facility for disposal.

SCHEDULE III
[SEE RULES 6 AND 9(3)]
LIST OF PRESCRIBED AUTHORITIES AND THE CORRESPONDING DUTIES

Sl. no.	Authority	Corresponding duties
1.	Ministry of Environment, Forest and Climate Change, Government of India	(i) Making policies concerning biomedical waste management in the country including notification of rules and amendments to the rules as and when required. (ii) Providing financial assistance for training and awareness programmes on biomedical waste management related activities to for the State Pollution Control Boards or Pollution Control Committees. (iii) Facilitating financial assistance for setting up or upgradation of common biomedical waste treatment facilities. (iv) Undertake or support operational research and assessment with reference to risks to environment and health due to biomedical waste and previously unknown disposables and wastes from new types of equipment. (v) Constitution of Monitoring Committee for implementation of the rules. (vi) Hearing Appeals and give decision made in Form-V against order passed by the prescribed authorities. (vii) Develop Standard manual for trainers and training. (viii) Notify the standards or operating parameters for new technologies for treatment of biomedical waste other than those listed in Schedule I.
2.	Central or State Ministry of Health and Family Welfare, Central Ministry for Animal Husbandry and Veterinary or State Department of Animal Husbandry and Veterinary	(i) Grant of license to health care facilities or nursing homes or veterinary establishments with a condition to obtain authorization from the prescribed authority for biomedical waste management. (ii) Monitoring, refusal or cancellation of license for health care facilities or nursing homes or veterinary establishments for violations of conditions of authorization or provisions under these rules. (iii) Publication of list of registered health care facilities with regard to biomedical waste generation, treatment and disposal. (iv) Undertake or support operational research and assessment with reference to risks to environment and health due to biomedical waste and previously unknown disposables and wastes from new types of equipment. (v) Coordinate with State Pollution Control Boards for organizing training programmes to staff of health care facilities and municipal workers on biomedical waste. (vi) Constitution of Expert Committees at National or State level for overall review and promotion of clean or new technologies for biomedical waste management. (vii) Organizing or Sponsoring of trainings for the regulatory authorities and health care facilities on biomedical waste management related activities. (viii) Sponsoring of mass awareness campaigns in electronic media and print media.

Contd…

Sl. no.	Authority	Corresponding duties
3.	Ministry of Defense	(i) Grant and renewal of authorization to Armed Forces health care facilities or common biomedical waste treatment facilities (Rule 9).
		(ii) Conduct training courses for authorities dealing with management of biomedical wastes in Armed Forces health care facilities or treatment facilities in association with State Pollution Control Boards or Pollution Control Committees or Central Pollution Control Board or Ministry of Environment, Forest and Climate Change.
		(iii) Publication of inventory of occupiers and biomedical waste generation from Armed Forces health care facilities or occupiers.
		(iv) Constitution of Advisory Committee for implementation of the rules.
		(v) Review of management of biomedical waste generation in the Armed Forces health care facilities through its Advisory Committee (Rule 11).
		(vi) Submission of annual report to Central Pollution Control Board within the stipulated time period (Rule 13).
4.	Central Pollution Control Board	(i) Prepare guidelines on biomedical waste management and submit to the Ministry of Environment, Forest and Climate Change.
		(ii) Co-ordination of activities of State Pollution Control Boards or Pollution Control Committees on biomedical waste.
		(iii) Conduct training courses for authorities dealing with management of biomedical waste.
		(iv) Lay down standards for new technologies for treatment and disposal of biomedical waste (Rule 7) and prescribe specifications for treatment and disposal of biomedical wastes (Rule 7).
		(v) Lay down criteria for establishing common biomedical waste treatment facilities in the country.
		(vi) Random inspection or monitoring of health care facilities and common biomedical waste treatment facilities.
		(vii) Review and analysis of data submitted by the State Pollution Control Boards on biomedical waste and submission of compiled information in the form of annual report along with its observations to Ministry of Environment, Forest and Climate Change.
		(viii) Inspection and monitoring of health care facilities operated by the Director General, Armed Forces Medical Services (Rule 9).
		(ix) Undertake or support research or operational research regarding biomedical waste.
5.	State Government of Health or Union Territory Government or Administration	(i) To ensure implementation of the rule in all health care facilities or occupiers.
		(ii) Allocation of adequate funds to Government health care facilities for biomedical waste management.
		(iii) Procurement and allocation of treatment equipment and make provision for consumables for biomedical waste management in Government health care facilities.
		(iv) Constitute State or District Level Advisory Committees under the District Magistrate or Additional District Magistrate to oversee the biomedical waste management in the Districts.
		(v) Advise State Pollution Control Boards or Pollution Control Committees on implementation of these Rules.
		(vi) Implementation of recommendations of the Advisory Committee in all the health care facilities.

Contd…

Sl. no.	Authority	Corresponding duties
6.	State Pollution Control Boards or Pollution Control Committees	(i) Inventorization of Occupiers and data on biomedical waste generation, treatment & disposal. (ii) Compilation of data and submission of the same in annual report to Central Pollution Control Board within the stipulated time period. (iii) Grant and renewal, suspension or refusal cancellation or of authorization under these rules (Rule 7, 8 and 10). (iv) Monitoring of compliance of various provisions and conditions of authorization. (v) Action against health care facilities or common biomedical waste treatment facilities for violation of these rules (Rule 18). (vi) Organizing training programmes to staff of health care facilities and common biomedical waste treatment facilities and State Pollution Control Boards or Pollution Control Committees Staff on segregation, collection, storage, transportation, treatment and disposal of biomedical wastes. (vii) Undertake or support research or operational research regarding biomedical waste management. (viii) Any other function under these rules assigned by Ministry of Environment, Forest and Climate Change or Central Pollution Control Board from time to time. (ix) Implementation of recommendations of the Advisory Committee. (x) Publish the list of Registered or Authorized (or give consent) Recyclers. (xi) Undertake and support third party audits of the common biomedical waste treatment facilities in their State.
7.	Municipalities or Corporations, Urban Local Bodies and Gram Panchayats	(i) Provide or allocate suitable land for development of common biomedical waste treatment facilities in their respective jurisdictions as per the guidelines of Central Pollution Control Board. (ii) Collect other solid waste (other than the biomedical waste from the health care facilities as per the Municipal Solid Waste (Management and Handling) Rules, 2000 or as amended time to time. (iii) Any other function stipulated under these Rules.

SCHEDULE IV
[SEE RULES 8(3) AND (5)]

PART–A

Label for Biomedical Waste Containers or Bags

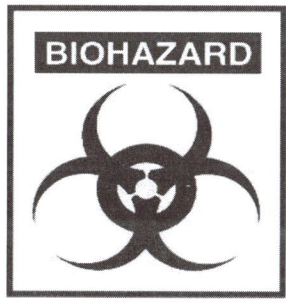

Handle with care

Cytotoxic Hazard Symbol

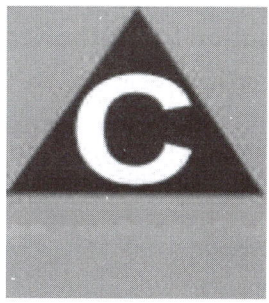

Handle with care

PART–B

Label for Transporting Biomedical Waste Bags or Containers

Day ....Month ....Year ....

Date of generation ....

Waste category number .... Waste quantity.....................................

Sender's Name and Address: Receiver's Name and Address:

Phone number .... Phone number ....

Fax number.. Fax number ....

Contact person .... Contact person ....

In case of emergency please contact:

Name and Address: Phone number

Note: Label shall be non-washable and prominently visible.

FORM–I
[(See Rules 4(o), 5(i) and 15(2)]

Accident Reporting

1. Date and time of accident:
2. Type of accident:
3. Sequence of events leading to accident:
4. Has the authority been informed immediately?
5. The type of waste involved in accident:
6. Assessment of the effects of the accidents on human health and the environment:
7. Emergency measures taken:
8. Steps taken to alleviate the effects of accidents:
9. Steps taken to prevent the recurrence of such an accident:
10. Does your facility has an Emergency Control policy? If yes, give details:

Date: ....   Signature:...........................

Place: ....   Designation: ....

FORM–II
[See Rule 10]

Application for Authorization or Renewal of Authorization

(To be submitted by occupier of health care facility or common biomedical waste treatment facility)

To

    The Prescribed Authority

    (Name of the State or UT Administration)

    Address

1. Particulars of Applicant:
   (i) Name of the Applicant:
       (In block letters & in full)

(ii) Name of the health care facility (HCF) or common biomedical waste treatment facility (CBWTF) :

(iii) Address for correspondence:

(iv) Tele No., Fax No.:

(v) E-mail:

(vi) Website Address:

2. Activity for which authorization is sought:

    Activity   Please tick

    Generation, segregation

    Collection

    Storage packaging

    Reception

    Transportation

    Treatment or processing or conversion

    Recycling

    Disposal or destruction use

    offering for sale, transfer

    Any other form of handling

3. Application for ☐ fresh or ☐ renewal of authorization (please tick whatever is applicable):

  (i) Applied for CTO/CTE   Yes/No

  (ii) In case of renewal previous authorization number and date:

(iii) Status of Consents:

    (a)   Under the Water (Prevention and Control of Pollution) Act, 1974:

    (b)   Under the Air (Prevention and Control of Pollution) Act, 1981:

        ----

4. (i) Address of the health care facility (HCF) or common biomedical waste treatment facility (CBWTF):

  (ii) GPS coordinates of health care facility (HCF) or common biomedical waste treatment facility (CBWTF):

5. Details of health care facility (HCF) or common biomedical waste treatment facility (CBWTF):

  (i) Number of beds of HCF:

  (ii) Number of patients treated per month by HCF:

  (iii) Number of health care facilities covered by CBMWTF: _____

  (iv) No. of beds covered by CBMWTF: _____

  (v) Installed treatment and disposal capacity of CBMWTF:_____kg/day

  (vi) Quantity of biomedical waste treated or disposed by CBMWTF:_____kg/day

  (vii) Area or distance covered CBMWTF:_

    (Please attach map, a map with GPS locations of CBMWTF and area of coverage.)

  (viii) Quantity of Biomedical waste handled, treated or disposed:

Category	Type of Waste	Quantity Generated or Collected, kg/day	Method of Treatment and Disposal (Refer Schedule- i)
Yellow	(a) Human anatomical waste: (b) Animal anatomical waste : (c) Soiled waste: (d) Expired or discarded medicines: (e) Chemical solid waste: (f) Chemical liquid waste : (g) Discarded linen, mattresses, beddings contaminated with blood or body fluid. (h) Microbiology, biotechnology and other clinical laboratory waste:		
Red	Contaminated waste (Recyclable)		
White (Translucent)	Waste sharps including metals:		
Blue	Glassware: Metallic body implants		

6. Brief description of arrangements for handling of biomedical waste (attach details):
   (i) Mode of transportation (if any) of biomedical waste:
   (ii) Details of treatment equipment (please give details such as the number, type and capacity of each unit)

                         No. of units   **Capacity of each unit**

Incinerators:
Plasma pyrolysis:
Autoclaves:
Microwave:
Hydroclave:
Shredder:
Needle tip cutter or destroyer:
Sharps encapsulation or concrete pit:
Deep burial pits:
Chemical disinfection:
Any other treatment equipment:

7. Contingency plan of common biomedical waste treatment facility (CBWTF)(attach documents):
8. Details of directions or notices or legal actions if any during the period of earlier authorization.
9. Declaration:
   I do hereby declare that the statements made and information given above are true to the best of my knowledge and belief and that I have not concealed any information.
   I do also hereby undertake to provide any further information sought by the prescribed authority in relation to these rules and to fulfill any conditions stipulated by the prescribed authority.

Date: Signature of the Applicant

Place: Designation of the Applicant

FORM–III

[See Rule 10]

Authorization

(Authorization for operating a facility for generation, collection, reception, treatment, storage, transport and disposal of biomedical wastes)

1. File number of authorization and date of issue……………………………………….
2. M/s an occupier or operator of the facility located at is hereby granted an authorization for;

Activity	**Please tick**
Generation, segregation	
Collection	
Storage packaging	
Reception	
Transportation	
Treatment or processing or conversion	
Recycling	
Disposal or destruction use offering for sale, transfer	
Any other form of handling	

3. M/s is hereby authorized for handling of biomedical waste as per the capacity given below;
   (i) Number of beds of HCF:
   (ii) Number healthcare facilities covered by CBMWTF:
   (iii) Installed treatment and disposal capacity:___kg/day
   (iv) Area or distance covered by CBMWTF:____
   (v) Quantity of Biomedical waste handled, treated or disposed:

Type of Waste	Category	Quantity permitted for handling
Yellow	Red	
White (Translucent)		
Blue		

3. This authorization shall be in force for a period of …………. years from the date of issue.
4. This authorization is subject to the conditions stated below and to such other conditions as may be specified in the rules for the time being in force under the Environment (Protection) Act, 1986.

Date …………….....   Signature: …...........…………

Place ……………..   Designation: …………………..

Terms and Conditions of Authorization

1. The authorization shall comply with the provisions of the Environment (Protection) Act, 1986 and the rules made there under.
2. The authorization or its renewal shall be produced for inspection at the request of an officer authorized by the prescribed authority.
3. The person authorized shall not rent, lend, sell, transfer or otherwise transport the biomedical wastes without obtaining prior permission of the prescribed authority.
4. Any unauthorized change in personnel, equipment or working conditions as mentioned in the application by the person authorized shall constitute a breach of his authorization.

5. It is the duty of the authorized person to take prior permission of the prescribed authority to close down the facility and such other terms and conditions may be stipulated by the prescribed authority.

Form–IV
[See Rule 13]
ANNUAL REPORT

[To be submitted to the prescribed authority on or before 30th June every year for the period from January to December of the preceding year, by the occupier of health care facility (HCF) or common biomedical waste treatment facility (CBWTF)]

Sl. no.	Particulars					
1.	Particulars of the Occupier	:				
	(i) Name of the authorized person (occupier or operator of facility)	:				
	(ii) Name of HCF or CBMWTF	:				
	(iii) Address for Correspondence	:				
	(iv) Address of Facility					
	(v) Tel. No, Fax. No	:				
	(vi) E-mail ID	:				
	(vii) URL of Website	:				
	(viii) GPS coordinates of HCF or CBMWTF	:				
	(ix) Ownership of HCF or CBMWTF	:	(State Government or Private or Semi Govt. or any other)				
	(x) Status of Authorization under the Biomedical Waste (Management and Handling) Rules	:	Authorization No.: ………………………… …….valid up to ………..				
	(xi) Status of Consents under Water Act and Air Act	:	Valid up to:				
2.	Type of Health Care Facility	:				
	(i) Bedded Hospital	:	No. of Beds:…..				
	(ii) Non-bedded hospital (Clinic or Blood Bank or Clinical Laboratory or Research Institute or Veterinary Hospital or any other)	:				
	(iii) License number and its date of expiry	:				

Contd…

Sl. no.	Particulars					
3.	Details of CBMWTF	:				
	(i) Number of healthcare facilities covered by CBMWTF	:				
	(ii) No. of beds covered by CBMWTF	:				
	(iii) Installed treatment and disposal capacity of CBMWTF:	:	____kg/day			
	(iv) Quantity of biomedical waste treated or disposed by CBMWTF	:	____kg/day			
4.	Quantity of waste generated or disposed in kg/annum (on monthly average basis)	:	Yellow category: Red category: White: Blue category: General solid waste:			
5.	Details of the storage, treatment, transportation, processing and disposal facility					
	(i) Details of the on-site storage facility disposal facilities	:	Size: Capacity: Provision of on-site storage: (cold storage or any other provision)			
			Type of treatment equipment	No. of units	Capacity kg/day	Quantity treated or disposed in kg per annum
			Incinerators			
			Plasma Pyrolysis			
			Autoclaves Microwave			
			Hydroclave Shredder			
			Needle tip cutter or destroyer	—		
			Sharps encapsulation or concrete pit	—		
			Deep burial pits:	—		
			Chemical disinfection:			
			Any other treatment equipment:			
	(ii) Quantity of recyclable wastes sold to authorized recyclers after treatment in kg/annum.	:	Red Category (like plastic, glass etc.)			
	(iii) No. of vehicles used for collection and transportation of biomedical waste	:				

Contd…

Sl. no.	Particulars				
	(iv) Details of incineration ash and ETP sludge generated and disposed during the treatment of wastes in kg/annum	Incineration Ash ETP Sludge		Quantity generated	Where disposed
	(v) Name of the Common Biomedical Waste Treatment Facility Operator through which wastes are disposed of	:			
	(vi) List of member HCF not handed over biomedical waste.				
6.	Do you have biomedical waste management committee? If yes, attach minutes of the meetings held during the reporting period.	:			
7.	Details trainings conducted on BMW				
	(i) Number of trainings conducted on BMW management.				
	(ii) Number of personnel trained				
	(iii) Number of personnel trained at the time of induction				
	(iv) Number of personnel not undergone any training so far				
	(v) Whether standard or manual for training is available?				
	(vi) Any other information				
8.	Details of the accident occurred during the year				
	(i) Number of accidents occurred				
	(ii) Number of the persons affected				
	(iii) Remedial action taken (Please attach details if any)				
	(iv) Any fatality occurred, details				
9.	Are you meeting the standards of air pollution from the incinerator? How many times in last year could not met the standards? Details of continuous online emission monitoring systems installed				

Contd…

Sl. no.	Particulars				
10.	Liquid waste generated and treatment methods in place. How many times you have not met the standards in a year?				
11.	Is the disinfection method or sterilization meeting the log 4 standards? How many times you have not met the standards in a year?				
12.	Any other relevant information	:	(Air Pollution Control Devices attached with the Incinerator)		

Certified that the above report is for the period from

....

....

....

Date: Name and Signature of the Head of the Institution
Place:

FORM–V

[See Rule 16]

Application for Filing Appeal against Order Passed by the Prescribed Authority

1. Name and address of the person applying for appeal:

2. Number, date of order and address of the authority which passed the order, against which appeal is being made (certified copy of order to be attached):

3. Ground on which the appeal is being made:

4. List of enclosures other than the order referred in para 2 against which appeal is being filed:

Date: ....

Signature ....
Name and Address.....................
[F. No. 3-1/2000-HSMD]
(Bishwanath Sinha)
Joint Secretary to the Government of India

Amendments 2000

BIOMEDICAL WASTE
(MANAGEMENT AND HANDLING)
RULES, 1998
AS AMENDED 2000 – RELEVANT PROVISIONS
BIOMEDICAL WASTE (MANAGEMENT AND HANDLING)
RULES, 1998
MINISTRY OF ENVIRONMENT & FORESTS
NOTIFICATION
New Delhi, 20th July, 1998

S.O. 630 (E). A notification in exercise of the powers conferred by Sections 6, 8 and 25 of the Environment (Protection) Act, 1986 (29 of 1986) was published in the Gazette vide S.O. 746 (E) dated 16 October, 1997 inviting objections from the public within 60 days from the date of the publication of the said notification on the Biomedical Waste (Management and Handling) Rules, 1998.

In exercise of the powers conferred by section 6, 8 and 25 of the Environment (Protection) Act, 1986 the Central Government hereby notifies the rules for the management and handling of biomedical waste.

1. **Short Title and Commencement:**

   (1) These rules may be called the Biomedical Waste (Management and Handling) Rules, 1998.

   (2) They shall come into force on the date of their publication in the official Gazette.

2. **Application:** These rules apply to all persons who generate, collect, receive, store, transport, treat, dispose, or handle biomedical waste in any form.

3. **Definitions:**

   In these rules unless the context otherwise requires

   (1) **"Act"** means the Environment (Protection) Act, 1986 (29 of 1986);

   (2) **"Animal House"** means a place where animals are reared/kept for experiments or testing purposes;

   (3) **"Authorization"** means permission granted by the prescribed authority for the generation, collection, reception, storage.

Biomedical Waste (Management and Handling) Rules, 1998

Transportation, treatment, disposal and/or any other form of handling of biomedical waste in accordance with these rules and any guidelines issued by the Central Government.

   (4) **"Authorized person"** means an occupier or operator authorized by the prescribed authority to generate, collect, receive, store, transport, treat, dispose and/or handle biomedical waste in accordance with these rules and any guidelines issued by the Central Government;

   (5) **"Biomedical waste"** means any waste, which is generated during the diagnosis, treatment or immunization of human beings or animals or in research activities pertaining thereto or in the production or testing of biologicals, and including categories mentioned in Schedule I;

   (6) **"Biologicals"** means any preparation made from organisms or microorganisms or product of metabolism and biochemical reactions intended for use in the diagnosis, immunization or the treatment of human beings or animals or in research activities pertaining thereto;

   (7) "Biomedical waste treatment facility" means any facility wherein treatment. disposal of biomedical waste or processes incidental to such treatment or disposal is carried out;

   (8) **"Occupier"** in relation to any institution generating biomedical waste, which includes a hospital, nursing home, clinic dispensary, veterinary institution, animal house, pathological laboratory, blood

bank by whatever name called, means a person who has control over that institution and/or its premises;

(9) **"Operator of a biomedical waste facility"** means a person who owns or controls or operates a facility for the collection, reception, storage, transport, treatment, disposal or any other form of handling of biomedical waste;

(10) **"Schedule"** means schedule appended to these rules;

4. **Duty of Occupier:** It shall be the duty of every occupier of an institution generating biomedical waste which includes a hospital, nursing home, clinic, dispensary, veterinary institution, animal house, pathological laboratory, blood bank by whatever name called to take all steps to ensure that such waste is handled without any adverse effect to human health and the environment.

5. **Treatment and Disposal**

(1) Biomedical waste shall be treated and disposed of in accordance with Schedule I, and in compliance with the standards prescribed in Schedule V.

(2) Every occupier, where required, shall set up in accordance with the time-schedule in Schedule VI, requisite biomedical waste treatment facilities like incinerator, autoclave, microwave system for the treatment of waste, or, ensure requisite treatment of waste at a common waste treatment facility or any other waste treatment facility.

6. **Segregation, Packaging, Transportation and Storage**

(1) Biomedical waste shall not be mixed with other wastes.

(2) Biomedical waste shall be segregated into containers/bags at the point of generation in accordance with Schedule II prior to its storage, transportation, treatment and disposal. The containers shall be labeled according to Schedule III.

(3) If a container is transported from the premises where biomedical waste is generated to any waste treatment facility outside the premises, the container shall, apart from the label prescribed in Schedule III, also carry information prescribed in Schedule IV.

(4) Notwithstanding anything contained in the Motor Vehicles Act, 1988, or rules thereunder, untreated biomedical waste shall be transported only in such vehicle as may be authorized for the purpose by the competent authority as specified by the government.

(5) No untreated biomedical waste shall be kept stored beyond a period of 48 hours

Provided that if for any reason it becomes necessary to store the waste beyond such period, the authorized person must take permission of the prescribed authority and take measures to ensure that the waste does not adversely affect human health and the environment.

7. **Prescribed Authority**

(1) The Government of every State and Union Territory shall establish a prescribed authority with such members as may be specified for granting authorization and implementing these rules. If the prescribed authority comprises of more than one member, a chairperson for the authority shall be designated.

(2) The prescribed authority for the State or Union Territory shall be appointed within one month of the coming into force of these rules.

(3) The prescribed authority shall function under the supervision and control of the respective Government of the State or Union Territory.

(4) The prescribed authority shall on receipt of Form 1 make such enquiry as it deems fit and if it is satisfied that the applicant possesses the necessary capacity to handle biomedical waste in accordance with these rules, grant or renew an authorization as the case may be.

(5) An authorization shall be granted for a period of three years, including an initial trial period of one year from the date of issue. Thereafter, an application shall be made by the occupier/operator for renewal. All such subsequent authorization shall be for a period of three years. A provisional authorization will be granted for the trial period, to enable the occupier/operator to demonstrate the capacity of the facility.

(6) The prescribed authority may after giving reasonable opportunity of being heard to the applicant and for reasons thereof to be recorded in writing, refuse to grant or renew authorization.

(7) Every application for authorization shall be disposed of by the prescribed authority within 90 days from the date of receipt of the application.

(8) The prescribed authority may cancel or suspend an authorization, if for reasons, to be recorded in writing, the occupier/operator has failed to comply with any provision of the Act or these rules :
Provided that no authorization shall be cancelled or suspended without giving a reasonable opportunity to the occupier/operator of being heard.

8. **Authorization**

(1) Every occupier of an institution generating, collecting, receiving, storing, transporting, treating, disposing and/or handling biomedical waste in any other manner, except such occupier of clinics, dispensaries, pathological laboratories, blood banks providing treatment/service to less than 1000 (one thousand) patients per month, shall make an application in Form 1 to the prescribed authority for grant of authorization.

(2) Every operator of a biomedical waste facility shall make an application in Form 1 to the prescribed authority for grant of authorization.

(3) Every application in Form 1 for grant of authorization shall be accompanied by a fee as may be prescribed by the Government of the State or Union Territory.

(4) The authorization to operate a facility shall be issued in Form
IV subject to conditions laid therein and such other conditions, as the prescribed authority.

9. **Advisory Committee**

The Government of every State/Union Territory shall constitute an advisory committee. The committee will include experts in the field of medical and health, animal husbandry and veterinary sciences, environmental management, municipal administration, and any other related department or organization including non-governmental organizations. The State Pollution Control Board/Pollution Control Committee shall be represented. As and when required, the committee shall advise the Government of the State/Union Territory and the prescribed authority about matters related to the implementation of these rules.

10. **Annual Report:** Every occupier/operator shall submit an annual report to the prescribed authority in Form 11 by 31 January every year, to include information about the categories and quantities of biomedical wastes handled during the preceding year. The prescribed authority shall send this information in a compiled form to the Central Pollution Control Board by 31 March every year.

11. **Maintenance of Records**

(1) Every authorized person shall maintain records related to the generation, collect ion, reception, storage, transportation, treatment, disposal and/or any form of handling of biomedical waste in accordance with these rules and any guidelines issued.

(2) All records shall be subject to inspection and verification by the prescribed authority at any time.

12. **Accident Reporting:** When any accident occurs at any institution or facility or any other site where biomedical waste is handled or during transportation of such waste, the authorized person shall report the accident in Form Ill to the prescribed authority forthwith.

13. **Appeal**

Any person aggrieved by an order made by the prescribed authority under these rules may, within 30 days from the date on which the order is communicated to him, prefer an appeal to such authority as the Government of State/Union Territory may think fit to constitute:

Provided that the authority may entertain the appeal after the expiry of the said period of 30 days if it is satisfied that the appellant was prevented by sufficient cause from filing the appeal in time.

COMMON DISPOSAL/INCINERATION SITES

Without prejudice to rule 5 of these rules, the Municipal Corporation, Municipal Boards or Urban Local Bodies, as the case may be, shall be responsible for providing suitable common disposal/incineration sites for the biomedical wastes generated in the area under their jurisdiction and in areas outside the jurisdiction of any municipal bodies. It shall be the responsibility of the occupier generating the waste to dispose it of.

SCHEDULE I
(See Rule 5)
CATEGORIES OF BIOMEDICAL WASTE

Waste Category No.	Waste Category [Type]	Treatment and Disposal [Option+]
Category No. I	**Human Anatomical Waste** (human tissues, organs, body parts)	incineration@/deep burial*
Category No. 2	**Animal Waste** (Animal tissues, organs, body parts carcasses, bleeding parts, fluid, blood and experimental animals used in research, waste generated by veterinary hospitals colleges, discharge from hospitals, animal houses)	incineration@/deep burial*
Category No. 3	**Microbiology & Biotechnology Waste** (Wastes from laboratory cultures, stocks or specimens of microorganisms live or attenuated vaccines, human and animal cell culture used in research and infectious agents from research and industrial laboratories, wastes from production of biologicals, toxins, dishes and devices used for transfer of cultures)	local autoclaving/microwaving/ incineration@
Category No. 4	**Waste sharps** (Needles, syringes, scalpels, blades, glass, etc. that may cause puncture and cuts. This includes both used and unused sharps)	disinfection (chemical treatment autoclaving/microwaving and mutilation/shredding)

Contd...

Waste Category No.	Waste Category [Type]	Treatment and Disposal [Option+]
Category No. 5	**Discarded Medicines and Cytotoxic drugs** (Wastes comprising of outdated, contaminated and discarded medicines)	incineration@/destruction and drugs disposal in secured landfills
Category No. 6	**Solid Waste** (Items contaminated with blood, and body fluids including cotton, dressings, soiled plaster casts, lines, beddings, other material contaminated with blood)	incineration@autoclaving/microwaving
Category No. 7	**Solid Waste** (Wastes generated from disposable items other than the waste [sharps] such as tubings, catheters, intravenous sets, etc.).	disinfection by chemical treatment@@ autoclaving/microwaving and mutilation/ shredding##
Category No. 8	**Liquid Waste** (Waste generated from laboratory and washing, cleaning, housekeeping and disinfecting activities)	disinfection by chemical treatment@@ and discharge
Category No. 9	**Incineration Ash** (Ash from incineration of any biomedical waste)	disposal in municipal landfill
Category No. 10	**Chemical Waste** (Chemicals used in production of biologicals, chemicals used in disinfection, as insecticides, etc.)	chemical treatment@@ and discharge into drains for liquids and secured landfill for solids.

@Chemicals treatment using at least 1% hypochlorite solution or any other equivalent chemical reagent. It must be ensured that chemical treatment ensures disinfection.

##Mutilation/shredding must be such so as to prevent unauthorized reuse.

@@There will be no chemical pretreatment before incineration. Chlorinated plastics shall not be incinerated.

*Deep burial shall be an option available only in towns with population less than five lakhs and in rural areas.

SCHEDULE II

(See Rule 6)

COLOR CODING AND TYPE OF CONTAINER FOR DISPOSAL OF BIOMEDICAL WASTES

Color Coding	Type of Container-I Waste Category	Treatment Options as per Schedule I
Yellow	Plastic bag Cat. 1, Cat. 2, and Cat. 3, Cat. 6.	Incineration/deep burial
Red	Disinfected container/plastic bag Cat. 3, Cat. 6, Cat.7.	Autoclaving/Microwaving/ Chemical Treatment
Blue/White translucent	Plastic bag/puncture proof Cat. 4, Cat. 7. Container	Autoclaving/Microwaving/ Chemical Treatment and destruction/shredding
Black	Plastic bag Cat. 5 and Cat. 9 and Cat. 10. (solid)	Disposal in secured landfill

Notes:

Color coding of waste categories with multiple treatment options as defined in Schedule I, shall be selected depending on treatment option chosen, which shall be as specified in Schedule I.

Waste collection bags for waste types needing incineration shall not be made of chlorinated plastics.

Categories 8 and 10 (liquid) do not require containers/bags.

Category 3 if disinfected locally need not be put in containers/bags.

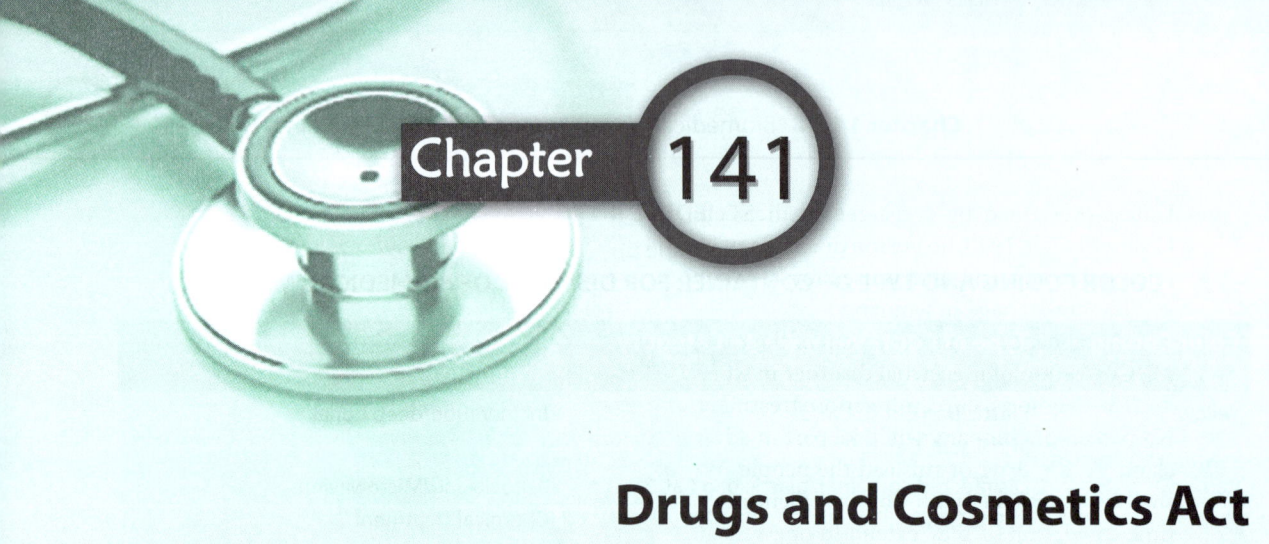

Chapter 141

Drugs and Cosmetics Act

This Act was originally known as the Drug Act and was passed in 1940. The original act was prepared in accordance to the recommendations of the Chopra Committee formed in 1930. The related Drugs Rules were passed in 1945. Since 1940, the act has undergone several amendments and is now known as the Drugs and Cosmetics Act, 1940.

The term **"drug"** as defined in the act includes a wide variety of substance, diagnostic and medical devices. The act defines **"cosmetic"** as any product that is meant to be applied to the human body for the purpose of beautifying or cleansing. The definition, however, excludes soaps. In 1964, the Act was amended to include Ayurveda and Unani drugs.

The Section 16 of the Act defines the standards of quality for drugs. The Section 17 defines "misbranding." A drug is considered misbranded if it claims to be of more therapeutic value than it actually is. The manufacturer of such a drug may be asked to suspend manufacture of the drug under Section 18. Section 27 deals with fake and adulterated drugs. The Act requires that ingredients of the drugs should be printed on the label.

The Section 22 defines the powers of the Drug Inspectors and Section 23 defines the strict procedure which should be followed by the inspectors during any raids.

The Act has been amended several times. The following are a list of amending acts:

- The Drugs (Amendment) Act, 1955 (11 of 1955).
- The Drugs (Amendment) Act, 1960 (35 of 1960).
- The Drugs (Amendment) Act, 1962 (21 of 1962).
- The Drugs and Cosmetics (Amendment) Act, 1964 (13 of 1964).
- The Drugs and Cosmetics (Amendment) Act, 1955 (19 of 1972).
- The Drugs and Cosmetics (Amendment) Act, 1982 (68 of 1982).
- The Drugs and Cosmetics (Amendment) Act, 1986.
- The Drugs and Cosmetics (Amendment) Act, 1995 (71 of 1995).
- The Drugs and Magic Remedies (Objectionable Advertisements) Act, 1955.
- An Act to control, the advertisement of drugs in certain cases, to prohibit the advertisement for certain purpose of remedies alleged to possess magic qualities and to provide for matters connected therewith.
- The Act defines drugs and registered medical practitioners besides defining magic remedy. According to Act the Magic remedy includes a *talisman mantra kavacha,* and any other charm of any kind which is alleged and possess miraculous powers for or in the diagnosis, cure, mitigation treatment or prevention of any disease in human beings or animals or for affecting or influencing in any way the structure or any organic function of human beings or animals.

- Unless prescribed by registered medical practitioners or after consultation with the Drugs and Cosmetics Act, 1940, no person or company, shall take any part in the publication of any advertisement referring to any drug that is used for:
  - ❖ The miscarriage in woman,
  - ❖ Maintenance or improvement of the capacity of human beings for sexual pleasures,
  - ❖ Correction of menstrual disorder in women, and
  - ❖ The diagnosis, cure, mitigation, treatment or prevention of any disease.
- No person or company will take part in advertisement which give false impression or makes a false claim for the drug or mislead the people. Whosoever contravenes any of the provision of this Act shall be punishable with imprisonment extended to six months or with fine, or with both for first time conviction. It may extend to one-year imprisonment or with fine or with both on subsequent convictions.
- The schedule for diseases specified under the Act are: appendicitis, atherosclerosis, blindness, blood poisoning, Bright's disease, cancer, cataract, deafness, diabetes, brain diseases or disorder, uterus diseases, disorder of menstrual flow, disorders of nervous system, prostatic gland disorders, dropsy, epilepsy, female disease (in general), fever (in general), fits, forms and structure of the female breast, gallbladder stones, kidney stones, bladder stones, gangrene, glaucoma, goiter, heart diseases, high or low blood pressure, hydrocele, hysteria, infantile paralysis, insanity, leprosy, leukoderma, lock jaw, locomotor ataxia, lupus, nervous debility, obesity, paralysis, plague, pleurisy, pneumonia, rheumatism, ruptures, sexual impotence, smallpox, stature of person, sterility of women, trachoma, TB, tumors, typhoid fever, ulcers of Gastrointestinal (GI) tract, venereal diseases including, AIDS.

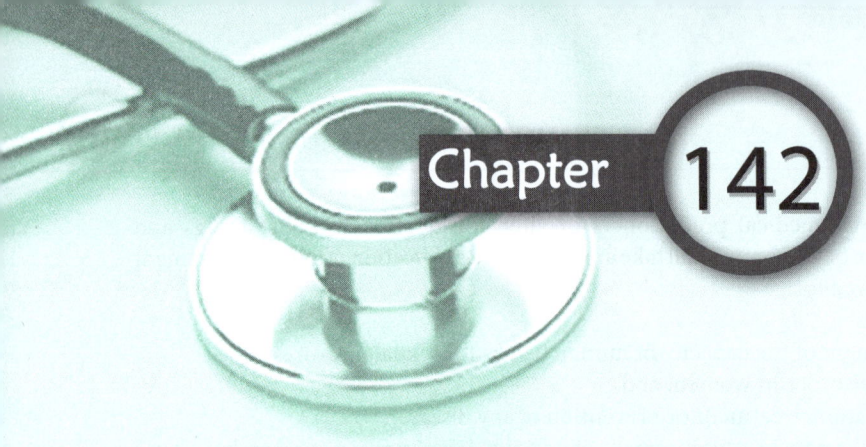

Chapter 142

Mental Health Act

[ACT NO. 14 OF 1987]

[22nd May, 1987]

*A*n Act to consolidate and amend the law relating to the treatment and care of mentally ill persons, to make better provision with respect to their property and affairs and for matters connected therewith or incidental thereto.

STATEMENT OF OBJECTS AND REASONS OF ACT 14 OF 1987

1. The attitude of the society towards persons afflicted with mental illness has changed considerably and it is now realized that no stigma should be attached to such illness as it is curable, particularly, when diagnosed at an early stage. Thus, the mentally ill persons are to be treated like any other sick persons and the environment around them should be made as normal as possible.

2. The experience of the working of Indian Lunacy Act, 1912 (4 of 1912) has revealed that it has become out-moded. With the rapid advance of medical science and the understanding of the nature of malady, it has become necessary to have fresh legislation with provisions for treatment of mentally ill persons in accordance with the new approach.

3. It is considered necessary—

   (i) To regulate admission to psychiatric hospitals or psychiatric nursing homes of mentally ill persons who do not have sufficient understanding to seek treatment on a voluntary basis, and to protect the rights of such persons while being detained

   (ii) To protect society from the presence of mentally ill persons who have become or might become a danger or nuisance to others

   (iii) To protect citizens from being detained in psychiatric hospitals or psychiatric nursing homes without sufficient cause

   (iv) To regulate responsibility for maintenance charges of mentally ill persons who are admitted to psychiatric hospitals or psychiatric nursing homes

   (v) To provide facilities for establishing guardianship or custody of mentally ill persons who are incapable of managing their own affairs

   (vi) To provide for the establishment of Central Authority and State Authorities for Mental Health Services

   (vii) To regulate the powers of the Government for establishing, licensing and controlling psychiatric hospitals and psychiatric nursing homes for mentally ill persons

(viii)   To provide for legal aid to mentally ill persons at State expense in certain cases.

4.   The main object of the Bill is to implement the aforesaid proposals.

Preamble: It is established law that preamble discloses the primary intention of the statute but does override the express provisions of the statute. Although a preamble of a statute is a key to interpretation of the provisions of the Act, but the intention of Legislature is not necessarily to be gathered from the preamble taken by itself, but to be gathered from the provisions of the Act. Where the language of the Act is clear, the preamble cannot be a guide, but where the object or meaning of the provisions of the Act is not clear then an aid from the preamble can be taken into consideration for purpose of explaining the provisions of the Act.

It is now well settled that the preamble of a statutory instrument cannot control the express clear language and sweep of the operating provisions of such an instrument. Nor can the express language of a statutory provision be curtailed or read down in the light of the preamble in the absence of any ambiguity in the enacted provisions.

CHAPTER I: PRELIMINARY

1.   **Short title, extent and commencement—**

    (i)   This Act may be called the Mental Health Act, 1987.

    (ii)   It extends to the whole of India.

    (iii)   It shall come into force on such date as the Central Government may, by notification, appoint and different dates may be appointed for different States and for different provisions of this Act, and any reference in any provision to the commencement of this Act in a State shall be construed as a reference to the coming into force of that provision in that state.

Comment: The Act repeals the Indian Lunacy Act, 1912 (4 of 1912), and the Lunacy Act, 1977 (Jammu and Kashmir Act 25 of 1977). The provisions of the Indian Lunacy Act 1912 and the Amending Act which compendiously called Lunacy Act, 1912–1926 were not absolutely exhaustive.

S.O. 43 (E), Dated 11th January, 1993—In exercise of the powers conferred by sub-section (3) of Section 1 of the Mental Health Act, 1987 (14 of 1987), the Central Government hereby appoints the 1st day of April, 1993 as the date on which the said Act shall come into force in all the States and Union Territories.

Rule of interpretation: It is an accepted proposition of law that Acts must be construed as a whole. Guidance with regard to the meaning of a particular word or phrase may be found in other words and phrases in the same section or in other sections although the utility of an extensive consideration of other parts of the same statute will vary from case to case.

In interpreting the provisions, the exercise undertaken by the Court is to make explicit the intention of the Legislature which enacted the legislation. It is not for the Court to reframe the legislation for the very good reason that the powers to "legislate" have not been conferred on the Court.

In order to sustain the presumption of constitutionality of a legislative measure, the Court can take into consideration matters of common knowledge, matters of common report, the history of the times and also assume every state of fact which can be conceived existing at the time of the legislation.

The principle of the interpretation that no word used by the Legislature in a legislation is useless, cannot be fitted into the situation where the question relates to the interpretation of an agreement. An agreement is not to be culled out from ambiguity.

Interpretation of statute-duty of the court: It is well settled that the Courts should read different provisions of an Act in a manner that no part thereof is held to be superfluous or surplus and that where language of statute leads to manifest contradictions the Court must construe them on the basis of which the said provisions can survive.

Generalia specialibus nonderogant: It is well-known proposition of law that when a matter falls under any specific provision, then it must be governed by that provision and not by the general provision (Generalia specialibus nonderogant).

Construction of work: It is settled view that in determining the meaning or connotation of words and expressions describing an article one should be construed in the sense in which they are understood. The reason is that it is they who are concerned with it and, it is the sense in which they understand it which constitutes the definitive index of the legislative intention.

2. **Definitions—**

    In this Act, unless the context otherwise requires:

    (a) **"Cost of maintenance".** In relation to a mentally ill person admitted in a psychiatric hospital or psychiatric nursing home, shall mean the cost of such items as the State Government may, by general or special order, specify in this behalf

    (b) **"District Court"** means, in any area for which there is a city Civil Court, that Court, and in any other area the principal Civil Court of original jurisdiction, and includes any other Civil Court which the State Government may, by notification, specify as the Court competent to deal with all or any of the matters specified in this Act

    (c) **"Inspecting Officer"** means a person authorized by the State Government or by the licensing authority to inspect any psychiatric hospital or psychiatric nursing home

    (d) **"License"** means a license granted under Section 8

    (e) **"Licensee"** means the holder of a license

    (f) **"Licensed psychiatric hospital"** or **"licensed psychiatric nursing home"** means a psychiatric hospital or psychiatric nursing home, as the case may be, licensed, or deemed to be licensed, under this Act

    (g) **"Licensing authority"** means such officer or authority as may be specified by the State Government to be the licensing authority to the purposes of this Act

    (h) **"Magistrate"** means

        (1) in relation to a metropolitan area within the meaning of Cl (k) of Section 2 of the Code of Criminal Procedure, 1973 (2 of 1974), a Metropolitan Magistrate

        (2) in relation to any other area, the Chief Judicial Magistrate, Sub-Divisional Judicial Magistrate or such other Judicial Magistrate of the first class as the State Government may, by notification, empower to perform the functions of a Magistrate under this Act:

    (i) **"Medical officer"** means a gazetted medical officer in the service of Government and includes a medical practitioner declared, by a general or special order of the State Government, to be a medical officer for the purposes of this Act

    (j) **"Medical officer in charge"** in relation to any psychiatric hospital or psychiatric nursing home, means the medical officer who, for the time being, is in charge of that hospital or nursing home

    (k) **"Medical practitioner"** means a person who possesses a recognized medical qualification as defined—

        (i) in Cl (h) of Section 2 of the Indian Medical Council Act, 1956 (102 of 1956), and whose name has been entered in the State Medical Register, as defined in Cl (k) of that section

        (ii) in Cl (h) of sub-section (1) of Section 2 of the Indian Medicine Central Council Act, 1970 (48 of 1970), and whose name has been entered in a State Register of Indian Medicine, as defined in Cl (j) of sub-section (1) of that section and

(iii) in Cl. (g) of sub-section (1) of Section 2 of the Homoeopathy Central Council Act, 1973 (59 of 1973), and whose name has been entered in a State Register of Homoeopathy, as defined in Cl (I) of sub-section (1) of that section

(l) **"Mentally ill person"** means a person who is in need of treatment by person of any mental disorder other than mental retardation

(m) **"Mentally ill prisoner"** means a mentally ill person for whose detention in, or removal to, a psychiatric hospital, psychiatric nursing home, jail or other place of safe custody, an order referred to in Section 27 has been made

(n) **"Minor"** means a person who has not completed the age of 18 years

(o) **"Notification"** means a notification published in the Official Gazette

(p) **"Prescribed"** means prescribed by rules made under this Act

(q) **"Psychiatric hospital"** or **"Psychiatric nursing home"** means a hospital, or as the case may be, a nursing home established or maintained by the Government or any other person for the treatment and care of mentally ill persons and includes a convalescent home established or maintained by the Government or any other person for such mentally ill persons but does not include any general hospital or general nursing home established or maintained by the Government and which provides also for psychiatric services

(r) **"Psychiatrist"** means a medical practitioner possessing a postgraduate degree or diploma in psychiatry, recognized by the Medical Council of India, constituted under Indian Medical Council Act, 1856 (102 of 1956), and includes, in relation to any State, any medical officer who, having regard to his knowledge and experience in psychiatry, has been declared by the Government of that State to be a psychiatrist for the purposes of this Act

(s) **"Reception order"** means an order made under the provision of this Act for the admission and detention of a mentally ill person in a psychiatric Hospital or psychiatric nursing home

(t) **"Relative"** includes any person related to the mentally ill person by blood, marriage or adoption

(u) **"State government"** in relation to a Union territory, means the Administrator thereof.

Interpretation of section: The Court can merely interpret the section it cannot re-write, recast or redesign the Section 1.

Relative—meaning of—Certainly the word "relative" used in Section 3 of the Lunacy Act (since repealed by this Act) has to be understood in a legal sense and it has to be understood in the setting where that word is used in the provisions of the statute, particularly, the provision enabling a relative to entertain a petition under Section 63 of the Lunacy Act 2.

CHAPTER II: MENTAL HEALTH AUTHORITIES

3. **Central authority for mental health services—**

   (1) The Central Government shall establish an authority for mental health with such designation as it may deem fit.

   (2) The Authority established under sub-section (1) shall be subject to the superintendence, direction and control of the Central Government.

   (3) The authority established under sub-section (1) shall:

       (a) be in charge of regulation, development, direction and co-ordination with respect to Mental Health Services under the Central Government and all other matters which, under this Act, are the concern of the Central Government or any officer or authority subordinate to the Central Government.

(b) supervise the psychiatric hospitals and psychiatric nursing homes and other Mental Health Service Agencies (including places in which mentally ill persons may be kept or detained) under the control of the Central Government.

(c) advise the Central Government on all matters relating to mental health and

(d) discharge such other functions with respect to matters relating to mental health as the Central Government may require.

4. **State authority for mental health services—**

(1) The State Government shall establish an authority for mental with such designation as it may deem fit.

(2) The Authority established under sub-section (1) shall be subject to the superintendence, direction and control of the State Government.

(3) **The authority established under sub-section (1) shall—**

(a) be in charge of regulation, development and co-ordination with respect to Mental Health Service under the State Government and all other matters which, under this Act, the concern of the State Government or any officer or authority subordination to the State Government:

(b) supervise the psychiatric hospitals and psychiatric nursing homes and other Mental Health Services Agencies (including places in which mentally ill persons may be kept or detained) under the control of the State Government.

(c) advise the State Government on all matters relating to mental health and

(d) discharge such other functions with respect to matters relating to mental health as the State Government may require.

CHAPTER III: PSYCHIATRIC HOSPITALS AND PSYCHIATRIC NURSING HOMES

5. **Establishment or maintenance of psychiatric hospitals and psychiatric nursing homes—**

(1) The Central Government may, in any part of India, or the State Government may, within the limits of its jurisdiction, established or maintain psychiatric hospitals or psychiatric nursing homes for the admission, and care of mentally ill persons at such places as it thinks fit and separate psychiatric hospitals and psychiatric nursing homes may be established or maintained for:

(a) those who are under the age of 16 years

(b) those who are addicted to alcohol or other drugs which lead to behavioral changes in a person

(c) those who have been convicted of any offence and

(d) those belonging to such other or category of persons as may be prescribed.

(2) Where a psychiatric hospital or psychiatric nursing home is established or maintained by the Central Government, any reference in this Act to the State Government shall, in relation to such hospital or nursing home, be construed as a reference to the Central Government.

6. **Establishment or maintenance of psychiatric hospitals or psychiatric nursing homes only with license—**

(1) On and after the commencement of this Act, no person shall established or maintain a psychiatric hospital or psychiatric nursing home unless he holds a valid license granted to him under this Act:

Provided that a psychiatric hospital or psychiatric nursing home (whether called asylum or by any other name) licensed by the Central Government or any State Government and maintained as such immediately before the commencement of this Act may continue to be maintained, and shall be deemed to be a licensed psychiatric hospital or licensed psychiatric nursing home, as the case may be, under this Act:

(a) for a period of three months from such commencement,

(b) if an application made in accordance with Section 7 for a license is pending on the expiry of the period specified in Cl. (a) till the disposal of such application.

(2) Nothing contained in sub-section (1) shall apply to a psychiatric hospital or psychiatric nursing home established or maintained by a Central Government or a State Government.

Comment—This section prohibits establishment or maintenance of any psychiatric hospital or psychiatric nursing home by any person, unless he holds a valid license granted to him under the Act.

7. **Application for license—**

(1) Every person, who holds, at the commencement of this Act, a valid license authorizing that person to establish or maintain any psychiatric hospital or psychiatric nursing home, shall, if the said person intends to establish or continue the maintenance of such hospital or nursing home after the expiry of the period referred to in Cl. (a) of the proviso to sub-section (1) of Section 6, make at least one month before the expiry of such period, an application to the licensing authority for the grant of a fresh license for the establishment or maintenance of such hospital or nursing home, as the case may be.

(2) A person, who intends to establish or maintain, after the commencement of this Act, a psychiatric hospital or psychiatric nursing home, shall, unless the said person already holds a valid license, make an application to the license authority for the grant of a license.

(3) Every application under sub-section (1) or sub-section (2) shall be in such form and be accompanied by such fee as may be prescribed.

8. **Grant or refusal of license—**

On receipt of an application under Section 7, the licensing authority shall make such inquiries as it may deem fit and where it is satisfied that:

(a) the establishment or maintenance of the psychiatric hospital or psychiatric nursing home or the continuance of the maintenance of any such hospital or nursing home established before the commencement of this Act is necessary

(b) the applicant is in a position to provide the minimum facilities prescribed for the admission, treatment and care of mentally ill persons and

(c) the psychiatric hospital or psychiatric nursing home, will be under the charge of medical officer who is a psychiatrist.

It shall grant a license to the applicant in the prescribed form, and where it is not so satisfied, the licensing authority shall, by order, refuse to grant the license applied for:

Provided that, before making any order refusing to grant a license, the licensing authority shall give to the applicant a reasonable opportunity of being heard and every order of refusal to grant a license shall set out therein the reasons for such refusal and such reasons shall be communicated to the applicant in such manner as may be prescribed.

9. **Duration and renewal of license—**

(1) A license shall not be transferable or heritable.

(2) Where a licensee is unable to function as such for any reason or where a licensee dies, the licensee or, as the case may be, the legal representative of such licensee shall forthwith report the matter in the prescribed manner to the licensing authority and notwithstanding anything contained in sub-section (I), the psychiatric hospital or psychiatric nursing home concerned may continue to be maintained and shall be deemed to be a licensed psychiatric hospital or licensed psychiatric nursing home, as the case may be:

(a) for a period of three months from the date of such report or in the case of the death of the licensee from the date of his death, or

(b) if an application made in accordance with sub-section (3) for a license is pending on the expiry of the period specified in Cl. (a), till the disposal of such application.

(3) The legal representative of the licensee referred to in sub-section (2) shall, if he intends to continue the maintenance of the psychiatric hospital or psychiatric nursing home after the expiry of the period referee to in sub-section (2), make, at least one month before the expiry of such period, an application to the licensing authority for the grant of a fresh license for the maintenance of such hospital or nursing home, as the case may be, and the provisions of Section 8 shall apply in relation to such application as they apply in relation to an application made under Section 7.

(4) Every license shall, unless revoked earlier under Section 11, be valid for a period of 5 years from the date on which it is granted.

(5) A license may be renewed from time to time, on an application made in that behalf to the licensing authority, in such form and accompanied by such fee, as may be prescribed, and every such application shall be made not less than one year before the date on which the period of validity of the license is due to expire:

Provided that the renewal of a license shall not be refused unless the licensing authority is satisfied that:

(i) The licensee is not in a position to provide in a psychiatric hospital or psychiatric nursing home, the minimum facilities prescribed for the admission, treatment and care therein mentally ill persons or

(ii) The licensee is not in a position to provide a medical officer which is a psychiatrist to take charge of the psychiatric hospital or psychiatric nursing home, or

(iii) The licensee has contravened any of the provisions of this Act or any rule made thereunder.

10. **Psychiatric hospital and psychiatric nursing home to be maintained in accordance with prescribed conditions—**

Every psychiatric hospital or psychiatric nursing home shall be maintained in such manner and object to such condition as may be prescribed.

11. **Revocation of license—**

(1) The licensing authority may, without prejudice to any other penalty that may be imposed on the licensee, by order in writing, revoke the license if it is satisfied that:

(a) the psychiatric hospital or psychiatric nursing home is not being maintained by the licensee in accordance with the provisions of this Act or the rules made thereunder or

(b) the maintenance of the psychiatric hospital or psychiatric nursing home is being carried on in a manner detrimental to the moral, mental or physical well-being of other in-patients thereof:

Provided that no such order shall be made except after giving the licensee a reasonable opportunity of being heard, and every such order shall set out therein the grounds for the revocation of the license and such grounds shall be communicated to the licensee in such manner as may be prescribed.

(2) Every order made under sub-section (1) shall contain a direction that the in-patients of the psychiatric hospital or psychiatric nursing home shall be transferred to such other psychiatric hospital or psychiatric nursing home as may be specified in that order and it shall also contain such provisions (including provisions by way of directions) as to the care and custody of such in-patients pending such transfer.

(3) Every order made under sub-section (1) shall take effect:

    (a) where no appeal has been preferred against such order under Section 12, immediately on the expiry of the period prescribed for such appeal and

    (b) where such appeal has been preferred and the same has been dismissed, from the date of the order of such dismissal.

12. Appeal—

(1) Any person aggrieved by an order of the licensing authority refusing to grant or renew a license, or revoking a license, may, in such manner and within such period as may be prescribed, prefer an appeal to the State Government:

Provided that the State Government may entertain an appeal preferred after the expiry of the prescribed period if it is satisfied that the appellant was prevented by sufficient cause from preferring the appeal in time.

(2) Every appeal under sub-section (1) shall be made in such form and accompanied by such fee as may be prescribed.

13. Inspection of psychiatric hospitals and psychiatric nursing homes and visiting of patients—

(1) An Inspecting Officer may, at any time, enter and inspect any psychiatric hospital or psychiatric nursing home and require the production of any records, which are required to be kept in accordance with the rules made in this behalf, for inspection:

Provided that any personal records of a patient so inspected shall be kept confidential except for the purposes of sub-section (3).

(2) The Inspecting Officer may interview in private any patient receiving treatment and care therein:

    (a) for the purpose of inquiring into any complaint made by or on behalf of such patient as to the treatment and care.

    (b) in any case, where the Inspecting Officer has reason to believe that any in-patient is not receiving proper treatment and care.

(3) Where the Inspecting Officer is satisfied that any in-patient in a psychiatric hospital or psychiatric nursing home is not receiving proper treatment and care, he may report the matter to the licensing authority and thereupon the licensing authority may issue such direction as it may deem fit to the medical officer-in-charge of the licensee of the psychiatric hospital, or, as the case may be, the psychiatric nursing home and every such medical officer-in-charge or licensee shall be bound to comply with such directions.

14. Treatment of out-patient—

Provision shall be made in every psychiatric hospital or psychiatric nursing homes for such facilities as may be prescribed for the treatment of every mentally ill person, patient or who, for the time being, is not undergoing treatment as in-patients.

CHAPTER IV: ADMISSION AND DETENTION IN PSYCHIATRIC HOSPITAL OR PSYCHIATRIC NURSING HOME

Part I—Admission on Voluntary Basis

15. **Request by major for admission as voluntary patient—**

Any persons (not being a minor), who considers himself to be a mentally ill person and desires to be admitted to any psychiatric nursing home for treatment, may request the medical officer in charge for being admitted as a voluntary patient.

16. **Request by guardian for admission of a ward—**

Where the guardian of a minor considers such minor to be a mentally ill person and desires to admit such minor in any psychiatric hospital or psychiatric nursing home for treatment, he may request the medical officer-in-charge for admitting such minor as a voluntary patient.

17. **Admission of, and regulation with respect to, voluntary patient—**

(1) On receipt of a request under Section 15 or Section 16, the medical officer-in-charge shall make such inquiry as he may deem fit within a period not exceeding twenty-four hours and if satisfied that the applicant or, as the case may be, the minor requires treatment as an in-patient in the psychiatric hospital or psychiatric nursing home, he may admit therein such application or, as the case may be, minor as a voluntary patient.

(2) Every voluntary patient admitted to a psychiatric hospital or psychiatric nursing home shall be bound to abide by such regulations as may be made by the medical officer-in-charge or the licensee of the psychiatric hospital or psychiatric nursing home.

18. **Discharge of voluntary patients—**

(1) The medical officer in charge of a psychiatric hospital or psychiatric nursing home shall, on a request made in that behalf:

(a) by any voluntary patient and

(b) by the guardian of the patient, if he is a minor voluntary patient, discharge, subject to the provisions of sub-section (3) and within 24 hours of the receipt of such request, the patient from the psychiatric hospital or psychiatric nursing home.

(2) Where a minor voluntary patient who is admitted as an in-patient in any psychiatric hospital or psychiatric nursing home attains majority, the medical officer in charge of such hospital or nursing home, shall, as soon as may be, intimate the patient that he has attained majority and that unless a request for his continuance as an in-patient is made by him within a period of one month of such intimation, he shall be discharged, and if, before the expiry of the said period, no request is made to the medical officer in charge for his continuance as an in-patient, he shall, subject to the provisions of sub-section (3), be discharged on the expiry of the said period.

(3) Notwithstanding anything contained in sub-section (1) or sub-section (2) where the medical officer in charge of a psychiatric hospital or psychiatric nursing home is satisfied that the discharge of a voluntary patient under sub-section (1) or sub-section (2) will not be in the interest of such voluntary patient, he shall, within seventy-two hours of the receipt of a request under sub-section (1), or, if no request under sub-section (2) has been made by the voluntary patient before the expiry of the period mentioned in that sub-section within seventy-two hours of such expiry constitute a Board consisting of two medical officers and seek its opinion as to whether such voluntary patient needs further treatment and if the Board is of the opinion that such voluntary patient needs further treatment in the psychiatric hospital or psychiatric nursing home, the medical officer shall not discharge the voluntary patient, but continue his treatment for a period not exceeding 90 days at a time.

Part II—Admission under Special Circumstances

19. Admission of mentally ill persons under certain special circumstances—

Any mentally ill person who does not, or is unable to, express his willingness for admission as a voluntary patient, may be admitted and kept as an inpatient in a psychiatric nursing hospital or psychiatric nursing home on an application made in that behalf by a relative or a friend of the mentally ill persons if the medical officers-in-charge is satisfied that in the interest of the mentally ill persons it is necessary so to do:

Part III—Reception Orders

20. Application for reception order—

(1) An application for a reception order may be made by:

    (a) the medical officer-in-charge of a psychiatric hospital or psychiatric nursing home, or

    (b) by the husband, wife or any other relative of the mentally ill person.

(2) Where a medical officer-in-charge of a psychiatric hospital or psychiatric nursing home in which a mentally ill-person is undergoing treatment under a temporary treatment order is satisfied that:

    (a) the mentally ill person is suffering from mental disorder of such a nature and degree that his treatment in the psychiatric hospital or as the case may be, psychiatric nursing home is required to be continued for more than six months, or

    (b) it is necessary in the interests of the health and personal safety of the mentally ill person or for the protection of others that such person shall be detained in a psychiatric hospital or psychiatric nursing home.

    He may make an application to the Magistrate within the local limits of whose jurisdiction the psychiatric hospital or, as the case may be, psychiatric nursing home is situated, for the detention of such mentally ill-person under a reception order in such psychiatric hospital or psychiatric nursing home, as the case may be.

(3) Subject to the provisions of sub-section (5), the husband or wife of a person who is alleged to be mentally ill or, where there is no husband or wife, or where the husband or wife is prevented by reason of any illness or absence from India or otherwise from making the application, any other relative of such person may make an application to the Magistrate within the local limits of whose jurisdiction the said person ordinarily resides, for the detention of the alleged mentally ill-person under a reception order in a psychiatric hospital or psychiatric nursing home.

(4) Where the husband or wife of the alleged mentally ill person is not the applicant, the application shall contain the reasons for the application not being made by the husband or wife and shall indicate the relationship of the applicant with the alleged mentally ill person and the circumstances under which the application is being made.

(5) No person—

    (i) who is a minor, or

    (ii) who, within 14 days before the date of the application, has not seen the alleged mentally ill person, shall make an application under this section.

(6) Every application under sub-section (3) shall be made in the prescribed form and shall be signed and verified in the prescribed manner and shall state whether any previous application had been made for inquiry into the mental condition of the alleged mentally ill person and shall be accompanied by two medical certificates from two medical practitioners of whom one shall be a medical practitioner in the service of Government.

Comment—This section details the procedure for disposal of application for reception order.

21. Form and contents of medical certificates—

Every medical certificate referred to in sub-section (6) of Section 20 shall contain a statement:

(a) that each of the medical practitioner referred to in that sub-section has independently examined the alleged mentally ill person and has formed his opinion on the basis of his own observations and from the particulars communicated to him

(b) that in the opinion of each such medical practitioner the alleged mentally ill person is suffering from mental disorder of such a nature and degree as to warrant the detention of such person in a psychiatric hospital or psychiatric nursing home and that such detention is necessary in the interests of the health and personal safety of that person or for the protection of others.

22. Procedure upon application for reception order—

(1) On receipt of an application under sub-section (2) of Section 20, the Magistrate may make a reception order, if he is satisfied that:

  (i) the mentally ill person is suffering from mental disorder of such a nature and degree that it is necessary to detain him in a psychiatric hospital or psychiatric nursing home for treatment or

  (ii) it is necessary in the interests of the mental and personal safety of the mentally ill person or for the protection of others that he should be so detained, and a temporary treatment order would not be adequate in the circumstances of the case and it is necessary to make a reception order.

(2) On receipt of an application under sub-section of Section 20, the Magistrate shall consider the statements made in the application and the evidence of mental illness as disclosed by the medical certificates.

(3) If the Magistrate considers that there are sufficient grounds for proceeding further, he shall personally examine the alleged mentally ill person unless, for reasons to be recorded in writing, he thinks that it is not necessary or expedient to do so.

(4) If the Magistrate is satisfied that a reception order may properly be made forthwith, he may make such order, and if the Magistrate is not so satisfied, he shall fix a date for further consideration of the application and may make such inquiries concerning the alleged mentally ill-person as he thinks fit.

(5) The notice of the date fixed under sub-section (4) shall be given to the applicant and to any other person to whom, in the opinion of the Magistrate such notice shall be given.

(6) If the Magistrate fixes a date under sub-section (4) for further consideration of the application, he may make such order as he thinks fit, for the proper care and custody of the alleged mentally ill person pending disposal of the application.

(7) On the date fixed under sub-section (4), or on such further date as may be fixed by the Magistrate, he shall proceed to consider the application in camera, in the presence of—

  (i) the applicant

  (ii) the alleged mentally ill person (unless the Magistrate in his discretion otherwise directs)

  (iii) the person who may be appointed by the alleged mentally ill person to represent him and

  (iv) such other person as the Magistrate thinks fit, and if the Magistrate is satisfied that the alleged mentally ill person, in relation to whom the application is made, is so mentally ill that in the interests of the health and personal safety of that person or for the protection of others it is necessary to detail him in a psychiatric hospital or psychiatric nursing home for treatment, he may pass a reception order for that purpose and if he is not so satisfied, he shall dismiss the application and any such order may provide for the payment of the costs of the inquiry by the applicant personally or from out of the estate of the mentally ill person, as the Magistrate may dccm appropriate.

(8)   If any application is dismissed under sub-section (7), the Magistrate shall record the reasons for such dismissal and a copy of the order shall be furnished to the applicant.

23. Powers and duties of police officers in respect of certain mentally ill persons—

(1)   Every officer-in-charge of a police station:

(i)   may take or cause to be taken into protection any person found wandering at large within the limits of his station whom he has reason to believe to be so mentally ill as to be incapable of taking care of himself, and

(ii)   shall take or cause to be taken into protection any person within the limits of his station whom he has reason to believe to be dangerous by reason of mental illness.

(2)   No person taken into protection under sub-section (1) shall be detained by the police without being informed, as soon as may be, of the grounds for taking him into such protection, or where, in the opinion of the officer taking the person into protection, such person is not capable of understanding those grounds, without his relatives or friends, if any, being informed of such grounds.

(3)   Every person who is taken into protection and detained under this section shall be produced before the nearest Magistrate within a period of twenty-four hours of taking him into such protection excluding the time necessary for the journey from the place where he was taken into such protection of the Court of the Magistrate and shall not be detained beyond the said period without the authority of the Magistrate.

24. Procedure on production of mentally ill person—

(1)   If a person is produced before the Magistrate under sub-section (3) of Section 23, and if in his opinion, there are sufficient grounds for proceeding further, the Magistrate shall:

(a)   examine the person to assess his capacity to understand.

(b)   cause him to be examined by a medical officer, and

(c)   make such inquiries in relation to such person as he may deem necessary.

(2)   After the completion of the proceeding under sub-section (1), the Magistrate may pass a reception order authorizing the detention of the said person as an in-patient in a psychiatric hospital or psychiatric nursing home:

(i)   if the medical officer certifies such person to be a mentally ill person, and

(ii)   if the Magistrate is satisfied that the said person is a mentally ill person and that in the interest of the health and personal safety of that person or for the protection of others, it is necessary to pass such order.

Provided that if any relative or friend of the mentally ill person desires that the mentally ill person be sent to any particular licensed psychiatric hospital or licensed psychiatric nursing home for treatment therein and undertakes in writing to the satisfaction of the Magistrate to pay the cost of maintenance of the mentally ill person in such hospital or nursing home, the Magistrate shall, if the medical officer in charge of such hospital or nursing home consents, make a reception order for the admission of the mentally ill person into that hospital or nursing home and detention therein:

Provided further that if any relative or friend of the mentally ill person enters into a bond, with or without sureties for such amount as the Magistrate may determine, undertaking that such mentally ill person will be properly taken care of and shall be prevented from doing any injury to himself or to others, the Magistrate may, instead of making a reception order, hand him over to the care of such relative or friend.

25. Order in case of mentally ill person cruelly treated or not under proper care and control—

(1) Every officer in charge of a police station is mentally ill and is not under proper care and control, or is mentally ill person, shall forthwith report the fact to the Magistrate within the local limits of whose jurisdiction the mentally ill person resides.

(2) Any private person who has reason to believe that any person is mentally ill and is not under proper care and control, or is ill-treated or neglected by any relative or other person having charge of such mentally ill person, may report the fact to the Magistrate within the local limits of whose jurisdiction the mentally ill person resides.

(3) If it appears to the Magistrate, on the report of a police officer or on the report or information derived from any other person, or otherwise that any mentally ill person within the local limits of his jurisdiction is not under proper care and control, or is ill-treated or neglected by any relative or other person having the charge of such mentally ill person, the Magistrate may cause the mentally ill person to be produced before him, and summon such relative or other person who is, or who ought to be in charge of, such mentally ill person.

(4) If such relative or any other person is legally bound to maintain the mentally ill person, the Magistrate may, by order, require the relative or the other person to take proper care of such mentally ill person and where such relative or other person willfully neglects to comply with the said order, he shall be punishable with fine which may extend to two thousand rupees.

(5) If there is no person legally bound to maintain the mentally ill person, or if the person legally bound to maintain the mentally ill person refuses or neglects to maintain such person, or if, for any other reason, the Magistrate thinks fit so to do, he may cause the mentally ill person to be produced before him and, without prejudice to any action that may be taken under sub-section (4), proceed in the manner provided in Section 24 as if such person had been produced before him under sub-section (3) of Section 23.

26. Admission as in-patient after inquisition—

If any District Court holding an inquisition under Chapter VI regarding any person who is found to be mentally ill is of opinion that it is necessary so to do in the interests of such person, it may, by order, direct that such person shall be admitted and kept as an in-patient in a psychiatric hospital or psychiatric nursing home and every such order may be varied from time to time or revoked by the District Court.

27. Admission and detention of mentally ill prisoner—

An order under Section 30 of the Prisoners Act, 1900 (3 of 1900) or under Section 144 of the Air Force Act, 1950 (45 of 1950), or under Section 145 of the Army Act 1950 (46 of 1950), or under Section 143 or Section 144 of the Navy Act, 1957 (62 of 1957), or under Section 330 or Section 335 of the Code of Criminal Procedure 1973 (2 of 1974), directing the reception of a mentally ill prisoner into any psychiatric hospital or psychiatric nursing home, shall be sufficient authority for the admission of such person in such hospital or, as the case may be, such nursing home or any other psychiatric hospital or psychiatric nursing home to which such person may be lawfully transferred for detention therein.

28. Detention of alleged mentally ill person pending report by medical officer—

(1)   When any person alleged to be a mentally ill person appears or is brought before a Magistrate under Section 23 or Section 25, the Magistrate may, by order in writing, authorize the detention of the alleged mentally ill person under proper medical custody in an observation ward of a general hospital or general nursing home or psychiatric hospital of psychiatric nursing home or in any other suitable place for such period not exceeding ten days as the Magistrate may consider necessary for enabling any medical officer to determine whether a medical certificate in respect of that alleged mentally ill person may properly be given under Cl. (a) of sub-section (2) of Section 24.

(2)   The Magistrate may, from time to time, for the purpose mentioned in sub-section (1), by order in writing, authorize such further detention of the alleged mentally ill person for periods not exceeding 10 days at a time as he may deem necessary:

Provided that no person shall be authorized to be detained under this sub-section for a continuous period exceeding 30 days in the aggregate.

Scope of the section: The provision which the Magistrate could probably have thought of to justify his action is Section 16 of the Lunacy Act (since repealed by this Act). No other provision gives him the power of detention before adjudging a person as lunatic. Section 16(1) confers jurisdiction on a Magistrate to deal with a person who is alleged to be lunatic when he is brought before the Magistrate under the provisions of Section 13 of Section 15. Such a person can be detained by an order of the Magistrate, "for such time not exceeding 10 days as may be, in his opinion necessary to enable the medical officer to determine whether such alleged lunatic is a person in respect of whom a medical certificate may be properly given". The proviso to sub-section (2) imposes a ban on the Magistrate against extension of the period of detention beyond a total period of 30 days.

29. Detention of mentally ill person pending his removal to psychiatric hospital or psychiatric nursing home—

Whenever any reception order is made by a Magistrate under Section 22, Section 23 or Section 25, he may by reasons to be recorded in writing, direct that the mentally ill person in respect of whom the order is made may be detained for such period not exceeding 30 days in such place as he may deem appropriate. Pending the removal of such person to a psychiatric hospital or psychiatric nursing home.

30. Time and manner of medical examination of mentally ill person—

Where any other order under this Chapter is required to be made on the basis of a medical certificate, such order shall not be made unless the person who has signed the medical certificate, or where such order is required to be made on the basis of two medical certificates, the signatory of the respective certificates, has certified that he has personally examined the alleged mentally ill person:

(i)   in the case of an order made on an application, not earlier than 10 clear days immediately before the date on which such application is made and

(ii)   in any other case, not earlier than 10 clear days immediately before the date of such order

(iii) provided that where a reception order is required to be made on the basis of two medical certificates such order shall not be made unless the certificates show that the signatory of each certificate examined the alleged mentally ill person independently of the signatory of the other certificate.

31. Authority for reception order

A reception order made under this Chapter shall be sufficient authority:

(i)   for the applicant or any person authorized by him, or

(ii)   in the case of a reception order made otherwise than on an application, for the person authorized so to do by the authority making this order.

To take the mentally ill person to the place mentioned in such order or for his admission and treatment as an in-patient in the psychiatric hospital or psychiatric nursing home specified in the order or, as the case may be, for his admission and detention, therein or in any psychiatric hospital or psychiatric nursing home to which he may be removed in accordance with the provisions of this Act, and the medical officer in charge shall be bound to comply with such order:

Provided that in any case where the medical officer-in-charge finds accommodation in the psychiatric hospital or psychiatric nursing home inadequate he shall, after according admission, intimate that fact to the Magistrate or the District Court which passed the order and thereupon the Magistrate or the District Court, as the case may be, shall pass such order as he or it may deem fit:

Provided further that every reception order shall cease to have effect:

(i)   on the expiry of 30 days from the date on which it was made, unless within that period, the mentally ill person has been admitted to the place mentioned therein

(ii)   on the discharge, in accordance with the provisions of this Act, of the mentally ill person.

32. Copy of reception order to be sent to medical officer-in-charge—

Every Magistrate or District Court making a reception order shall forthwith send a certified copy thereof together with copies of the requisite medical certificates and the statement of particulars to the medical officer in charge of the psychiatric hospital or psychiatric nursing home to which the mentally ill person is to be admitted.

33. Restriction as to psychiatric hospitals and psychiatric nursing homes into which reception order may direct admission—

No Magistrate or District Court shall pass a reception order for the admission as an in-patient to, or for the detention of any mentally ill person, as an in-patient to, or for the detention of any mentally ill person, in any psychiatric hospital or psychiatric nursing home outside the State in which the Magistrate or the District Court exercises jurisdiction:

Provided that an order for admission or detention into or in a psychiatric hospital or psychiatric nursing home situated in any other State may be passed if the State Government has by general or special order and after obtaining the consent of the Government of such other State, authorized the Magistrate or the District Court in that behalf.

34. Amendment of order or document—

If, after the admission of any mentally ill person to any psychiatric hospital or psychiatric nursing home under a reception order, it appears that the order under which he was admitted or detained or any of the documents on the basis of which such order was made defective or incorrect, the same may, at any time thereafter be amended with the permission of the Magistrate or the District Court, by the person or persons who signed the same and upon such amendment being made, the order shall have effect and shall be deemed always to have had effect as if it had been originally made as so amended, or, as the case be, the documents upon which it was made had been originally furnished, also amended.

35. Power to appoint substitute for person upon whose application reception order has been made—

(1)   Subject to the provisions of this section the Magistrate may, by order in writing (hereinafter referred to the orders of substitution), transfer the duties and responsibilities under this Act, of the person on whose application a reception order was made, to any other person who is willing to undertake the same and such other person shall thereupon be deemed for the purposes of this Act to be the person on whose application the reception order was made and all references in this Act to the latter person shall be construed accordingly:

Provided that no such order of substitution shall absolve the person upon whose application the reception order was made or, if he is dead, his legal representatives, from any liability incurred before the date of the order of substitution.

(2)   Before making any order of substitution, the Magistrate shall send a notice to the person on whose application the reception order was made if he is alive, and to any relative of the mentally ill person who, in the opinion of the Magistrate, shall have notice.

(3)   The notice under sub-section (2) shall specify the name of the person in whose favor it is proposed to make the order of substitution and the date (which shall be not less than 20 days from the date of issue of the notice) on which objections, if any, to the making of such order shall be considered.

(4)   On the date specified under sub-section (3), or on any subsequent date to which the proceedings may be adjourned, the Magistrate shall consider any objection made by any person to whom notice was sent or by any other relative of the mentally ill person, and shall receive all such evidence as may be produced by or on behalf of any such person or relative and after making such inquiry as the Magistrate may deem fit make or refrain from making the order of substitution:

Provided that, if the person on whose application the reception order was made is dead and any other person is willing and is, in the opinion of the Magistrate, fit to undertake the duties and responsibilities under this Act of the former person, the Magistrate shall, subject to the provisions contained in the proviso to sub-section (1), make an order to that effect.

(5)   In making any substitution order under this section, the Magistrate shall give preference to the person who is the nearest relative of the mentally ill person, unless, for reasons to be recorded in writing the Magistrate considers that giving such preference will not be in the interests of the mentally ill person.

(6)   The Magistrate may make such order for the payment of the costs of an inquiry under this section by any person or from out of the estate of the mentally ill person as he thinks fit.

(7)   Any notice under sub-section (2) may be sent by post to the last known address of the person for whom it is intended.

Proviso—A proviso to a section is not independent of the section calling for independent of the section calling for independent consideration or construction detached from the construction to be placed on the main section as it is merely subsidiary to the main section and is to be construed in the light of the section itself.

It is settled that a proviso cannot expand or limit the clear meaning of the main provision.

36. Officers competent to exercise powers and discharge function of Magistrate under certain sections—
In any area where a Commissioner of Police has been appointed, all the powers and functions of the Magistrate under Sections 23, 24, 25 and 28 may be exercised or discharged by the Commissioner of Police and all the functions of an officer-in-charge of a police station under this Act may be discharged by any police officer not below the rank of an Inspector.

Commissioner, if includes "deputy" or "assistant": It is clear that in the present case the Deputy Commissioner who acted in the matter had no power under Section 17 of the Lunacy Act (since repealed by this Act). In any case, no such power could be conferred upon him even by the State Government. Because Lunacy Act, (since repealed by this Act) has not recognized conferment of such power upon any Deputy or Assistant to the Commissioner.

CHAPTER V: INSPECTION, DISCHARGE, LEAVE OF ABSENCE AND REMOVAL OF MENTALLY ILL PERSONS

Part I—Inspection

37. Appointment of visitors—

(1) The State Government or the Central Government, as the case may be, shall appoint for every psychiatric hospital and every psychiatric nursing home, not less than five visitors, of whom at least one shall be a medical officer, preferably a psychiatrist and two social workers.

(2) The head of the Medical Services of the State or his nominee preferably a psychiatrist be an ex officio visitor of all the psychiatrist hospital and psychiatric nursing homes in the State.

(3) The qualifications of persons to be appointed as visitors under sub-section (1) and the terms and conditions of their appointment shall be such as may be prescribed.

38. Monthly inspection by visitors—

Not less than three visitors shall at least once in every month, make a joint inspection of every part of the psychiatric hospital or psychiatric nursing home in respect of which they have been appointed and examine every minor admitted as a voluntary patient under Section 17 and, as far as circumstances will permit, every other mentally ill person admitted therein and the order for the admission of and subsequent to the joint inspection immediately preceding, and shall enter in a book kept for that purpose such remarks as they deem appropriate in regard to the management and condition of such hospital or nursing home and of the in-patient thereof:

Provided that the visitors shall not be entitled to inspect any personal records of an in-patient which in the opinion of the medical officer-in-charge are confidential in nature:

Provided further that if any of the visitors does not participate in the joint inspection of the psychiatric hospital or psychiatric nursing home in respect of which he was appointed a visitor for three consecutive months, he shall cease to hold office as such visitor.

39. Inspection of mentally ill prisoners—

(1) Notwithstanding anything contained in Section 38, where any person is detained under the provisions of Section 144 of the Air Force Act, 1950 (45 of 1950), or Section 145 of the Army Act, 1950 (46 of 1950), or Section 143 or Section 144 of the Navy Act 1957 (62 of 1957) or Section 330 or Section 335 of the Code of Criminal Procedure 1973 (2 of 1974)—

    (i) the Inspector-General of Prisons, where such person is detained in a jail

    (ii) all or any three of the visitors including at least one social worker appointed under sub-section (1) of Section 37, where such person is detained, in a psychiatric hospital or psychiatric nursing home, shall, once in every three months visit such person at the place where he is detained, in order to assess the state of mind of such person and make a report thereon to the authority under whose order such person is so detained.

(2) The State Government may empower any of its officers to discharge all or any of the functions of the Inspector-General of Prisons under Sub-section (1).

(3) The medical officer in charge of a psychiatric hospital or psychiatric nursing home wherein any person referred to in sub-section (1) is detained, shall once in every six months, make a special report regarding the mental and physical condition of such person to the authority under whose order such person is detained.

(4)   Every person who is detained in jail under the provisions of various Acts referred to in sub-section (1) shall be visited at least once in every three months by a psychiatrist, or where a psychiatrist is not available, by a medical officer empowered by the State Government in this behalf and such psychiatrist or, as the case may be, such medical officer shall make a special report regarding the mental and physical condition of such person to the authority under whose order such person is detained.

Part II—Discharge

40. Order of discharge by medical officer in charge—

Notwithstanding anything contained in Chapter IV, the medical officer-in-charge of a psychiatric hospital or psychiatric nursing home may, on the recommendation of two medical practitioners one of whom shall preferably be a psychiatrist, by order in writing, direct the discharge of any person other than a voluntary patient detained or undergoing treatment therein as an in-patient, and such person shall thereupon be discharged from the psychiatric hospital or psychiatric nursing home:

Provided that no order under this sub-section shall be made in respect of a mentally ill prisoner otherwise than as provided in Section 30 of the Prisoner Act, 1900 (3 of 1900), or in any other relevant law.

Where any order of discharge is made under sub-section (1) in respect of a person who had been detained or is undergoing treatment as in-patient in pursuance of an order off any authority, a copy of such hospital/nursing home.

41. Discharge of mentally ill persons on application—

Any person detained in a psychiatric hospital or psychiatric nursing home under an order and in pursuance of an application made under this Act, shall be discharged on an application made in that behalf to the medical officer in charge by the person on whose application the order was made:

Provided that no person shall be discharged under this section if the medical officer in charge certifies in writing that the person is dangerous and unfit to be at large.

42. Order of discharge on the undertaking of relatives or friends, etc. for due care of mentally ill persons—

(1)   Where any relative of friend of a mentally ill person detained in a psychiatric hospital or psychiatric nursing home under Section 22, Section 24 or Section 25 desires that such person shall be delivered over to his care and custody, he may make an application to the medical officer-in-charge who shall forward it together with his remarks thereon to the authority under whose orders the mentally ill person is detained.

(2)   Where an application is received under sub-section (1), the authority shall, on such relative or friend furnishing a bond, with or without sureties, for such amounts as such authority may specify in this behalf, undertaking to take proper care of such mentally ill person, and ensuring that the mentally ill person shall be prevented from causing injury to himself or to others, make an order of discharge and thereupon the mentally ill person shall be discharged.

43. Discharge of person on his request

(1)   Any person (not being a mentally ill prisoner) detained in pursuance of an order made under this Act who feels that he has recovered from his mental illness, may make an application to the Magistrate, where necessary under the provisions of this Act, for his discharge from the psychiatric hospital or psychiatric nursing home.

(2)   An application made under sub-section (1) shall be supported by a certificate either from the medical officer in-charge of the psychiatric hospital or psychiatric nursing home where the applicant is undergoing treatment or from a psychiatrist.

(3)   The Magistrate may, after making such inquiry as he may deem fit, pass an order discharging the person or dismissing the application.

44. Discharge of person subsequently found on inquisition to be of sound mind—

If any person detained in a psychiatric hospital or psychiatric nursing home in pursuance of a reception order made under this Act is subsequently found, on an inquisition held in accordance with the provisions of Chapter VI, to be of sound mind or capable of taking care of himself and managing his affairs, the medical officer-in-charge shall forthwith, on the production of a copy of such finding duly certified by the District Court, discharge such person from such hospital or nursing home.

Part III—Leave of Absence

45. Leave of absence—

(1)   An application for leave of absence on behalf of any mentally ill person (not being a mentally ill prisoner) undergoing treatment as an inpatient in any psychiatric hospital or psychiatric nursing home may be made to the medical officer in charge:

(i)   in the case of a person who was admitted on the application of the husband or wife, by the husband or wife of such mentally ill person, or where by reason of mental or physical illness, absence from India or otherwise, the husband or wife is not in a position to make such application, by any other relative of the mentally ill person duly authorized by the husband or wife, or

(ii)   in the case of any other person, by the person on whose application the mentally ill person was admitted.

    Provided that no application under this sub-section shall be made by a person who has not attained the age of majority.

(2)   Every application under sub-section (1) shall be accompanied by a bond, with or without sureties for such amount as the medical officer-in-charge may specify, undertaking:

(i)   to take proper care of the mentally ill person,

(ii)   to prevent the mentally ill person from causing injury to himself or to others, and

(iii)   to bring back the mentally ill person to the psychiatric hospital, or, as the case may be, psychiatric nursing home, on the expiry of the period of leave.

(3)   On receipt of an application under sub-section (1), the medical officers in charge may grant leave of absence to the mentally ill persons for such period as the medical officers-in-charge may deem necessary and subject to such condition as may, in the interests of the protection of others, be specified in the order:

    Provided that the total number of days for which leave of absence may be granted to a patient under this sub-section shall not exceed 60 days.

(4)   Where the mentally ill persons is not brought back to the psychiatric hospital or psychiatric nursing home on the expiry of the leave granted to him under this section the medical officer-in-charge shall forthwith report that fact to the Magistrate within the local limits of whose jurisdiction such hospital or nursing home is situate and the Magistrate may, after making such inquiry as he may deem fit, make an order directing him to be brought back to the psychiatric hospital or psychiatric nursing home, as the case may be.

(5) Nothing contained in this section shall apply to a voluntary patient referred to in Section 15 or Section 16 and the provisions of Section 18 shall apply to him.

46. Grant of leave of absence by Magistrate—

(1) Where the medical officer in charge refuses to grant leave of absence to a mentally ill person under Section 45, the applicant may apply to the Magistrate within the local limits of whose jurisdiction the psychiatric hospital or psychiatric nursing home wherein the mentally ill person is detained is situate, for the grant of leave of absence to the mentally ill person and the Magistrate may if he is satisfied that it is necessary so to do, and on the applicant entering into a bond in accordance with the provisions of sub-section (2), by order grant leave of absence to the mentally ill person for such period and subject to such conditions as may be specified in the order.

(2) Every bond referred to in sub-section (1) shall be with or without sureties and for such amount as the Magistrate may decide and shall contain the undertaking referred to in sub-section (2) of Section 45.

(3) The Magistrate shall forward a copy of the order to the medical officer-in-charge and on receipt of such order the medical officer-in-charge shall entrust the mentally ill person to the person on whose application the leave of absence was granted under this section.

Part IV—Removal

47. Removal of mentally ill person from one psychiatric hospital or psychiatric nursing home to any other psychiatric hospital or psychiatric nursing home—

(1) Any mentally ill person other than a voluntary patient referred to in Section 15 or Section 16 may, subject to any general or special order of the State Government, be removed from any psychiatric hospital or psychiatric nursing home to any other psychiatric hospital or psychiatric nursing home within the State, or to any other psychiatric hospital or psychiatric nursing home in any other State with the consent of the Government of that other State:

Provided that no mentally ill person admitted to a psychiatric hospital or psychiatric nursing home under an order made in pursuance of an application made under the Act shall be so removed unless intimation thereof has been given to the applicant.

(2) The State Government may make such general or special order as it thinks fit directing the removal of any mentally ill prisoner from the place where he is for the time being detained, to any psychiatric hospital, psychiatric nursing home, jail or other place of safe custody in the State or to any psychiatric hospital, psychiatric nursing home, jail or other place of safe custody in any other State with the consent of the Government of that other State.

48. Admission, detention and retaking in certain cases—

Every person brought into a psychiatric hospital or psychiatric nursing home under any order made under this Act, may be detained or, as the case may be, admitted as an in-patient therein until he is removed or is discharged under any law, and in case of his escape from such hospital or nursing home he may, by virtue of such order, be retaken by any police officer or by the medical officer-in-charge or any officer or servant of such hospital or nursing home, or by any other person authorized in that behalf by the medical officer-in-charge and conveyed to, and received and detained or, as the case may be, kept as an in-patient in such hospital or nursing home:

Provided that in the case of a mentally ill person (not being a mentally ill prisoner) the power to retake as aforesaid under this section shall not be exercisable after the expiry of a period of one month from the date of his escape.

49. Appeal from orders of Magistrate—

Any person aggrieved by any order of a Magistrate, passed under any of the foregoing provisions may, within 60 days from the date of the order, appeal against that order to the District Court within the local limits of whose jurisdiction the Magistrate exercised the powers, and decision of the District Court on such appeal shall be final.

CHAPTER VI: JUDICIAL INQUISITION REGARDING ALLEGED MENTALLY ILL PERSON POSSESSING PROPERTY, CUSTODY OF HIS PERSON AND MANAGEMENT OF HIS PROPERTY

50. Application for judicial inquisition

(1)   Where an alleged mentally ill person is possessed of property, an application for holding an inquisition into the mental condition of such person may be made either–

    (i)   by any of his relatives

    (ii)   by a public curator appointed under the Indian Succession Act, 1925 (39 of 1925)

    (iii)   by the Advocate-General of the State in which the alleged mentally ill person resides

    (iv)   where the property of the alleged mentally ill person comprises land or interest in land, or where the property or part thereof is of such a nature as can lawfully be entrusted for management to a Court of Wards established under any law for the time being in force in the State, by the Collector of the District in which such land is situate, to the District Court within the local limits of whose jurisdiction the alleged mentally ill person resides.

(2)   On receipt of an application under sub-section (1), the District Court shall, by personal service or by such other mode of service as it may deem fit, serve a notice on the alleged mentally ill person to attend at such place and at such time as may be specified in the notice or shall, in like manner, serve a notice on the person having the custody of the alleged mentally person to produce such person at the said place and at the said time, for being examined by the District Court or by any other person from whom the District Court may call for a report concerning the mentally ill person:

Provided that, if the alleged mentally ill person is a woman, who according to the custom prevailing in the area where she resides or according to the religion to which she belongs, ought not to be compelled to appear in public, the District Court may cause her to be examined by issuing a commission as provided in the Code of Civil Procedure, 1908 (5 of 1908).

(3)   A copy of the notice under sub-section (2) shall also be served upon the applicant and upon any relative of the alleged mentally ill person or other person who, in the opinion of the District Court, shall have notice of judicial inquisition to be held by it.

(4)   For the purpose of holding the inquisition applied for, the District Court may appoint two or more persons to act as assessors.

51. Issues on which finding should be given by district court after inquisition—

On completion of the inquisition, the District Court shall record its findings on:

(1)   whether the alleged mentally ill person is in fact mentally ill or not

(2)   where such person is mentally ill, whether he is incapable of taking care of himself and managing his property, or incapable of managing his property only.

52. Provision for appointing guardian of mentally ill person and for manager of property—

(1) Where the District Court records a finding that the alleged mentally ill person is in fact mentally ill and is incapable of taking care of himself and of managing his property, it shall make an order for the appointment of a guarding under Section 53 to take care of his person and of a manager under Section 54 for the management of his property.

(2) Where the District Court records a finding that the alleged mentally ill person is in fact mentally ill and is incapable of managing his property but capable of taking care of himself, it shall make an order under Section 54 regarding the management of his property.

(3) Where the District Court records a finding that the alleged mentally ill person is not mentally ill, it shall dismiss the application.

(4) Where the District Court deems fit, it may appoint under sub-section (1) the same person to be the guardian and manager.

53. Appointment of guardian of mentally ill person—

(1) Where the mentally ill person is incapable of taking care of himself, the District Court or, where a direction has been issued under sub-section (2) of Section 54, the Collector of the District, may appoint any suitable person to be his guardian.

(2) In the discharge of his functions under sub-section (1), the Collector shall be subject to the supervision and control of the State Government or of any authority appointed by it in that behalf.

54. Appointment of manager for management of property of mentally ill person—

(1) Where the property of the mentally ill person who is incapable of managing it is such as can be taken charge of by a Court of Wards under any law for the time being in force, the District Court shall authorize the Court of Wards to take charge of such property, and thereupon notwithstanding anything contained in such law, the Court of Wards shall assume the management of such property in accordance with that law.

(2) Where the property of the mentally ill person consists in whole or in part of land or of any interest in land which cannot be taken charge of by the Court of Wards, the District Court may, after obtaining the consent of the Collector of the District in which the land is situate, direct the Collector to take charge of the person and such part of the property or interest therein of the mentally ill person as cannot be taken charge of by the Court of Wards.

(3) Where the management of the property of the mentally ill person cannot be entrusted to the Court of Wards or to the Collector under sub-section (1) or sub-Section (2), as the case may be, the District Court shall appoint any suitable person to be the manager of such property.

55. Appointment of manager by collector—

Where the property of a mentally ill person has been entrusted to the Collector by the District Court under sub-section (2) of Section 54, he may, subject to the control of the State Government or of any authority appointed by it in that behalf, appoint any suitable person for the management of the property of the mentally ill person.

56. Manager of property to execute bond—

Every person who is appointed as the manager of the property of a mentally ill person by the District Court or by the Collector shall, if so required by the appointing authority, enter into a bond for such sum, in such form and with such sureties as that authority may specify, to account for all receipts from the property of the mentally ill person.

57. Appointment and remuneration of guardians and managers

(1) No person, who is the legal heir of a mentally ill person shall be appointed under Section 53, 54 or 55 to be the guardian of such mentally ill person or, as the case may be, the manager of his property unless the District Court or, as the case may be, the Collector, for reasons to be recorded in writing, considers that such appointment is for the benefit of the mentally ill person.

(2) The guardian of a mentally ill person or the manager of the property or both appointed under this Act shall be paid, from out of the property of the mentally ill person, such allowance as the appointing authority may determine.

58. Duties of guardian and manager—

(1) Every person appointed as a guardian of a mentally ill person or manager of his property, or of both, under this Act shall have the care of the mentally ill person or his property or of both, and be responsible for the maintenance of the mentally ill person and of such members of his family as are dependent on him.

(2) Where the person appointed as guardian of a mentally ill person is different from the person appointed as the manager of his property, the manager of his property shall pay to the guardian of the mentally ill person such allowance as may be fixed by the authority appointing the guardian for the maintenance of the mentally ill person and of such members of his family as are dependent on him.

59. Powers of manager—

(1) Every manager under this Act shall, subject to the provisions of this Act, exercise the same powers in regard to the management of the property of the mentally ill person in respect of which he is appointed as manager, as the mentally ill person would have exercised as owner of the property had he not been mentally ill and shall realize all claims due to the estate of the mentally ill person and pay all debts and discharge all liabilities legally due from that estate:

Provided that the manager shall not mortgage, create any charge on, or, transfer by sale, gift, exchange or otherwise, any immoveable property of the mentally ill person or lease out any such property for a period exceeding 5 years, unless he obtains the permission of the District Court in that behalf.

(2) The District Court may, on an application made by the manager, grant him permission to mortgage. Create a charge on, or, transfer by sale, gift, exchange or otherwise, any immoveable property of the mentally ill person or to lease out any such property for a period exceeding 5 years, subject to such conditions or restrictions as that Court may think fit to impose.

(3) The District Court shall cause notice of every application for permission to be served on any relative or friend of the mentally ill person and after considering objections, if any, received from the relative or friend and after making such inquiries as it may deem necessary, grant or refuse permission having regard to the interests of the mentally ill person.

60. Manager to furnish inventory and annual accounts—

(1) Every manager appointed under this Act shall, within a period of six months from the date of his appointment, deliver to the authority, which appointed him, an inventory of the immoveable property belonging to the mentally ill person and of all assets and other moveable property received on behalf of the mentally ill person, together with a statement of all claims due to and all debts and liabilities due by, such mentally ill person.

(2) Every such manager shall also furnish to the said appointing authority within a period of three months of the close of every financial year, an account of the property and assets in his charge, the sums received and disbursed on account of the mentally ill person and the balance remaining with him.

61. Manager's power to execute conveyances under orders of district court—

Every manager appointed under this Act, may, in the name and on behalf of the mentally ill person:

(i)   Execute all such conveyance and instruments of transfers by way of sale, mortgage or otherwise of property of the mentally ill person as may be permitted by the District Court and

(ii) Subject to the orders of the District Court, exercise all powers vested in that behalf in the mentally ill person, in his individual capacity or in his capacity as a trustee or as a guardian.

62. Manager to perform contracts directed by district court—

Where the mentally ill person had, before his mental illness, contracted to sell or otherwise dispose of his property or any portion thereof, and if such contract is, in the opinion of the District Court, of such a nature as ought to be performed, the District Court may direct the manager appointed under this Act to perform such contract and to do such other acts in fulfillment of the contract as the Court considers necessary and thereupon the manager shall be bound to act accordingly.

63. Disposal of business premises—

Where a mentally ill person had been engaged in business before he became mentally ill, the District Court may, if it appears to be for the benefit of the mentally ill person to dispose of his business premises, direct the manager appointed under this Act in relation to the property of such person to sell and dispose of such premises and to apply the sale proceeds thereof in such manner as the District Court may direct and thereupon the manager shall be bound to act accordingly.

64. Manager may dispose of leases—

Where a mentally ill person is entitled to a lease or under lease, and it appears to the manager appointed under this Act in relation to the property of such person that it would be for the benefit of the mentally ill person to dispose of such leas or under lease, such manager may, after obtaining the orders of the District Court, surrender, assign or otherwise dispose of such lease or under lease to such person for such consideration and upon such terms and conditions as the Court may direct.

65. Power to make order concerning any matter connected with mentally ill person—

The District Court may, on an application made to mentally ill person or his property, make such order, subject to the provisions of this Chapter, in relation to that matter as in the circumstances it thinks fit.

66. Proceeding if accuracy of inventory or accounts is impugned—

If any relative of the mentally ill person or the collector impugns, by a petition to the District Court, the accuracy of the inventory or statement referred to in sub-section (1), or, as the case may be, any annual account referred to in sub-section (2) of Section 60, the Court may summon the manager and summarily inquire into the matter and make such order thereon as it thinks fit.

Provided that the District Court may, in its discretion, refer such petition to any Court subordinate to it, or to the Collector in any case where the manager was appointed by the Collector and the petition is not presented by the Collector.

67. Payment into public treasury and investment of proceeds of estate—

All sums received by a manager on account of any estate in excess of what may be required for the current expenses of the mentally ill person or for the management of his property, shall be paid into the public treasury on account of the estate, and shall be invested from time to time in any of the securities specified in Section 20 of the Indian Trusts Act, 1882 (2 of 1982), unless the authority which appointed him, for reasons to be recorded in writing, directs that, in the interests of the mentally ill person such sums be otherwise invested or applied.

68. Relative may sue for account

Any relative of a mentally ill person may, with the leave of the District Court, sue for an account from any manager appointed under this Act, or from any such person after his removal from office or trust, or from his legal representative in the case of his death, in respect of any property then or formerly under his management or of any sum of money or other property received by him on account of such property.

69. Removal of managers and guardians—

(1)   The manager of the property of a mentally ill person may, for sufficient cause and for reasons to be recorded in writing, be removed by the authority which appointed him and such authority may appoint a new manager in his place.

(2)   Any manager removed under sub-section (1) shall be bound to deliver the charge of all property of the mentally ill person to the new manager and to account for all moneys received or disbursed by him.

(3)   The District Court may, for sufficient cause, remove any guardian of a mentally ill person and appoint in his place a new guardian.

70. Dissolution and disposal of property of partnership on a member becoming mentally ill—

(1)   Where a person, being a member of a partnership firm, is found to be mentally ill, the District Court may, on the application of any other partner for the dissolution of partnership or on the application of any person who appears to that Court to be entitled to seek such dissolution, dissolve the partnership.

(2)   Upon the dissolution under sub-section (1), or otherwise, in due course of law, of a partnership firm to which that sub-section applies, the manager appointed under this Act may, in the name and on behalf of the mentally ill person, join with the other partners in disposing of the partnership property upon such terms, and shall do all such acts for carrying into effect the dissolution of the partnership, as the District Court may direct.

71. Power to apply property for maintenance of mentally ill person without appointing manager in certain cases—

(1)   Notwithstanding anything contained in the foregoing provisions, the District Court may, instead of appointing a manager of the estate, order that in the case of cash, the cash and in the case of any other property the produce thereof, shall be realized and paid or delivered to such person as may be appointed by the District Court in this behalf, to be applied for the maintenance of the mentally ill person and of such members of his family as are dependent on him.

(2)   A receipt given by the person appointed under sub-section (1) shall be valid discharge to any person who pays money or delivers any property of the mentally ill person to the person so appointed.

72. Power to order transfer of stock, securities or shares belonging to mentally ill person in certain cases—

Where any stock or Government securities or any share in a company (transferable within India or the dividends of which are payable therein) is or are standing in the name of, or vested in, a mentally ill person beneficially entitled thereto, or in the manager appointed under this Act or in a trustee for him, and the manager dies intestate, or himself becomes mentally ill, or is out of the jurisdiction of the District Court, or it is uncertain whether the manager is living or dead, or he neglects or refuses to transfer the stock, securities or shares, or to receive and pay over thereof the dividends to a new manager appointed in his place, within 14 days after being required by the Court to do so, then the District Court may direct the company or Government concerned to make such transfer, or to transfer the same, and to receive and pay over the dividends in such manner as it may direct.

73. **Power to order transfer of stock, securities or shares of mentally ill person residing out of India—**

Where any stock or Government securities or share in a company is or are standing in the name of, or vested in, any person residing out of India, the District Court upon being satisfied that such person has been declared to be mentally ill and that his personal estate has been vested in a person appointed for the management thereof, according to the law of the place where he is residing, may direct the company or Government concerned to make such transfer of the stock, securities or shares or of any part thereof, to or into the name of the person so appointed or otherwise, and also to receive and pay over the dividends and proceeds, as the District Court thinks fit.

74. **Power to apply property for mentally ill person's maintenance in case of temporary mental illness—**

If it appears to the District Court that the mental illness of a mentally ill person is in its nature temporary, and that it is expedient to make provision for a temporary period, for his maintenance for the maintenance of such members of his family as are dependent on him, the District Court may, in like manner as under Section 71, direct his property or a sufficient part thereof to be applied for the purpose specified therein.

75. **Action taken in respect of mentally ill person to be set aside if district court finds that his mental illness has ceased—**

    (1) Where District Court has reason to believe that any person who was found to be mentally ill after inquisition under this Chapter has ceased to be mentally ill, it may direct any Court subordinate to it to inquire whether such person has ceased to be mentally ill.

    (2) An inquiry under sub-section (1) shall, so far as may be, conducted in the same manner as an inquisition conducted under this Chapter.

    (3) If after an inquiry under this section, it is found that the mental illness of a person has ceased, the District Court shall order all actions taken in respect of the mentally ill person under this Act to be set aside on such terms and conditions as that Court thinks fit to impose.

76. **Power of district court to make regulations—**

The District Court may, from time to time, make regulations for the purpose of carrying out the provisions of this Chapter.

CHAPTER VII: LIABILITY TO MEET COST OF MAINTENANCE OF MENTALLY ILL PERSONS DETAINED IN PSYCHIATRIC HOSPITAL OR PSYCHIATRIC NURSING HOME

77. **Cost of maintenance to be borne by government in certain cases—**

The cost of maintenance of a mentally ill person detained as an in-patient in any psychiatric hospital or psychiatric nursing home shall, unless otherwise provided for by any law for the time being in force, be borne by the Government of the State wherein the authority which passed the order in relation to the mentally ill person is subordinate, if:

    (1) That authority which made the order has not taken an undertaking from any person to bear the cost of maintenance of such mentally ill person, and

    (2) No provision for bearing the cost of maintenance of such a District Court under this Chapter.

78. **Application to district court for payment of cost of maintenance out of estate of mentally ill person or from a person legally bound to maintain him—**

    (1) Where any mentally ill person detained in a psychiatric hospital or psychiatric nursing home has an estate or where any person legally bound to maintain such person has the means to maintain such person, the Government liable to pay the cost of maintenance of such person under Section 78 or any local authority liable to bear the cost of maintenance of such mentally ill person under any law for the time being in force, may make an application to the District Court within whose jurisdiction the estate of the mentally ill person is situate or the person legally bound to maintain the mentally ill person and having the means therefor resides, for an order authorizing it to apply the estate of the mentally ill person to the cost of maintenance or, as the case may be, directing the person legally bound to maintain the mentally ill person and having the means therefor to bear the cost of maintenance of such mentally ill person.

    (2) An order made by the District Court under sub-section (1) shall be enforced in the same manner, shall have the same force and effect and be subject to appeal, as a decree made by such Court in a suit in respect of the property or person mentioned therein.

79. **Persons legally bound to maintain mentally ill person not absolved from such liability—**

    Nothing contained in the foregoing provisions shall be deemed to absolve a person legally bound to maintain a mentally ill person from maintaining such mentally ill person.

CHAPTER VIII: PROTECTION OF HUMAN RIGHTS OF MENTALLY ILL PERSONS

80. **Protection of human rights of mentally ill persons—**

    (1) No mentally ill person shall be subjected during treatment to any indignity (whether physical or mental) or cruelty.

    (2) No mentally ill person under treatment shall be used for purposes of research, unless:

    (i) such research is of direct benefit to him for purposes of diagnosis or treatment, or

    (ii) such person, being a voluntary patient, has given his consent in writing or where such person (whether or not a voluntary patient) is incompetent, by reason of minority or otherwise, to give valid consent, the guardian or other person competent to give consent on his behalf, has given his consent in writing, for such research.

    (ii) subject to any rules made in this behalf under Section 94 for the purpose of preventing vexatious or defamatory communications or communications prejudicial to the treatment of mentally ill persons, no letters or other communications sent by or to a mentally ill person under treatment shall be intercepted, detained or destroyed.

CHAPTER IX: PENALTIES AND PROCEDURE

81. **Penalty for establishment or maintenance of psychiatric hospital or psychiatric nursing home in contravention—**

    (1) Any person who establishes or maintains a psychiatric hospital or psychiatric nursing home in contravention of the provisions of Chapter III shall, on conviction, be punishable with imprisonment for a term which may extend to three months, or with fine which may extend to two hundred rupees, or with both, and in the case of a second or subsequent offence, with imprisonment for a term which may extend to six months, or with fine which may extend to one thousand rupees, or with both.

(2) Whoever, after conviction under sub-section (1) continues to maintain a psychiatric hospital or psychiatric nursing home in contravention of the provisions of Chapter III shall, on conviction, be punishable with fine which may extend to one hundred rupees, for every day after the first day during which the contravention is continued.

82. Penalty for improper reception of mentally ill person—

Any person who receives or detains or keeps a mentally ill person in a psychiatric hospital or psychiatric nursing home otherwise than in accordance with the provision of this Act, shall, on conviction, be punishable with imprisonment for a term which may extend to 2 years or with fine which may extend to one thousand rupees, or with both.

83. Penalty for contravention of Sections 60 and 69—

Any manager appointed under this Act to manage the property of a mentally ill person who contravenes the provisions of Section 60 or sub-section (2) of Section 69, shall, on conviction, be punishable with fine which may extend to two thousand rupees and may be detained in a civil prison till he complies with the said provisions.

84. General provision for punishment of other offences—

Any person who contravenes any of the provisions of this Act or of any rule or regulation made thereunder, for the contravention of which no penalty is expressly provided, in this Act, shall, on conviction, be punishable with imprisonment for a term which may extend to six months, or with fine which may extend to five hundred rupees, or with both.

85. Offences by companies—

(1) Where an offence under this Act has been committed by a company, every person who, at the time of offence was committed, was in charge of, and was responsible to, the company for the conduct of the business of the company, as well as the company, shall be deemed to be guilty of the offence and shall be liable to be proceeded against and punished accordingly.

(2) Notwithstanding anything contained in sub-section (1), where an offence under this Act has been committed by a company and it is proved that the offence has been committed with the consent or connivance of, or is attributable to any neglect on the part of, any director, manager, secretary or other officer of the company, such director, manager, secretary or other officer shall also be deemed to be guilty of that offence and shall be liable to be proceeded against and punished accordingly.

Penal provision: Penal provision is to be construed rigidly.

86. Sanction for prosecutions—

Notwithstanding anything contained in the Code of Criminal Procedure, 1973 (2 of 1974), no Court shall take cognizance of any offence punishable under Section 82, except with the previous sanction of the licensing authority.

CHAPTER X: MISCELLANEOUS

87. Provision as to bonds—

The provisions of Chapter XXXIII of the Code of Criminal Procedure, 1973 (2 of 1974) shall, as far as may be apply to bonds taken under this Act.

Comment—This section makes provision as to bonds taken under this Act.

88. Report by medical officer—

The medical officer-in-charge of a psychiatric hospital or psychiatric nursing home shall, as soon as may be, after any mentally ill person detained therein has been discharged make a report in respect of his mental and physical condition to the authority under whose orders such person had been so detained.

89. Pension, etc. of mentally ill person payable by government—

(1) Where any sum is payable in respect of pay, pension, gratuity or any allowance to any person by any Government and the person to whom the sum is payable is certified by a Magistrate under this Act to be a mentally ill person, the officer under whose authority such sum would be payable, may pay to the person having charge of the mentally ill person so much of the said sum as he thinks fit, having regard to the cost of maintenance of such person and may pay to such member of the family of the mentally ill person as are dependent on him for maintenance, the surplus, if any, or such part thereof as he thinks fit, having regard to the cost of maintenance of such members.

(2) Where there is any further surplus amount available out of the funds specified in sub-section (1) after making payments as provided in that sub-section, the Government shall hold the same to be dealt with as follows namely:

    (i) where the mentally ill person is certified to have ceased to be mentally ill person by the District Court within the local limits of whose jurisdiction such person resides or is kept or detains, the whole of the surplus amount shall be paid back to that person

    (ii) where the mentally ill person dies before payment, the whole of the surplus amount shall be paid over to those of his heirs who are legally entitled to receive the same

    (iii) where the mentally ill person dies during his mental illness without leaving any person legally entitled to succeed to his estate, the whole of the surplus amount shall, with the prior permission of the District Court, be utilized for such charitable purpose as may be approved by the District Court.

(3) The Central Government or the State Government, as the case may be, shall be discharged of all liability in respect of any amount paid in accordance with this section.

90. Legal aid to mentally ill person at state expense in certain cases—

(1) Where a mentally ill person is not represented by a legal practitioner in any proceeding under this Act before a District Court or a Magistrate and it appears to the District Court or Magistrate that such person has not sufficient means to engage a legal practitioner, the District Court or Magistrate shall assign a legal practitioner to represent him at the expense of the State.

(2) Where a mentally ill person having sufficient means to engage a legal practitioner is not represented by a legal practitioner in any proceeding under this Act before a District Court or a Magistrate and it appears to the District Court or Magistrate, having regard to all the circumstances of the case, that such person ought to be represented by a legal practitioner, the District Court, or Magistrate may assign a legal practitioner to represent him and direct the State to bear the expenses with respect thereto and recover the same from out of the property of such person.

(3) The High Court may, with the previous approval of the State Government, make rules providing for:

    (a) The mode of selecting legal practitioners for the purpose of Sub-section (1) and (2)

    (b) The facilities to be allowed to such legal practitioners

    (c) The fees payable to such legal practitioners by the Government and generally for carrying out the purpose of sub-sections (1) and (2).

91. Protection of action taken in good faith—

(1) No suit, prosecution or other legal proceeding shall lie against any person for anything which is in good faith done or intended to be done in pursuance of this Act or any rules, regulations or orders made thereunder.

(2) No suit or other legal proceeding shall lie against the Government for any damage caused or likely to be caused for anything which is in good faith done or intended to be done in pursuance of this Act or any rules, regulations or orders made thereunder.

92. Construction of reference to certain laws, etc.—

(1) Any reference in this Act to a law which is not in force in any area shall, in relation to that area, be construed as a reference to the corresponding law, if any, in force in that area.

(2) Any reference in this Act to any officer or authority shall, in relation to any area in which there is no offer or authority with the same designation, be construed as a reference to such officer or authority as may be specified by the Central Government by notification.

Social welfare legislation—In construing social welfare legislation, the Courts should adopt a beneficent rule of construction and in any event, that construction should be preferred which fulfils the policy of the legislation. Construction to be adopted should be more beneficial to the purposes in favor of and in whose interest the Act has been passed.

93. Power of Central Government and State Government to make rules—

(1) The Central Government may, by notification, make rules providing for the qualifications of persons who may be appointed as Mental Health Authority under Section 3 and the terms and conditions subject to which they may be appointed under that section and all other matters relating to such authority.

(2) Subject to the provisions of sub-section (1), the State Government, with the previous approval of the Central Government may, by notification, make rules for carrying out the provisions of this Act: Provided that the first rules shall be made by the Central Government by notification.

(3) In particular, and without prejudice to the generality of the foregoing power, rules made under sub-section (2) may provide for all or any of the following matters, namely:

   (i) The qualifications of persons who may be appointed as Mental Health Authority and the terms and conditions subject to which they may be appointed under Section 4 and all other matters relating to such authority

   (ii) The class or category of persons for whom separate psychiatric hospitals and psychiatric nursing homes may be established and maintained under Cl. (d) of sub-section (1) of Section 5

   (iii) The form in which,—

      (a) an application, may be made for grant or renewal of a license and the fee payable in respect thereof under Section 7 or as the case may be, Section 9

      (b) a license may be granted for the establishment or maintenance of a psychiatric hospital or a psychiatric nursing home under Section 8

      (c) an application may be made for a reception order under Section 20

      The manner in which an order refusing to grant, or revoking, a license shall be communicated under Section 8 or, as the case may be Section 11

      The manner in which a report may be made to the licensing authority under sub-section (2) of Section 9

      The minimum facilities referred to in the proviso to sub-section (5) of Section 9 including—

      Psychiatrist-patient ratio

      Other medical or paramedical staff

      Space requirement

      Treatment facilities and

      Equipment:

- The manner in which and the conditions subject to which a psychiatric hospital or psychiatric nursing home shall be maintained under Section 10.
- The form and manner in which and the period within which an appeal against any order refusing to grant or renew a license or revoking a license shall be preferred and the fee payable in respect thereof under Section 12.

- The manner in which records shall be maintained under sub-section (1) of Section 13.
- The facilities to be provided under Section 14 of the treatment of a mentally ill person as an outpatient
- The manner in which application for a reception order shall be signed and verified under sub-section (6) of Section 20
- The qualification of persons who may be appointed as visitors and the terms and conditions on which they may be appointed, under Section 37 and their functions
- Prevention of vexatious or defamatory communications and other matters referred to in sub-section (3) of Section 81
- Any other matter which is required to be, or may be, prescribed.

Rules of construction—It is well-settled canon of construction that the rules made under a statute must be treated exactly as if they were in the Act and are of the same effect as if contained in the Act. There is another principle equally fundamental to the rules of construction, namely, that the rules shall be consistent with the provision of the Act.

94. Rules made by Central Government or the State Government to be laid before the legislature—

(1) Every rule made by the Central Government under this Act shall be laid, as soon as may be after it is made, before each House of Parliament, while it is in session, for a total period of 30 days which may be comprised in one session or in two or more successive sessions, and if, before the expiry of the session immediately following the session or the successive sessions aforesaid, both Houses agree in making any modification in the rule or both Houses agree that the rule should not be made, the rule shall thereafter have effect only if such modified form or be of no effect, as the case may be so, however, that any such modification or annulment shall be without prejudice to the validity of anything previously done under that rule.

(2) Every rule made by the State Government under this Act shall be laid, as soon as may be after it is made, before the State Legislature.

95. Effect of act on other laws—

The provisions of this Act shall have effect notwithstanding anything inconsistent therewith contained in any other law for the time being in force and to the extent of such inconsistency that other law shall be deemed to have no effect.

96. Power to remove difficulty—

If any difficulty arises in giving effect to the provisions of this Act in any State, the State Government may, by order, do anything not inconsistent with such provisions which appears to it to be necessary or expedient for the purpose of removing the difficulty:

Provided that no order shall be made under this section in relation to any State after the expiry of 2 years from the date on which this Act comes into force in that State.

97. Repeal and saving

(1) The Indian Lunacy Act, 1912 (4 of 1912) and the Lunacy Act, 1977 [Jammu and Kashmir Act 25 of 1977 (1920 AD)] are hereby repealed.

(2) Notwithstanding such repeal, anything done or any action taken under either of the said Acts shall, in so far as such thing or action is not inconsistent with the provisions of this Act, be deemed to have been done or taken under the corresponding provisions of this Act and shall continue in force until superseded by anything done or any action taken under this Act.

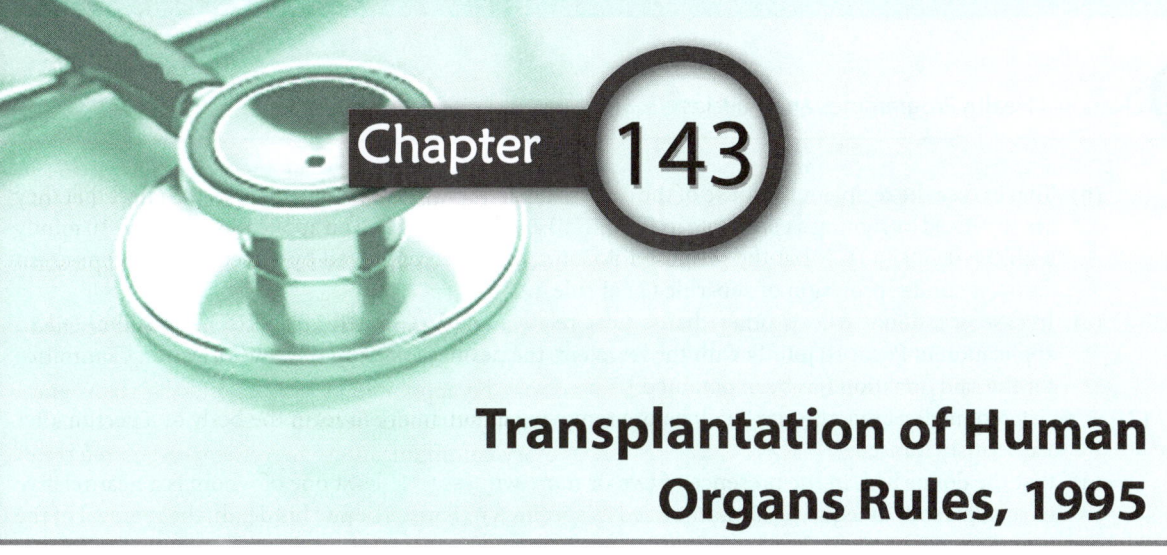

Chapter 143

Transplantation of Human Organs Rules, 1995

GSR NO. 51(E), in exercise of the powers conferred by sub-section (1) if section 24 of the Transplantation of Human Organs Act, 1994 (42 of 1994), the Central Government hereby makes the following rules, namely:-

1. **Short title and commencement:**
   (1) These rules may be called the Transplantation of Human Organs Rules, 1995.
   (2) They shall come into force on the date of their publication in the Official Gazette.

2. **Definitions:**
   (a) "Act" means the Transplantation of Human Organs Act, 1994 (42 of 1994);
   (b) "Form" means a form annexed to these Rules;
   (c) "Section" means a section of the Act;
   (d) "National Accreditation Board for Laboratories" (NABL) means a Board set up by the Quality Council of India (set up by the Government of India) for undertaking assessment and accreditation of testing and calibration of laboratories in accordance with the international standard ISO/IEC/17025 and ISO 15189;
   (e) The Registered Medical Practitioner, as defined in clause (n) of section 2 of Transplantation of Human Organs Act, 1994 includes an allopathic doctor with MBBS or equivalent degree under the Medical Council of India Act.
   (f) Words and expressions used and not defined in these Rules, but defined in the Act, shall have the same meanings respectively assigned to them in the Act.

3. **Authority for removal of human organ:-** Any donor may authorize the removal, before his death, of any human organ of his body for therapeutic purposes in the manner and so such conditions as specified in [4][Forms 1(A), 1(B) and 1(C).

4. **Duties of the Medical Practitioner:**
   (1) A registered medical practitioner shall, before removing a human organ from the body of a donor before his death, satisfy himself–
   (a) that the donor has given his authorization in Form 1(A) or 1(B) or 1(C).
   (b) that the donor is in proper state of health and is fit to donate the organ, and the registered medical practitioner shall sign a certificate as specified in Form 2.
   (c) that the donor is a near relative of the recipient as certified in Form 3, who has signed Form 1(A) or 1(B) as applicable to the donor and that the donor has submitted an application in Form 10 jointly with the recipient and that the proposed donation has been approved by the concerned competent authority and that the necessary documents as prescribed and medical tests, if required, to determine the factum of near relationship, have been examined to the satisfaction of the Registered Medical Practitioner, i.e., In charge of transplant center.

(d) That in case the recipient is spouse of the donor, the donor has given a statement to the effect that they are so related by signing a certificate in Form 1(B) and has submitted an application in Form 10 jointly with the recipient and that the proposed donation has been approved by the concerned competent authority under provision of sub-rule (2) of rule 4A.

(e) In case of a donor who is other than a near relative and has singed Form 1(C) and submitted an application in Form 10 jointly with the recipient, the permission from the Authorization Committee for the said donation has been obtained.]

(2) A registered medical practitioner shall, before removing a human organ form the body of a person after his death satisfy himself:

(a) that the donor had, in the presence of two or more witnesses (at least one of whom is a near relative of such person), unequivocally authorized as specified in Form 5 before his death, the removal of the human organ of his body, after his death, for therapeutic purposes and there is no reason to believe that the donor had subsequently revoked the authority aforesaid;

(b) that then person lawfully in possession of the dead body has signed a certificate as specified in Form 6.]

(3) A registered medical practitioner shall, before removing a human organ from the body of a person in the event of his brain stem death, satisfy himself:

(a) that a certificate as specified in Form 8 has been signed by all the members of the Board of Medical Experts referred to in sub-section (6) of section 3 of the Act;

(b) that in the case of brain stem death of a person of less than 18 years of age, a certificate specified in Form 8 has been signed by all the members of the Board of Medical Experts referred to in sub-section (6) of section 3 of the Act and an authority as specified in Form 9 has been signed by either of the parents of such person.

4A. Authorization committee:

(1) The medical practitioner who will be part of the organ transplantation team for carrying out transplantation operation shall not be a member of the Authorization committee constituted under the provision of clauses (a) and (b) of sub-section (4) of section 9 of the Act.

(2) Where the proposed transplantation is between a married couple, the Registered Medical Practitioner, i.e., in charge of transplant center must evaluate the factum and duration of marriage and ensure that documents such as marriage certificate, marriage photograph, etc. Are kept for records along with the information on the number of age of children and family photograph depicting the entire immediately family, birth certificate of children containing particulars of parents.

(3) When the proposed donor or recipient or both are not Indian Nationals/citizens whether 'near relatives' or otherwise, Authorization Committees shall consider all such requests.

(4) When the proposed donor and the recipient are not "near relatives", as defined under clause (i) of section 2 of the Act, the Authorization Committee shall evaluate that—

(i) there is no commercial transaction between the recipient and the donor and that no payment or money or money's worth as referred to the Act, has been made to the donor or promised to be made to the donor or any other person;

(ii) the following shall specifically be assessed by the Authorization Committee:

(a) an explanation of the link between them and the circumstances which led to the offer being made;

(b) reasons why the donor wished to donate;

(c) documentary evidence of the link, e.g., proof that they have lived together, etc.

(d) old photographs showing the donor and recipient together;

(iii) that there is no middleman or tout involved;

(iv) that financial status of the donor and the recipient is probed by asking them to give appropriate evidence of their vocation and income for the previous three financial years. Any gross disparity between the status of the two must be evaluated in the backdrop of the objective of preventing commercial dealing;

(v) that the donor is not a drug addict or known person with criminal record;

(vi) that the next of the kin of the proposed unrelated donor is interviewed regarding awareness about his or her intention to donate an organ, the authenticity of the link between the donor and the recipient and the reasons for donation. Any strong views or disagreement or objection such kin shall also be recorded and taken note of.

5. **Preservation of organs**: The organ removed shall be preserved according to current and accepted scientific methods in order to ensure viability for the purpose of transplantation.

Provided that the eye-ball removed shall be preserved in the following three steps, namely:

(i) short-term preservation;

(ii) medium-term preservation;

(iii) long-term preservation; and suitable media shall be used for preservation.

6. The donor and the recipient shall make jointly an application to grant approval for removal and transplantation of human organ, to the concerned competent authority or Authorization Committee as specified in Form 10. The Authorization Committee shall take a decision on such application in accordance with the guidelines in the rule 6A.

6A. Composition of Authorization Committees:

(1) There shall be one State Level Authorization Committee.

(2) Additional authorization committees may be set up at various levels as per norms given below, namely—

(i) no member from transplant team of the institution should be a member of the respective Authorization committee. All Foreign Nationals (related and unrelated) should go to "Authorization Committee" as abundant precaution needs to be taken in such cases;

(ii) Authorization Committee should be Hospital based in Metro and big cities if the number of transplants exceeds 25 in a year at the respective transplantation centers. In small towns, there are State or District Level Committees if transplants are less than 25 in a year in the respective districts.

(A) Composition of Hospital Based Authorization Committees: (To be constituted by the State Government and in case of Union Territory by the Central Government):

(a) the senior most person officiating as Medical Director or Medical Superintendent of the Hospital;

(b) two senior medical practitioners from the same hospital who are not part of the transplant team;

(c) two members being persons of high integrity, social standing and credibility, who have served in high ranking Government positions, such as in higher judiciary, senior cadre of police service or who have served as a reader or professor in University Grants Commission approved University or are self- employed professionals of repute such as lawyers, chartered accountants and doctors (of Indian Medical Association) etc.; and

(d) Secretary (Health) or nominee and Director Health Services or nominee.

(B) Composition of state or District Level Authorization Committees: (To be constituted by the State Government and in case of Union territory by the Central Government).

- (a) a Medical Practitioner officiating as Chief Medical Officer or any other equivalent post in the main/major Government Hospital of the District;
- (b) two senior medical practitioners to be chosen from the pool of such medical practitioners who are residing in the concerned District and who are not part of any transplant team;
- (c) two senior citizens, non-medical background (one lady) of high reputation and integrity to be chosen from the pool of such citizens residing in the same district, who have served in high ranking Government positions, such as in higher judiciary, senior cadre of police service or who have served as a reader or professor in University grants Commission approved University or are self- employed professionals of repute such as lawyers, chartered accountants and doctors (of Indian Medical Association) etc. and
- (d) Secretary (Health) or nominee and Director Health Services or nominee.

(**Note:** Effort should be made to have most of the members' *ex-officio* so that the need to change the composition of committee is less frequent.)

6B. The State level committees shall be formed for the purpose of providing approval or no objection certificate to the respective donor and recipient to establish the legal and residential status as a domicile state. It is mandatory that if donor, recipient and place of transplantation are from different states, then the approval or "no objection certificate" from the respective domicile State Government should be necessary. The institution where the transplant is to be undertaken in such case the approval of Authorization committee is mandatory.

6C. The quorum of the Authorization Committee should be minimum four. However, quorum ought not to be considered as complete without the participation of the chairman. The presence of Secretary (Health) or Nominee and Director of Health Services or nominee is mandatory.

6D. The format of the Authorization Committee approval should be uniform in all the institutions in a State. The format may be notified by respective State Government.

6E. Secretariat of the Committee shall circulate copies of all applications received from the proposed donors to all members of the Committee. Such applications should be circulated along with all annexures, which may have been filed along with the applications. At the time of the meeting, the Authorization committee should take note of all relevant contents and documents in the course of its decision making process and in the event any documents in the course of its decision making process and in the event any document or information is found to be inadequate or doubtful, explanation should be sought from the applicant and if it is considered necessary that any fact or information requires to be verified in order to confirm its veracity or correctness, the same be ascertained through the concerned officer(s) if the State/Union territory Government.

6F. The Authorization committee shall focus its attention on the following, namely:-

- (a) Where the proposed transplant is between persons related genetically, Mother, Father, Brother, Sister, Son or Daughter Above the age of 18 years), the concerned competent authority shall evaluate:
  - (i) results of tissue typing and other basic tests;
  - (ii) documentary evidence of relationship e.g. relevant birth certificates and marriage certificate, certificate from Sub-divisional Magistrate/Metropolitan Magistrate/or Sarpanch of the Panchayat;
  - (iii) documentary evidence of identity and residence of the proposed donor, e.g., Ration Card or Voters Identity Card or Passport or Driving License or PAN Card or Bank Account and family

photograph depicting the proposed donor and the proposed recipient along with another near relative;

(iv) if in its opinion, the relationship is not conclusively established after evaluating the above evidence, it may in its discretion direct further medical tests as prescribed as below:

    (a) the test for Human Leukocyte Antigen (HLA), Human Leukocyte Antigen-B alleles to be performed by the serological and/or Polymerase chain reaction (PCR) based Deoxyribonucleic acid (DNA) methods.

    (b) test for Human Leukocyte Antigen-DR beta genes to be performed using the Polymerase Chain reaction (PCR) based Deoxyribonucleic acid (DNA) methods.

    (c) the tests referred to in sub-rules (i) to (ii) shall be got done from a laboratory accredited with National Accreditation Board for Laboratories (NABL).

    (d) where the tests referred to in (i) to (iii) above do not establish a genetic relationship between the donor and the recipient, the same tests to be performed on both or at least one parent, preferably both parents. If parents are not available, same tests to be performed on such relatives of donor and recipient as are available and are willing to be tested failing which, genetic relationship between the donor and the recipient will be deemed to have not been established.

(b) The papers for approval of transplantation would be processed by the registered medical practitioner and administrative division of the Institution for transplantation, while the approval will be granted by the Authorization Committee.

(c) Where the proposed transplant is between a married couple (except foreigners, whose cases should be dealt by Authorization Committee):

The concerned competent authority or authorization committee as the case may be must evaluate all available evidence to establish the factum and duration of marriage and ensure the documents such as marriage certificate, marriage photograph is placed before the committee along with the information on the number and age of children and a family photograph depicting the entire immediate family, birth certificate of children containing the particulars of parents.

(d) Where the proposed transplant is between individuals who are not "near relatives" the authorization committee shall evaluate;-

    (i) that there is no commercial transaction between the recipient and the donor. That no payment of money or money's worth as referred to in the sections of the Act, has been made to the donor or promised to be made to the donor or any other person. In this connection, the Authorization Committee shall take into consideration:-

        (a) an explanation of the link between them and the circumstances which led to the offer being made;

        (b) documentary evidence of the link, e.g., proof that they have lived together, etc.

        (c) reasons why the donor wishes to donate; and

        (d) old photographs showing the donor and the recipient together.

    (ii) that there is no middleman/tout involved;

    (iii) that financial status of the donor and the recipient is probed by asking them to give appropriate evidence of their vocation and income for the previous three financial years. Any gross disparity between the status of the two, must be evaluated in the backdrop of the objective of preventing commercial dealing;

    (iv) that the donor is not a drug addict or a known person with criminal record;

    (v) that the next of kin of the proposed unrelated donor is interviewed regarding awareness about his/her intention to donate an organ, the authenticity of the link between the donor and the recipient and the reasons for donation. Any strong view of disagreement or objection of such kin may also be recorded and taken note of; and

(e) When the proposed donor or the recipient or both are foreigners:

    (i) a senior Embassy official of the country of origin has to certify the relationship between the donor and the recipient.

    (ii) Authorization Committee shall examine the cases of Indian donors consenting to donate organs to a foreign national (who is a near relative), including a foreign national of India origin, with greater caution. Such cases should be considered rarely on case to case basis.

(f) In the course, of determining eligibility of the applicant to donate, the applicant should be personally interview by the Authorization Committee and minutes of the interview should be recorded. Such interviews with the donors should be videographed.

(g) In case where the donor is a woman greater precautions ought to be taken. Her identity and independent consent should be confirmed by a person other than the recipient. Any document with regard to the proof of the residence or domicile and particulars of parentage should be relatable to the photo identity of the applicant in order to ensure that the documents pertain to the same person, who is the proposed donor and in the event of any inadequate or doubtful information to this effect, the Authorization committee may in its discretion seek such other information or evidence as may be expedient; and desirable in the peculiar facts of the case.

(h) The Authorization Committee should state in writing its reason for rejecting/approving the application of the proposed donor and all approvals should be subject to the following conditions:

    (i) that the approved proposed donor would be subjected to all such medical test as required at the relevant stages to determine his biological capacity and compatibility to donate the organ in question.

    (ii) further that the psychiatrist clearance would also be mandatory to certify his mental condition, awareness, absence of any overt or latent psychiatric disease and ability to give free consent.

    (iii) all prescribed forms have been and would be filled up by all relevant persons involved in the process of transplantation.

    (iv) all interviews to be video recorded.

(i) The authorization committee shall expedite its decision making process and use its discretion judiciously and pragmatically in all such cases where, the patient requires immediate transplantation.

(j) Every authorized transplantation center must have its own website. The Authorization Committee is required to take final decision within 24 hours of holding the meeting for grant of permission of rejection for transplant. The decision of the Authorization committee should be displayed on the notice board of the hospital or institution immediately and should reflect on the website of the hospital or institution within 24 hours of taking the decision. Apart from this, the website of the hospital or institution must update its website regularly in respect of the total number of the transplantations done in that hospital or institution along with the details of each transplantation. The same data should be accessible for compilation, analysis and further use by respective State Governments and Central Government.

7. **Registration of hospital:**

(1) An application for registration shall be made to the Appropriate Authority as specified in Form 11. The application shall be accompanied by a fee or rupees one thousand payable to the Appropriate Authority by means of a bank draft or postal order.

(2) The Appropriate Authority shall, after holding an inquiry and after satisfying itself that the applicant has complied with all the requirements, grant a certificate of registration as specified in Form 12 and shall be valid for a period of 5 years form the date of its issue and shall be renewable.

(3) Before a hospital is registered under the provisions of this rule, it shall be mandatory for the hospital to nominate a transplant coordinator.

8. **Renewal of registration:**

(1) An application for the renewal of a certificate of registration shall be made to the Appropriate Authority within a period of three months prior to the date of expiry of the original certificate of registration and shall be accompanied by a fee of rupees five hundred payable to the Appropriate Authority by means of a bank draft or postal order.

(2) A renewal certificate of registration shall be as specified in Form 13 and shall be valid for a period of 5 years.

(3) If, after an inquiry including inspection of the hospital and scrutiny of its past performance and after giving an opportunity to the applicant, the Appropriate Authority is satisfied that the application, since grant of certificate of registration under sub-rule (2) of rule 7 has not complied with the requirements of this Act and the Rules made thereunder and conditions subject to which the certificate of registration has been granted, shall, for reasons to be recorded in writing, refuse to grant renewal of the certificate of registration.

9. **Conditions for grant of certificate of registration**: No hospital shall be granted a certificate of registration under this Act unless it fulfills the following requirement of manpower, equipment, specialized services and facilities as laid down below—

(A) **General Manpower Requirement Specialized Services and Facilities:**

1. 24-hours availability of medical and surgical, (senior and junior) staff.

2. 24-hours availability of nursing staff, (general and specially trained).

3. 24-hours availability of Intensive Care Units with adequate equipment, staff and support system, including specialists in anesthesiology, intensive care.

4. 24-hours availability of laboratory with multiple discipline testing facilities including but not limited to Microbiology, Bio-Chemistry, pathology and Hematology and Radiology departments with trained staff.

5. 24-hours availability of Operation Theater facilities (OT facilities) for planned and emergency procedures with adequate staff, support system and equipment.

6. 24-hours availability of communication system, with power backup, including but not limited to multiple line telephones, public telephone system, fax, computers and paper photo-imaging machine.

7. Experts, (other than the experts required for the relevant transplantation) of relevant and associated specialties including but not limited to and depending upon the requirements, the experts in internal medicine, diabetology, gastroenterology, nephrology, neurology, pediatrics, gynecology, immunology and cardiology etc. should be available to the transplantation center.

(B) **Equipment:** Equipment as per current and expected scientific requirements specific to organ or organs being transplanted. The transplant center should ensure the availability of the accessories, spare-parts and back-up/maintenance/service support system in relation to all relevant equipment.

(C) **Experts and their qualifications:**

(a) **Kidney Transplantation**

M.S. (Gen.) Surgery or equivalent qualification with 3 years post M.S. training in a recognized center in India or abroad and having attended to adequate number of renal transplantation as an active member of team.

(b) **Transplantation of liver and other abdominal organs**

M.S. (Gen.) Surgery or equivalent qualification with adequate post M.S. training in an established center with a reasonable experience of performing liver transplantation as an active member of team.

(c) **Cardiac, Pulmonary, Cardio-Pulmonary Transplantation**

M.Ch. Cardiothoracic and vascular surgery or equivalent qualification in India or abroad with at least 3-year experience as an active member of the team performing an adequate number of open heart operations per year and well-versed with Coronary by-pass surgery and Heart-Valve surgery.

(d) **Cornea Transplantation**

M.D./M.S. ophthalmology or equivalent qualification with one-year post M.D./M.S. training in a recognized hospital carrying out Corneal transplant operations]

10. Appeal: (1) Any person aggrieved by an order of the Authorization Committee under sub-section (6) of section9, or by an order of the Appropriate Authority under subsection (2) of section 15 and section 16 of the Act, may, within 30 days from the date of receipt of the order, prefer an appeal to the Central Government.

(2) Every appeal shall be in writing and shall be accompanied by a copy of the order appealed against.

FORM 1(A)

[To be completed by the prospective related donor]
[See rule 3]

To be affixed and attested by Notary Public after it is affixed.

Photograph of the Donor
(Attested by Notary Public)

My full name is …………………………………………….....................................And this is my photograph

My permanent home address is

…………………………………………….......................................   Tel:……………………......

My present home address is

…………………………………………….......................................   Tel:……………………......

Date of birth ……………………………………………........................   (day/month/year)

- Ration/consumer Card number and Date of issue & place

  ……………………………..

  (Photocopy attached)

  and/or

- Voter's I-Card number, date of issue, Assembly Constituency

  …………………………….

  (Photocopy attached)

  and/or

- Passport number and country of issue ……………………………………... (Photocopy attached)

  …………………………….

  (Photocopy attached)

  and/or

- Driving License number, Date of issue, licensing authority

  …………………………….

  (Photocopy attached)

  and/or

- PAN …………………………………………...

  and/or

- Other proof of identity and address ……………………………………...

  I hereby authorize removal for therapeutic purposes/consent to donate my ……………………………………………. (state which organ) to my relative (specify son/daughter/father/mother/brother/sister), whose name is ………………………………………….. and who was born on ……………………………. (day/month/year) and whose particulars are as follows:

> To be affixed and attested by Notary Public after it is affixed.

Photograph of the Recipient

(Attested by Notary Public)

- Ration/consumer Card number and Date of issue & place

  ....

  (Photocopy attached)

  and/or

- Voter's I-Card number, date of issue, Assembly Constituency

  ....

  (Photocopy attached)

  and/or

- Passport number and country of issue ....

  ....

  (Photocopy attached)

  and/or

- Driving License number, Date of issue, licensing authority

  ....

  (Photocopy attached)

  and/or

- PAN ....

  and/or

- Other proof of identity and address ....

I solemnly affirm and declare that sections 2, 9, and 19 of the transplantation of Human Organs Act, 1994 have been explained to me and I confirm that: -

1. I understand the nature of criminal offences referred to in the sections.
2. No payment of money or money's worth as referred to in the sections of the Act has been made to me or will be made to me or any other person.

3. I am giving the consent and Authorization to remove my .... (organ) of my own free will without any undue pressure, inducement, influence or allurement.

4. I have been given a full explanation of the nature of the medical procedure involved and the risks involved for me in the removal of my .... (organ). That explanation was given by .... (name of registered medical practitioner).

5. I understand the nature of that medical procedure and of the risks to me as explained by that practitioner.

6. I understand that I may withdraw my consent to the removal of that organ at any time before the operation takes place.

7. I state that particulars filled by me in the form are true and correct to my knowledge and nothing material has been concealed by me.

....

Signature of the prospective donor   Date

Note: To be sworn before Notary Public, who while attesting shall ensure that the person/persons swearing the affidavit(s) signs(s) on the Notary Register, as well.

• Wherever applicable.

FORM 1(B)
[To be completed by the prospective spousal donor]
(See rule 3)

To be affixed and
attested by Notary
Public after it is
affixed.

Photograph of the Donor
(Attested by Notary Public)

My full name is ……………………………………...and this is my photograph

My permanent home address is

……………………………………….....................................   Tel:…………………......

My present home address is

……………………………………….....................................   Tel:…………………......

Date of birth ……………………………………….........................   (day/month/year)

I authorize to remove for therapeutic purposes/consent to donate my ………………….. (state which organ)
to my husband/wife …………………………….whose full name is …………………………………………….
was born on …………………. (day/month/year) and whose particulars are as follows:

To be affixed and attested by Notary Public after it is affixed.	Photograph of the Recipient (Attested by Notary Public)

- Ration/consumer Card number and Date of issue & place

  ....

  (Photocopy attached)

  and/or

- Voter's I-Card number, date of issue, Assembly Constituency

  ....

  (Photocopy attached)

  and/or

- Passport number and country of issue ....

  ....

  (Photocopy attached)

  and/or

- Driving License number, Date of issue, licensing authority

  ....

  (Photocopy attached)

  and/or

- PAN ....

  and/or

- Other proof of identity and address ....

I submit the following as evidence of being married to the recipient:-

(a) A Certified copy of a marriage certificate.

OR

(b) An affidavit of a "near relative" confirming the status of marriage to be sworn before Class-I Magistrate/ Notary Public.

(c) Family photographs.

(d) Letter from member of Gram Panchayat/Tehsildar/Block Development Officer/MLA/MP certifying factum and status of marriage.

OR

(e) Other credible evidence.

I solemnly affirm and declare that Section 2, 9 and 19 of The Transplantation of Human Organs Act, 1994 have been explained to me and I confirm that: -

1. I understand that nature of criminal offences referred to in the sections.
2. No payment of money or money's worth as referred to in the sections of the Act has been made to me or will be made to me or any other person.
3. I am giving the consent and Authorization to remove my .... (organ) of my own free will without any undue pressure, inducement, influence or allurement.
4. I have been given a full explanation of the nature of the medical procedure involved and the risks involved for me in the removal of my
.... (organ). That explanation was given by
...............................(name of registered medical practitioner).
5. I understand the nature of that medical procedure and of the risks to me as explained by that practitioner.
6. I understand that I may withdraw my consent to the removal of that organ at any time before the operation takes place.
7. I state that particulars filled by me in the form are true and correct to my knowledge and noting material has been concealed by me.

....

Signature of the prospective donor   Date

Note- To be sworn before Notary Public, who while attesting shall ensure that the person/persons swearing the affidavit(s) signs (s) on the Notary Register, as well.

• Tick wherever applicable.

FORM 1(C)
[To be completed by the prospective spousal donor]
(See rule 3)

<table>
<tr><td>To be affixed and attested by Notary Public after it is affixed.</td><td>Photograph of the Donor
(Attested by Notary Public)</td></tr>
</table>

My full name is ……………………………………............................………And this is my photograph

My permanent home address is

……………………………….............................…….......................   Tel:……………………......

My present home address is

……………………………….............................…….......................   Tel:……………………......

Date of birth ……………………………………….......................   (day/month/year)

- Ration/consumer Card number and Date of issue & place

    ………………………………..

    (Photocopy attached)

                                    and/or

- Voter's I-Card number, date of issue, Assembly Constituency

    ………………………………..

    (Photocopy attached)

                                    and/or

- Passport number and country of issue ……………………………………...

    ………………………………..

    (Photocopy attached)

                                    and/or

- Driving License number, Date of issue, licensing authority

  ....

  (Photocopy attached)

  and/or

- PAN ....

  and/or

- Other proof of identity and address ....

- Details of last 3-year income and vocation of donor ....

  ....

  ....

I hereby authorize removal for therapeutic purposes/consent to donate my ....
(state which organ) to a person whose full name is .... and who was born on
.... (day/month/year) and whose particulars are as follows:

To be affixed and
attested by Notary
Public after it is
affixed.

Photograph of the Recipient
(Attested by Notary Public)

- Ration/consumer Card number and Date of issue & place

  ....

  (Photocopy attached)

  and/or

- Voter's I-Card number, date of issue, Assembly Constituency

  ....

  (Photocopy attached)

  and/or

- Passport number and country of issue ....

  ....

  (Photocopy attached)

  and/or

- Driving License number, Date of issue, licensing authority

  ……………………............

  (Photocopy attached)

  and/or

- PAN …………………………………………...

  and/or

- Other proof of identity and address …………………………………………..

I solemnly affirm and declare that sections 2, 9, and 19 of the transplantation of Human Organs Act, 1994 have been explained to me and I confirm that: -

1. I understand the nature of criminal offences referred to in the sections.
2. No payment of money or money's worth as referred to in the sections of the Act has been made to me or will be made to me or any other person.
3. I am giving the consent and Authorization to remove my ………………………….. (organ) of my own free will without any undue pressure, inducement, influence or allurement.
4. I have been given a full explanation of the nature of the medical procedure involved and the risks involved for me in the removal of my

   ……………………………. (organ). That explanation was given by

   …………………………….. (name of registered medical practitioner).
5. I understand the nature of that medical procedure and of the risks to me as explained by that practitioner.
6. I understand that I may withdraw my consent to the removal of that organ at any time before the operation takes place.
7. I state that particulars filled by me in the form are true and correct to my knowledge and nothing material has been concealed by me.

……………………………………………　　　　　　　　　　　　　………………..

Signature of the prospective donor　　　　　　　　　　　　　　　　　　Date

Note- To be sworn before Notary Public, who while attesting shall ensure that the person/persons swearing the affidavit(s) signs(s) on the Notary Register, as well.

- Tick wherever applicable.

[1][FORM 2
[To be completed by the concerned medical practitioner]
[Refer rule 4(1) (b)]

I, Dr. .... possessing qualification of .... registered as medical practitioner at Serial no. .... by the .... Medical Council, certify that I have examined Shri/Smt./Km .... S/o, W/o, D/o Shri .... aged ....who has given in- formed consent about donation of the organ, namely (name of the organ .... to Shri/Smt./Km .... who is a "near relative" of the donor/other that near relative of the donor, who had been approved by the Authorization Committee/ Registered Medical Practitioner, i.e., in-charge of transplant center (as the case may be) and that the said donor is in proper state of health and is medically fit to be subjected to the procedure of organ removal.

Place ....
Date ....

....
Signature of Doctor Seal

To be affixed (pasted and
attested by the doctor
concerned. The signatures
and seal should partially
appear on photograph
and document without
disfiguring the face in
photograph.

To be affixed (pasted and
attested by the doctor
concerned. The signatures
and seal should partially
appear on photograph
and document without
disfiguring the face in
photograph.

Photograph of the Donor
(Attested by Doctor)

Photograph of the recipient
(Attested by the Doctor)

FORM 3
[See rule 4(1) (c)]

I, Dr./Mr./Mrs.. ..…………………… working as ..………………… at ..………………………………. and possessing qualification of .………………….... certify that Shri/Smt. Km. ..…………………………………. S/o, D/o, W/o Shri/Smt. ..…………………………………… aged ..……………... the donor and Shri/Smt. ..………………………. S/o, D/o, W/o, Shri/Smt..……………... aged ..……………. the proposed recipient of the organ to be donated by the said donor are related to each other as brother/sister/mother/father/sons/daughter as per their statement and the fact of this relationship has been established/not established by the results of the tests for Antigenic Products of the Human Major Histocompatibility Complex. The results of the test are attached.

Place ..…………………………

Signature
(To be signed by the Head of the Laboratory)

Date ..…………………………..

Seal

FORM 6
[See rule 4(2) (b)]

I, ... S/o, W/o, D/o Shri ....aged.................. resident of ....
having lawful possession of the dead body of Shri/Smt/Km.
....S/o, W/o, D/o Shri .... aged ....
resident of .... having known that the deceased has not expressed any objection to his/her organ/
organs being removed for therapeutic purposes after his/her death and also having reasons to believe that no
near relative of the said deceased person has objection to any of his/her organs being used for therapeutic
purposes, authorize removal of his/her body organs, namely, ...

Signature
Person in lawful possession of the dead body
Address……………………………………......

Date ....
Place ....

FORM 8

[See rule 4(3) (a) and (b)]

We, the following members of the Board of Medical Experts after careful personal examination, hereby certify
that Shri/Smt/Km. .... aged about .... S/o, W/o, D/o, Shri ………...................
resident of .... is dead on account of permanent and irreversible cessation of all functions of the
brain stem. The tests carried out by us and the findings therein are recorded in the brain-stem death certificate
annexed hereto.

Date ……………..   Signature……………...

1. R.M.P., incharge of the hospital in which brain stem death has occurred.
2. R.M.P., nominated from the panel of names approved by the Appropriate Authority.
3. Neurologist/Neurosurgeon nominated from the panel of names approved by the Appropriate Authority.
4. R.M.P., treating the aforesaid deceased person.

BRAIN STEM DEATH CERTIFICATE

(A) Patient Details:

1. Name of the Patient Shri/Smt/Km. ……...

    S/o. / W/o. / D/o. Shri …………………………………………………….......................

    Sex…… ....   Age……….......................................

2. Home Address

    ....

    ....

    ....

    ....

3. Hospital Number...

4. Name and address of next of kin or person responsible for the patient (if none exists, this must be specified)

    ....

    ....

    ....

    ....

5. Has the patient or next of kin agreed to any transplant?

    ....

    ....

6. Is this a Police Case? Yes………No………...

(B) Preconditions:

1. **Diagnosis:** Did the patient suffer from any illness or accident that led to irreversible brain damage? Specify

    Details………………………………………………………………….......................................

    ....

Date and time of accident/onset of illness ....

Date and onset of non-responsible coma ....

2. **Findings of Board of Medical Experts:**

   1. The following reversible cause of coma have been excluded:
      Intoxication (Alcohol)
      Depressant Drugs
      Relaxants (Neuromuscular blocking agents)

First Medical Examination		Second Medical Examination	
1st	2nd	1st	2nd

      Primary hypothermia
      Hypovolemic shock
      Metabolic of endocrine disorders
      Test for absence of brain stem functions
   2. Coma
   3. Cessation of spontaneous breathing
   4. Pupillary size
   5. Pupillary light reflexes
   6. Doll's head eye movements
   7. Corneal reflexes (Both sizes)
   8. Motor response in any cranial nerve distribution, any responses to stimulation of face, limb or trunk
   9. Gag reflex
   10. Cough (Tracheal)
   11. Eye movements on caloric testing bilaterally
   12. Apnea tests as specified
   13. Were any respiratory movements seen?

Date and time of first testing: ....

Date and time of second testing: ....

This is to certify that the patient has been carefully examined twice after an interval of about 6 hours and on the basis of findings recorded above,

Shri/Smt/Km. .... is declared brain steam dead.

Signature ....

1. Medical Administrator Incharge of the hospital.
2. Authorized Specialist.
3. Neurologist/Neurosurgeon.
4. Medical Officer treating the patient.

N.B. I. The Minimum time interval between the first testing and second testing will be 6 hours.

II.   No. 2 and No. 3 will be co-opted by the Administrator in charge of the hospital from the panel of experts approved by the Appropriate Authority.

FORM 9
[See rule 4(3) (a) (b)]

I, Shri/Smt. ....S/o. W/o, Shri .... resident of .... hereby authorize removal of the organ/organs, namely, ...for therapeutic purpose from the dead body of my son/daughter Shri/Km. ....aged .... Whose brain stem death has been duly certified in accordance with the law.

Signature ....

Name ....

Place ....

Date ....

FORM 10
APPLICATION FOR APPROVAL FOR TRANSPLANTATION (LIVE DONOR)
[To be completed by the proposed recipient and the proposed donor]
[See Rule 4(1) (a) (b)]

To be self-attested across the affixed photograph	To be self-attested across the affixed photograph

Photograph of the Doctor
(Self-attested)

Photograph of the recipient
(Self-attested)

Whereas I .... S/o, D/o, W/o, Shri/Smt. .... aged............................for therapeutic................... residing at .... have been advised by my doctor .... that I am suffering from... and may be benefited by transplantation of .... into my body.

And whereas I .... S/o, D/o, W/o, Shri/Smt. .... aged .... residing at .... by the following reason(s):

(a) by virtue of being a near relative, i.e.,

....

(b) by reason of affection/attachment/other special reason as explained below:-

....

....

I would therefore like to donate my (name of the organ) ....

to Shri/Smt. ....We .... and ....

(Donor)   (Recipient)

hereby apply to Authorization Committee for permission for such transplantation to be carried out.

We solemnly affirm that the above decision has been taken without any undue pressure, inducement, influence or allurement and that all possible consequences and options of organ transplantation have been explained to us.

Instructions for the applications:

1. Form 10 must be submitted along with the completed Form 1(A), or Form 1(B) or Form 1 (C) as may be applicable.
2. The applicable form, i.e. Form 1(A) or Form 1(B) or Form 1(C), as the case may be, should be accompanied with all documents mentioned in the applicable form and all relevant queries set out in the applicable form must be adequately answered.
3. Completed Form 3 to be submitted along with the laboratory report.
4. The doctor's advice recommending transplantation must be enclosed with the application.
5. In addition to above, in case the proposed transplant is between unrelated persons, appropriate evidence of vocation and income of the donor as well as the recipient for the last 3 years must be enclosed with this application. It is clarified that the evidence of income does not necessarily mean the proof of income-tax returns, keeping in view that the applicant(s) in a given case may not be filing income-tax returns.
6. The application shall be accepted for consideration by the Authorization Committee only if it is complete in all respects and any omission of the documents or the information required in the forms mentioned above, shall render the application incomplete.
7. As per the Supreme Court's judgment dt. 31-3-2005, the approval/No Objection Certificate from the concerned State/Union Territory Government or Authorization Committees is mandatory from the domicile State/Union Territory of donor as well as recipient. It is understood that final approval for transplantation should be granted by the Authorization Committee/Registered Medical Practitioner, i.e., in charge of transplant center (as the case may be) where transplantation should be done.

We have read and understood the above instructions.

Signature of the Prospective Donor   Signature of the Prospective Recipient

Date ....   Date...

Place ....   Place...

FORM 11
APPLICATION FOR REGISTRATION OF HOSPITAL TO CARRY OUT ORGAN TRANSPLANTATION

To

The Appropriate Authority for organ transplantation............. (State or Union Territory) We hereby apply to be recognized as an institution to carry out organ transplantation.

The required data about the facilities available in the hospital are as follows: -

(A) Hospital

1.　Name ....
2.　Location...
3.　Govt./Pvt...
4.　Teaching/Nonteaching...........................
5.　Approached by:

Road:	Yes	No
Rail:	Yes	No
Air:	Yes	No

6.　Total bed strength: ....
7.　Name of the disciplines in the hospital..........................
8.　Annual budget ....
9.　Patient turnover/year ....

(B) Surgical Team

1.　No. of beds ....
2.　No. of permanent staff members with their designations..............
3.　No. of temporary staff with their designations.........................
4.　No. of operations done per year. ....
5.　Trained persons available for transplantation (Please specify organ for transplantation)

(C) Medical Team

1.　No. of beds ....
2.　No. of permanent staff members with their designations.................................
3.　No. of temporary staff members with their designations................................
4.　Patient turnover per year ....
5.　No. of potential transplant candidates admitted per year. ....

(D) Anesthesiology

    1. No. of permanent staff members with their designations.................

    2. No. of temporary staff members with their designations ....

    3. Name and No. of operations performed ....

    4. Name and No. of equipment available ....

    5. Total No. of operation theatres in the hospital ....

    6. No. of emergency operation theatres ....

    7. No. of separate transplant operation theatres ....

(E) ICU/HDU Facilities

    1. ICU/HDU facilities: Present ....   Not present...............

    2. No. of ICU beds ....

    3. Trained Nurses ....

       Technicians ....

    4. Name and number of equipment in ICU ....

(F) Other Supportive Facilities

    Data about facilities available in the hospital. ....

(G) Laboratory Facilities

    1. No. of permanent staff with their designations. ....

    2. No. of temporary staff with their designations. ....

    3. Names of the investigations carried out in the department. ....

    4. Name and number of equipment available. ....

(H) Imaging Services

    1. No. of permanent staff with their designations. ....

    2. No. of temporary staff with their designations. ....

    3. Names of the investigations carried out in the department. ....

    4. Name and number of equipment available. ....

(I) Hematology Services

    1. No. of permanent staff with their designations. ....

    2. No. of temporary staff with their designations. ....

    3. Names of the investigations carried out in the department. ....

    4. Name and number of equipment available. ....

(J) Blood Bank Facilities   Yes ....   No ....
(K) Dialysis Facilities   Yes. ....   No ....
(L) Other Personnel

    1.   Nephrologist   Yes/No
    2.   Neurologist   Yes/No
    3.   Neurosurgeon   Yes/No
    4.   Urologist   Yes/No
    5.   GI Surgeon   Yes/No
    6.   Pediatrician   Yes/No
    7.   Physiotherapist   Yes/No
    8.   Social worker   Yes/No
    9.   Immunologists   Yes/No
   10. Cardiologist   Yes/No

The above said information is true to the best of my knowledge and I have no objection to any scrutiny of our facility by authorized personnel. A Bank Draft/Cheque of ₹1,000/- is being enclosed.

Head of the Institution.

FORM 12
CERTIFICATE OF REGISTRATION

This is to certify that .... hospital located at .... has been inspected by the Appropriate Authority and certificate of registration is granted for performing the organ transplantation of the following organs:

    1. ....
    2. ....
    3. ....
    4. ....

This certificate of registration is valid for a period of 5 years from the date of issue.

Signature ....   Signature ....

FORM 13
[See sub-rule 8(2)]
OFFICE OF THE APPROPRIATE AUTHORITY

This is with reference to the application, dated ……………………….. from ……………………. (Name of the hospital) for renewal of certificate of registration for performing organ transplantation, under the Act.

After having considered the facilities and standards of the above said hospital, the Appropriate Authority hereby renews the certificate of registration of the said hospital for the purpose of performing organ transplantation for a period of 5 years.

Appropriate authority…………………………

Place ………………..
Date ……………..…

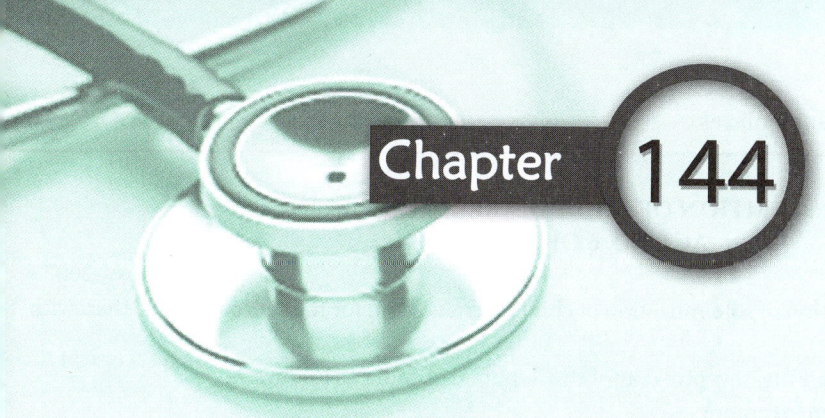

Chapter 144

Prohibition of Child Marriage Act

ARRANGEMENT OF SECTIONS

THE PROHIBITION OF CHILD MARRIAGE ACT, 2006
ACT NO. 6 OF 2007

[10th January, 2007.]

An Act to provide for the prohibition of solemnization of child marriages and for matters connected therewith or incidental thereto.

Be it enacted by Parliament in the Fifty-seventh Year of the Republic of India as follows:—

1. **Short title, extent and commencement.—**
   (1) This Act may be called the Prohibition of Child Marriage Act, 2006.
   (2) It extends to the whole of India except the State of Jammu and Kashmir; and it applies also to all citizens of India without and beyond India:
   Provided that nothing contained in this Act shall apply to the Renoncants of the Union territory of Pondicherry.
   (3) It shall come into force on such date[1] as the Central Government may, by notification in the Official Gazette, appoint; and different dates may be appointed for different States and any reference in any provision to the commencement of this Act shall be construed in relation to any State as a reference to the coming into force of that provision in that State.

2. **Definitions.—**In this Act, unless the context otherwise requires,—
   (a) "child" means a person who, if a male, has not completed 21 years of age, and if a female, has not completed 18 years of age;
   (b) "child marriage" means a marriage to which either of the contracting parties is a child;
   (c) "contracting party", in relation to a marriage, means either of the parties whose marriage is or is about to be thereby solemnized;
   (d) "Child Marriage Prohibition Officer" includes the Child Marriage Prohibition Officer appointed under sub-section (1) of section 16;
   (e) "district court" means, in any area for which a Family Court established under section 3 of the Family Courts Act, 1984 (66 of 1984) exists, such Family Court, and in any area for which there is no Family Court but a city civil court exists, that court and in any other area, the principal civil court of original jurisdiction and includes any other civil court which may be specified by the State Government, by notification in the Official Gazette, as having jurisdiction in respect of the matters dealt with in this Act;
   (f) "minor" means a person who, under the provisions of the Majority Act, 1875 (9 of 1875), is to be deemed not to have attained his majority.

3. **Child marriages to be voidable at the option of contracting party being a child.—**
   (1) Every child marriage, whether solemnized before or after the commencement of this Act, shall be voidable at the option of the contracting party who was a child at the time of the marriage:
   Provided that a petition for annulling a child marriage by a decree of nullity may be filed in the district court only by a contracting party to the marriage who was a child at the time of the marriage.
   (2) If at the time of filing a petition, the petitioner is a minor, the petition may be filed through his or her guardian or next friend along with the Child Marriage Prohibition Officer.
   (3) The petition under this section may be filed at any time but before the child filing the petition completes 2 years of attaining majority.

---

[1]1st November, 2007, *vide* notification No. S.O. 1850(E), dated 30th October, 2007, *see* Gazette of India, Extraordinary, Part II, sec. 3(*ii*).

(4) While granting a decree of nullity under this section, the district court shall make an order directing both the parties to the marriage and their parents or their guardians to return to the other party, his or her parents or guardian, as the case may be, the money, valuables, ornaments and other gifts received on the occasion of the marriage by them from the other side, or an amount equal to the value of such valuables, ornaments, other gifts and money:

Provided that no order under this section shall be passed unless the concerned parties have been given notices to appear before the district court and show cause why such order should not be passed.

4. **Provision for maintenance and residence to female contracting party to child marriage.**—

   (1) While granting a decree under section 3, the district court may also make an interim or final order directing the male contracting party to the child marriage, and in case the male contracting party to such marriage is a minor, his parent or guardian to pay maintenance to the female contracting party to the marriage until her remarriage.

   (2) The quantum of maintenance payable shall be determined by the district court having regard to the needs of the child, the lifestyle enjoyed by such child during her marriage and the means of income of the paying party.

   (3) The amount of maintenance may be directed to be paid monthly or in lump sum.

   (4) In case the party making the petition under section 3 is the female contracting party, the district court may also make a suitable order as to her residence until her remarriage.

5. **Custody and maintenance of children of child marriages.**—

   (1) Where there are children born of the child marriage, the district court shall make an appropriate order for the custody of such children.

   (2) While making an order for the custody of a child under this section, the welfare and best interests of the child shall be the paramount consideration to be given by the district court.

   (3) An order for custody of a child may also include appropriate directions for giving to the other party access to the child in such a manner as may best serve the interests of the child, and such other orders as the district court may, in the interest of the child, deem proper.

   (4) The district court may also make an appropriate order for providing maintenance to the child by a party to the marriage or their parents or guardians.

6. **Legitimacy of children born of child marriages.**—Notwithstanding that a child marriage has been annulled by a decree of nullity under section 3, every child begotten or conceived of such marriage before the decree is made, whether born before or after the commencement of this Act, shall be deemed to be a legitimate child for all purposes.

7. **Power of district court to modify orders issued under section 4 or section 5.**—The district court shall have the power to add to, modify or revoke any order made under section 4 or section 5 and if there is any change in the circumstances at any time during the pendency of the petition and even after the final disposal of the petition.

8. **Court to which petition should be made.**—For the purpose of grant of reliefs under sections 3, 4 and 5, the district court having jurisdiction shall include the district court having jurisdiction over the place where the defendant or the child resides, or where the marriage was solemnized or where the parties last resided together or the petitioner is residing on the date of presentation of the petition.

9. **Punishment for male adult marrying a child.**—Whoever, being a male adult above 18 years of age, contracts a child marriage shall be punishable with rigorous imprisonment which may extend to 2 years or with fine which may extend to one lakh rupees or with both.

10. **Punishment for solemnizing a child marriage.**—Whoever performs, conducts, directs or abets any child marriage shall be punishable with rigorous imprisonment which may extend to 2 years and shall be liable to fine which may extend to 1 lakh rupees unless he proves that he had reasons to believe that the marriage was not a child marriage.

11. **Punishment for promoting or permitting solemnization of child marriages.**—

    (1) Where a child contracts a child marriage, any person having charge of the child, whether as parent or guardian or any other person or in any other capacity, lawful or unlawful, including any member of an organization or association of persons who does any act to promote the marriage or permits it to be solemnized, or negligently fails to prevent it from being solemnized, including attending or participating in a child marriage, shall be punishable with rigorous imprisonment which may extend to 2 years and shall also be liable to fine which may extend up to one lakh rupees:
    Provided that no woman shall be punishable with imprisonment.

    (2) For the purposes of this section, it shall be presumed, unless and until the contrary is proved, that where a minor child has contracted a marriage, the person having charge of such minor child has negligently failed to prevent the marriage from being solemnized.

12. **Marriage of a minor child to be void in certain circumstances.**—Where a child, being a minor—

    (a) is taken or enticed out of the keeping of the lawful guardian; or

    (b) by force compelled, or by any deceitful means induced to go from any place; or

    (c) is sold for the purpose of marriage; and made to go through a form of marriage or if the minor is married after which the minor is sold or trafficked or used for immoral purposes, such marriage shall be null and void.

13. **Power of court to issue injunction prohibiting child marriages.**—

    (1) Notwithstanding anything to the contrary contained in this Act, if, on an application of the Child Marriage Prohibition Officer or on receipt of information through a complaint or otherwise from any person, a Judicial Magistrate of the first class or a Metropolitan Magistrate is satisfied that a child marriage in contravention of this Act has been arranged or is about to be solemnized, such Magistrate shall issue an injunction against any person including a member of an organization or an association of persons prohibiting such marriage.

    (2) A complaint under sub-section (1) may be made by any person having personal knowledge or reason to believe, and a non-governmental organization having reasonable information, relating to the likelihood of taking place of solemnization of a child marriage or child marriages.

    (3) The Court of the Judicial Magistrate of the first class or the Metropolitan Magistrate may also take *suomotu* cognizance on the basis of any reliable report or information.

    (4) For the purposes of preventing solemnization of mass child marriages on certain days such as *Akshaya Trutiya*, the District Magistrate shall be deemed to be the Child Marriage Prohibition Officer with all powers as are conferred on a Child Marriage Prohibition Officer by or under this Act.

    (5) The District Magistrate shall also have additional powers to stop or prevent solemnization of child marriages and for this purpose, he may take all appropriate measures and use the minimum force required.

    (6) No injunction under sub-section (1) shall be issued against any person or member of any organization or association of persons unless the Court has previously given notice to such person, members of the organization or association of persons, as the case may be, and has offered him or them an opportunity to show cause against the issue of the injunction:
    Provided that in the case of any urgency, the Court shall have the power to issue an interim injunction without giving any notice under this section.

(7) An injunction issued under sub-section (1) may be confirmed or vacated after giving notice and hearing the party against whom the injunction was issued.

(8) The Court may either on its own motion or on the application of any person aggrieved, rescind or alter an injunction issued under sub-section (1).

(9) Where an application is received under sub-section (1), the Court shall afford the applicant an early opportunity of appearing before it either in person or by an advocate and if the Court, after hearing the applicant rejects the application wholly or in part, it shall record in writing its reasons for so doing.

(10) Whoever knowing that an injunction has been issued under sub-section (1) against him disobeys such injunction shall be punishable with imprisonment of either description for a term which may extend to 2 years or with fine which may extend to one lakh rupees or with both:

Provided that no woman shall be punishable with imprisonment.

14. Child marriages in contravention of injunction orders to be void.—Any child marriage solemnized in contravention of an injunction order issued under section 13, whether interim or final, shall be void *ab initio*.

15. Offences to be cognizable and non-bailable.—Notwithstanding anything contained in the Code of Criminal Procedure, 1973 (2 of 1974), an offence punishable under this Act shall be cognizable and non-bailable.

16. Child Marriage Prohibition Officers.—

(1) The State Government shall, by notification in the Official Gazette, appoint for the whole State, or such part thereof as may be specified in that notification, an officer or officers to be known as the Child Marriage Prohibition Officer having jurisdiction over the area or areas specified in the notification.

(2) The State Government may also request a respectable member of the locality with a record of social service or an officer of the Gram Panchayat or Municipality or an officer of the Government or any public sector undertaking or an office bearer of any non-governmental organization to assist the Child Marriage Prohibition Officer and such member, officer or office bearer, as the case may be, shall be bound to act accordingly.

(3) It shall be the duty of the Child Marriage Prohibition Officer—

(a) to prevent solemnization of child marriages by taking such action as he may deem fit;

(b) to collect evidence for the effective prosecution of persons contravening the provisions of this Act;

(c) to advise either individual cases or counsel the residents of the locality generally not to indulge in promoting, helping, aiding or allowing the solemnization of child marriages;

(d) to create awareness of the evil which results from child marriages;

(e) to sensitize the community on the issue of child marriages;

(f) to furnish such periodical returns and statistics as the State Government may direct; and

(g) to discharge such other functions and duties as may be assigned to him by the State Government.

(4) The State Government may, by notification in the Official Gazette, subject to such conditions and limitations, invest the Child Marriage Prohibition Officer with such powers of a police officer as may be specified in the notification and the Child Marriage Prohibition Officer shall exercise such powers subject to such conditions and limitations, as may be specified in the notification.

(5) The Child Marriage Prohibition Officer shall have the power to move the Court for an order under sections 4, 5 and 13 and along with the child under section 3.

17. **Child Marriage Prohibition Officers to be public servants.**—The Child Marriage Prohibition Officers shall be deemed to be public servants within the meaning of section 21 of the Indian Penal Code (45 of 1860).

18. **Protection of action taken in good faith.**—No suit, prosecution or other legal proceedings shall lie against the Child Marriage Prohibition Officer in respect of anything in good faith done or intended to be done in pursuance of this Act or any rule or order made thereunder.

19. **Power of State Government to make rules.**—

    (1) The State Government may, by notification in the Official Gazette, make rules for carrying out the provisions of this Act.

    (2) Every rule made under this Act shall, as soon as may be after it is made, be laid before the State Legislature.

20. **Repeal and savings.**—

    (1) The Child Marriage Restraint Act, 1929 (19 of 1929) is hereby repealed.

    (2) Notwithstanding such repeal, all cases and other proceedings pending or continued under the said Act at the commencement of this Act shall be continued and disposed of in accordance with the provisions of the repealed Act, as if this Act had not been passed.

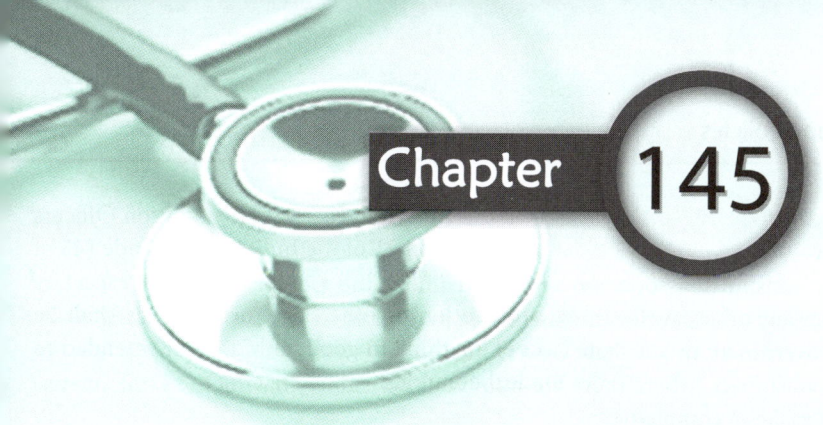

Chapter 145

Consumer Protection Act

(Act No. 68 of 1986)

*A*n Act to provide for better protection of the interests of consumers and for that purpose to make provision *for the establishment of consumer councils and other authorities for the settlement of consumers' disputes and for matters connected therewith.*

Be it enacted by Parliament in the Thirty-seventh Year of the Republic of India as follows:—

CHAPTER I: PRELIMINARY

1. **Short title, extent, commencement and applications—**

    (1) This Act may be called the Consumer Protection Act, 1986.

    (2) It extends to the whole of India except the State of Jammu and Kashmir.

    (3) It shall come into force on such date as the Central Government may, by notification, appoint and different dates may be appointed for different States and for different provisions of this Act.

    (4) Save as otherwise expressly provided by the Central Government by notifications, this Act shall apply to all goods and services.

2. **Definitions—**

    (1) In this Act, unless the context otherwise requires,—

    (a) **"Appropriate laboratory"** means a laboratory or organization—

        (i) recognized by the Central Government

        (ii) recognized by a State Government, subject to such guidelines as may be prescribed by the Central Government in this behalf or

        (iii) any such laboratory or organization established by or under any law for the time-being in force, which is maintained, financed or aided by the Central Government or a State Government for carrying out analysis or test of any goods with a view to determining whether such goods suffer from any defect.

    (aa) **"Branch office"** means—

        (i) any establishment described as a branch by the opposite party, or

        (ii) any establishment carrying on either the same or substantially the same activity as that carried on by the head office of the establishment

(b) **"Complainant"** means—
   (i) a consumer or
   (ii) any voluntary consumer association registered under the Companies Act, 1956 (1 of 1956), or under any other law for the time being in force or
   (iii) the Central Government or any State Government,
   (iv) one or more consumers, where there are numerous consumers having the same interest who or which makes a complaint.

(c) **"Complaint"** means any allegation in writing made by a complainant that—
   (i) an unfair trade practice or a restrictive trade practice has been adopted by any trader
   (ii) [the goods bought by him or agreed to be bought by him] suffer from one or more defect
   (iii) [the services hired or availed of or agreed to be hired or availed of by him] suffer from deficiency in any respect
   (iv) a trader has charged for the goods mentioned in the complaint a price in excess of the price fixed by or under any law for the time being in force or displayed on the goods or any package containing such goods
   (v) goods which will be hazardous to life and safety when used, are being offered for sale to the public in contravention of the provisions of any law for the time being in force requiring traders to display information in regard to the contents, manner and effect of use of such goods, with a view to obtaining any relief provided by or under this Act.

(d) **"Consumer"** means any person who—
   (i) buys any goods for a consideration which has been paid or promised or partly paid and partly promised, or under any system of deferred payment and includes any user of such goods other than the person who buys such goods for consideration paid or promised or partly paid or partly promised, or under any system of deferred payment when such use is made with the approval of such person, but does not include a person who obtains such goods for resale or for any commercial purpose or
   (ii) [hires or avails of] any services for a consideration which has been paid or promised or partly paid and partly promised, or under any system of deferred payment and includes any beneficiary of such services other than the person who hires or avails of] the services for consideration paid or promised, or partly paid and partly promised, or under any system of deferred payments, when such services are availed of with the approval of the first-mentioned person
   Explanation—For the purposes of sub-clause (i), "commercial purpose" does not include use by a consumer of goods bought and used by him exclusively for the purpose of earning his livelihood, by means of self-employment.

(e) **"Consumer dispute"** means a dispute where the person against whom a complaint has been made, denies or disputes the allegations contained in the complaint

(f) **"Defect"** means any fault, imperfection or shortcoming in the quality, quantity, potency, purity or standard which is required to be maintained by or under any law for the time being in force or [under any contract, express or] implied, or as is claimed by the trader in any manner whatsoever in relation to any goods

(g) **"Deficiency"** means any fault, imperfection, shortcoming or inadequacy in the quality, nature and manner of performance which is required to be maintained by or under any law for the time being in force or has been undertaken to be performed by a person in pursuance of a contract or otherwise in relation to any service

(h) **"District forum"** means a Consumer Disputes Redressal Forum established under clause (a) of Section 9

(i) **"Goods"** means goods as defined in the Sale of Goods Act, 1930 (3 of 1930)

(j) **"Manufacturer"** means a person who—

   (i) makes or manufactures any goods or parts thereof or

  (ii) does not make or manufacture any goods but assembles parts thereof made or manufactured by others and claims the end product to be goods manufactured by himself or

 (iii) puts or causes to be put his own mark on any goods made or manufactured by any other manufacturer and claims such goods to be goods made or manufactured by himself.

    Explanation—Where a manufacturer dispatches any goods or part thereof to any branch office maintained by him, such branch office shall not be deemed to be the manufacturer even though the parts so dispatched to it are assembled at such branch office and are sold or distributed from such branch office.

[(jj) **"Member"** includes the President and a member of the National Commission or a State Commission or a District Forum, as the case may be]

(k) **"National Commission"** means the National Consumer Disputes Redressal Commission established under clause (c) of Section 9

(l) **"Notification"** means a notification published in the Official Gazette

(m) **"Person"** includes—

   (i) a firm whether registered or not

  (ii) a Hindu undivided family

 (iii) a co-operative society

 (iv) every other association of persons whether registered under the Societies Registration Act, 1860 (22 of 1860) or not

(n) **"Prescribed"** means prescribed by rules made by the State Government, or as the case may be, by the Central Government under this Act

[(nn) **"Restrictive trade practice"** means any trade practice which requires a consumer to buy, hire or avail of any goods or, as the case may be, services as a condition precedent for buying, hiring or availing of other goods or services]

(o) **"Service"** means service of any description which is made available to potential users and includes the provision of facilities in connection with banking, financing, insurance, transport, processing, supply of electrical or other energy, board or lodging or both, [housing construction], entertainment, amusement or the purveying of news or other information, but does not include the rendering of any service free of charge or under a contract of personal service.

(p) **"State Commission"** means a Consumer Disputes Redressal Commission established in a State under clause (b) of Section 9

(q) **"Trader"** in relation to any goods means a person who sells or distributes any goods for sale and includes the manufacturer thereof, and where such goods are sold or distributed in package form, includes the packer thereof

(r) **"Unfair trade practice"** means a trade practice which, for the purpose of promoting the sale, use or supply of any goods or for the provision of any service, adopts any unfair method or unfair or deceptive practice including any of the following practices, namely,—

(1) the practice of making any statement, whether orally or in writing or by visible representation which,—

   (i) falsely represents that the goods are of a particular standard, quality, quantity, grade, composition, style or model

   (ii) falsely represents that the services are of a particular standard, quality or grade

   (iii) falsely represents any re-built, second-hand, renovated, reconditioned or old goods as new goods

   (iv) represents that the goods or services have sponsorship, approval, performance, characteristics, accessories, uses or benefits which such goods or services do not have

   (v) represents that the seller or the supplier has a sponsorship or approval or affiliation which such seller or supplier does not have

   (vi) makes a false or misleading representation concerning the need for, or the usefulness of, any goods or services

   (vii) gives to the public any warranty or guarantee of the performance, efficacy or length of life of a product or of any goods that is not based on an adequate or proper test thereof:
Provided that where a defense is raised to the effect that such warranty or guarantee is based on adequate or proper test, the burden of proof of such defense shall lie on the person raising such defense

   (viii) makes to the public a representation in a form that purports to be—

     (a) a warranty or guarantee of a product or of any goods or services or

     (b) a promise to replace, maintain or repair an article or any part thereof or to repeat or continue a service until it has achieved a specified result, if such purported warranty or guarantee or promise is materially misleading or if there is no reasonable prospect that such warranty, guarantee or promise will be carried out.

   (ix) materially misleads the public concerning the price at which a product or like products or goods or services, have been or are, ordinarily sold or provided, and, for this purpose, a representation as to price shall be deemed to refer to the price at which the product or goods or services has or have been sold by sellers or provided by suppliers generally in the relevant market unless it is clearly the price at which the product has been sold or services have been provided by the person by whom or on whose behalf the representation is made

   (x) gives false or misleading facts disparaging the goods, services or trade of another person.
Explanation—For the purposes of clause (1), a statement that is—

     (a) expressed on an article offered or displayed for sale, or on its wrapper or container or

     (b) expressed on anything attached to, inserted in, or accompanying, an article offered or displayed for sale, or on anything on which the article is mounted for display or sale or

     (c) contained in or on anything that is sold, sent, delivered, transmitted or in any other manner whatsoever made available to a member of the public, shall be deemed to be a statement made to the public by, and only by, the person who had caused the statement to be so expressed, made or contained.

(2) permits the publication of any advertisement whether in any newspaper or otherwise, for the sale of supply at a bargain price, of goods or services that are not intended to be offered for sale or supply at the bargain price, or for a period that is, and in quantities that are, reasonable, having regard to the nature of the market in which the business is carried on, the nature and size of business, and the nature of the advertisement.

Explanation—For the purposes of clause (2), **"Bargaining price"** means—

    (a)   a price that is stated in any advertisement to be a bargain price, by reference to an ordinary price or otherwise, or

    (b)   a price that a person who reads, hears or sees the advertisement, would reasonably understand to be a bargain price having regard to the prices at which the product advertised or like products are ordinarily sold

  (3) permits—

    (a)   the offering of gifts, prizes or other items with the intention of not providing them as offered or creating impression that something is being given or offered free of charge when it is fully or partly covered by the amount charged in the transaction as a whole

    (b)   the conduct of any contest, lottery, games of chance or skill, for the purpose of promoting, directly or indirectly, the sale, use or supply of any product or any business interest

  (4) permits the sale or supply of goods intended to be used, or are of a kind likely to be used, by consumers, knowing or having reason to believe that the goods do not comply with the standards prescribed by competent authority relating to performance, composition, contents, design, constructions, finishing or packaging as are necessary to prevent or reduce the risk of injury to the person using the goods

  (5) (1) permits the hoarding or destruction of goods, or refuses to sell the goods or to make them available for sale or to provide any service, if such-hoarding or destruction or refusal raises or tends to raise or is intended to raise, the cost of those or other similar goods or services.

    (2)   Any reference in this Act to any other Act or provision thereof which is not in force in any area to which this Act applies shall be construed to have a reference to the corresponding Act or provision thereof in force in such area.

3.   Act not in derogation of any other law—

The provisions of this Act shall be in addition to and not in derogation of the provisions of any other law for the time being in force.

CHAPTER II: CONSUMER PROTECTION COUNCILS

4.   The central consumer protection council—

  (1) The Central Government may, by notification, establish with effect from such date as it may specify in such notification, a council to be known as the Central Consumer Protection Council (hereinafter referred to as the Central Council).

  (2) The Central Council shall consist of the following members, namely,—

    (a)   the Minister in charge of [consumer affairs] in the Central Government, who shall be its Chairman, and

    (b)   such number of other official or non-official members representing such interests as may be prescribed.

5.   Procedure for meetings of the central council—

  (1) The Central Council shall meet as and when necessary, but [at least one meeting] of the council shall be held every year.

  (2) The Central Council shall meet at such time and place as the Chairman may think fit and shall observe such procedure in regard to the transaction of its business as may be prescribed.

6. **Objects of the Central Council—**

   The objects of the Central Council shall be to promote and protect the rights of the consumers such as—

   (a) the right to be protected against the marketing of goods and services which are hazardous to life and property

   (b) the right to be informed about the quality, quantity, potency, purity, standard and price of goods or services, as the case may be, so as to protect the consumer against unfair trade practices

   (c) the right to be assured, wherever possible, access to a variety of goods and services at competitive prices

   (d) the right to be heard and to be assured that consumers' interests will receive due consideration at appropriate forums

   (e) the right to seek redressal against unfair trade practices or restrictive trade practices or unscrupulous exploitation of consumers and

   (f) the right to consumer education.

7. **The State Consumer Protection Councils—**

   (1) The State Government may, by notification, establish with effect from such date as it may specify in such notification, a council to be known as the Consumer Protection Council (hereinafter referred to as the State Council).

   (2) The State Council shall consist of the following members, namely,—

       (a) the Minister in-charge of consumer affairs in the State Government who shall be its Chairman

       (b) such number of other official or non-official members representing such interests as may be prescribed by the State Government.

   (3) The State Council shall meet as and when necessary but not less than two meetings shall be held every year.

   (4) The State Council shall meet at such time and place as the Chairman may think fit and shall observe such procedure in regard to the transaction of its business as may be prescribed by the State Government.

8. **Objects of the State Council—**

   The objects of every State Council shall be to promote and protect within the State the rights of the consumers laid down in clauses (a) to (f) of Section 6.

CHAPTER III: CONSUMER DISPUTES REDRESSAL AGENCIES

9. **Establishment of consumer disputes redressal agencies—**

   There shall be established for the purposes of this Act, the following agencies, namely,—

   (a) a Consumer Disputes Redressal Forum to be known as the **"District Forum"** established by the State Government in each district of the State by notification:

   Provided that the State Government may, if it deems fit, establish more than one District Forum in a district

   (b) a Consumer Disputes Redressal Commission to be known as the "State Commission" established by the State Government in the State by notification and

   (c) a National Consumer Disputes Redressal Commission established by the Central Government by notification.

10. **Composition of the district forum—**

(1) Each District Forum shall consist of—

   (a) a person who is, or has been, or is qualified to be a District Judge, who shall be its President

   (b) two other members, who shall be persons of ability, integrity and standing, and have adequate knowledge or experience of, or have shown capacity in dealing with, problems relating to economics, law, commerce, accountancy, industry, public affairs or administration, one of whom shall be a woman.

   (1A) Every appointment under sub-section (1) shall be made by the State Government on the recommendation of a selection committee consisting of the following, namely,—

      (i) the President of the State Commission-Chairman,

      (ii) Secretary, Law Department of the State-Member,

      (iii) Secretary in charge of the Department dealing with consumer affairs in the State-Member.

(2) Every member of the District Forum shall hold office for a term of 5 years or up to the age of 65 years, whichever is earlier, and shall not be eligible for reappointment:

   Provided that a member may resign his office in writing under his hand addressed to the State Government and on such resignation being accepted, his office shall become vacant and may be filled by the appointment of a person possessing any of the qualifications mentioned in sub-section (1) in relation to the category of the member who has resigned.

(3) The salary or honorarium and other allowances payable to, and the other terms and conditions of service of the members of the District Forum shall be such as may be prescribed by the State Government.

11. **Jurisdiction of the district forum—**

(1) Subject to the other provisions of this Act, the District Forum shall have jurisdiction to entertain complaints where the value of the goods or services and the compensation, if any, claimed [does not exceed rupees five lakhs].

(2) A complaint shall be instituted in a District Forum within the local limits of whose jurisdiction—

   (a) the opposite party or each of the opposite parties, where there are more than one, at the time of the institution of the complaint, actually and voluntarily resides or [carries on business, or has a branch office or] personally works for gain or

   (b) any of the opposite parties, where there are more than one, at the time of the institution of the complaint, actually and voluntarily resides, or carries on business or has a branch office, or personally works for gain:

   Provided that in such case either the permission of the District Forum is given, or the opposite parties who do not reside, or carry on business or have a branch office, or personally work for gain, as the case may be, acquiesce in such institution or

   (c) the cause of action, wholly or in part, arises.

12. **Manner in which complaint shall be made—**

   A complaint in relation to any goods sold or delivered or agreed to be sold or delivered or any service provided or agreed to be provided, may be filed with a District Forum, by—

   (a) the consumer to whom such goods are sold or delivered or agreed to be sold or delivered or such service provided or agreed to be provided

   (b) any recognized consumer association whether the consumer to whom the goods sold or delivered or service provided or agreed to be provided is a member of such association or not or

    (c)   one or more consumers, where there are numerous consumers having the same interest, with the permission of the District Forum, on behalf of, or for the benefit of, all consumers so interested or

    (d)   the Central or the State Government.

13. Procedure on receipt of complaint—

  (1) The District Forum shall, on receipt of a complaint, if it relates to any goods—

    (a)   refer a copy of the complaint to the opposite party mentioned in the complaint directing him to give his version of the case within a period of 30 days or such extended period not exceeding 15 days as may be granted by the District Forum

    (b)   where the opposite party on receipt of a complaint referred to him under clause (a) denies or disputes the allegations contained in the complaint, or omits or fails to take any action to represent his case within the time given by the District Forum, the District Forum shall proceed to settle the consumer dispute in the manner specified in clauses (c) to (g)

    (c)   where the complaint alleges a defect in the goods which cannot be determined without proper analysis or test of the goods, the District Forum shall obtain a sample of the goods from the complainant, seal it and authenticate it in the manner prescribed and refer the sample so sealed to the appropriate laboratory along with a direction that such laboratory make an analysis with a view to finding out whether such goods suffer from any defect alleged in the complaint or suffer from any other defect and to report its findings thereon to the District Forum within a period of 45 days of the receipt of the reference or within such extended period as may be granted by the District Forum

    (d)   before any sample of the goods is referred to any appropriate laboratory under clause (c), the District Forum may require the complainant to deposit to the credit of the Forum such fees as may be specified, for payment to the appropriate laboratory for carrying out the necessary analysis or test in relation to the goods in question

    (e)   the District Forum shall remit the amount deposited to its credit under clause (d) to the appropriate laboratory to enable it to carry out the analysis or test mentioned in clause (c) and on receipt of the report from the appropriate laboratory, the District Forum shall forward a copy of the report along with such remarks as the District Forum may feel appropriate to the opposite party

    (f)   if any of the parties disputes the correctness of the findings of the appropriate laboratory, or disputes the correctness of the methods of analysis or test adopted by the appropriate laboratory, the District Forum shall require the opposite party or the complainant to submit in writing his objections in regard to the report made by the appropriate laboratory

    (g)   the District Forum shall thereafter give a reasonable opportunity to the complainant as well as the opposite party of being heard as to the correctness or otherwise of the report made by the appropriate laboratory and also as to the objection made in relation thereto under clause (f) and issue an appropriate order under Section 14.

  (2) The District Forum shall, if the complaint received by it under Section 12 relates to goods in respect of which the procedure specified in sub-section (1) cannot be followed, or if the complaint relates to any services,—

    (a)   refer a copy of such complaint to the opposite party directing him to give his version of the case within a period of 30 days or such extended period not exceeding 15 days as may be granted by the District Forum

(b) where the opposite party, on receipt of a copy of the complaint, referred to him under clause (a) denies or disputes the allegations contained in the complaint, or omits or fails to take any action to represent his case within the time given by the District Forum, the District Forum shall proceed to settle the consumer dispute,—

    (i) on the basis of evidence brought to its notice by the complainant and the opposite party, where the opposite party denies or disputes the allegation contained in the complaint, or

    (ii) on the basis of evidence brought to its notice by the complainant where the opposite party omits or fails to take any action to represent his case within the time given by the Forum.

(3) No proceedings complying with the procedure laid down in sub-sections (1) and (2) shall be called in question in any court on the ground that the principles of natural justice have not been complied with.

(4) For the purposes of this section, the District Forum shall have the same powers as are vested in a civil court under the Code of Civil Procedure, 1908 (5 of 1908) while trying a suit in respect of the following matters, namely,—

    (i) the summoning and enforcing attendance of any defendant or witness and examining the witness on oath

    (ii) the discovery and production of any document or other material object producible as evidence

    (iii) the reception of evidence on affidavits

    (iv) the requisitioning of the report of the concerned analysis or test from the appropriate laboratory or from any other relevant source

    (v) issuing of any commission for the examination of any witness and

    (vi) any other matter which may be prescribed.

(5) Every proceeding before the District Forum shall be deemed to be a judicial proceeding within the meaning of Sections 193 and 228 of the Indian Penal Code (45 of 1860), and the District Forum shall be deemed to be a civil court for the purposes of Section 195 and Chapter XXVI of the Code of Criminal Procedure, 1973 (2 of 1974).

(6) Where the complainant is a consumer referred to in sub-clause (iv) of clause (b) of sub-section (1) of Section 2, the provisions of Rule 8 of Order I of Schedule I to the Code of Civil Procedure, 1908 (5 of 1908) shall apply subject to the modification that every reference therein to a suit or decree shall be construed as a reference to a complaint or the order of the District Forum thereon.

14. Finding of the district forum—

(1) If, after the proceeding conducted under Section 13, the District Forum is satisfied that the goods complained against suffer from any of the defects specified in the complaint or that any of the allegations contained in the complaint about the services are proved, it shall issue an order to the opposite party directing him to do one or more of the following things, namely,—

    (a) to remove the defect pointed out by the appropriate laboratory from the goods in question

    (b) to replace the goods with new goods of similar description which shall be free from any defect

    (c) to return to the complainant the price, or, as the case may be, the charges paid by the complainant

    (d) to pay such amount as may be awarded by it as compensation to the consumer for any loss or injury suffered by the consumer due to the negligence of the opposite party.

    (e) to remove the defects or deficiencies in the services in question

    (f) to discontinue the unfair trade practice or the restrictive trade practice or not to repeat them

    (g) not to offer the hazardous goods for sale

    (h) to withdraw the hazardous goods from being offered for sale

    (i) to provide for adequate costs to parties.

[(2) Every proceeding referred to in sub-section (1) shall be conducted by the President of the District Forum and at least one member thereof sitting together:

Provided that where the member, for any reason, is unable to conduct the proceeding till it is completed, the President and the other member shall conduct such proceeding de novo:

(2A) Every order made by the District Forum under sub-section (1) shall be signed by its President and the member or members who conducted the proceedings:

Provided that where the proceeding is conducted by the President and one member and they differ on any point or points, they shall state the point or points on which they differ and refer the same to the other member for hearing on such point or points and the opinion of the majority shall be the order of the District Forum.

(3) Subject to the foregoing provisions, the procedure relating to the conduct of the members of the District Forum, its sittings and other matters shall be such as may be prescribed by the State Government.

15. Appeal—

Any person aggrieved by an order made by the District Forum may prefer an appeal against such order to the State Commission within a period of 30 days from the date of the order, in such form and manner as may be prescribed:

Provided that the State Commission may entertain an appeal after the expiry of the said period of 30 days if it is satisfied that there was sufficient cause for not finding it within that period.

16. Composition of the State Commission—

(1) Each State Commission shall consist of—

   (a) a person who is or has been a Judge of a High Court, appointed by the State Government, who shall be its President:

      Provided that no appointment under this clause shall be made except after consultation with the Chief Justice of the High Court.

   (b) two other members, who shall be persons of ability, integrity and standing and have adequate knowledge or experience of, or have shown capacity in dealing with, problems relating to economics, law, commerce, accountancy, industry, public affairs or administration, one of whom shall be a woman:

      Provided that every appointment under this clause shall be made by the State Government on the recommendation of a selection committee consisting of the following, namely,—

      (i) President of the State Commission-Chairman,

      (ii) Secretary of the Law Department of the State-Member,

      (iii) Secretary in-charge of the department dealing with consumer affairs in the State-Member.

(2) The salary or honorarium and other allowances payable to, and the other terms and conditions of service of the members of the State Commission shall be such as may be prescribed by the State Government.

(3) Every member of the State Commission shall hold office for a term of 5 years or up to the age of 67 years, whichever is earlier and shall not be eligible for reappointment.

(4) Notwithstanding anything contained in sub-section (3), a person appointed as a President or as a member before the commencement of the Consumer Protection (Amendment) Act, 1993, shall continue to hold such office as President or member, as the case may be, till the completion of his term.

17. **Jurisdiction of the State Commission—**

Subject to the other provisions of this Act, the State Commission shall have jurisdiction—

(a) to entertain—

    (i) complaints where the value of the goods or services and compensation, if any, claimed exceeds rupees five lakhs but does not exceed rupees twenty lakhs and

    (ii) appeals against the orders of any District Forum within the State and

(b) to call for the records and pass appropriate orders in any consumer dispute which is pending before or has been decided by any District Forum within the State where it appears to the State Commission that such District Forum has exercised a jurisdiction not vested in it by law, or has failed to exercise a jurisdiction so vested or has acted in exercise on its jurisdiction illegally or with material irregularity.

18. **Procedure applicable to State Commission—**

The provisions of Sections 12, 13 and 14 and the rules made thereunder for the disposal of complaint by the Districts Forum shall, with such modification as may be necessary, be applicable to the disposal of disputes by the State Commission:

18A. Vacancy in the office of the President—When the office of the President of the District Forum or of the State Commission, as the case may be, is vacant or when any such President is, by reason of absence or otherwise, unable to perform the duties of his office, the duties of the office shall be performed by such person, who is qualified to be appointed as President of the District Forum or, as the case may be, of the State Commission, as the State Government may appoint for the purpose.

19. **Appeals—**

Any person aggrieved by an order made by the State Commission in exercise of its powers conferred by sub-clause (i) of clause (a) of Section 17 may prefer an appeal against such order to the National Commission within a period of 30 days from the date of the order in such form and manner as may be prescribed:

Provided that the National Commission may entertain an appeal after the expiry of the said period of 30 days if it is satisfied that there was sufficient cause for not filing it within that period.

20. **Composition of the National Commission—**

(1) The National Commission shall consist of—

    (a) a person who is or has been a Judge of the Supreme Court, to be appointed by the Central Government, who shall be its President:

        Provided that no appointment under this clause shall be made except after consultation with the Chief Justice of India

    (b) four other members who shall be persons of ability, integrity and standing and have adequate knowledge or experience of, or have shown capacity in dealing with, problems relating to economics, law, commerce, accountancy, industry, public affairs or administration, one of whom shall be a woman:

        Provided that every appointment under this clause shall be made by the Central Government on the recommendation of a selection committee consisting of the following, namely,—

        (a) a person who is a Judge of the Supreme Court, to be nominated by the Chief Justice of India—Chairman,

        (b) the Secretary in the Department of Legal Affairs in the Government of India—Member.

(2) The salary or honorarium and other allowances payable to and the other terms and conditions of service of the members of the National Commission shall be such as may be prescribed by the Central Government.

(3) Every member of the National Commission shall hold office for a term of 5 years or up to the age of 70 years, whichever is earlier and shall not be eligible for re-appointment.

(4) Notwithstanding anything contained in sub-section (3), a person appointed as a President or as a member before the commencement of the Consumer Protection (Amendment) Act, 1993, shall continue to hold such office as President or member, as the case may be, till the completion of his term.

21. **Jurisdiction of the National Commission—**

Subject to the other provisions of this Act, the National Commission shall have jurisdiction—

(a) to entertain
   (i) complaints where the value of the goods or services and compensation, if any, claimed exceeds rupees [twenty lakhs] and
   (ii) appeals against the orders of any State Commission and

(b) to call for the records and pass appropriate orders in any consumer dispute which is pending before or has been decided by any State Commission where it appears to the National Commission that such State Commission has exercised a jurisdiction not vested in it by law, or has failed to exercise a jurisdiction so vested, or has acted in the exercise of its jurisdiction illegally or with material irregularity.

22. **Power of and procedure applicable to the National Commission—**

The National Commission shall, in the disposal of any complaints or of any proceedings before it, have

(a) the powers of a civil court as specified in sub-sections (4), (5) and (6) of Section 13

(b) the power to issue an order to the opposite party directing him to do any one or more of the things referred to in clauses (a) to (i) of sub-section (1) of Section 14, and follow such procedure as may be prescribed by the Central Government.

23. **Appeal—**

Any person, aggrieved by an order made by the National Commission in exercise of its powers conferred by sub-clause (i) of clause (a) of Section 21, may prefer an appeal against such order to the Supreme Court within a period of 30 days from the date of the order:

Provided that the Supreme Court may entertain an appeal after the expiry of the said period of 30 days if it is satisfied that there was sufficient cause for not filing it within that period.

24. **Finality of order—**

Every order of a District Forum, State Commission or the National Commission shall, if no appeal has been preferred against such order under the provisions of this Act, be final.

24A. **Limitation period—**

(1) The District Forum, the State Commission or the National Commission shall not admit a complaint unless it is filed within 2 years from the date on which the cause of action has arisen.

(2) Notwithstanding anything contained in sub-section (1), a complaint may be entertained after the period specified in sub-section (1), if the complainant satisfies the District Forum, the State Commission or the National Commission, as the case may be, that he had sufficient cause for not filing the complaint within such period:

Provided that no such complaint shall be entertained unless the National Commission, the State Commission or the District Forum, as the case may be, records its reasons for condoning such delay.

24B. Administrative control—

(1) The National Commission shall have administrative control over all the State Commissions in the following matters, namely,—

   (i) calling for periodical returns regarding the institution, disposal, pendency of cases

   (ii) issuance of instructions regarding adoption of uniform procedure in the hearing of matters, prior service of copies of documents produced by one party to the opposite parties, furnishing of English translation of judgments written in any language, speedy grant of copies of documents

   (iii) generally overseeing the functioning of the State Commissions or the District Fora to ensure that the objects and purposes of the Act are best served without in any way interfering with their quasi-judicial freedom.

(2) The State Commission shall have administrative controls over all the District Fora within its jurisdiction in all matters referred to in sub-section (1).

25. Enforcement of orders by the forum, the State Commission or the National Commission—

Every order made by the District Forum, the State Commission or the National Commission, may be enforced by the District Forum, the State Commission or the National Commission as the case may be, in the same manner as if it were a decree or order made by a court in a suit pending therein and it shall be lawful for the District Forum, the State Commission or the National Commission to send, in the event of its inability to execute it, such order to the court within the local limits of whose jurisdiction—

(a) in the case of an order against a company, the registered office of the company is situated, or

(b) in the case of an order against any other person, the place where the person concerned voluntarily resides or carries on business or personally works for gain, is situated, and thereupon, the court to which the order is so sent, shall execute the order as if it were a decree or order sent to it for execution.

26. Dismissal of frivolous or vexatious complaints—

Where a complaint instituted before the District Forum, the State Commission or, as the case may be, the National Commission, is found to be frivolous or vexatious, it shall, for reasons to be recorded in writing, dismiss the complaint and make an order that the complainant shall pay to the opposite party such cost, not exceeding ten thousand rupees, as may be specified in the order.

27. Penalties—

Where a trader or a person against whom a complaint is made [or the complainant] fails or omits to comply with any order made by the District Forum, the State Commission or the National Commission, as the case may be, such trader or person [or complainant] shall be punishable with imprisonment for a term which shall not be less than one month but which may extend to 3 years, or with fine which shall not be less than two thousand rupees but which may extend to ten thousand rupees, or with both:

Provided that the District Forum, the State Commission or the National Commission, as the case may be, may, if it is satisfied that the circumstances of any case so require, impose a sentence of imprisonment or fine, or both, for a term lesser than minimum term and the amount lesser than the minimum amount, specified in this section.

CHAPTER IV: MISCELLANEOUS

28. Protection of action taken in good faith—

No suit, prosecution or other legal proceedings shall lie against the members of the District Forum, the State Commissions or the National Commission or any officer or person acting under the direction of the District Forum, the State Commission or the National Commission for executing any order made by it or in respect of anything which is in good faith done or intended to be done by such member, officer or person under this Act or under any rule or order made thereunder.

29. Power to remove difficulties—

(1) If any difficulty arises in giving effect to the provisions of this Act, the Central Government may, by order in the Official Gazette, make such provisions not inconsistent with the provisions of this Act as appear to it to be necessary or expedient for removing the difficulty:

Provided that no such order shall be made after the expiry of a period of 2 years from the commencement of this Act.

(2) Every order made under this section shall, as soon as may be after it is made, be laid before each House of Parliament.

29A. Vacancies or defects in appointment not to invalidate orders—

No act or proceeding of the Districts Forum, the State Commission or the National Commission shall be invalid by reason only of the existence of any vacancy amongst its members or any defect in the constitution thereof.

30. Power to make rules—

(1) The Central Government may, by notification, make rules for carrying out the provisions contained in [clause (a) of sub-section (1) of Section 2], clause (b) of sub-section (2) of Section 4, sub-section (2) of section 5, clause (vi) of sub-section (4) of section 13, section 19, sub-section (2) of Section 20 and Section 22 of this Act.

(2) The State Government may, by notification, make rules for carrying out the provisions contained in [clause (b) of sub-section (2) and sub-section (4) of Section 7], sub-section (3) of Section 10, clause (c) of sub-section (1) of Section 13, sub-section (3) of Section 14, Section 15 and sub-section (2) of Section 16.

31. Laying of rules—

(1) Every rule made by the Central Government under this Act shall be laid, as soon as may be after it is made, before each House of Parliament, while it is in session, for a total period of 30 days which may be comprised in one session or in two or more successive sessions, and if, before the expiry of the session immediately following the session or the successive sessions aforesaid, both Houses agree in making any modification in the rule or both Houses agree that the rule should not be made, the rule shall thereafter have effect only in such modified form or be of no effect, as the case may be so, however, that any such modification or annulment shall be without prejudice to the validity of anything previously done under that rule.

(2) Every rule made by a State Government under this Act shall be laid as soon as may be after it is made, before the State Legislature.

THE CONSUMER PROTECTION ACT, 2019: AMENDMENTS

The 2019 Act was notified on 15th July 2020 and brought into effect on 20th July 2020 and has established consumer councils etc. to settle consumer's grievances and matters connected there with it. This Act was enacted basically to resolve a large pendency of consumer complaints in Consumer Forums and Courts across the country. The Act defined the jurisdiction of the Consumer Disputes Redressal Commission (CDRCs). Under the new Act the National CDRC is empowered to hear complaints worth more than ₹10 crores and the State CDRC was given jurisdiction for the value of more than ₹1 crore but less than ₹10 crore. This empowered the District CDRC to entertain complaints where the value of goods or service is up to ₹1 crore.

The features of the new Act were as under:-

Commencement of E-filing: The New Act lays down provisions permitting consumers to file complaints electronically or through the process of E-filing. The proceedings and Evidence can be done through video-conferencing thereby giving procedural ease and reducing hassle for the consumers. Further, a consumer can also file the complaint from wherever he resides rather than relying on territorial jurisdiction. Inclusion of Unfair Trade practices: The 2019 Act introduces Unfair Trade Practices definition, and gives privacy to Consumers for information they share in confidence. Any disclosure has to be made in accordance with the provisions of any other law. Procedure for Appeal altered: The Opposing Party has to deposit 50% of the amount ordered by the District Commission before filing an appeal to the State Consumer Disputes Redressal Commission, as opposed to the earlier maximum amount of ₹25,000/-, as the old ceiling has been made redundant. Inclusion of E-commerce transactions: Under the 2019 Act E-commerce transactions are included for adjudication under direct sales. Mediation as an ADR: Under the 2019 Act Mediation has been introduced as an alternate mode of dispute resolution. Augmented Penalties: In the New Act, the CCPA imposes a penalty of up to ₹1,000,000 on a producer or an endorser, for a false or deceiving advertisement, as also a sentence for imprisonment for up to 2 years is provided for. A repeat offender may get penalized ₹5,000,000 and face imprisonment of up to 5 years.

Way ahead with the 2019 Act

As consumers cannot examine the goods in move-away selling, the vendor has all-encompassing obligations to disclose information about his products and the consumer has the right of withdrawal in many cases, which is really a good protection for the consumer. The 2019 Act establishes central regulator viz the Central Consumer Protection Authority (CCPA), to tackle issues related to consumer rights, unfair trade practices, misleading advertisements and imposes penalties for selling damaged or simulated products. Therefore, it is believed that the new Act gives stringent measures and stiffens existing rules to safeguard the consumer.

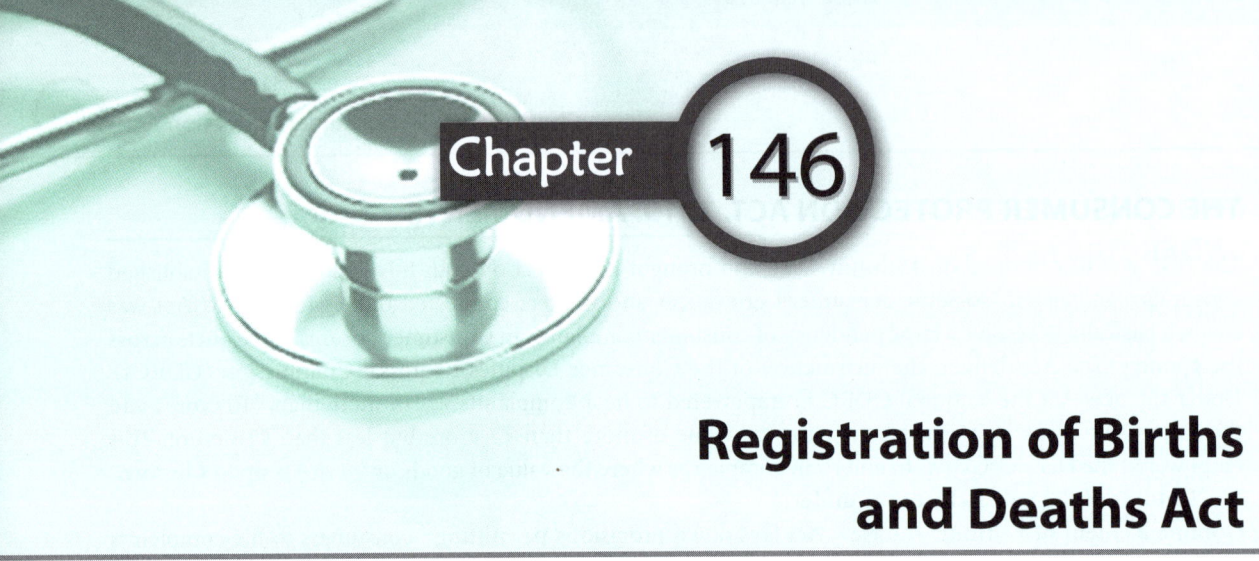

Registration of Births and Deaths Act

The Registration of Births and Deaths (Amendment) Bill, 2012 was introduced in Rajya Sabha on May 7, 2012 by Mr. Salman Khurshid, Minister of Law and Justice.

SHORT TITLE AND COMMENCEMENT

1. (a) This Act may be called the Registration of Births and Deaths (Amendment) Act, 212.
    (b) It shall come into force on such date as the Central Government may, by notification in the official Gazette, appoint.

AMENDMENT OF LONG TITLE

2. In the Registration of Births and Deaths Act, 1969 (hereinafter referred to as the principal Act), in the long title, for the words "Births and Deaths", the words "Births, Marriages and Deaths" shall be substituted.

AMENDMENT OF SECTION 1

3. In Section 1 of the principal Act, in sub-section (1), for the words "Births and Deaths", the words "Births, Marriages and Deaths" shall be substituted.

SUBSTITUTION OF REFERENCE TO CERTAIN EXPRESSIONS BY CERTAIN OTHER EXPRESSIONS

4. Throughout the principal Act (except Sections 8, 9, 10 and 20), for the words "births and deaths", "births or deaths", "every birth and of every death" wherever they occur, the words "births, marriages and deaths", "births or marriages or deaths" and "every birth, every marriage and of every death", as the case may be, shall respectively be substituted; and such other consequential amendments as the rules of grammar may require shall also be made.

INSERTION OF NEW SECTION 1A

5. After Section 1 of the principal Act, the following section shall be inserted, namely:—

APPLICATION OF PROVISIONS RELATING TO REGISTRATION OF MARRIAGES UNDER THIS ACT

"1A.(1) Every person shall get his marriage registered under this Act or the Anand Marriage Act, 1909 or under any other law for the time being in force (including State Act).

(2) The parties to the marriage, whose marriage has been registered under this Act, shall not be required to get their marriage registered under the Anand Marriage Act, 1909 or any other law for the time being in force (including State Act).

(3) The provisions of this Act shall not apply to any person who has registered his marriage under any other law for the time being in force including a State Act providing for registration of marriages or with any other authority under that law and nothing contained in this Act shall affect the validity of the marriages registered under that law."

AMENDMENT OF SECTION 2

6. In Section, 2 of the principal Act, in sub-section (1), after clause (d), the following clause shall be inserted, namely:—

'(da) "marriage" means and includes a marriage solemnized between a male and a female belonging to any caste or religion or tribe under any law for the time being in force and includes marriages solemnized under any custom or usage in any form or manner recognized by law or the marriage registered under any law for the time being in force and also includes remarriage.

AMENDMENT OF SECTION 7

7. In Section 7 of the principal Act, after sub-section (2), the following sub-section shall be inserted, namely:—

"(2A) Every Registrar shall, on payment of prescribed fees, enter in the register maintained for the purpose, all information given to him under Section 8 or Section 8A or Section 9 and shall also take steps to inform himself carefully of every marriage which takes place in his jurisdiction and to ascertain and register the particulars required to be registered."

INSERTION OF NEW SECTIONS 8A AND 8B

8. After Section 8 of the principal Act, the following section shall be inserted, namely:—

PERSONS REQUIRED TO REGISTER MARRIAGES

"8A.(1) For the purposes of facilitating the proof of marriages, the parties to the marriages, who intend to get their marriage registered under this Act shall, either themselves, or from the persons specified below, give or cause to be given, either orally or in writing, according to the best of their knowledge and belief, within such time as may be prescribed, information and requisite documents and fees to the Registrar of the several particulars required to be entered in the forms prescribed by the State Government under sub-Section (1) of Section 16, —

(a) in respect of marriage in a house, whether residential or non-residential, not being any place referred to in clauses (b) and (c), the head of the house, and in the absence of any such person, the oldest adult male person present therein during the said period;

(b) in respect of marriage in a temple, church, mosque, synagogue or such other religious place, the priest or such other person, by whatever name called, officiating such marriage or the trustee or any other person in charge thereof;

(c) in respect of marriage in a place specifically used for conducting marriages, including marriage halls, choultry, chatram, hotels or such other place, the person in charge thereof;

(d) in respect of marriage in an open place or field or ground, the headman

or other corresponding officer in the case of a village and the officer in charge of the local police station elsewhere;

(e) in any other place, such person as may be prescribed.

(2) Notwithstanding anything contained in sub-section (1), the State Government, having regard to the conditions obtaining in a registration division, may, by order, require that for such period as may be specified in the order, any person specified by the State Government by designation in this behalf, shall give or cause to be given information regarding marriages in a house referred to in clause (a) of sub-section (1) instead of the persons specified in that clause.

(3) Without prejudice to the provisions contained in this Act, the State Government may make rules providing that the parties to a marriage may have particulars relating to their marriage entered in such manner and subject to such conditions as may be prescribed.

REFUSAL TO REGISTER MARRIAGE

8B. The Registrar shall not refuse to register any marriage for which a duly filled up and signed form has been received by him except on such grounds as may be prescribed:

Provided that different grounds may be specified by rules for different class or classes of persons to marriage.

INSERTION OF NEW SECTION 10A

9. After Section 10 of the principal Act, the following section shall be inserted, namely:—

DUTY OF CERTAIN PERSONS TO INFORM MARRIAGES

"10A.(1) Upon the request made by parties to the marriage who intend to get their marriage registered under this Act, it shall be the duty of the persons referred to in clauses (a) to (e) of sub-section (1) of Section 8A to give necessary information and documents relating to such marriage to the Registrar within such time and in such manner as may be prescribed.

(2) In any area, the State Government, having regard to the facilities available therein in this behalf, may require that a certificate as to marriage shall be obtained by the Registrar from such person and in such form as may be prescribed."

SUBSTITUTION OF NEW SECTION FOR SECTION 13

10. For Section 13 of the principal Act, the following section shall be substituted, namely:—

DELAYED REGISTRATION OF BIRTHS' MARRIAGES OR DEATHS

"13. (1) Any birth or marriage or death, as the case may be, of which information is given to the Registrar after the expiry of the period specified therefor, but within 30 days of its occurrence, shall be registered on payment of such late fee as may be prescribed.

(2) Any birth or marriage or death, as the case may be, of which delayed information is given to the Registrar after 30 days but within one year of its occurrence shall be registered only with the written permission of the prescribed authority and on payment of the prescribed fee and the production of an affidavit made before a notary public or any other officer authorized in this behalf by the State Government.

(3) Any birth or marriage or death, as the case may be, which has not been registered within one year of its occurrence, shall be registered only on an order made by a Magistrate of the first class after verifying the correctness of the birth or marriage or death and on payment of the prescribed fee.

(4) The provisions of this section shall be without prejudice to any action that may be taken against a person for failure on his part to register any birth or marriage or death within the time specified therefor and any such birth or marriage or death, as the case may be, may be registered during the pendency of any such action."

SUBSTITUTION OF NEW SECTION FOR SECTION 15

11. For Section 15 of the principal Act, the following section shall be substituted, namely:—

CORRECTION OR CANCELLATION OF ENTRY IN THE REGISTER OF BIRTHS OR MARRIAGES OR DEATHS

"15. If it is proved to the satisfaction of the Registrar that any entry of a birth or marriage or death in any register kept by him under this Act is erroneous in form or substance, or has been fraudulently or improperly made, he may, subject to such rules as may be made by the State Government with respect to the conditions on which and the circumstances in which such entries may be corrected or cancelled, correct the error or cancel the entry by suitable entry in the margin, without any alteration of the original entry, and shall sign the marginal entry and add thereto the date of the correction or cancellation."

SUBSTITUTION OF NEW SECTION FOR SECTION 17

12. For Section 17 of the principal Act, the following section shall be substituted, namely: —

SEARCH OF BIRTHS, MARRIAGES AND DEATHS REGISTER

"17. (1) Subject to any rules made in this behalf by the State Government, including rules relating to the payment of fees and postal charges, any person may—

(a) cause a search to be made by the Registrar for any entry in a register of births, marriages and deaths; and

(b) obtain an extract from such register relating to any birth or marriage or death:

Provided that no extract relating to any death, issued to any person, shall disclose the particulars regarding the cause of death as entered in the register.

(2) All extracts given under this section shall be certified by the Registrar or any other officer authorized by the State Government to give such extracts as provided in Section 76 of the Indian Evidence Act, 1872, and shall be admissible in evidence for the purpose of proving the birth or marriage or death to which the entry relates."

SUBSTITUTION OF NEW SECTION FOR SECTION 21

13. For Section 21 of the principal Act, the following section shall be substituted, namely: —

POWER OF REGISTRAR TO OBTAIN INFORMATION REGARDING BIRTH OR MARRIAGE OR DEATH

"21. The Registrar may either orally or in writing require any person to furnish any information within his knowledge in connection with a birth or marriage or death in the locality within which such person resides and that person shall be bound to comply with such requisition."

AMENDMENT OF SECTION 23

14. In Section 23 of the principal Act,—
    (i) in sub-section (1), in clause (a), for the word and figures "Sections 8 and 9", the words, figure and letter "Section 8 or Section 8A or Section 9" shall be substituted;
    (ii) after sub-section (3), the following sub-section shall be inserted, namely:—
    "(3A) Any person who contravenes the provisions of sub-section (1) of Section 10A, shall be punishable with fine which may extend to fifty rupees."

INSERTION OF NEW SECTION 29A

15. After Section 29 of the principal Act, the following section shall inserted, namely:—

REGISTRATION OF MARRIAGES NOT TO AFFECT RIGHTS OF PARTIES TO MARRIAGE

"29A. The provisions of this Act relating to registration of marriage shall be in addition to, and not in derogation of, any other law for the time being in force and the registration of marriages of the parties under this Act shall not be deemed to affect any right recognized or acquired by any such party under any law, custom or usage.

AMENDMENT OF SECTION 30

16. In Section 30 of the principal Act,—
    (i) after clause (a), the following clauses shall be inserted, namely:-—
        (aa) the fees under sub-section (2A) of Section 7;
    (ii) after clause (b), the following clauses shall be inserted, namely:—
        "(ba) the period within which information should be given to the Registrar under sub-section (1) of Section 8A;

(bb) the persons under clause (e) of sub-section (1) of Section 8A;

(bc) the manner and the conditions under sub-section (3) of Section 8A; (bd) the grounds under Section 8B;"

(iii) after clause (c), the following clauses shall be inserted, namely:—

"(ca) the time and the manner for giving information under sub-section (1) of Section 10A;

(cb) the persons from whom and the form in which certificate shall be obtained."

INSERTION OF NEW SECTION 30A

17. After Section 30 of the principal Act, the following section shall be inserted, namely:—

POWER OF CENTRAL GOVERNMENT TO MAKE RULES

"30A. (1) The Central Government may, by notification in the Official Gazette, make such provisions for implementation of the provisions of this Act and for carrying out the purposes of this Act.

(2) The Central Government may, by notification in the Official Gazette, direct that any of the provisions of this Act specified in the notification—

(a) shall not apply to any marriages solemnized under any Act for the time being in force or any customs or usage recognized in law;

(b) shall apply to any marriages solemnized under any Act for the time being in force or any customs or usage recognized in law, with such exceptions, modifications and adaptations as may be specified in the notification."

AMENDMENT OF SECTION 31

18. In Section 31 of the principal Act, after sub-section (2), the following sub-section shall be inserted, namely:—

"(3) Nothing contained in sub-sections (1) and (2) shall apply to any matter or law relating to marriages including the Anand Marriage Act, 1909 or any State law or to any rules or notification or order making provisions for registration of marriages in any State."

STATEMENT OF OBJECTS AND REASONS

1. The Registration of Births and Deaths (Amendment) Bill, 2012 seeks to amend the Registration of Births and Deaths Act, 1969 (18 of 1969) so as to provide for registration of marriages irrespective of religion professed and practiced by the parties to the marriage. At present the Registration of Births and Deaths Act, 1969 provides only for the regulation of registration of births and deaths and for matters connected therewith.

2. The Hon'ble Supreme Court in Seema *Vs.* Ashwani Kumar (AIR 2006 SC 1158) in its judgment dated 14-02-2006 has directed the Government that marriages of all persons who are citizens of India belonging to various religious denominations should be made compulsorily registrable in their respective States where such marriages are solemnized and, *inter alia,* directed that as and when the Central Government enacts a comprehensive statute, the same shall be placed before that Court for scrutiny.

3. The Committee on Empowerment of Women (2006–2007) in its Twelfth Report (Fourteenth Lok Sabha) on Plight of Indian Women Deserted by Non Resident Indian (NRI) Husbands presented to Lok Sabha on the 13th August, 2007, has, *inter alia,* expressed the view that all marriages, irrespective of religion should be compulsorily registered and desired that the Government to make registration of all marriages mandatory, making the procedure simpler, affordable and accessible.

4. The 18th Law Commission of India in its 205th Report titled "Proposal to Amend the Prohibition of Child Marriage Act, 2006 and other Allied Laws", *inter alia,* recommended that "registration of marriages within a stipulated period, of all the communities, *viz.* Hindu, Muslim, Christian, etc., should be made mandatory by the Government". Further, the 18th Law Commission in its 211th Report titled "Laws on Registration of Marriage and Divorce—A proposal for Consolidation and Reform", has recommended for Parliamentary legislation on compulsory registration of marriages which will bring country-wide uniformity in the substantive law relating to registration and will be helpful in achieving the desired goal.

5. The Registration of Births and Deaths Act, 1969, *inter alia,* provides for Registration establishments consisting of Registrar-General, Chief Registrar and registration division, District Registrars and Registrars. It also provides procedures for registration of births and deaths and for maintenance of records and statistics. Further, by virtue of the powers conferred under Section 30 of the aforesaid Act, rules for compulsory registration of births and deaths have been framed by the State Governments and Union territory Administrations. Therefore, it is proposed to amend the aforesaid Act suitably to include registration of marriages as well within its scope so that the existing administrative machinery would also be able to carry out registration of marriages in accordance with the specified procedures and be able to maintain necessary records and statistics for registration of marriages also.

6. Having regard to the aforesaid directions of the Supreme Court, report of the Committee on Empowerment of Women and recommendations of the Law Commission referred to in the foregoing paragraphs, it is proposed to amend the Registration of Births and Deaths Act, 1969 to provide for compulsory registration of marriages without affecting in any manner the State law making provisions for compulsory registration of marriages in their respective States. For this purpose, suitable provisions are incorporated in the Bill to avoid any duplication of registration of marriages under the proposed Central law and the State law. It is also proposed to provide in the Bill that the Registration of Births and Deaths Act, 1969 (after the enactment of proposed amendments) shall not apply to any person who has registered his marriage under any other law for the time being in force including a State Act providing for registration of marriages or with any other authority under that law and nothing contained in this Act shall affect the validity of the marriages registered under that law. Further, the parties to the marriage, whose marriage has been registered under this Act shall not be required to get their marriage registered under the Anand Marriage Act, 1909 or any other law for the time being in force. Moreover, the registration of marriages thereunder shall not affect any right recognized or acquired by any party to marriage under any law, custom or usage.

7. The proposed Bill will provide for registration of marriages of all persons who are citizens of India belonging to various religious denominations and be beneficial to women, as the registration certificate would provide evidentiary value in matrimonial and maintenance cases and prevent unnecessary harassment meted out to them. It will also provide evidentiary value in the matters of age of parties, custody of children and the right of children born out of such marriages.

8. The Bill seeks to achieve the above objects.

ANNEXURE

EXTRACTS FROM THE REGISTRATION OF BIRTHS AND DEATHS ACT, 1969 (18 of 1969)

*   *   *   *   *

An Act to provide for the regulation of registration of births and deaths and for matters connected therewith.

*   *   *   *   *

CHAPTER I: PRELIMINARY

Short title, extent and commencement—

1. (1) This Act may be called the Registration of Births and Deaths Act, 1969.

*   *   *   *   *

Definitions—

2. (1) In this Act, unless the context otherwise requires,—

*   *   *   *   *

Delayed registration of births and deaths—

13. (1) Any birth or death of which information is given to the Registrar after the expiry of the period specified therefor, but within 30 days of its occurrence, shall be registered on payment of such late fee as may be prescribed.

(2) Any birth or death of which delayed information is given to the Registrar after 30 days but within one year of its occurrence shall be registered only with the written permission of the prescribed authority and on payment of the prescribed fee and the production of an affidavit made before a notary public or any other officer authorized in this behalf by the State Government.

(3) Any birth or death which has not been registered within one year of its occurrence, shall be registered only on an order made by a magistrate of the first class or a Presidency Magistrate after verifying the correctness of the birth or death and on payment of the prescribed fee.

(4) The provisions of this section shall be without prejudice to any action that may be taken against a person for failure on his part to register any birth or death within the time specified therefor and any such birth or death may be registered during the pendency of any such action.

*   *   *   *   *

Correction or cancellation of entry in the register of births and deaths—

15. If it is proved to the satisfaction of the Registrar that any entry of a birth or death in any register kept by him under this Act is erroneous in form or substance, or has been fraudulently or improperly made, he may, subject to such rules as may be made by the State Government with respect to the conditions on which and the circumstances in which such entries may be corrected or cancelled, correct the error or cancel the entry by suitable entry in the margin, without any alteration of the original entry, and shall sign the marginal entry and add thereto the date of the correction of cancellation.

*   *   *   *   *

17. (1) Subject to any rules made in this behalf by the State Government, including rules relating to the payment of fees and postal charges, any person may—

(a) cause a search to be made by the Registrar for any entry in a register of births and deaths; and

(b) obtain an extract from such register relating to any birth or death:

Provided that no extract relating to any death, issued to any person, shall disclose the particulars regarding the cause of death as entered in the register.

(2) All extracts given under this section shall be certified by the Registrar or any other officer authorized by the State Government to give such extracts as provided in Section 76 of the Indian Evidence Act, 1872, and shall be admissible in evidence for the purpose of proving the birth or death to which the entry relates.

*   *   *   *   *

Power of registrar to obtain information regarding births or deaths—

21. The Registrar may either orally or in writing require any person to furnish any information within his knowledge in connection with a birth or death in the locality within which such person resides and that person shall be bound to comply with such requisition.

*   *   *   *   *

Penalties—

23. (1) Any person who—

(a) fails without reasonable cause to give any information which it is his duty to give under any of the provisions of Sections 8 and 9; or

*   *   *   *   *

RAJYA SABHA

————

A

BILL

further to amend the Registration of Births and Deaths Act, 1969.

————

(Shri Salman Khurshid, Minister of Law and Justice)

GMGIPMRND—719RS(S3)—03-05-2012.

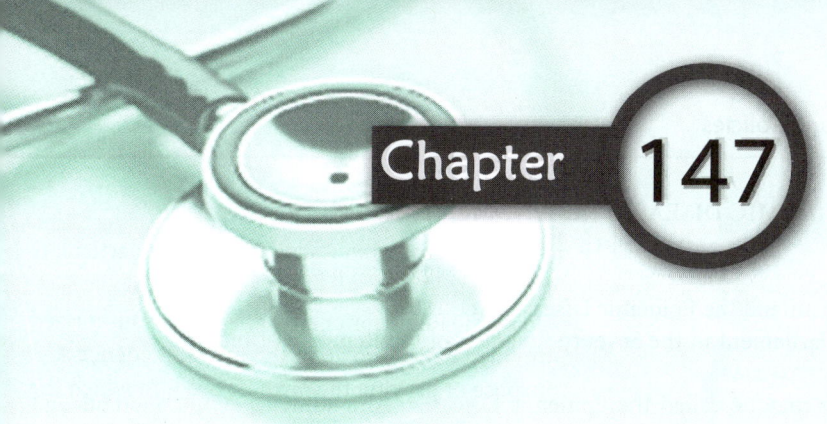

Chapter 147

Epidemic Diseases Act

[ACT NO. 3 OF 1897]

[4th February, 1897]

An act to provide for the better prevention of the spread of dangerous epidemic diseases.

Whereas it is expedient to provide for the better prevention of the spread of dangerous epidemic disease; it is hereby enacted as follows:—

1. **Short title and extent**— This Act may be called the Epidemic Diseases Act, 1897.

2. It extends to the whole of India except the territories Part B States.

2A. **Powers of Central Government**—When the Central Government is satisfied that India or any part thereof is visited by, or threatened with, an outbreak of any dangerous epidemic disease and that the ordinary provisions of the law for the time being in force are insufficient to prevent the outbreak of such disease or the spread thereof, the Central Government may take measures and prescribe regulations for the inspection of any ship or vessel leaving or arriving at any port in the territories to which this Act extends and for such detention thereof, or of any person intending to sail therein, or arriving thereby, as may be necessary.

3. **Penalty**—Any person disobeying any regulation or order made under this Act shall be deemed to have committed an offence punishable under Section 188 of the Indian Penal Code (45 of 1860).

4. **Protection to persons acting under Act**—No suit or other legal proceeding shall lie against any person for anything done or in good faith intended to be done under this Act.

This act was further amended and the amendments done in 2020 are as follows:

THE EPIDEMIC DISEASES (AMENDMENT) ACT, 2020
No. 34 of 2020

[28th September, 2020.]

An Act further to amend the Epidemic Diseases Act, 1897.

Be it enacted by Parliament in the Seventy-first Year of the Republic of India as follows:—

1. (1) This Act may be called the Epidemic Diseases (Amendment) Act, 2020.

   (2) It shall be deemed to have come into force on the 22nd day of April, 2020.

Short title and commencement.

3 of 1897.

2. In section 1 of the Epidemic Diseases Act, 1897 (hereinafter referred to as the principal Act), in sub-section (2), the words, figures and letters "except the territories which, immediately before the 1st November, 1956, were comprised in Part B States" shall be omitted.

Amendment of section 1.

Insertion of new section 1A.

Definitions.

3. After section 1 of the principal Act, the following section shall be inserted, namely:—

   '1A. In this Act, unless the context otherwise requires,—

   (a) "act of violence" includes any of the following acts committed by any person against a healthcare service personnel serving during an epidemic, which causes or may cause—

   (i) harassment impacting the living or working conditions of such healthcare service personnel and preventing him from discharging his duties;

   (ii) harm, injury, hurt, intimidation or danger to the life of such healthcare service personnel, either within the premises of a clinical establishment or otherwise;

   (iii) obstruction or hindrance to such healthcare service personnel in the discharge of his duties, either within the premises of a clinical establishment or otherwise; or

   (iv) loss or damage to any property or documents in the custody of, or in relation to, such healthcare service personnel;

   (b) "healthcare service personnel" means a person who while carrying out his duties in relation to epidemic related responsibilities, may come in direct contact with affected patients and thereby is at the risk of being impacted by such disease, and includes—

   (i) any public and clinical healthcare provider such as doctor, nurse, paramedical worker and community health worker;

   (ii) any other person empowered under the Act to take measures to prevent the outbreak of the disease or spread thereof; and

   (iii) any person declared as such by the State Government, by notification in the Official Gazette;

   (c) "property" includes—

   (i) a clinical establishment as defined in the Clinical Establishments (Registration and Regulation) Act, 2010;

23 of 2010.

(*ii*) any facility identified for quarantine and isolation of patients during an epidemic;

(*iii*) a mobile medical unit; and

(*iv*) any other property in which the healthcare service personnel have direct interest in relation to the epidemic;

(*d*) the words and expressions used herein and not defined, but defined in the Indian Ports Act, 1908, the Aircraft Act, 1934 or the Land Ports Authority of India Act, 2010, as the case may be, shall have the same meaning as assigned to them in that Act.'

15 of 1908.
22 of 1934.
31 of 2010.

Amendment of section 2A.

4. In section 2A of the principal Act, for the portion beginning with the words "the Central Government may take measures" and ending with the words "as may be necessary", the following shall be substituted, namely:— "the Central Government may take such measures, as it deems fit and prescribe regulations for the inspection of any bus or train or goods vehicle or ship or vessel or aircraft leaving or arriving at any land port or port or aerodrome, as the case may be, in the territories to which this Act extends and for such detention thereof, or of any person intending to travel therein, or arriving thereby, as may be necessary.".

Insertion of new section 2B.

Prohibition of violence against healthcare service personnel and damage to property.

5. After section 2A of the principal Act, the following section shall be inserted, namely:— "2B. No person shall indulge in any act of violence against a healthcare service personnel or cause any damage or loss to any property during an epidemic.".

Amendment of section 3.

6. Section 3 of the principal Act shall be renumbered as sub-section (*1*) thereof, and after sub-section (*1*) as so renumbered, the following sub-sections shall be inserted, namely:— "(*2*) Whoever,—

(*i*) commits or abets the commission of an act of violence against the healthcare service personnel; or

(*ii*) abets or causes damage or loss to any property,

shall be punished with imprisonment for a term which shall not be less than three months, but which may extend to five years, and with fine, which shall not be less than fifty thousand rupees, but which may extend to two lakh rupees.

45 of 1860.

(*3*) Whoever, while committing an act of violence against the healthcare service personnel, causes grievous hurt as defined in section 320 of the Indian Penal Code to such person, shall be punished with imprisonment for a term which shall not be less than six months, but which may extend to seven years and with fine, which shall not be less than one lakh rupees, but which may extend to five lakh rupees.".

7. After section 3 of the principal Act, the following sections shall be inserted, namely:— Insertion of new sections 3A, 3B, 3C, 3D and 3E.

2 of 1974.

'3A. Notwithstanding anything contained in the Code of Criminal Procedure, 1973,— Cognizance, investigation and trial of offences.

     (*i*) an offence punishable under sub-section (*2*) or sub-section (*3*) of section 3 shall be cognizable and non-bailable;

     (*ii*) any case registered under sub-section (*2*) or sub-section (*3*) of section 3 shall be investigated by a police officer not below the rank of Inspector;

     (*iii*) investigation of a case under sub-section (*2*) or sub-section (*3*) of section 3 shall be completed within a period of thirty days from the date of registration of the First Information Report;

     (*iv*) in every inquiry or trial of a case under sub-section (*2*) or sub-section (*3*) of section 3, the proceedings shall be held as expeditiously as possible, and in particular, when the examination of witnesses has once begun, the same shall be continued from day to day until all the witnesses in attendance have been examined, unless the Court finds the adjournment of the same beyond the following day to be necessary for reasons to be recorded, and an endeavor shall be made to ensure that the inquiry or trial is concluded within a period of one year:

Provided that where the trial is not concluded within the said period, the Judge shall record the reasons for not having done so:

Provided further that the said period may be extended by such further period, for reasons to be recorded in writing, but not exceeding six months at a time.

Composition of certain offences. 3B. Where a person is prosecuted for committing an offence punishable under sub-section (*2*) of section 3, such offence may, with the permission of the Court, be compounded by the person against whom such act of violence is committed.

Presumption as to certain offences. 3C. Where a person is prosecuted for committing an offence punishable under sub-section (*3*) of section 3, the Court shall presume that such person has committed such offence, unless the contrary is proved.

Presumption of culpable mental state. 3D. (1) In any prosecution for an offence under sub-section (*3*) of section 3 which requires a culpable mental state on the part of the accused, the Court shall presume the existence of such mental state, but it shall be a defence for the accused to prove the fact that he had no such mental state with respect to the act charged as an offence in that prosecution.

     (2) For the purposes of this section, a fact is said to be proved only when the Court believes it to exist beyond reasonable doubt and not merely when its existence is established by a preponderance of probability.

Explanation.—In this section, "culpable mental state" includes intention, motive, knowledge of a fact and the belief in, or reason to believe, a fact.

Compensation for acts of violence.

3E. (1) In addition to the punishment provided for an offence under sub-section (2) or sub-section (3) of section 3, the person so convicted shall also be liable to pay, by way of compensation, such amount, as may be determined by the Court for causing hurt or grievous hurt to any healthcare service personnel.

(2) Notwithstanding the composition of an offence under section 3B, in case of damage to any property or loss caused, the compensation payable shall be twice the amount of fair market value of the damaged property or the loss caused, as may be determined by the Court.

(3) Upon failure to pay the compensation awarded under sub-sections (1) and (2), such amount shall be recovered as an arrear of land revenue under the Revenue Recovery Act, 1890:

1 of 1890.

Repeal and savings.

8. (1) The Epidemic Diseases (Amendment) Ordinance, 2020 is hereby repealed.

Ord. 5 of 2020.

(2) Notwithstanding such repeal, anything done or any action taken under the Epidemic Diseases Act, 1897, as amended by the said Ordinance, shall be deemed to have been done or taken under the corresponding provisions of the said Act as amended by this Act.

3 of 1897.

————

DR. G. NARAYANA RAJU,
Secretary to the Govt. of India.

Notes

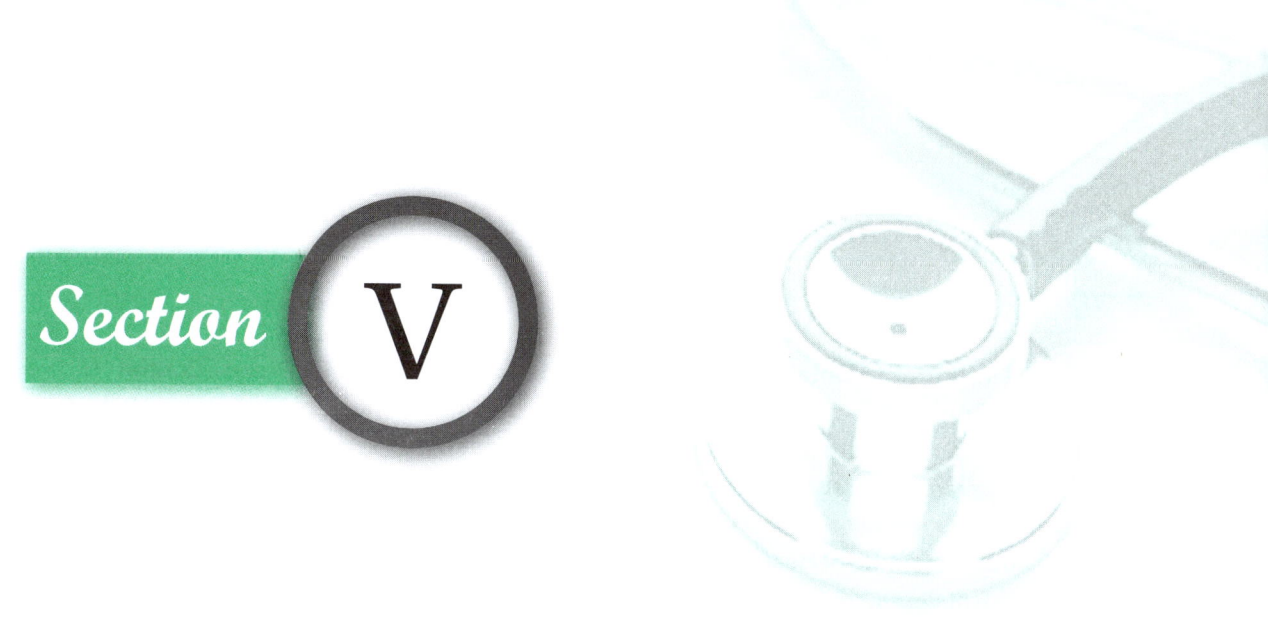

Section **V**

NATIONAL HEALTH INSTITUTES

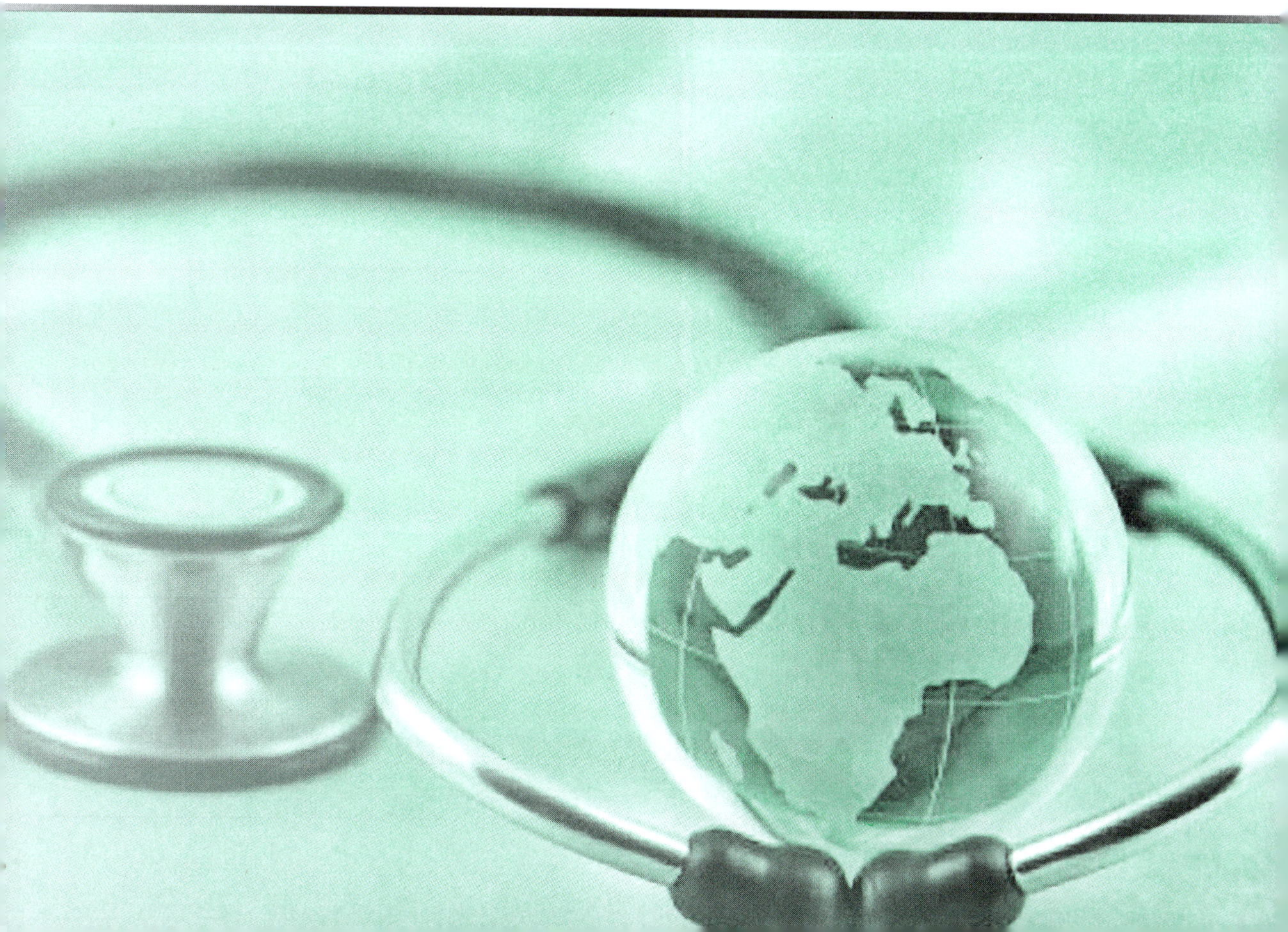

Contents

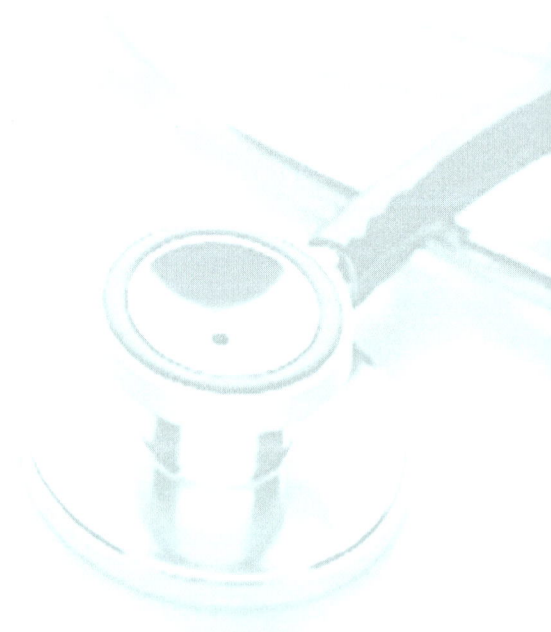

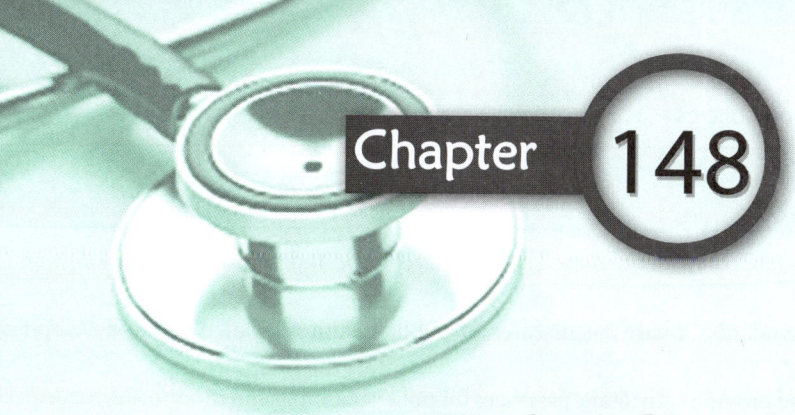

Chapter 148

National Institute of Mental Health and Neurosciences

INTRODUCTION

The National Institute of Mental Health and Neurosciences (NIMHANS) is a multidisciplinary institute for patient care and academic pursuit in the field of mental health and neurosciences.

NIMHANS is synonymous with providing high standards of clinical care, quality training and cutting-edge research in the frontier areas. Combined priorities for comprehensive patient care, manpower development and research, stem from the commitment to an integrated and multidisciplinary approach which addresses societal needs. The advances in genomics, computational neuroscience, mathematical modeling, neuroimaging, molecular biology and a host of new disciplines including public health, are being translated to help humanity in need and promote the growth of knowledge.

A special feature of this Institute since its inception is the combination of research and training with promotive, preventive and curative aspects of clinical services in Mental Health and Neurosciences.

The manpower development programmes at NIMHANS reflect the strides in fusing together and nurturing behavioral sciences, neurosciences, basic biological sciences and ancient health systems.

The Institute provides inputs to the Central and State Governments in areas including the establishment of new psychiatric facilities, improvement of existing facilities and strategizing a national programme for mental health.

The Institute has emerged as the nodal center for evolving national policies in the field of mental health, neurosciences and injury. This exemplifies a unique model of successful partnership between the Union and State Governments (Ministry of Health and Family Welfare).

NIMHANS has made significant progress and is a center for excellence in mental health and neuroscience in the country. NIMHANS has produced more than 1,000 psychiatrists, about 600 clinical psychologists and psychiatric nurses so far—who are working in both national and international contexts.

The Central Government recognized its eminent academic position, growth and contributions, and declared it a 'Deemed University' in 1994. In 2012, NIMHANS was conferred the status of an 'Institute of National Importance'.

VISION

To be a world leader in the area of mental health and neurosciences and evolve state-of-the-art approaches to patient care through translational research.

MISSION

- Test establish the highest standards of evidence-based care for psychiatric and neurological disorders and rehabilitation.
- Develop expertise and set standards of care for diseases of public health relevance in the developing world.
- Work with the government and provide consultancy services for policy planning and monitoring strategies in the field of mental health and neurosciences and facilitate execution of national health programme.
- Human resource capacity building by training in diverse fields related to mental health and neurosciences.
- Develop and strengthen inter-disciplinary, inter-institutional and international collaboration with universities and research institutes across the globe to foster scientific research, training in advanced technology and exchange of ideas in the areas of mental health and neurosciences.
- Strive to enhance equitable accessibility of primary care in mental health and neurological disorders to all sections of society and ages including the vulnerable population.
- Evolve and monitor the strategies for disaster management and psycho-social rehabilitation in different cultural and ethnic groups.
- Promote mental health literacy and eliminate the stigma attached to the mental and neurological Illnesses by taking the measures and the delivery system to the centers of primary health care honoring the human rights and dignity.
- Integrate allopathic and oriental medicine into health care delivery and promote evidence-based research.
- Integrate physical and metaphysical aspects of neuroscience research to promote yoga and its application to positive mental health.
- Participate in broad field of neuroscience and behavioral research applicable to human ethics, organ transplantation, stem cell research, space science, and nuclear science.

Milestones	
1847	Bangalore Lunatic Asylum was founded. Dr. Charles Irving Smith, a British medical practitioner in Bengaluru, played a pivotal role in the establishment of the asylum.
1925	The Bengaluru asylum was renamed the Mysore Government Mental Hospital, an important step towards developing a medical approach to mental illness.
1935	Insulin Coma Therapy (ICT), developed by Austrian-American psychiatrist Manfred J Sakel, was introduced in the Mysore Government Mental Hospital by Dr. MV Govindaswamy, the then medical superintendent of the Mysore Government Mental Hospital, as in the UK (1935) and the US (1936).
1936	The second highest hillock in Bengaluru was allotted for the hospital, which was earlier housed in a building on Avenue Road, where the State Bank of Mysore head office stands today. Maharaja of Mysore, Krishnaraja Wadiyar laid the foundation stone for constructing the hospital in May, 1936.
1940	A well-equipped laboratory and medical library were started. The Hospital was recognized as a teaching institution for MBBS, BA Hons. in Psychology, and LMP.
1942	The first leucotomy operation in the country was performed on 21st September 1942 by Dr MV Govindaswamy and Dr. BN Balakrishna Rao at the hospital.

Contd…

Milestones	
1945	Following the recommendations of the Mental Health Advisory Committee of the Indian Council for Medical Hygiene under Sir AL Mudaliar in 1945 and Bhore Committee in 1946, the Government of India sanctioned the establishment of the All India Institute of Mental Health on 1st April 1954. On 6th August 1954, Rajkumari Amrit Kaur, the then Union Health Minister inaugurated the AIIMH and Dr MV Govindaswamy was appointed as the Director on 15th September 1954.
1955	The first postgraduate courses, Diploma in Psychological Medicine (DPM) and Diploma in Medical Psychology (DMP) were started.
1961	Children's Pavilion comprising a child guidance clinic and a children's ward was opened.
1966	New postgraduate courses in psychiatry (MD psychological Medicine), Neurology (DM Neurology), Neurosurgery (MCh Neurosurgery) and Post Graduate Diploma in Psychiatric Social Work (DPSW) in affiliation with Bangalore University. Five special clinics: Anxiety Clinic, Behavior Disorder Clinic, Headache Clinic, Hysteria Clinic and Mental Deficiency Clinic started functioning from the same year.
1971	Occupational Therapy and Rehabilitation Center with different sections was inaugurated.
1973	The Neurocenter, with a separate blood bank and a well-equipped neuroradiology section was inaugurated.
1974	The Mental Hospital established by the Government of Mysore and the All India Institute of Mental Health established by the Government of India were amalgamated on 27th December 1974, resulting in the formation of the National Institute of Mental Health and Neurosciences (NIMHANS). Community Psychiatry Unit was also launched in the same year.
1975	Neuropathology Museum storing human brain specimens for academic and research purposes was inaugurated. Community mental health services were launched at Sakalwara. A unique facility of family wards was also opened.
1979	The Central Animal Research Facility (CARF) was started as an aid to research and teaching.
1982	Electron Microscopy Lab in the Neuropathology Department was established.
1994	Recognizing its eminent academic position, NIMHANS was declared a Deemed University, with academic autonomy.
1995	The Human Brain Bank was established with financial aid from the Department of Science and Technology (DST), Department of Biotechnology (DBT), and Indian Council for Medical Research (ICMR).
2002	Advanced Center for Ayurveda to augment clinical service and research activity was started.
2007	The Neurobiology Research Center (NRC), a sophisticated common research facility, was opened.
2011	Inventa, a critical care ventilator, was developed by NIMHANS.
2011	The NIMHANS Center for well-being at BTM Layout was started, with an aim to provide promotive and preventive services in the area of mental health.
2012	NIMHANS was declared an Institute of National Importance, vide the Gazette of India Notification dated 14th September 2012 by the Government of India. Center for Public Health (CPH) was established to provide inputs for strengthening public health components in formulating policies and programme development focusing on problems, priorities, challenges and solutions, in the same year.
2014	ICMR Advanced Center for Translational Research was started.

2014 NIMHANS Integrated Centre for Yoga (NICY)

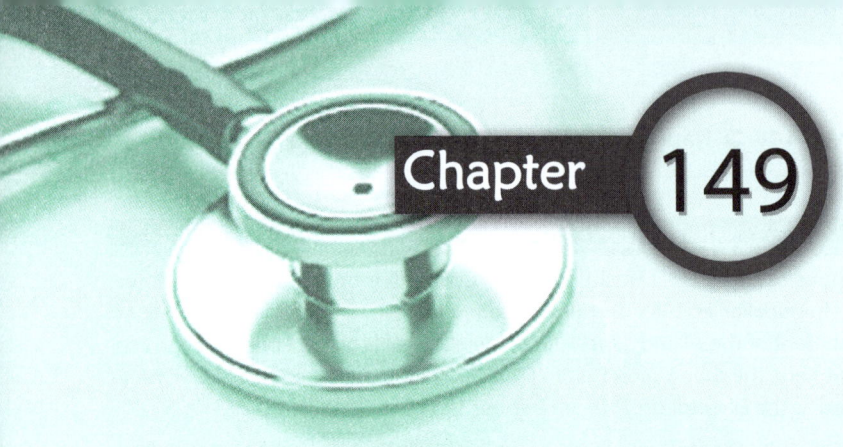

Chapter 149

Central Bureau of Health Intelligence

Efficient health information is key to healthy and prosperous world.

ORGANIZATION

Established in 1961, **Central Bureau of Health Intelligence (CBHI)** is the National Nodal Institute in the Directorate General of Health Services (Dte. GHS), Ministry of Health and Family Welfare, Government of India. CBHI headquarter is located at Nirman Bhavan, New Delhi. CBHI is the National Nodal Institution for Health Intelligence in India.

CBHI is headed by **Director**, has four divisions viz.
  i. CB Policy and Infrastructure—headed by a Joint Director
 ii. Training, Collaboration and Research—headed by a Joint Director
iii. Information and Evaluation—headed by a Joint Director and
 iv. Administration—headed by Director/Deputy Director Administration

It has Six Health Information **Field Survey Units (FSUs)** located in different Regional Offices of Health and Family Welfare (ROHFW) of GOI at **Bangalore, Bhopal, Bhubaneswar, Jaipur, Lucknow and Patna;** each headed by a Deputy Director with Technical and Support staff, who function under the supervision of Regional Director (HFW/GOI).

Regional Health Statistics Training Center (RHSTC) of CBHI at Mohali, Punjab (near Chandigarh) and Other Training Centers viz. (i) Medical Record Department and Training Center of **Safdarjung Hospital,** New Delhi and (ii) **JIPMER Puducherry;** conduct CBHI in service Training Courses.

CBHI headed by Deputy Director General and Director.

CBHI headed by Deputy Director General and Director, has four divisions viz.

- Policy and Infrastructure
- Training, Collaboration and Research
- Information and Evaluation
- Administrative along with Six Health Information Field Survey Units (FSUs) located at Bangalore, Bhopal, Bhubaneswar, Jaipur, Lucknow and Patna and Regional Health Statistics Training Center (RHSTC) at Mohali, Punjab (near Chandigarh).

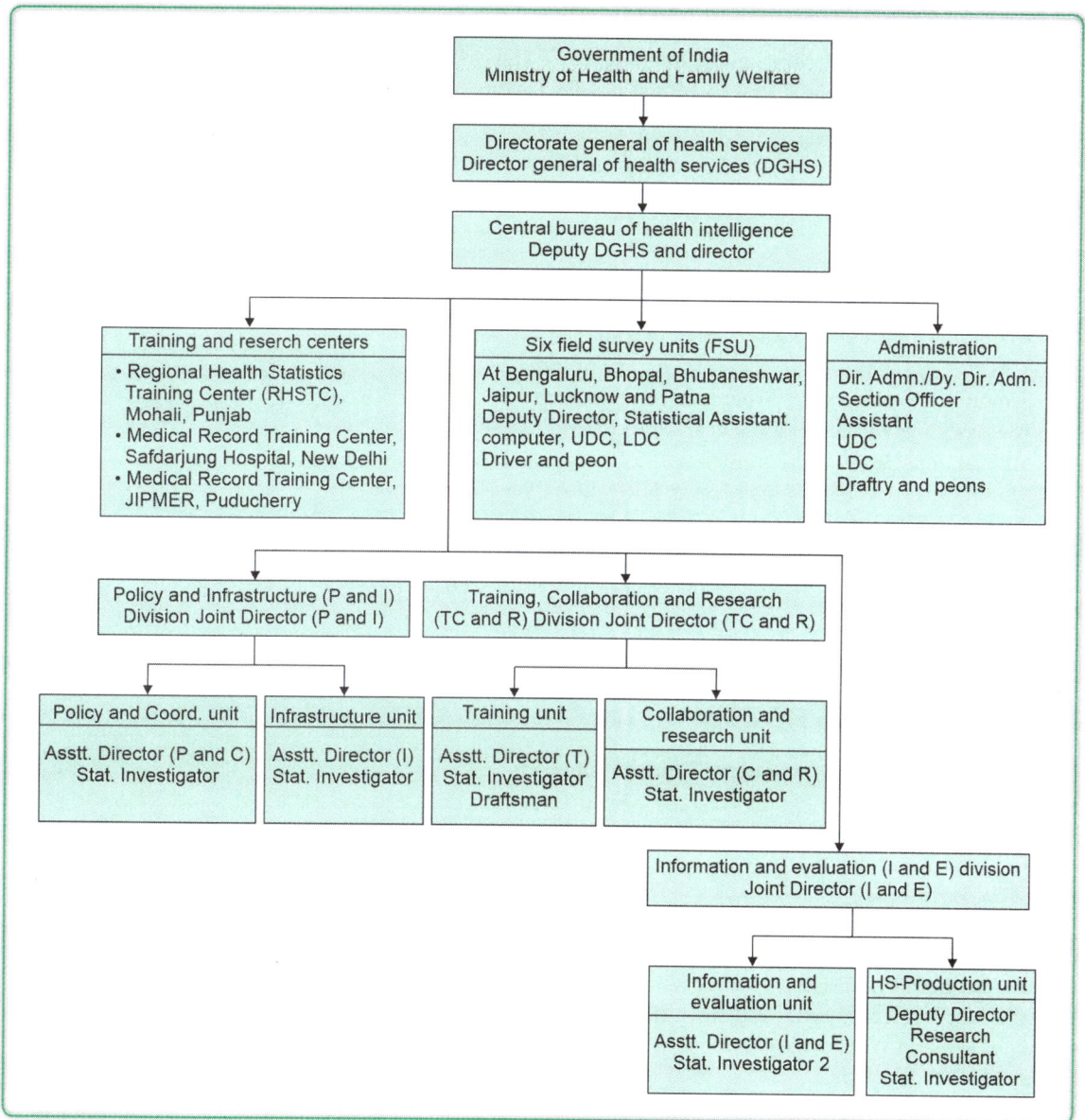

OBJECTIVES

CBHI is the National Nodal Institution for Health Intelligence in the country with broad objectives to:

- Maintain and Disseminate the (i) National Health Profile (NHP), (ii) Health Sector Policy Reform Options Database (HS-PROD), (iii) Inventory and GIS Mapping of Government Health Facilities in India, etc.
- Review the Progress of Health Sector Millennium Development Goal (MDG) in India.

- Annual Road Safety Profile of India.
- Facilitate Capacity Building and Human Resource Development
- Need Based Operational Research for Efficient Health Information System (HIS) as well as use of Family of International Classification in India and South East Asia Region.

CBHI LINKAGE AND COORDINATION

- All 19 Regional Offices of Health and FW/GOI
- All 35 States/UTS
- Planning Commission, Government of India
- Census Commission and Registrar General of India
- Union M/o Statistics and Programme Implementation
- Medical, Nursing and Paramedical Councils and Institutions
- All National Health Programmes
- Union Ministries of Railways, Labor, HRD, Rural Development, etc.
- Public Health, Medical Care and Research Institutions (including ICMR) from Government and Non-Government Sectors.
- WHO and other UN Agencies Concerned with Health and Socio-economic Development.
- European Commission
- Other concerned Departments/Institutions/Non-Government Organizations.

MAJOR ACTIVITIES OF CBHI

Maintain and disseminate the National Health Profile on:
- **Demography**
  - Population Statistics
  - Vital Statistics
- **Socio-Economic**
  - Education
  - Social indicators
  - Economic indicators
  - Employment housing and amenities
  - Drinking Water and sanitation
  - Health legislation
- **Health Status**
  - **Morbidity and Mortality**
    - i. Communicable diseases
    - ii. Non communicable diseases
    - iii. Reproductive and child health
    - iv. Disability
- **Health Finance**
  - Five-Year Plan Outlay
  - Health Expenditures and Financing Agents

- **Human Resources in Health Sector, including AYUSH**
- **Health infrastructure, including AYUSH**
  - Education Infrastructure (medical, nursing and paramedical)
  - Health Care Service Infrastructure

Maintain website: www.cbhidghs.nic.in with information on CBHI, the Annual Publication "National Health Profile (NHP)," National Recommendations on Health Information System (HIS), National Recommendations on Improving and Strengthening the use of ICD 10 and Medical Record System, CBHI Training Calendar and Application Forms, Module and Work Book on ICD-10, Formats for (monthly/annually) Health Data Reporting from States/UTs to CBHI, Road Safety Profile (2008) of India for WHO Global Report and various other Publications of CBHI. This website also has provisions for on-line data transmission by the States/UTs to CBHI.

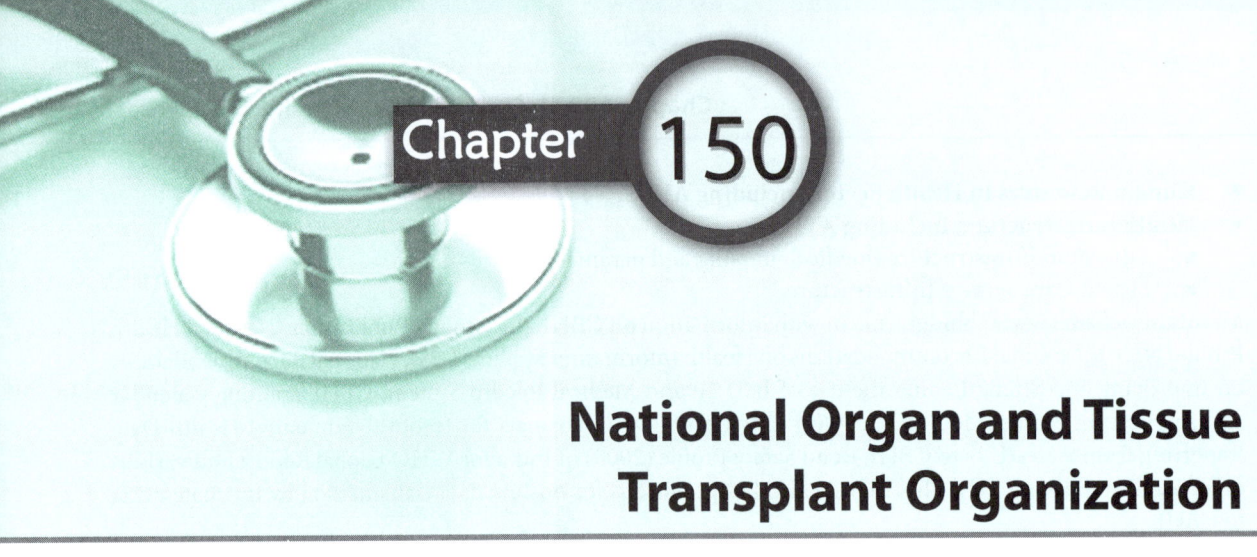

Chapter 150

National Organ and Tissue Transplant Organization

INTRODUCTION

National organ and tissue transplant organization (NOTTO) is a National level organization set up under Directorate General of Health Services, Ministry of Health and Family Welfare, Government of India located at 4th and 5th Floor of Institute of Pathology (ICMR) Building in Safdarjung Hospital, New Delhi. It has following two divisions:

- "National Human Organ and Tissue Removal and Storage Network"
- "National Biomaterial Center"

NATIONAL HUMAN ORGAN AND TISSUE REMOVAL AND STORAGE NETWORK

This has been mandated as per the Transplantation of Human Organs (Amendment) Act 2011. The network will be established initially for Delhi and gradually expanded to include other States and Regions of the country. Thus, this division of the NOTTO is the nodal networking agency for Delhi and shall network for Procurement Allocation and Distribution of Organs and Tissues in Delhi.

Functions/Activities

National Network division of NOTTO would function as apex center for All India activities of coordination and networking for procurement and distribution of organs and tissues and registry of organs and tissues donation and transplantation in the country. The following activities would be undertaken to facilitate organ transplantation in the safest way in shortest possible time and to collect data to develop and publish National registry.

At National Level

- Lay down policy guidelines and protocols for various functions.
- Network with similar regional and state level organizations.
- All registry data from States and Regions would be compiled and published.
- Creating awareness, promotion of organ donation and transplantation activities.
- Coordination from procurement of organs and tissues to transplantation when organ is allocated outside the region.

- Dissemination of information to all concerned organizations, hospitals and individuals.
- Monitoring of transplantation activities in the Regions and States and maintaining data-bank in this regard.
- To assist in data management for organ transplant surveillance and organ transplant and Organ Donor registry.
- Consultancy support on the legal and non-legal aspects of donation and transplantation.
- Coordinate and organize trainings for various cadre of workers.

For Delhi and NCR

- Maintaining the waiting list of terminally ill patients requiring transplants.
- Networking with transplant centers, retrieval centers and tissue banks.
- Co-ordination for all activities required for procurement of organs and tissues including medico legal aspects.
- Matching of recipients with donors.
- Allocation, transportation, storage and distribution of organs and tissues within Delhi and National Capital Territory region.
- Post-transplant patients and living donor follow-up for assessment of graft rejection, survival rates, etc.
- Awareness, advocacy and training workshops and other activities for promotion of organ donation.

NATIONAL BIOMATERIAL CENTER (NATIONAL TISSUE BANK)

The Transplantation of Human Organs (Amendment) Act 2011 has included the component of tissue donation and registration of tissue Banks. It becomes imperative under the changed circumstances to establish National Level Tissue Bank to fulfill the demands of tissue transplantation including activities for procurement, storage and fulfill distribution of biomaterials.

The main thrust and objective of establishing the center is to fill up the gap between 'Demand' and 'Supply' as well as 'Quality Assurance' in the availability of various tissues.

The center will take care of the following tissue allografts:

- Bone and bone products, e.g., deep frozen bone allograft, freeze dried bone allograft, dowel allograft, AAA Bone, Dura mater, fascia lata, fresh frozen human amniotic membrane, high temperature treated board cadaveric joints like knees, hips and shoulders, cadaveric cranium bone graft, loose bone fragment, different types of bovine allograft, used in orthodontics.
- Skin graft
- Cornea
- Heart valves and vessels
  Other tissues shall be gradually included.

Activities

- Coordination for tissue procurement and distribution
- Donor tissue screening
- Removal of tissues and storage
- Preservations of tissue
- Laboratory screening of tissues
- Tissue tracking

- Sterilization
- Records maintenance, data protection and confidentiality
- Quality management in tissues
- Patient information on tissues
- Development of guidelines, protocols and standard operating procedures
- Trainings
- Assisting as per requirement in registration of other tissue banks.

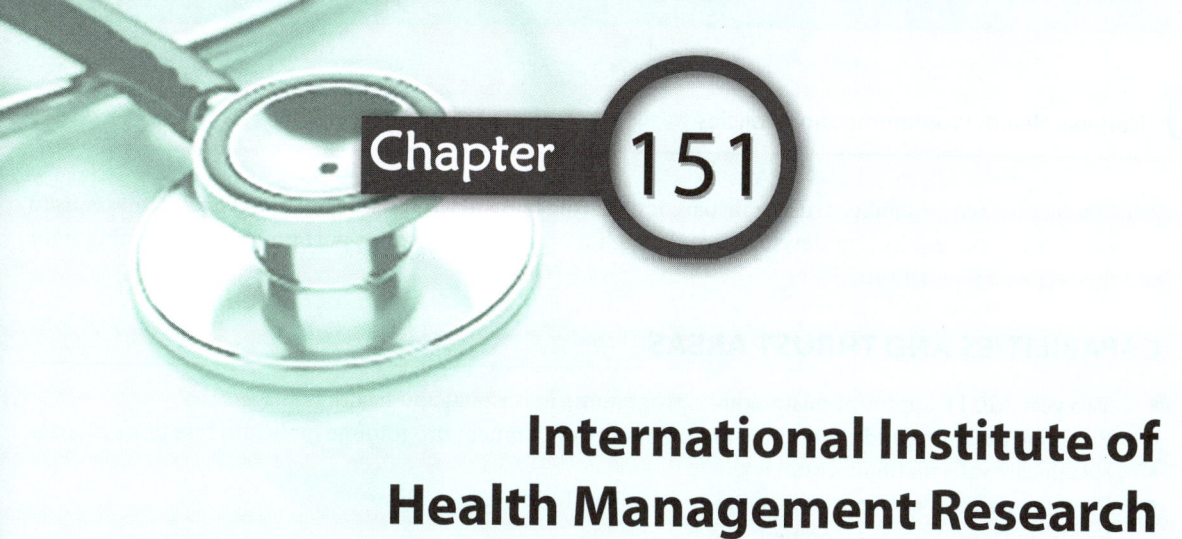

Chapter 151

International Institute of Health Management Research

INTRODUCTION

The International Institute of Health Management Research, New Delhi is part of the Society for Indian Institute of Health Management Research (IIHMR), which was established in October 1984 under the Societies Registration Act 1958. IIHMR Delhi was set up in 2008 with a focus on national and international health to cater to the growing needs of the country and the Asia-Pacific region. Our chief goals are to play a major role in promoting and conducting research in policy analysis and formulation, strategy development and effective implementation of policies, training and capacity development and preparing professionals for the health care sector. We undertake capacity building of health professionals in a big way through our executive training programmes. The Institute offers a two-year full-time postgraduate programme with specialization in hospital management, health management and health care IT. To meet the educational challenges of the rapidly growing health sector in India, IIHMR Delhi provides students with a managerial and technical foundation for careers in consulting, health care systems, hospital management, public health management, Health IT and health insurance.

The institute has three main activities:

- Research that have high relevance to health policies and programmes of India and Asia-Pacific Region.
- Postgraduate programme (PGDHM) with specialization in health management, hospital management and health care information technology.
- Management development programmes to improve management practices in health and related systems and embarked upon developing knowledge and skills of management among health managers, planners, decision-makers, trainers and research scientists at the national and international levels management development programmes.

MISSION

The IIHMR Delhi is an institution dedicated to the improvement in standards of health through better management of health care and related programmes. It seeks to accomplish this through management research, training, consultation and institutional networking in a national and global perspective.

VISION OF THE PROMOTING BODY

The IIHMR is a premier institute in health management education, training, research, programme management and consulting in the health care sector globally. The Institute is known as a learning organization with its core values as quality, accountability, trust, transparency, sharing knowledge and information. The Institute aims to contribute for social equity and development through its commitment to support programmes aiming poor and the deprived population.

CAPABILITIES AND THRUST AREAS

- Two year AICTE approved postgraduate programme in hospital and health management.
- Planning, designing and conducting management development programme for health care professionals.
- Health care information technology.
- Planning and management of hospital and primary health care services.
- Institutional capacity development and networking.
- Project planning, management and evaluation.
- Operations research.
- Economic and financial analysis.
- Survey research.
- Social assessment.
- Quality assurance and accreditation.
- Health insurance
- E-learning.

The organizational structure is given in the Flowchart 1.

Flowchart 1: Organizational structure

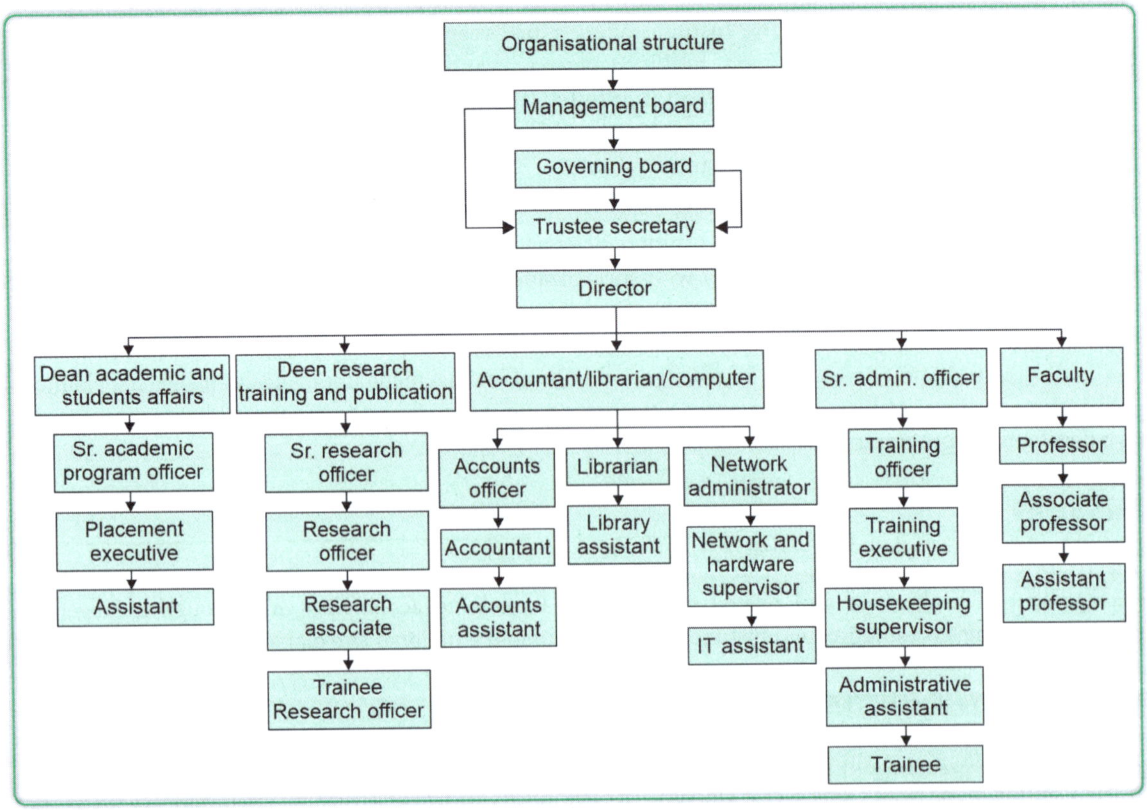

Chapter 152

National Institute of Health and Family Welfare

INTRODUCTION

The National Institute of Health and Family Welfare (NIHFW), was established on 9th March, 1977 by the merger of two national level institutions, viz. the National Institute of Health Administration and Education (NIHAE) and the National Institute of Family Planning (NIFP). The NIHFW, an autonomous organization, under the Ministry of Health and Family Welfare, Government of India, acts as an 'apex technical institute' as well as a 'think tank' for the promotion of health and family welfare programmes in the country.

The Institute addresses a wide range of issues on health and family welfare from a variety of perspectives through the departments of communication, community health administration, education and training, epidemiology, management sciences, medical care and hospital administration, population genetics and human development, planning and evaluation, reproductive bio-medicine, statistics and demography and social sciences.

VISION

NIHFW is to be seen as an Institute of global repute in public health and family welfare management.

MISSION

To act as think tank, catalyst and innovator for management of public health and related health and family welfare programmes by pursuing multiple functions of education and training, research and evaluation, consultancy and advisory services as well as provision of specialized services through interdisciplinary teams.

CORE VALUES

- Excellence
- Equity
- Convergence
- Market orientation
- Sustainability

AREAS OF WORK

- Health and related policies
- Public health management
- Health sector reforms
- Health economics and financing
- Population optimization
- Reproductive health
- Hospital management
- Communication for health
- Training technology in health

AREAS OF CONCERN

- Rural health (Theme 2005: National Rural Health Mission)
- Health of urban slum dwellers
- Tribal health
- Decentralization
- Inter and intersectoral coordination
- Community ownership
- NGOS
- Public-private partnership
- Human resources for health
- Financial management
- Social/community health insurance
- Care of elderly
- Gender sensitivity and care of girl child
- Adolescent health
- Emergency contraception
- Population education
- Medical ethics
- Health legislations
- Medical waste management
- HMIS
- Health informatics
- Quality in health care
- Replicating best practices

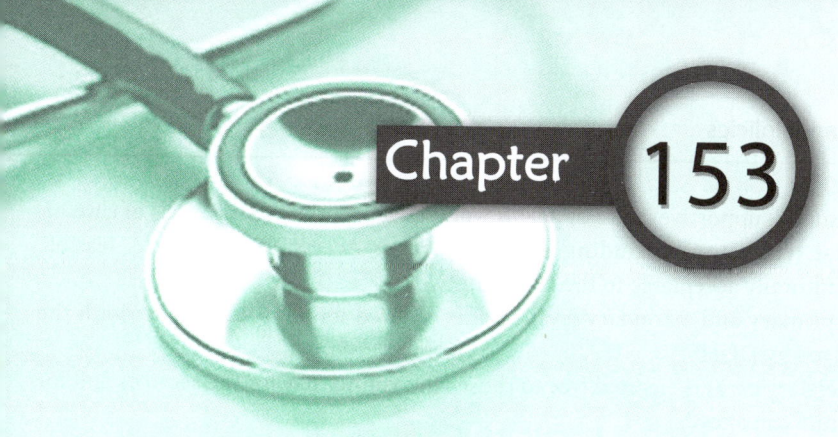

Chapter 153

Directorate General of Health Services

INTRODUCTION

The Directorate General of Health Services (DGHS) is a repository of technical knowledge concerning public health, medical education and health care. It is an attached organization of the Ministry of Health and Family Welfare. The Dte. GHS is headed by Director General of Health Services (DGHS), a secretary level officer of central health services, who renders technical advice on all medical and public health matters to Ministry of Health and Family Welfare. The Directorate co-ordinates with the Health Directorates of all States/UTs for implementation of various National Health Programmes through its Regional Offices of Health and Family Welfare. The Dte. GHS oversees the functioning of Central Government Hospitals and their management. It also addresses health concerns of the people through its Subordinate Offices/Institutes spread all over the country.

VISION

Providing evidence-based technical support for policy formulation and programme implementation in matters of public health, health care and medical education to the Government for achieving an acceptable standard of health for the people of India.

MISSION

Developing the Directorate General Health Services as a core agency so as to contribute in developing the health system with quality, excellence, equity and righteousness with participation of the people, communities and all stakeholders for health and well-being of all.

GUIDING PRINCIPLES

The over-arching principles would be:
- Equitable distribution of health care irrespective of age, gender, caste, creed, religion, etc.
- **Community participation:** Whole of society approach with community and civil society equal partners and take responsibility for their health and well-being.
- **Intersectoral collaboration:** Whole of Government approach with advocacy and action for health in policies of all sectors beyond health.

- **Health team approach:** Mutually supportive cadre of health workers appropriate to the levels of care.
- **Use of appropriate medical technology including essential drugs:** Accessible, affordable, feasible medical technology that is culturally acceptable to the community.
- Free Basic Health services (primary and secondary level care) is ensured for all in accordance with the public health standards evolved by DGHS.
- Advanced health services (tertiary care) is ensured free to those who cannot pay for the services and for others, at a cost the community can afford.

OBJECTIVES

The broad objectives of Directorate General of Health Services would be:
- To formulate evidence-based policies and strategies and to plan and implement programmes based on transparent, innovative, inclusive policies.
- To address social and cultural determinants to ensure every citizen has the right to health and well-being.
  - Guarantee food security to provide essential nutrition, especially for mother and child
  - Ensure potable water, sanitation facilities and proper housing
- To provide technical support to the Department of Health and Family Welfare in developing the strategies for credible free universal health care including free essential drugs, accessible to all citizens. Prioritize special groups that need attention; mother, child, destitute and geriatric population.
- To take effective measures to prevent, mitigate and eliminate/eradicate communicable diseases of public health importance and to prevent, mitigate and or contain public health emergencies due to biological including zoonotic, chemical and radiological hazards.
- To promote health through behavioral change with involvement of community, civil society, community based organizations, media, etc. to address issues related to non-communicable diseases such as cancer, cardiovascular disease, stroke, mental illnesses, alcoholism and other substance abuse.
- To ensure emergency medical services coverage for all that would include medical, surgical (including trauma), pediatric and obstetric emergencies.
- Address climate change issues impacting health.
- Lay down specific standards and norms for safety and quality assurance of all aspects of health care.
- To develop and ensure availability of human resources in health sector appropriate to the level of care.
- To manage information related to health status, health infrastructure and health services.
- To monitor progress and evaluate health outcome/impact through pre-determined health indicators, norms and benchmarks.
- To provide technical guidance and advice to the state health departments in responding to the challenges in meeting any of the objectives stated above.

DIVISIONS

The 'Divisions' are smaller units within the Directorate and are comprised of one or more branches/sections. The Section in the Directorate is the basic work unit responsible for attending to items of work allotted to it. It is generally headed by a section officer and includes 'Cell', 'Unit'.
- **Central Bureau of Health Intelligence:** To centralize collection, compilation, analysis, evaluation synthesis and dissemination of all information on health statistics for the nation.
- **Central Drugs Standard Control Organization Division:** Administrative work of all CDSCO, RDTL, CDTL, CDL.

- **Central Health Education Bureau Division:** Health education and health education material. Training of Health Personnel in Health Education. Publicity work relating to National Health Programme.
- **Expanded Programme on Immunization Division:** All administrative/Technical matter related to CRI Kasauli and BCG, Guindy, Chennai.
- **Emergency Medical Relief Division:** Emergency Medical Relief. Grievance redressal
- **Hindi Section**
  - Implementation of official language policy. Translation from English to Hindi and vice-versa.
- **Leprosy Division**
  - Release of funds as grant in aid to State Leprosy Societies. Provide drugs to States Government through WHO for MDT National Leprosy Eradication Programme including CLTRI/RLTRI.
- **Medical Education Division**
  - All India Entrance Exam for admission to MBBS/BDS/PG courses.
  - All work related to LHMC and SSKH, KSH, CIP Ranchi, AIIH and PH.
- **Medical Grants Division**
  - Implementation of Transplantation of Human Organ Act 1994 and Rules 1995 in the Union Territories including NCT Delhi.
- **Medical Hospital Division**
  - All budgetary matters. Human Resource and Planning. Work related to Safdarjung Hospital, New Delhi, Dr. R.M.L. Hospital S and CE Kolkata, AIIPMR Mumbai, Trauma Center, Burns.
  - Framing and amendment of RR of Group A, B, C posts in the Central Hospitals.
- **Medical Store Organization Division**
  - All administrative matter related to seven GMSDs.
- **Non-Communicable Diseases Division**
  - National programme for prevention and control of Deafness.
  - National programme for prevention and control of cancer, palliative care.
  - National programme of health care of elderly.
- **Order and Maintenance Division**
  - Election matter/JCM/office council/ISTM training. Coordination matter of Subordinate Offices and Dte. GHS (HQ).
  - Annual Report to CIC. RTI matter of Dte. GHS and Subordinate offices. Receiving application for General Public.
- **Public Health (Central Drugs Laboratory) Division**
  - All work related to NCDC, NVBDCP, CDEC
- **Procurement Division**
  - Handling procurement of Equipment above ₹50 lakhs Policy.
- **Regional Directorate Division**
  - All administrative work related to ROH and FW. Complaint cases against staff of ROH and FW.
- **Tuberculosis Division**
  - Implementation of National TB Control Programme in the Country. Release of funds as grants-in-aids to State TB society. All administrative matter of NTI, Bengaluru. Establishment/development of State Drugs Center.

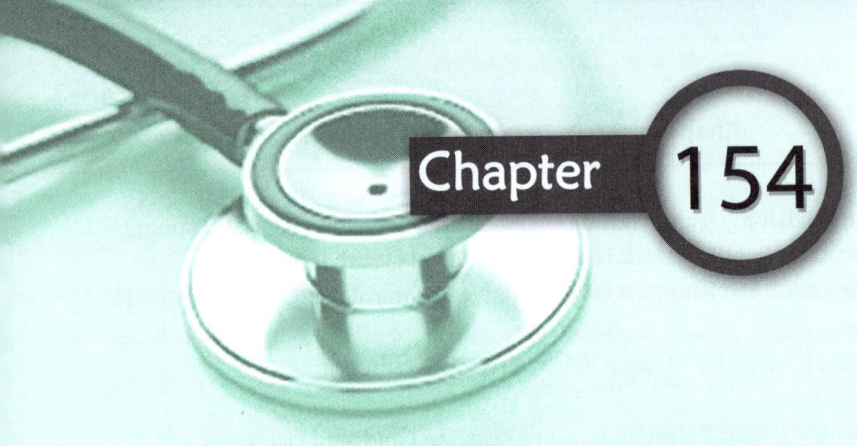

Chapter 154

National Health Systems Resource Center

INTRODUCTION

National Health Systems Resource Center (NHSRC) has been set up under the National Rural Health Mission (NRHM) of Government of India to serve as an apex body for technical assistance.

Established in 2007, the National Health Systems Resource Center's mandate is to assist in policy and strategy development in the provision and mobilization of technical assistance to the states and in capacity building for the Ministry of Health and Family Welfare (MoHFW) at the center and in the states. The goal of this institution is to improve health outcomes by facilitating governance reform, health systems innovations and improved information sharing among all stake holders at the national, state, district and sub-district levels through specific capacity development and convergence models.

It has a 21-member Governing Board, chaired by the Secretary, MoHFW, Government of India with the Mission Director, NRHM as the Vice Chairperson of the board and the Chairperson of its Executive Committee. Of the 21 members, 11 are ex-officio senior health administrators, four from the states. Ten are public health experts from academics and civil society. The Executive Director, NHSRC is the Member Secretary of both the board and the Executive Committee. NHSRC's annual governing board meet sanctions its work agenda and its budget.

The NHSRC is also a World Health Organization Collaborating Center for Priority Medical Devices and Health Technology Policy.

The NHSRC currently consists of eight divisions—Community Processes, Public Health Planning, Human Resources for Health, Quality Improvement in Health care, Health care Financing, Health care Technology, Health Informatics and Public Health Administration.

The NHSRC has a regional office in the north-east region of India. The North East Regional Resource Center (NERRC) has functional autonomy and implements a similar range of activities.

VISION

We are committed to facilitate the attainment of universal access to equitable, affordable and quality health care, which is accountable and responsive to the needs of the people of India.

MISSION

Technical support and capacity building for strengthening public health systems in India.

POLICY STATEMENT

The NHSRC is committed to lead as professionally managed technical support organization to strengthen public health system and facilitate creative and innovative solutions to address the challenges that this task faces.

In the above process, we shall build extensive partnerships and network with all those organizations and individuals who share the common values of health equity, decentralization and quality of care to achieve its goals.

The NHSRC is set to provide the knowledge-centered technical support by continually improving its processes, people and management practices.

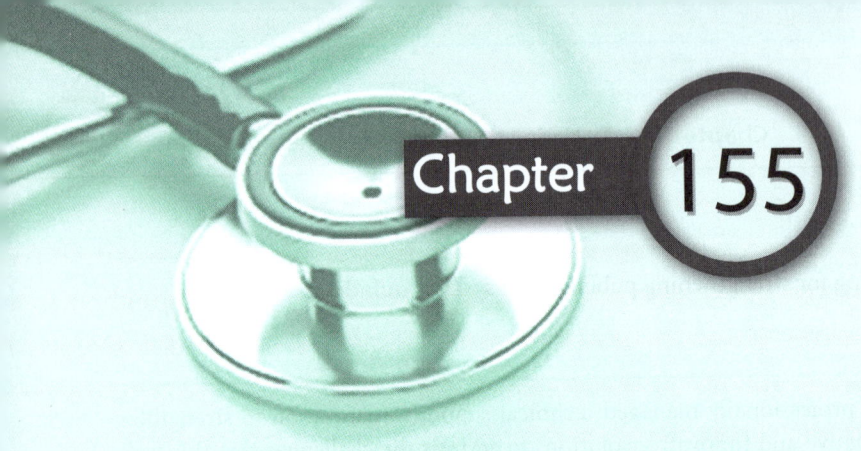

Chapter 155

National Center for Disease Control

INTRODUCTION

The National Institute of Communicable Diseases (NICD) had its origin as Central Malaria Bureau, established at Kasauli (Himachal Pradesh) in 1909 and following expansion was renamed in 1927 as the Malaria Survey of India. The organization was shifted to Delhi in 1938 and called as the Malaria Institute of India (MII). In view of the drastic reduction achieved in the incidence of malaria under National Malaria Eradication Programme (NMEP), Government of India decided to reorganize and expand the activities of the institute to cover other communicable diseases. Thus, on July 30, 1963 the erstwhile MII was renamed as NICD to shoulder these additional responsibilities.

The institute was established to function as a national center of excellence for control of communicable diseases. The function of the institute also included various areas of training and research using multi-disciplinary integrated approach. The institute was, in addition, expected to provide expertise to the States and Union Territories (UTs) on rapid health assessment and laboratory based diagnostic services. Surveillance of communicable diseases and outbreak investigation also formed an indispensable part of its activities.

The NICD campus at Delhi covers an approximate area of 15.35 acres which includes the former official residence of Commander in Chief of the Indian Army and now houses the administrative block, library, divisions of epidemiology and parasitic diseases. The Institute is one of its unique kind in the city of Delhi having so much of green area with about 80% as open area. The Institute has got three large sprawling lawns with well-maintained plants as well as a number of smaller garden islands. The headquarters of the directorate of National Anti Malaria Programme (NAMP), now named as National Vector Borne Disease Control Programme (NVBDCP) is also located in the NCDC campus. The facilities available in the campus include research laboratories, a large lecture hall, well-equipped conference and seminar rooms, animal house, fish hatcheries and two hostels with a total capacity to accommodate about 125 trainees and a well-maintained canteen. The campus has the facilities of play grounds for volleyball, badminton, etc. as well as for indoor facilities like carom, gymnasium, etc.

The Institute is under administrative control of the Director General of Health Services, Ministry of Health and Family Welfare, Government of India. The Director, an officer of the Public Health sub-cadre of Central Health Service, is the administrative and technical head of the Institute.

The Institute has its headquarters in Delhi and has 8 out-station branches located at Alwar (Rajasthan), Bengaluru (Karnataka), Kozhikode (Kerala), Coonoor (Tamil Nadu), Jagdalpur (Chattisgarh), Patna (Bihar), Rajahmundry (Andhra Pradesh) and Varanasi (Uttar Pradesh).

There are several technical divisions at the headquarters of the institute, i.e. Center for Epidemiology and Parasitic Diseases (Department of Epidemiology, Department of Parasitic Disease) Division of Microbiology, Division of Zoonosis, Center for HIV/AIDS and related diseases, Center for Medical Entomology and Vector Management, Division of Malariology and Coordination, Division of Biochemistry and Biotechnology.

In each division there are several sections and laboratories dealing with different communicable diseases. The divisions have well-equipped laboratories with modern equipment capable of undertaking tests using latest technology. The activities of each division are supervised by an officer-in-charge, supported by medical and non-medical scientists, research officers and other technical and paramedical staff. Every division is equipped with its own independent seminar room. The institute has a 24×7 disease monitoring cell operating round the clock to respond to enquiries related to disease outbreak along with video-conferencing facility to interact with the network of disease surveillance centers in the states and districts. The branches are also well equipped and staffed to carry out field studies, training activities and research.

VISION

The vision of the institute broadly covers three areas viz. services, trained health manpower development and research.

SERVICES

The institute takes leading role in undertaking investigations of disease outbreaks all over the country employing epidemiological and diagnostic tools. It also provides referral diagnostic services to individuals, community, medical colleges, research institutions and state health directorates. The service component provided by the institute also includes making available scientific research material, teaching aids, storage and supply of vaccines and quality control of biologicals. A brief of different services provided are mentioned below:

Outbreak Investigations

The institute investigates and recommends control measures for the outbreak of various communicable diseases in the States/UTs all over the country as well as to some neighboring countries in the South-East Asia Region. The institute also undertakes monitoring of outbreaks through-out the country, especially during its early rising phase by collecting information from the states and districts. The institute conducts emergency preparedness training for the officials in the state as well as investigates rumors in cases of diseases that have been considered as eradicated, e.g., smallpox case rumors.

Referral Services

- **Referral diagnostic services:** The institute provides referral diagnostic services for various communicable diseases of microbial origin especially for those for which diagnostic facilities are ordinarily not available in hospitals and medical colleges. These include:
    - **Viral diseases:** Poliomyelitis, measles, coxsackievirus, other enteroviruses, hepatitis virus, AIDS, rabies, arboviral infections, rubella, cytomegalovirus, etc.
    - **Bacterial diseases:** Meningitis, diphtheria, acute respiratory infections, cholera and newer entero-pathogens, plague, anthrax, brucellosis, rickettsiosis, etc.
    - **Mycotic diseases:** Common fungal infections, superficial as well as deep.
    - **Parasitic diseases:** Malaria, kala-azar, leptospirosis, hydatidosis.

Other Services

The Institute also provides other important services some of which are as follows:

- **Quality control of biologicals:** The institute routinely provides quality control services for various vaccines like BCG, OPV and diagnostic test kits for AIDS, hepatitis, meningitis, etc.
- **Storage and supply of vaccines and other biological materials:** The institute stores reagents, test kits and vaccines on behalf of the Directorate General of Health Services (DGHS) and distributes to various state health directorates and medical colleges on request. It also provides larvivorous fishes for the biological control of mosquitoes to various public health agencies.
- **Entomological investigations:** Includes identification of arthropods of medical importance especially during disease out-break situations.
- **Evaluation of chemical compounds:** The institute undertakes laboratory and field evaluation of insecticides/biocides to meet the requirements of the registration committee of Central Insecticide Board.
- Assessment of biochemical parameters to establish clinical diagnosis, e.g., thyroid function tests, etc.

TRAINED HEALTH MANPOWER DEVELOPMENT

This component of the mandate of the institute is addressed through the following activities

- **Training:** Special emphasis is given to trained health manpower development that is essential for the successful implementation of different health programmes in the country. Besides the regular training programmes, numerous short-term training activities are conducted every year. The course curricula of these training programmes are designed to develop the necessary need-based skills. The participants to these courses come from different States/Union Territories of India. In addition, trainees from some of the neighboring countries like Bangladesh, Bhutan, Sri Lanka, Myanmar and Nepal also participate in some of the training programmes. The institute also conducts separate training programmes specifically designed for international participants. Some of these courses are sponsored by international agencies like WHO, UNICEF, World Bank and USAID. The institute has developed training modules on different communicable diseases based on its field experiences, which are extensively used during training programmes at NICD. The trainees in various epidemiology courses are exposed to the application of computers and related software in epidemiology and disease surveillance.
- **Expert group meetings:** The institute organizes meetings for formulation of guidelines for surveillance, management, prevention and control of various communicable and non-communicable diseases. The meetings are attended by experts of the respective field, senior administrators of health services of the states, programme managers from medical, veterinary, agriculture and animal husbandry departments.
- **Supply of teaching and research material:** The institute provides teaching material on various communicable diseases in the form of slides, charts, maps, procedure manuals, pamphlets, books, etc. to medical colleges and teaching institutions. Various bacterial and fungal isolates, cell lines, slides of malaria, filaria, kala-azar, rabies, diphtheria, meningococcus, live cultures and preserved materials of arthropods are also provided to medical colleges and research institutions on request.
- **Fellowships:** Scientists, research workers and health professionals, from India and abroad on WHO fellowships are placed in the institute for training and exchange of technical knowledge.

RESEARCH

Applied integrated research in various aspects of communicable as well as some aspects of non-communicable diseases has been one of the prime functions of the Institute. To achieve this, the institute is actively engaged in research in the following broad areas.

- Applied research in the field of bacteriology, virology, mycology, parasitology, immunology, biotechnology, epidemiology, entomology and quality testing of vaccines and other biologicals with an aim of improving diagnostic capabilities of diseases of public health importance and providing laboratory support to the investigation and control of disease out breaks. The important diseases include cholera, polio, measles, yaws, diphtheria, meningitis, tetanus, hepatitis, AIDS, rubella, rabies, dengue, Japanese encephalitis, kala-azar, guinea worm, malaria, filaria, plague, leptospirosis, anthrax, etc.
- Applied field based research through longitudinal surveillance studies of various epidemic prone diseases.
- Laboratory and field oriented research in the transmission dynamics of arthropod borne diseases with the ultimate objective of vector control.
- Evaluation of new formulations of insecticides and biocides and screening of indigenous herbs to evaluate their insecticidal properties. Studies on biological hazards of pesticides.
- In vitro cultures of organisms, development of reagents, rapid diagnostic tests including molecular techniques using modern equipment and latest technology.
- Research on hormonal disorders.

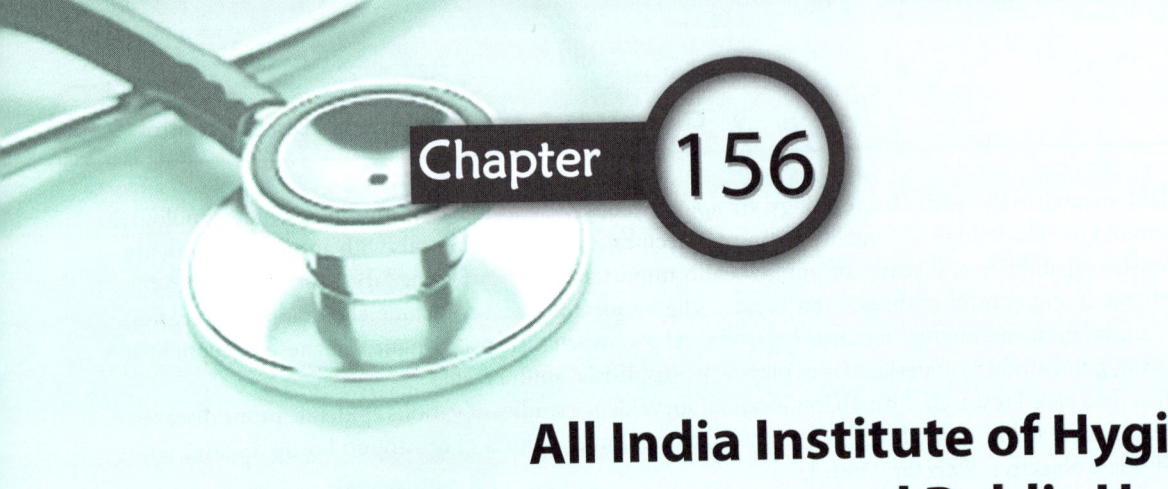

Chapter 156

All India Institute of Hygiene and Public Health

INTRODUCTION

All India Institute of Hygiene and Public Health (AIIH&PH), established in 1932 as the first school of public health in South-East Asia region, has been a pioneer institute of its kind dedicated to teaching, training, and research in various disciplines of public health and allied sciences to ensure capacity building in the area of public health. The teaching, training, and research at AIIH&PH have the unique support of its field laboratories, namely, Urban Health Center, Chetla and Rural Health Unit and Training Center, Singur.

The wider canvas available to the institute has been signified not only by its field laboratories, but also by the diverse disciplines such as biochemistry and nutrition, epidemiology, health promotion and education, maternal and child health, microbiology, occupational health, public health administration, public health nursing, environmental sanitation and sanitary engineering, preventive and social medicine, behavioral sciences, and statistics operating here.

The achievements and contributions of the institute have been commensurate with the prime status attached to the institute by its founders. The list of regular courses offered by the institute indicates that the Institute has been following a holistic approach to the issue of public health.

The institute has been conducting a number of short courses/training programmes for different categories and groups of health force on a regular basis in coordination with State Governments/Central Ministries/ International agencies, etc.

GOALS

- Conducting need based regular courses of high quality covering all aspects of public health.
- Designing and implementing need based short courses, and training programmes for augmenting and supplementing public health workforce.
- Informing, educating, and empowering people about health issues.
- Conducting research for new insights and innovative solutions to community health problems.
- Evolving best practices and setting standards in the field of public health.
- Evaluation of effectiveness, accessibility, and quality of personal and population-based health services.
- Playing a leadership role in the field of public health through evidence-based policy advocacy.
- Compliance with common statutory provisions.

MISSION

- To develop competent workforce for public health services through teaching, training, and research in the relevant fields on a regular basis.
- To strive for solutions based on harmonious blend of capacity development, knowledge dissemination, and community engagement taking the best technological advances into consideration to improve community health and hence quality of life for all.
- To develop model centers for health services to community, ensuring universal coverage for primary health care.

VISION

To be a center of excellence globally for education, training and research in the field of public health.

Chapter 157

National Institute of Disaster Management

INTRODUCTION

The National Institute of Disaster Management (NIDM) was constituted under an Act of Parliament with a vision to play the role of a premier institute for capacity development in India and the region. The efforts in this direction that began with the formation of the National Center for Disaster Management (NCDM) in 1995 gained impetus with its redesignation as the National Institute of Disaster Management (NIDM) for training and capacity development. Under the Disaster Management Act 2005, NIDM has been assigned nodal responsibilities for human resource development, capacity building, training, research, documentation and policy advocacy in the field of disaster management.

Both as a national center and then as the national institute, NIDM has performed a crucial role in bringing disaster risk reduction to the forefront of the national agenda. It is our belief that disaster risk reduction is possible only through promotion of a "Culture of Prevention" involving all stakeholders. We work through strategic partnerships with various ministries and departments of the central, state and local governments, academic, research and technical organizations in India and abroad and other bilateral and multilateral international agencies.

The NIDM provides technical support to the State Governments through the Disaster Management Centers (DMCs) in the Administrative Training Institutes (ATIs) of the States and Union Territories. Presently NIDM is supporting thirty such centers. Six of these centers are being developed as centers of excellence in the specialized areas of flood risk management, earthquake risk management, cyclone risk management, drought risk management, landslides risk management and management of industrial disasters. Eleven larger states (Andhra Pradesh, Bihar, Gujarat, Karnataka, Madhya Pradesh, Maharashtra, Rajasthan, Tamil Nadu, Uttar Pradesh, West Bengal and Odisha) have been provided with additional centers to cater their needs in this area.

In the backdrop of the International Decade for Natural Disaster Reduction (IDNDR), a National Center for Disaster Management was established in 1995 in the Indian Institute of Public Administration (IIPA) by the Ministry of Agriculture and Cooperation, the nodal ministry for disaster management in the country. The center was upgraded as the National Institute of Disaster Management (NIDM) on 16th October 2003, following the transfer of the subject of disaster management to the Ministry of Home Affairs. The Institute was inaugurated by Hon'ble Union Home Minister on 11th August, 2004.

The institute has achieved the status of a statutory organization under the National Disaster Management Act 2005. Section 42(8) of the Act has made the institute responsible for 'planning and promoting training and research in the area of disaster management, documentation and development of national level information base relating to disaster management policies, prevention mechanisms and mitigation measures'.

Section 42(9) of the Act has assigned the following specific functions to the institute:

- Develop training modules, undertake research and documentation in disaster management and organize training programmes.
- Formulate and implement a comprehensive human resource development plan covering all aspects of disaster management.
- Provide assistance in national level policy formulation.
- Provide required assistance to the training and research institutes for development of training and research programmes for stakeholders including government functionaries and undertake training of faculty members of the state level training institutes.
- Provide assistance to the State Governments and State training institutes in the formulation of State level policies, strategies, disaster management framework and any other assistance as may be required by the state governments or state training institutes for capacity-building of stakeholders, Government including its functionaries, civil society members, corporate sector and people's elected representatives.
- Develop educational materials for disaster management including academic and professional courses.
- Promote awareness among stakeholders including college or school teachers and students, technical personnel and others associated with multi-hazard mitigation, preparedness and response measures.
- Undertake, organize and facilitate study courses, conferences, lectures, seminars within and outside the country to promote the aforesaid objects.
- Undertake and provide for publication of journals, research papers and books and establish and maintain libraries in furtherance of the aforesaid objects.
- Do all such other lawful things as are conducive or incidental to the attainment of the above objects, and
- Undertake any other function as may be assigned to it by the Central Government.

VISION

- To be a premier institute of excellence for training and research on disaster risk mitigation and management in India and to be recognized as one of the leading institutions at the International level in the field.
- To strive relentlessly towards making a disaster free India by developing and promoting a culture of prevention and preparedness at all levels.

MISSION

- To work as a think tank for the Government by providing assistance in policy formulation and;
- To facilitate in reducing the impact of disasters through:
  - Planning and promoting training and capacity building services including strategic learning.
  - Research, documentation and development of national level information base.
  - System development and expertise promotion for effective disaster preparedness and mitigation.
  - Promoting awareness and enhancing knowledge and skills of all stakeholders.
  - Strengthening institutional mechanisms for training and capacity building of all stakeholders.
  - Networking and facilitating exchange of information, experience and expertise.

STRATEGIC PLAN

To build a national hub to share and learn and to create a critical mass of institutions, trainers and trained professionals.

- To undertake quality research covering both natural and human induced disasters, with a multi-hazard approach.
- To work as a National Resource Center for the Central and State Governments in the country through effective knowledge management and sharing of best practices.
- To professionalize disaster risk reduction and emergency management in India and other neighboring countries by developing an independent cadre of professionally trained emergency and mitigation managers.
- To promote formal training and education for disaster management in India and in the region.
- To build working partnerships with the government, universities, NGOs, corporate bodies and other national and international institutes of eminence.
- To link learning and action by building a synergy between institutions and professionals in the sector.

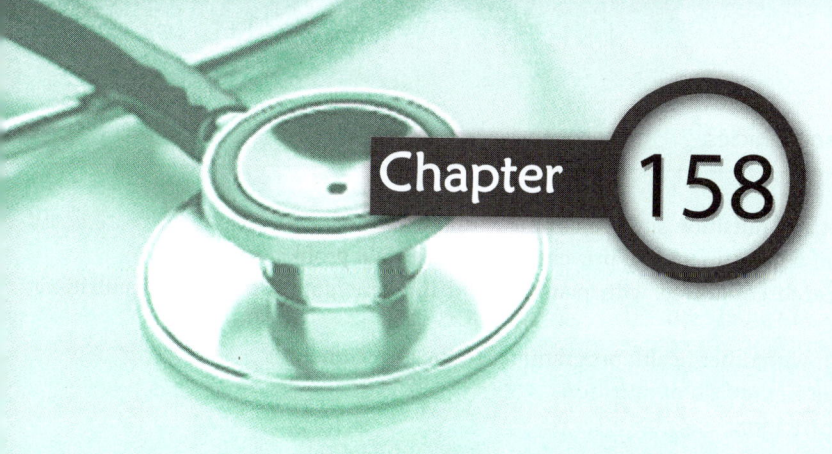

Chapter 158

National Institute of Nutrition

INTRODUCTION

National Institute of Nutrition (NIN) was founded by Sir Robert McCarrison in the year 1918 as 'Beri-Beri' enquiry unit in a single room laboratory at the Pasteur Institute, Coonoor, Tamil Nadu. Within a short span of seven years, this unit blossomed into a "Deficiency Disease Enquiry" and later in 1928, emerged as full-fledged "Nutrition Research Laboratories" (NRL) with Dr. McCarrison as its first Director. It was shifted to Hyderabad in 1958.

At the time of its golden jubilee in 1969, it was renamed as National Institute of Nutrition (NIN). The following centers also started functioning at NIN in later years:

- Food and Drug Toxicology Research Center (FDTRC) in 1971
- National Nutrition Monitoring Bureau (NNMB) in 1972
- National Center for Laboratory Animal Sciences (NCLAS) in 1976
- The institute is located on the salubrious campus of Osmania University with spacious buildings surrounded by lush green vegetation. The Institute's strength lies in the dedicated and devoted scientists belonging to diverse disciplines such as medicine, pediatrics, obstetrics and gynecology, biochemistry, pathology, community health, social sciences, dietetics, statistics, communication and other related areas.

The institute has been recognized by many national and international agencies as center for conducting advanced as well as adhoc training courses in nutrition and laboratory animal sciences. In addition, several reputed universities have recognized NIN as a Center for PhD programmes in different disciplines.

It possesses sophisticated equipment and swell-equipped modern facilities and for clinical, laboratory and community-based research. Nutrition Wards with adequate inpatient and outpatient facilities are available at hospitals viz., Niloufer Hospital for Women and Children, Government Maternity Hospital and Osmania General Hospital to carry out research in clinical nutrition.

The institute's library, well-stocked with books and journals is considered as one of the best science libraries in India. In addition, computer facilities are available for sophisticated data analysis and information retrieval from database.

The "Nutrition Museum" of the institute is an important teaching tool which highlights different aspects of food and nutrition and also covers the work undertaken at the institute.

OBJECTIVES

- To identify various dietary and nutrition problems prevalent among different segments of the population in the country.

- To continuously monitor diet and nutrition situation of the country.
- To evolve effective methods of management and prevention of nutritional problems.
- To conduct operational research connected with planning and implementation of national nutrition programmes.
- To dovetail nutrition research with other health programmes of the government.
- Human resource development in the field of nutrition.
- To disseminate nutrition information.
- To advise governments and other organizations on issues relating to nutrition.

VISION

To achieve optimal nutrition of vulnerable segments of population such as women of reproductive age, children, adolescent girls and elderly by 2020.

MISSION

To enable food and nutrition security conducive to good health, growth and development and increase productivity through dedicated research so as to achieve the national nutrition goals set by Government of India in the national nutrition policy.

ACTIVITIES OF NIN

The activities of NIN are given in Flowchart 1.

Flowchart 1: Activities of NIN

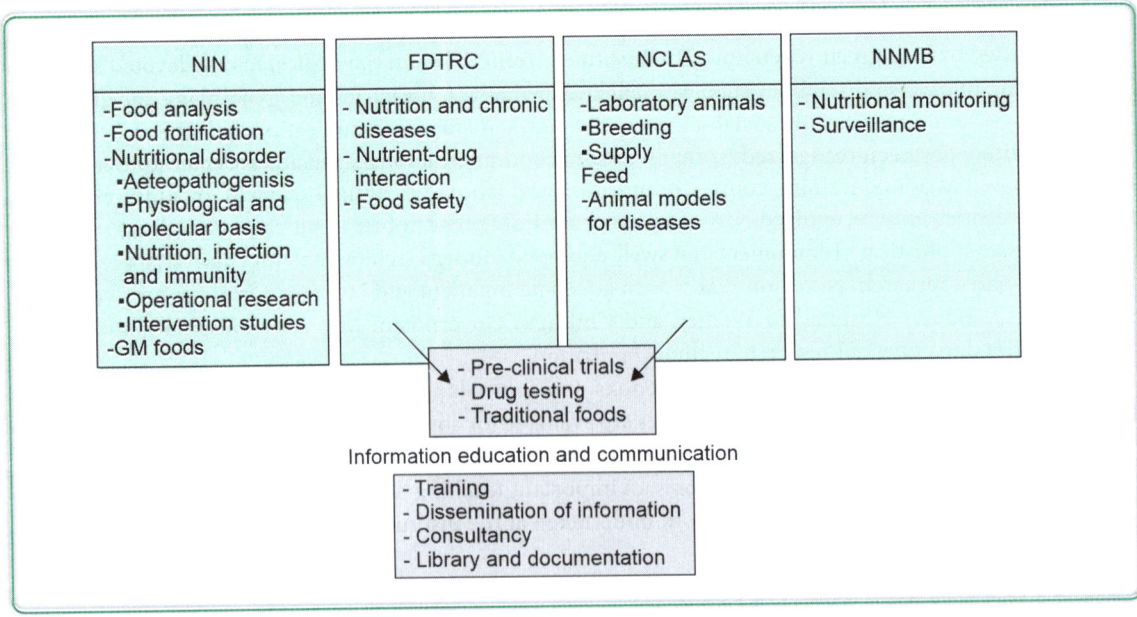

Chapter 159

National Institute of Occupational Health

INTRODUCTION

The National Institute of Occupational Health (NIOH) is the premier institute, under the aegis of the ICMR under the Department of Health Research, Ministry of Health and Family Welfare, Government of India.

The need for research in Occupational Health in the country was first appreciated by Indian Research Fund Association (IRFA), the forerunner of the Indian Council of Medical Research (ICMR). IRFA set up an Industrial Health Advisory Committee (IHAC) under the chairmanship of Col. Bozman in 1945. As per the recommendations of this Committee, in 1947, an Industrial Health Research Unit was created at the All India Institute of Hygiene and Public Health, Calcutta. In 1956, the IHAC recommended to the Government of India that priority should be given for the establishment of an Institute of Occupational Health Research during the Second Five Year Plan.

The National Institute of Occupational Health (NIOH), Ahmedabad, was established by the Indian Council of Medical Research, New Delhi. The Institute started functioning as "Occupational Health Research Institute" (OHRI) at the B. J. Medical College, Ahmedabad, in the year 1966. The OHRI was rechristened as "National Institute of Occupational Health" (NIOH) in 1970 and moved to the present premises. To cater local needs of the Southern and Eastern regions, the Institute established two Regional Occupational Health Centers (ROHC) at Bangalore (1977) and Calcutta (1980).

Occupational Health is a sustained activity aimed at promotion and maintenance of highest degree of physical, mental and social well-being of workers in all occupations. The National Institute of Occupational Health (NIOH) has been established with the following objectives:

- To promote intensive research to evaluate environmental stresses/factors at the workplace.
- To promote the highest quality of occupational health through fundamental and applied research.
- To develop control technologies and health programmes through basic and fundamental research and to generate human resources in the field.

The institute functions as a **WHO Collaborative** and Reference Center for Occupational Health. The institute has represented in many important functions of the Government of India, including the Ministry of Health and Family Welfare, Ministry of Labor, Ministry of Environment and Forests, Ministry of Agriculture, etc., to generate data and provide guidance and recommendations on issues related to occupational and environmental health.

To fulfill the objective of generating human resources in the field, the Institute has **collaborations** with well recognized organizations/institutions/universities, etc.

Since its inception, the institute is devoted to the cause of working class of people and aims to provide "Occupational Health" to the workers engaged in all occupations and minimize deterioration of workplace environment through: Research, education, service and render assistance to the regulatory authorities to take necessary policy decisions for the control of occupational health related problems.

The research activities of the institute are primarily based on national priorities and needs and envisage a multidisciplinary approach, encompassing epidemiological studies, experimental studies, ergonomics and intervention technologies, wherever necessary. The major contribution of the institute can be seen in the form of peer-reviewed publications, reports and large number of know-how influencing policy decisions through expert advice, research, development of modules for control of occupational diseases and help development of manpower through education and training.

VISION

To create safe work environment through intensive research, technology development and knowledge dissemination of quality support system, in order to improve upon the health and well-being of the workers.

THRUST AREA

- Occupational and environmental epidemiology
- Toxicology (metal, pesticide, reproductive, geno and neurobehavioral)
- Environmental pollution (air, water, noise, thermal)
- Operational research
- Women health
- Agricultural health
- Human resource development
- Control of health hazards
- Biological health hazards.

MISSION

To emerge as an international ranking center of excellence:
- Research and technology center
- Academic center.

PURPOSE AND FUNCTIONS

- To promote intensive research and activities in occupational and environmental health; to devote quality endeavors in fundamental and applied research.
- To study the occupational dynamics, the changing environmental contexts, and ascertain safe limits of human exposure to evolve guidelines of health programmes for their control.
- To apply basic data in devising new technique(s) adopting to local needs and conditions for clinical, experimental and intervention purposes.

- To internalize and externalize core competence to transfer knowledge and skill for relevant needs of the government, judiciary, industry and other stakeholders.
- To establish inter-organizational coordination for cooperative research and occupational health delivery.

GOALS

- To pursue excellence in research and establish linkage of the emerging occupational, environmental and lifestyle health issues, and devise models and approaches in predicting the burden of diseases and disorders.
- To create national level programmes for representative generation of database, and guidelines on physical factors, toxic chemicals and biological agents of environmental and occupational origin.
- To build capability for skill development and make available the pool of human resources to be deployed.
- To transfer knowledge and technology to contribute in resolving problems of workplaces and assist in national decision making.

VALUES

- Strive accomplish our mission and goals by the guiding principles of value of health and well-being of workers.
- Accomplish "Research to Reality and Research to Application".
- Achieve symbiotic relationships with the host communities.
- Open up avenues of communication and build human resources to face the challenges.

IMPERATIVES

The imperatives of the national endeavor in occupational and environmental health are driven by:
- The changing economic scenario that the organized industries have their dominating presence with islands of excellence in occupational health, with vastly deprived informal and the farming sectors.
- Surge in technological advances brings in newer challenges of man-machine compatibility, and lifestyle concerns.
- Vivid transformation of the demographic trend that women and younger workforce are fast becoming active contributors in economic activities.
- Public sensitization is vivid today than it was before, thus raising social awareness on the soft occupational and environmental health issues that are visible in the work environment; and
- Requirement of regulatory compliance that medium and large industrial enterprises fall under statutory jurisdiction, while vast farming and other informal sectors remain grossly out of the ambit of OHS regulatory provisions.

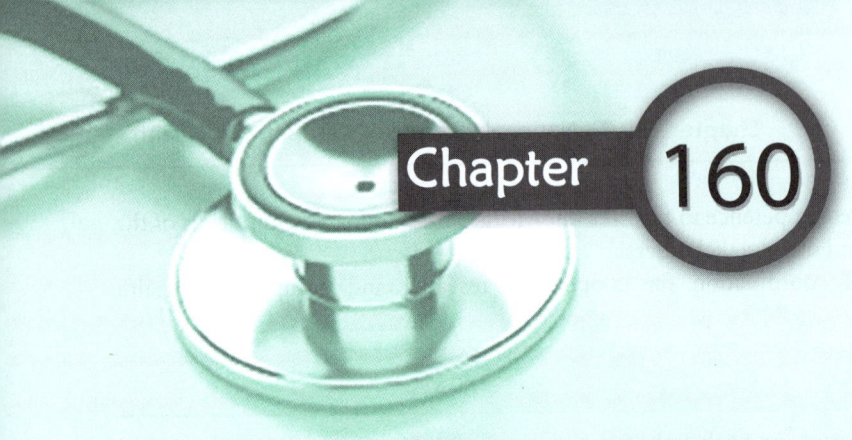

Chapter 160

National Institute of Homeopathy

INTRODUCTION

National Institute of Homeopathy (NIH) was established on 10th December 1975 in Kolkata (Presently Kolkata) as an autonomous organization under the Ministry of Health and Family Welfare, Government of India, presently under the Ministry of AYUSH, Government of India. The institute was affiliated to the University of Kolkata up to session 2003–04 and from 2004 to 2005 has been affiliated to the West Bengal University of Health Sciences, Kolkata. This Institute, conducts the degree course in Homeopathy, i.e., Bachelor of Homeopathic Medicine and Surgery [BHMS] since 1987 and Postgraduate course, i.e. Doctor of Medicine in Homeopathy [MD (Hom.)] since 1998. At present PG course is offered in six subjects viz. Organon of medicine, materia medica, repertory, homeopathic pharmacy, practice of medicine and pediatrics.

The institute is functioning in its own campus measuring about 16 acres of land at Block-GE, Sector-III, Salt Lake City, Kolkata - 700 106, from August 1986 onwards. The institute has an academic building/ administrative block, hospital (IPD/OPD) and under graduate hostels for boys and girls. Construction of the Phase-1 of the 8-storied academic-cum-library building situated in the main campus at block GE is about to be completed. The first Phase (G + 3 floors) of the new Academic-cum-Library building with all modern amenities is completed and has been operational; 8 departments are shifted to new building, the second phase of construction is near completion. The extension of hospital building (G + 3) is near completion for extension of hospital bed strength from existing 100–250 beds. There are two other campuses, one measuring about 9.5 acres located in Block-JC, Salt Lake, Kolkata, where residential quarters for the staff of the institute, international hostel and post graduate hostel are situated. Another campus measuring about 25 acres having a herbal plant garden and a peripheral OPD is located in Kalyani, Dist. Nadia, West Bengal, about 50 km away from the main campus. Government of India has declared the NIH, as the center for traditional medicine in South-East Asian region countries under Delhi Declaration.

GOALS

- To facilitate accessible and affordable quality education that leverages the students with scholarly and professional skills, moral principles, and global perspective.
- To augment both faculty and student research addressing basic and regional problems.
- To integrate a national and international perspective into our fundamental five-fold missions of teaching, research, extension, training and consultancy.

- To cultivate adaption of ethics, morality, healthy practice in professional life by installing habit of continual learning.
- To explore for knowledge and wisdom in order to build a wealth of academic resources indispensable for a sustainable development to accomplish the status of a leading research-intensive institution; and to engage in transferring of knowledge to the community in order to strengthen and elevate the community potential, and to increase the competitiveness of India in homeopathy at the global level.

National Institute of Homeopathy is located in the most planned and developed area of Salt Lake city of Kolkata. It is functioning in its own campus, situated on a plot of land measuring about 16 acres at Block-GE, Sector-III, Salt Lake, Kolkata-700106. Construction of the first phase (G + 3) of the new Academic-cum-Library building has been completed. A well-built hospital is also within the campus. The hospital is being expanded from its present bed strength of 100–250.

For undergraduate students, boys' hostel [(UG) (300 accommodation)], girls' hostel (112 accommodation) and an auditorium with 500 seating capacity are available in the campus. Quarters for Residential Medical Officers are also available in the campus.

The residential campus of the institute is located on a plot of land measuring about 10 acres at JC block, Salt Lake, Kolkata-700098, in close vicinity to the main campus. An International Hostel with all modern facilities for accommodating students from abroad, separate PG hostels for boys and girls along with 24 residential quarters for the employees of the institute is also available in the same campus.

Herbal Garden stretched over land area about of 25 acres at Kalyani (about 60 km from Kolkata) is maintained by the institute, envisaged for acclimatizing exotic species of plants, and to build a repository of authentic specimens of medicinal plants for use by students and researchers.

THE HERB GARDEN-KALYANI

There is a Herb Garden (about 25 acres) at Kalyani, about 60 km away from the institute, envisaged for acclimatizing exotic species which are generally imported in order to save foreign exchange and to build up repository of authentic specimens of medicinal plants for use by students and researchers.

The herb garden has maintained 90 different species of medicinal plants including 10 exotic species, which are high altitude, and cold climate plants. These exotic species have been successfully acclimatized in the genetic plain of West Bengal. Further studies are in progress. Besides maintaining plantation of indigenous medicinal plants recommended by Central Assistance Scheme 3 species have been introduced during the period under report, i.e. *Ocimum killimandscaricum, Sambucus javanica, Stereospermum, Suaveolens. Achillea millefolium, Echinacea purpurea* and *Conium maculatum* are notable among the exotic species which has been introduced during the period under report.

AIMS

- To promote the growth and development of homeopathy.
- To produce graduates and post graduates in homeopathy.
- To conduct research on various aspects of homeopathy.
- To provide medical care through homeopathy to the suffering humanity.
- To provide and assist in providing services and facilities for research, evaluation, training, consultation, and guidance related to homeopathy.
- To conduct experiments and develop patterns of teaching in undergraduate and postgraduate education on various aspects of homeopathy.

MISSION

The mission of NIH is to foster excellence in Homeopathic Medical Education and Research, to educate and train undergraduate, postgraduate students and research scholars of homeopathy in accordance with highest professional standards and ethical values unfettered by the barriers of nationality, language, culture, plurality, religion and to meet the health care needs of the community through dissemination of knowledge and service.

VISION

National Institute of Homeopathy, Kolkata, aspires to be the India's most energetic and responsive organization, offering unparalleled educational opportunities in homeopathy for learner community seeking the highest quality undergraduate, postgraduate, and continuing personal or professional enrichment in higher education and selected professions that will lead to formation of scholarly community serving the nation by advancing, sharing and applying knowledge, and by facilitating the development of thoughtful, creative, adaptable, contributing and human citizens.

MANAGEMENT

The chief executive of the institute is the Director. The management of the institute is under the control of a governing body constituted by the Dept. of AYUSH, Ministry of Health and Family Welfare, Government of India. The financial matters are supervised by the Standing Finance Committee, constituted by the Government of India.

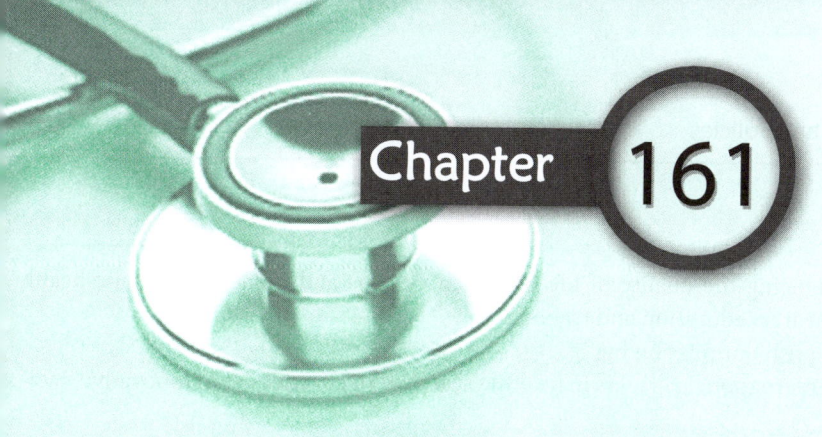

Chapter 161

National Institute of Epidemiology

INTRODUCTION

The National Institute of Epidemiology (NIE) was established on July 2, 1999 by merging the Central JALMA Institute for Leprosy (CJIL Field Unit), Avadi with the Institute for Research in Medical Statistics (IRMS), Chennai. The broad objectives of the institute cover development of human resources in epidemiology and biostatistics, networking of the various ICMR and non-ICMR Institutes at the national level for epidemiological purposes, and consultancy. The institute has the distinction of being the WHO Collaborating Center for Epidemiology of Leprosy and identified as a Technical Resource Group for Epidemiology of HIV by National AIDS Control Organization.

The institute carries out a variety of research activities which include areas such as interventional studies, disease modeling, health systems research, evaluation of health schemes and disease control programmes, issues of statistical methodology, epidemiological investigations and clinical trials of traditional remedies. The institute is recognized by the Sree Chitra Tirunal Institute for Medical Sciences and Technology (Deemed University), Thiruvananthapuram for the 2-year Field Epidemiology Training Programme (FETP-INDIA) leading to Master of Applied Epidemiology (MAE) degree. The institute has been conducting training programmes annually in bio-statistics, controlled clinical trials and basic epidemiology for medical doctors, PG medical students and para-medical workers. It also conducts WHO-SEARO 10 day regional workshops on surveillance, epidemic preparedness and response periodically. The institute is recognized by the University of Madras for research leading to PhD degree in the areas of epidemiology and bio-statistics. The institute has expertise in the areas of bio-statistics, epidemiology, epidemiology of communicable diseases namely leprosy, tuberculosis and other diseases, controlled clinical trials, maternal and child health, health surveys, data processing, etc. The institute has a good library, a well-equipped computing facility and a field practice area covering well characterized 5,00,000 population.

VISION

To be a catalyst for a vibrant national health system through responsive research, education and training in epidemiology and public health.

MISSION

To effectively contribute in enhancing the quality of life of Indian citizens and influencing public health practice and policies through research, education and training.

The institute will strive to accomplish our mission by:

- Working with national and international partners in health research with effective use of innovative state-of-art technologies.
- Aligning our research with all key stakeholders to generate and implement evidence-based health strategies for an effective and efficient National health system.
- Setting standards in public health education that would emphasize professionalism as a core competency.
- Strengthening human resources for National public health services through education and training and building bridges between educational and research institutions.

INSTITUTIONAL GOALS

The strategic goals to support the vision and mission of the organization are as follows:

- Co-ordinate DHR/ICMR multi-centric studies
- Develop faculty capacity to assume national leadership position in niche areas
- Develop institutional expertise in new areas
  - Bioinformatics
  - Health economics
  - Health policy
  - Organize periodic theme-based scientific conferences/meetings
- **Upgrade institutional facilities**
  - **Library:** State of the art facility for scientists and dissemination of health information
  - **Laboratory:** Infrastructure to provide support to epidemiological studies and public health
  - **Information technology:** Novel field based data collection and data management systems and health informatics
- **Promote PhD programmes**
- **Disseminate evidence in technical for a**
  - Research publications
  - Policy briefs
  - e-bulletin/Newsletter/journal
- Provide opportunities for internship to external students in areas of available institutional expertise
- Offer consultancy in the areas of available expertise
- **Disseminate health information to public**
  - Organize library services for children and youth
    - ❖ Conduct programmes on health days for public awareness and for health outreach
    - ❖ Write columns in newspapers periodically
    - ❖ Build public health museum
- Develop collaborative projects in AYUSH.

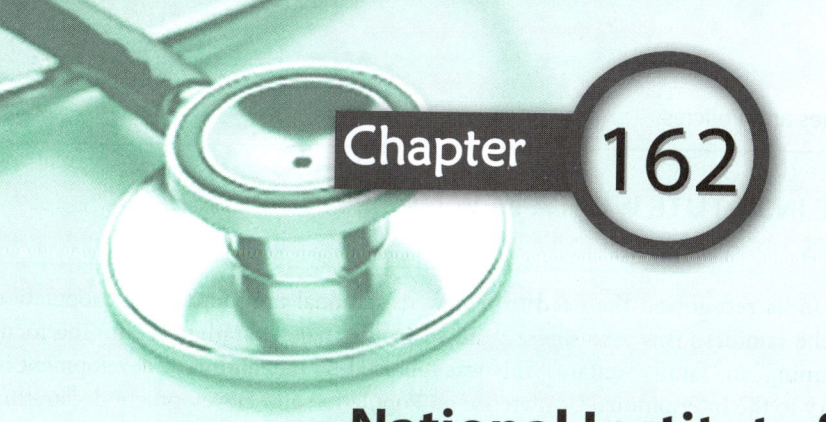

Chapter 162

National Institute for Research in Reproductive Health

INTRODUCTION

National Institute for Research in Reproductive Health (NIRRH), formerly known as Institute for Research in Reproduction is a premier research institute of the Indian Council of Medical Research (ICMR). It is situated in the vicinity of a number of hospitals and research institutes in central Mumbai. Since its inception in 1970, it has been making vigorous efforts to improve the reproductive health of people through research, education and health care services. The institute is affiliated to the University of Mumbai which awards degrees to the MSc and PhD students in the areas of biotechnology, life sciences, biochemistry and applied biology. The institute is one of the few centers in India, which can boast of a team of basic, clinical and operational research scientists and state-of-art laboratories equipped with modern facilities to carry out research on various components of reproductive health. Research programmes have also been initiated in new emerging areas such as stem cell biology, toxicology and transgenesis. The Institute is a WHO collaborating center for Research and Training in Reproductive Health. Collaborations are undertaken with national and international organizations in a global effort to promote research and dissemination of information on reproductive health matters.

CENTERS

- Biomedical Informatics Center
- Genetic Research Center
- National Center for Primate Breeding and Research
- National Center for Preclinical Reproductive and Genetic Toxicology.

The institute had a humble beginning in 1954 in the form of a Contraceptive Testing Unit. In 1970 it matured into an institute having a space of its own in the heart of Central Mumbai with a unique identity which was then named as the 'Institute for Research in Reproduction' (IRR).

Over the years, the Institute has made significant strides to develop newer contraceptives, both for the male and the female; generate information on the safety, efficacy and acceptability of available contraceptives in Indian population; and elucidate basic mechanisms underlying reproductive physiology. The Institute has also undertaken a number of studies on the social and behavioral aspects of fertility regulation with an aim to increase informed choices for women and to enable increased male participation in reproductive health matters. Reproductive tract infections (RTIs) including sexually transmitted infections (STIs) among women has also been the focus of research. The Institute has added new research areas and modern technological innovations to its plethora of already existing expertise, leading to several significant research contributions including the birth of India's first scientifically documented test tube baby.

RESURGENCE OF THE INSTITUTE WITH A NEW NAME AND RENEWED RESEARCH INTERESTS

In 1977 the Government of India recognized the need to review its national programmes on population stabilization and welfare of the families. This assessment resulted in the major paradigm shift. The focus was shifted from "family planning" to "family welfare". This was followed by the landmark development in 1994 when India as a signatory to the International Conference on Population and Development declaration re-oriented the family welfare programme to Reproductive and Child Health (RCH) programme. The institute also responded to the above paradigm shift by widening the spectrum of its research activities. To make this major shift visible and reflected in the name of the institute, its name was changed from Institute for Research in Reproduction to **National Institute for Research in Reproductive Health (Flowchart 1)**. The new name also reflects the national status accorded to the institute in recognition of its scientific contributions. The institute has also expanded its research mandate to reflect the initiation of multidisciplinary and comprehensive research avenues on almost all components of reproductive health as could be seen below:

The mandate of the institute is to:

- Conduct biomedical, clinical, operational and socio-behavioral research on various aspects of reproductive health.
- Collaborate with national and international research organizations in a global effort to promote multilateral exchange in reproductive health.
- Develop human resources by training in specialized areas of reproductive health.
- Incorporate research results into policy and programmes.
- Serve as one of the nuclei for various national level facilities.

Flowchart 1: Mandate of National Institute for Research in Reproductive Health (NIRRH)

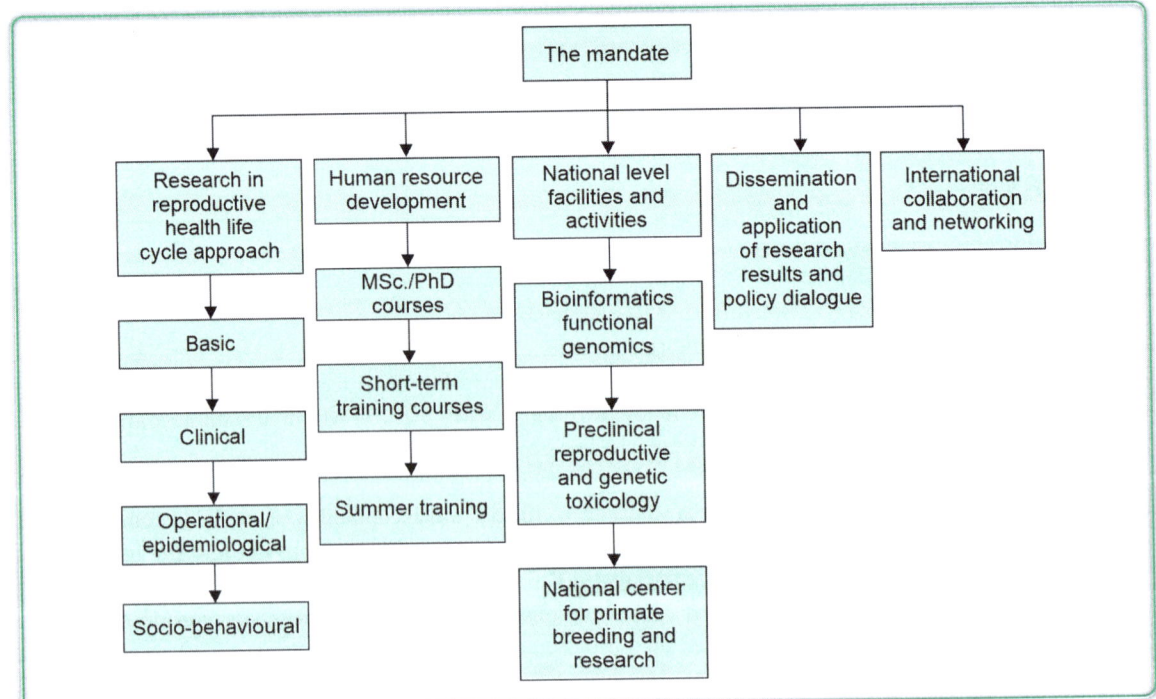

DEPARTMENTS

- Biochemistry
- Biostatistics
- Clinical research
- Gamete immunobiology
- Infectious diseases biology
- Innate immunity
- Infertility and reproductive endocrinology
- Molecular and Cellular biology
- Molecular endocrinology
- Molecular immunodiagnostics
- Molecular immunology
- Neuroendocrinology
- Operational research
- Primate biology
- Stem cell biology
- Structural biology

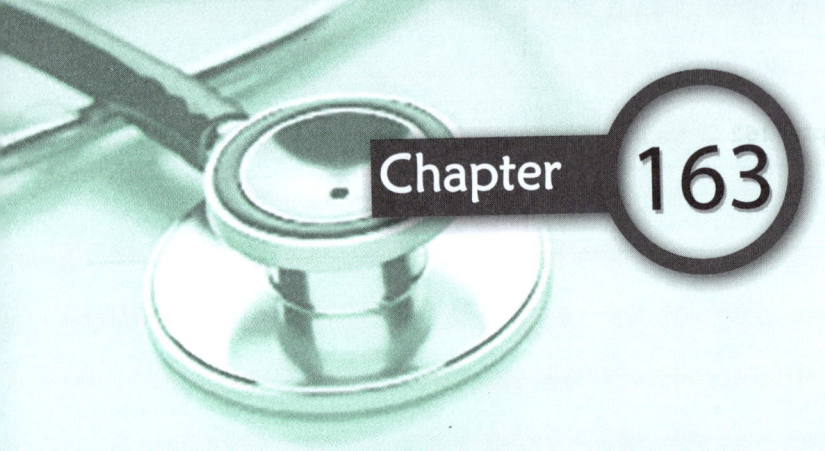

Chapter 163

National Institute of Medical Statistics

INTRODUCTION

National Institute of Medical Statistics (NIMS) is one of the permanent institutes of Indian Council of Medical Research (ICMR), New Delhi and known as NIMS.

The institute came into existence in the year 1977 with the mandate of the institute to provide technical expertise on research methodology, programme evaluation, mathematical modeling, data analysis, etc. It also provides technical assistance to institutes throughout India. Institute for research in medical statistics (IRMS), an institute of Indian Council of Medical Research, established in 1977 will be known as NIMS from 9th November 2005.

The institute has completed 32 years of its scientific and research existence. The institute has grown from a Division of Biostatistics in Indian Council of Medical Research to this height. During this period, it supported biomedical researches of the national relevance, developing research methodologies, evaluating national programmes and organizing need-based training programmes for biostatisticians and biomedical scientists. The institute has significantly contributed to sampling methodologies such as generalized estimation under successive sampling. It has also attempted to investigate the role of some sampling designs in case control studies for estimating relative risk. The Institute has completed number of projects of National importance viz. PHC facility survey in 90 demographically weak districts of India, Post survey check of national family health survey. It also functions as UP unit of National Nutrition Monitoring Bureau (NNMB). The institute has been designated as the nodal agency by Government of India to provide technical support to end line evaluation survey of eight India population project.

THRUST AREAS

- To provide latest methodologies in field of biostatistics for project planning with a component of research.
- Conduct need-based training programmes in medical statistics for the on job personnel of various institutions.
    - Involved in biomedical research
    - Seeking help in
        - Clinical trials
        - Statistical computing
- To provide consultancy to various users, researchers and scientists.

Notes

INTERNATIONAL RECOGNITION

- Clinical Trial Registry, India (CTRI) recognized as a primary register of International Clinical Trial Registry platform.
- Member of Global Reference Group for HIV estimation Technical Advisory Committee.
- Member of Science and Technology Group for HIV/AIDS in Asia Pacific Region.

RECOGNITION FOR DOCTORATE/MASTERS BY A UNIVERSITY

The NIMS is affiliated as an approved research center for PhD in Medical Statistics by the Guru Gobind Singh Indraprastha University, Delhi.

THE ROLE NIMS PLAYS TOWARD SCIENTIFIC RESEARCH IN INDIA

The tremendous involvement in the areas of medical statistics, biomedical and bio-behavioral research, surveillance of communicable and non-communicable diseases, epidemiology, nutrition research, reproductive and child health and cancer research necessitated the renaming of the IRMS as NIMS. The move will enhance not only the status of the institute but will also enable it to develop E-database of health sector reforms in India apart from strengthening its resources base and capacity building.

The institute provides statistical back up for designing and analysis of disease surveillance clinical trials of drugs and vaccines, and RCH. It provided valuable inputs to the estimation of HIV infection in India. It has examined access and utilization of AYUSH in general population and population covered under CGHS. Exercising surveillance of ICMRs various research programmes for ensuring statistical adequacy and validity is one the important areas from its mandate. Organizing training programmes in the areas of research methodology in biomedical research has been the feature of the institute. In fact, it is the only Institute of Medical Statistics in India.

MAJOR ACHIEVEMENTS

- India's only institute to coordinate and standardize the collection of medical and health statistics in the country.
- Establishment of India's first Clinical Trials Registry, in collaboration with DST and WHO.
- Chair, National Family Health Survey.
- Assisted NACO in HIV sentinel surveillance and estimation of HI IV burden in the country.
- Integrated Behavioral and Biological Assessment on National Highways (IBBA-NH) among truckers for HIV epidemic in the country.
- Identified as the National Nodal Agency for the implementation of IDSP-NCD risk factor survey.